SPORTS MEDICINE

SECOND EDITION

SPORTS MEDICINE

SECOND EDITION

RICHARD H. STRAUSS, M.D.

EDITOR

Associate Professor of Preventive Medicine and Internal Medicine
Team Physician
The Ohio State University
Columbus, Ohio

W.B. SAUNDERS COMPANY
Harcourt Brace Jovanovich, Inc.
Philadelphia London Toronto Montreal Sydney Tokyo

W. B. SAUNDERS COMPANY
Harcourt Brace Jovanovich, Inc.

The Curtis Center
Independence Square West
Philadelphia, PA 19106

Library of Congress Cataloging-in-Publication Data

Sports medicine / [editor] Richard H. Strauss.—2nd ed.
p. cm.
Includes bibliographical references and index.
ISBN 0-7216-3734-5
1. Sports medicine. 2. Exercise—Physiological aspects.
I. Strauss, Richard H.
[DNLM: 1. Sports medicine. QT 260 S763]
RC1210.S676 1991
617.1′027—dc20
DNLM/DLC 91-15435

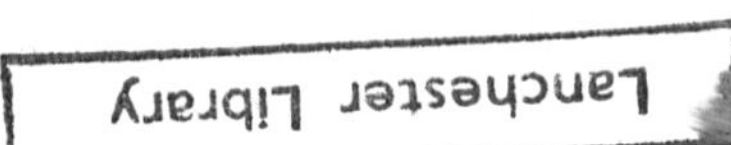

Editor: Edward H. Wickland, Jr.
Designer: Paul Fry
Production Manager: Linda R. Garber
Manuscript Editors: Carol DiBerardino and Mary Ellen Ford
Illustration Coordinator: Brett MacNaughton
Indexer: Angela Holt

Listed here is the latest translated edition of this book together with the language of the translation and the publisher.

Italian (*1st Edition*)—Verduce Editore, Rome, Italy

Sports Medicine, Second Edition ISBN 0-7216-3734-5

Printed in the United States of America

Last digit is the print number: 9 8 7 6 5 4 3 2 1

CONTRIBUTORS

MARVIN M. ADNER, MD

Clinical Professor, Medicine, Boston University School of Medicine, Boston, Massachusetts; Associate Chief of Medicine, Director of Hematology, Framingham Union Hospital, Framingham, Massachusetts

HEMATOLOGY

RAUL ARTAL, MD

Professor of Obstetrics and Gynecology and Exercise Science, University of Southern California School of Medicine, Los Angeles, California; Staff, Women's Hospital, LAC/USC Medical Center, Los Angeles, California

EXERCISE DURING PREGNANCY

WILMA FOWLER BERGFELD, MD, FACP

Head, Clinical Research, Department of Dermatology; Head, Dermatopathology, Department of Pathology, Cleveland Clinic Foundation, Cleveland, Ohio

THE SKIN

ROBERT A. BRUCE, MD

Clinical Associate Professor, Department of Ophthalmology, The Ohio State University, Columbus, Ohio; Staff, The Ohio State University Hospitals; Grant Medical Center; Mt. Carmel Medical Center; Children's Hospital; St. Anthony Medical Center, Columbus, Ohio

EAR, NOSE, THROAT, AND EYE

MICHAEL BUCHAL, MS

Exercise Physiologist, Cardiac Rehabilitation and Exercise Laboratories, Division of Cardiology, William Beaumont Hospital, Royal Oak, Michigan

EXERCISE PRESCRIPTION

ROBERT C. CANTU, MD, MA

Chief, Neurosurgery Service; Chairman, Department of Surgery; Director, Service of Sports Medicine, Emerson Hospital, Concord, Massachusetts

THE NERVOUS SYSTEM

NANCY CLARK, MS, RD

Nutritionist, Sports Medicine Brookline, Boston, Massachusetts

NUTRITION

GLEN M. DAVIS, PhD, FACSM

Department of Biological Sciences, Cumberland College of Health Sciences, The University of Sydney, Sydney, Australia

SPORTS AND RECREATION FOR THE PHYSICALLY DISABLED

PAUL G. DYMENT, MD

Professor of Pediatrics, University of Vermont, Portland, Maine; Chief of Pediatrics, Maine Medical Center, Portland, Maine

CHILDREN AND SPORTS; THE PREPARTICIPATION SCREENING EXAMINATION OF THE YOUNG ATHLETE

E. RANDY EICHNER, MD

Professor of Medicine, Director, Special Hematology Lab, University of Oklahoma Health Sciences Center, Oklahoma City, Oklahoma; Attending Physician, Oklahoma Memorial Hospital, Department of Veterans Affairs Medical Center, Oklahoma City, Oklahoma

CHRONIC FATIGUE AND STALENESS

KATHLEEN A. ELLICKSON, PhD

Clinical Assistant Professor of Psychiatry, The Ohio State University College of Medicine, Columbus, Ohio

PSYCHOLOGICAL ASPECTS OF EXERCISE AND SPORT

CARLOS ALBERTO VAZ FRAGOSO, MD

Director, Pulmonary Function Laboratory, Danbury Hospital, Danbury, Connecticut

THE RESPIRATORY SYSTEM

BARRY A. FRANKLIN, PhD

Associate Professor of Physiology, Wayne State University School of Medicine, Detroit, Michigan; Director, Cardiac Rehabilitation and Exercise Laboratories, Division of Cardiology, William Beaumont Hospital, Royal Oak, Michigan

EXERCISE PRESCRIPTION

JAMES G. GARRICK, MD

Medical Director, Center for Sports Medicine, Saint Francis Memorial Hospital, San Francisco, California

ORTHOPEDIC PREPARTICIPATION SCREENING EXAMINATION OF THE YOUNG ATHLETE

ROBERT C. GOLDSZER, MD

Assistant Professor, Harvard Medical School, Boston Massachusetts; Staff, Department of Internal Medicine, Brigham and Women's Hospital, Boston, Massachusetts

RENAL ABNORMALITIES DURING EXERCISE

SEYMOUR GORDON, MD

Clinical Professor of Health Sciences, Oakland University, Rochester, Michigan; Medical Director, Cardiac Rehabilitation and Exercise Laboratories, Division of Cardiology, William Beaumont Hospital, Royal Oak, Michigan

EXERCISE PRESCRIPTION

RALPH W. HALE, MD

Professor and Chairman, Department of Obstetrics and Gynecology, University of Hawaii, John A. Burns School of Medicine, Honolulu, Hawaii; Chief, Ob-Gyn Service, Kapiolani Medical Center for Women and Children, Honolulu, Hawaii

FACTORS IMPORTANT TO WOMEN ENGAGED IN VIGOROUS PHYSICAL ACTIVITY

WILLIAM L. HASKELL, PhD

Professor of Medicine, Stanford University School of Medicine, Stanford, California

CARDIOVASCULAR BENEFITS AND RISKS OF EXERCISE: THE SCIENTIFIC EVIDENCE

THOMAS N. HELM, MD

Chief Resident, Cleveland Clinic Foundation, Cleveland, Ohio

THE SKIN

ROBERT S. HILLMAN, MD

Professor of Medicine, University of Vermont, Burlington, Vermont; Chairman, Department of Medicine, Maine Medical Center, Portland, Maine

TRAVEL

VICTORIA HOLLINGSWORTH, MA

Manager, Cardiac Catheterization Laboratories, Division of Cardiology, William Beaumont Hospital, Royal Oak, Michigan

EXERCISE PRESCRIPTION

CHARLES S. HOUSTON, MD

Professor of Medicine (Emeritus), University of Vermont, Burlington, Vermont

ALTITUDE SICKNESS

PEKKA KANNUS, MD, PhD

Visiting Research Fellow and Physician, Department of Orthopaedics and Rehabilitation, University of Vermont, Burlington, Vermont; Chief Resident Physician of Sports Medicine, Tampere Research Station of Sports Medicine, University of Tampere, Tampere, Finland

PREVENTION OF SPORTS INJURIES

JOHN H. KENNELL, MD

Professor of Pediatrics, Case Western Reserve University School of Medicine, Cleveland, Ohio; Chief, Division of Child Development, Rainbow Babies and Childrens Hospital; Staff, MacDonald Hospital for Women, Cleveland, Ohio

SPORTS PARTICIPATION FOR THE CHILD WITH A CHRONIC HEALTH PROBLEM

ERIC P. KINDWALL, MD

Associate Professor, Hyperbaric Medicine, Medical College of Wisconsin, Milwaukee, Wisconsin; Staff, Froedtert Memorial Lutheran Hospital; Associate Staff, Children's Hospital of Wisconsin; Staff, Milwaukee County Medical Complex, Milwaukee, Wisconsin

MEDICAL ASPECTS OF SCUBA AND BREATH-HOLD DIVING

BRUCE C. PATON, MD, FRCP (Ed)

Clinical Professor of Surgery, University of Colorado Health Sciences Center, Denver, Colorado; Staff, Porter Memorial Hospital, Swedish Medical Center, University Hospital, Denver, Colorado

COLD INJURIES

PER RENSTROM, MD, PhD

Professor of Orthopaedics and Sports Medicine, Department of Orthopaedics and Rehabilitation, University of Vermont, Burlington, Vermont; Attending at Medical Center Hospital of Vermont, Burlington, Vermont; Fanny Allen Hospital, Winooski, Vermont

PREVENTION OF SPORTS INJURIES

DOUGLAS A. RUND, MD

Professor and Chairman, Department of Emergency Medicine, The Ohio State University, Columbus, Ohio; Chief of Service, Emergency Medicine, The Ohio State University Hospitals, Columbus, Ohio

MANAGEMENT OF EMERGENCIES

WAYNE RUSIN, MD

Staff, Theda Clark Hospital, Neenah, Wisconsin; St. Elizabeth's Hospital, Appleton, Wisconsin

SPORTS PARTICIPATION FOR THE CHILD WITH A CHRONIC HEALTH PROBLEM

DAVID E. SCHULLER, MD

Professor and Chairman, Department of Otolaryngology, The Ohio State University, Columbus, Ohio; Director, Arthur G. James Cancer Hospital and Research Institute; Staff, The Ohio State University Hospitals; Staff, Children's Hospital, Columbus, Ohio

EAR, NOSE, THROAT, AND EYE

ROY J. SHEPHARD, MD, PhD, DPE, FACSM, FFIMS

Director, School of Physical and Health Education; Professor of Applied Physiology, Department of Preventive Medicine and Biostatistics, University of Toronto, Ontario, Canada; Consultant: Toronto Rehabilitation Centre and Gage Research Institute, Toronto-Western Hospital, Toronto, Canada

SPORTS AND RECREATION FOR THE PHYSICALLY DISABLED

ARTHUR J. SIEGEL, MD

Assistant Professor of Medicine, Harvard Medical School, Boston, Massachusetts; Medical Director, Hahnemann Hospital, Boston, Massachusetts

RENAL ABNORMALITIES DURING EXERCISE; EXERCISE AND AGING

HARVEY B. SIMON, MD

Assistant Professor of Medicine, Harvard Medical School, Boston, Massachusetts; Physician, Infectious Disease Unit and Cardiovascular Health Center, Massachusetts General Hospital, Boston, Massachusetts

IMMUNE MECHANISMS AND INFECTIOUS DISEASES IN EXERCISE AND SPORTS

JAMES S. SKINNER, PhD

Professor, Department of Exercise Science and Physical Education; Director, Exercise and Sport Research Institute, Arizona State University, Tempe, Arizona

PHYSIOLOGY OF EXERCISE AND TRAINING

ROBERT P. SMITH, MD

Clinical Associate Professor of Medicine, University of Vermont, Burlington, Vermont; Associate Vice President for Medical Education, Maine Medical Center, Portland, Maine

TRAVEL

STEPHEN N. SULLIVAN, MD, FRCPUK, FRCPC

Professor of Medicine, University of Western Ontario, London, Ontario, Canada; Head of Gastroenterology, King Fahad Hospital, Riyadh, Saudi Arabia

THE GASTROINTESTINAL SYSTEM

RICHARD H. STRAUSS, MD

Associate Professor of Preventive and Internal Medicine, The Ohio State University, Columbus, Ohio; Team Physician, The Ohio State University, Columbus, Ohio

DRUGS IN SPORTS; MEDICAL ASPECTS OF SCUBA AND BREATH-HOLD DIVING

JOHN R. SUTTON, MD, FRACP, FRCP(C)

Professor of Medicine and Exercise Physiology and Head, Department of Biological Sciences, Cumberland College of Health Sciences, The University of Sydney, Sydney, Australia

DIABETES AND EXERCISE; HEAT ILLNESS

DAVID M. SYSTROM, MD

Instructor in Medicine, Harvard Medical School, Boston, Massachusetts; Assistant in Medicine, Pulmonary and Critical Care Unit, Massachusetts General Hospital, Boston, Massachusetts

THE RESPIRATORY SYSTEM

JEFFREY L. TANJI, MD

Assistant Professor, Department of Family Practice, University of California, Davis, Sacramento, California; Staff, University of California, Davis, Medical Center, Sacramento, California

HYPERTENSION

PAUL D. THOMPSON, MD

Associate Professor of Medicine, Brown University, Providence, Rhode Island; Director of Preventive Cardiology, The Miriam Hospital, Providence, Rhode Island

CARDIAC EVALUATION OF THE YOUNG OR OLD, COMPETITIVE OR RECREATIONAL ATHLETE

GERALD C. TIMMIS, MD

Clinical Professor of Health Sciences, Oakland University, Rochester, Michigan; Medical Director of Clinical Research, Division of Cardiology, William Beaumont Hospital, Royal Oak, Michigan

EXERCISE PRESCRIPTION

STEVEN P. VAN CAMP, MD

Professor, College of Professional Studies, San Diego State University, San Diego, California

CLINICAL EXERCISE TESTING

CHARLES E. YESALIS, ScD

Professor of Health Policy and Administration and Exercise and Sport Science, Pennsylvania State University, University Park, Pennsylvania

DRUGS IN SPORTS

JEFFREY P. YORK, MD

Assistant Professor, Division of Urology, The Ohio State University, Columbus, Ohio; Staff, The Ohio State University Medical Center and Grant Medical Center, Columbus, Ohio

THE GENITOURINARY SYSTEM IN THE MALE

PREFACE

This book is unusual in that it is devoted to nontraumatic medical problems in sports and exercise. Many of the reasons that physically active persons visit their physicians fall in the realm of general medicine, including cardiology, dermatology, and nutrition. These patients seek advice on how to optimize their health and fitness as well as help in overcoming specific medical problems.

This volume is intended for the primary physician and for physicians in other specialties who desire a comprehensive view of nontraumatic sports medicine. Each chapter is written by a recognized authority in the field and provides both practical medical applications and the underlying scientific information.

Athletes generally are interesting patients to work with. They are basically healthy and highly motivated to return to competition as quickly as possible. The physician can speed their return to sports activity by appropriate treatment but must also advise them when return is optimal—when play is safe but without requiring an unnecessarily long convalescence. Such advice depends, in part, on the rigors of the particular sport.

Medical problems among athletes are grouped by organ system, with topics ranging from acne in football players to anemia and proteinuria in runners. Factors for optimizing performance and fitness are covered, as are nutrition, drugs, and ergogenic aids, applied psychology, and travel. Considerations important to physically active women are discussed in detail, including participation during pregnancy. A synopsis of exercise physiology is included.

Organized sports competition begins in grade school for some, with soccer, Little League baseball, Pop Warner football, or swimming. An experienced pediatrician discusses physical and psychosocial factors to consider for the well-being of growing children. When they are advised by an informed physician, children with chronic health problems often find exercise and sports more enjoyable and their disease less limiting than was feared. Specific guidelines for the physical evaluation of young sports participants are included.

For the older sports participant, cardiovascular benefits and risks of exercise are covered in detail and exercise testing and prescription are described. An internist discusses aspects of aging and sports, from cancer to sexuality.

Opportunities for physically disabled adults to participate in sports have expanded dramatically as a result of technical advances and social acceptance of the importance of exercise for this group. The interested physician will find special coverage of such considerations in this book.

The environment is, at times, an overwhelming factor in physical performance and even survival. Heat illness, particularly prominent in recreational runners, can be avoided.

In cold environments, hypothermia can kill and frostbite can maim. At high altitudes, pulmonary edema may occur and may require rapid return to a lower elevation. Holding one's breath in a swimming pool while scuba diving can lead to air embolism. This book first stresses how to stay out of trouble and then describes the treatment of specific environmentally caused problems.

We believe that this book will be useful not only to physicians but also to medical students, sports scientists, athletic trainers, nurses, and others who need information about nontraumatic sports medicine.

Richard H. Strauss, M.D.

CONTENTS

SECTION I

DISORDERS OF THE CARDIOVASCULAR SYSTEM

1

CARDIAC EVALUATION OF THE YOUNG OR OLD, COMPETITIVE OR RECREATIONAL ATHLETE

Paul D. Thompson, MD

Exercise-related sudden death in an apparently healthy person is usually due to heat stroke or a cardiac abnormality. The incidence of death during exercise is extremely low, but even the remote possibility of such an event produces considerable concern for sports participants, sports officials, and physicians caring for athletes. This chapter presents clinical principles for the cardiac evaluation of competitive and recreational athletes. The first principle is that "abnormal" cardiac findings in endurance athletes are usually variants of normal.

PRINCIPLE 1 *"Abnormal" cardiac findings in endurance athletes are usually variants of normal*

Consequently, we will first present the normal cardiovascular response to exercise, the normal adaptations to exercise training, and the clinical consequences of these adaptations. We will also discuss the incidence and pathology of exercise-related deaths so that the clinical examination can be designed to exclude conditions that may be lethal after vigorous exertion. Throughout, we will illustrate clinical principles with cases from our experience and the literature.

THE ACUTE CARDIOVASCULAR RESPONSE TO EXERCISE

Exercise requires an increase in oxygen uptake ($\dot{V}O_2$) to supply energy for the exercising muscles. The Fick equation for cardiac output ($\dot{Q}$) may be rearranged as follows:

$$\dot{V}O_2 = \dot{Q} \times \text{(arterial-venous oxygen difference)}$$

Oxygen uptake during exercise can be increased by an increase in $\dot{Q}$, an increase in the arterial-venous oxygen difference (A-V O_2 difference), or both.[1] $\dot{Q}$ increases during upright exercise because of increases in heart rate and stroke volume. The A-V O_2 difference also increases because of greater oxygen extraction across the exercising muscle bed, shunting of blood flow from inactive to active tissue, and an increase in arterial hemoglobin concentration from a loss of plasma volume.[2] The maximal exercise capacity is expressed as the maximal oxygen uptake ($\dot{V}O_{2max}$) and is determined by the maximal $\dot{Q}$ and A-V O_2 difference.[1]

Mechanical efficiency varies among individuals, but in general the "external" work rate[3] or the work performed on the environment determines the $\dot{V}O_2$ during exercise. The $\dot{Q}$ response to exercise is also closely coupled to the increase in oxygen uptake and therefore to the external work rate. In contrast, the heart rate and blood pressure response to exercise is linearly related to the degree of internal stress (expressed as a percentage of $\dot{V}O_{2max}$) that an external work load represents for the individual.[4] Consequently, identical external work loads may produce different heart rate and blood pressure responses in different subjects.

The initial increase in heart rate during exercise is largely due to a reduction in resting vagal tone.[5] Additional increases during exercise result from cardiac sympathetic stimulation. The blood pressure response (ΔP) to exercise is a consequence of the increase in cardiac output ($\Delta\dot{Q}$) and the decrease in total peripheral resistance (ΔR) according to the equation $\Delta P = \Delta\dot{Q} \times \Delta R$.[6] The decrease in peripheral resistance is primarily due to vasodilatation in the exercising muscle and is under local control.[7] In normal subjects, the increase in $\dot{Q}$ exceeds the decrease in peripheral resistance so that systolic and mean blood pressure increase with exercise.

The product of heart rate and systolic blood pressure, or the rate-pressure product (RPP), correlates directly with myocardial oxygen demand.[8] Since the increases in heart rate and blood pressure are related to the percentage of $\dot{V}O_{2max}$ required by an exercise task, identical external work rates can require different "internal" work rates[3] or myocardial oxygen demands depending on the person's maximum exercise capacity. At rest, 70% to 80% of arterial oxygen is extracted by the myocardium. Additional myocardial needs, therefore, must be met by increased flow. In healthy subjects, the increased flow is achieved by a reduction in coronary artery vasomotor tone.[9] In individuals with obstructive coronary lesions, however, vasodilatation is impeded and cardiac ischemia results.

Recent evidence suggests that coronary lesions need not be markedly stenotic to produce exercise ischemia. Normal coronary arteries vasodilate with exercise, but atherosclerotically diseased vessels may vasoconstrict. This paradoxical response is not limited to severely diseased segments, but also occurs in arteries showing only early endothelial irregularities. The mechanism for this abnormal vasoconstriction is not certain but likely relates to endothelial injury and the absence of vasodilators produced by normal endothelium.[10]

CASE 1

A 34-year-old runner developed an inferior wall myocardial infarction 1 mile into a planned 15-mile run. Examination revealed bilateral Achilles tendon thickening consistent with xanthomata and a definite right elbow xanthoma. His serum cholesterol level was 350 mg/dL with an HDL cholesterol level of 64 mg/dL and a triglyceride level of 97 mg/dL. Coronary arteriography 1 month after the infarct showed normal coronary arteries except for atherosclerotic plaque in the right coronary artery. He was treated with nifedipine, preexercise nitroglycerin, niacin, and cholestyramine and has been asymptomatic during 3 years of follow-up. This case illustrates the possibility that ischemic syndromes can occur with noncritical coronary artery lesions. The mechanism in this case could be a resolving coronary thrombosis or a spasm-induced infarct.

CARDIOVASCULAR ADAPTATIONS TO EXERCISE TRAINING

The major physiologic adaptation to exercise training is an increase in maximal exercise capacity or in $\dot{V}O_{2max}$. The increase in $\dot{V}O_{2max}$ is due to increases in both maximal $\dot{Q}$ and the maximal A-V O_2 difference.[1] Maximal heart rate does not increase and may even fall, so that the higher $\dot{Q}$ is achieved by an increase in maximal stroke volume.[4] The increase in $\dot{V}O_{2max}$ means that the same work load after exercise training represents less stress, expressed as percent $\dot{V}O_{2max}$. Consequently, the heart rate and blood pressure responses to the same external work load and the myocardial oxygen demand are less after training.

Changes in $\dot{V}O_{2max}$ do not indicate all of the adaptations that occur with exercise training. $\dot{V}O_{2max}$ measures maximal power or work load per minute. Endurance capacity, the ability to perform submaximal work for prolonged periods, also increases with exercise training, but has rarely been quantified in training studies.[2] Such increases in endurance capacity probably result from enhanced skeletal muscle oxidative capacity.[2]

Because the major effect of training is increased exercise capacity, athletes who complain of a decrease in exercise performance require a complete evaluation. Nevertheless, physical fatigue and/or psychological factors, often from overtraining, are responsible for most complaints of reduced exercise capacity in well-trained endurance athletes.

PRINCIPLE 2 *Physical fatigue and/or psychological factors are responsible for most complaints of reduced exercise capacity in endurance athletes*

On the other hand, we are aware of several young athletes with cardiomyopathies who first presented with decreased exercise performance despite adequate training. Therefore, even if overtraining or psychological fatigue is suspected, such a conclusion requires frequent reevaluation. Also, physical work capacity or $\dot{V}O_{2max}$ depends on both cardiac factors (heart rate and stroke volume) and extracardiac factors (arterial oxygen content, systemic shunting, and muscle oxygen extraction). Extracardiac factors, such as decreased oxygen-carrying capacity from anemia, limit exercise tolerance and should be considered in athletes who develop effort intolerance.

ALTERATIONS IN CARDIAC RATE AND RHYTHM

Endurance exercise training reduces resting heart rate and slows atrioventricular (AV) nodal conduction. These changes have generally been attributed to enhanced vagal tone.[11] Enhanced vagal tone is unlikely to be the entire explanation, however, since the heart rates of endurance athletes are lower at rest than those of control subjects even after autonomic influence has been eliminated by large doses of atropine and propranolol.[12] Nevertheless, endurance athletes commonly have heart rates between 40 and 50 beats/min and an occasional endurance athlete will have a resting heart rate in the mid-30s range. Marked variation in the sinus rate with respiration, so-called sinus arrhythmia, also occurs with increased vagal tone and occurs in 13% to 69% of athletes.[13] Increased vagal tone can produce first-degree AV block and second-degree Wenckebach AV block. Ambulatory monitoring of athletes may even demonstrate prolonged sinus pauses with nodal and even ventricular escape rhythms on the electrocardiogram (ECG).[13] These ectopic pacemakers arise because vagal inhibition of the sinus mechanism shifts the pacemaker to a lower focus. A rare athlete can demonstrate third-degree or complete heart block. The most extreme of these rhythm "abnormalities" are seen only in well-trained endurance athletes. All normal variants of rate and rhythm disappear with the exercise-induced withdrawal of vagal tone, and the appearance of conduction abnormalities during exercise in athletes is distinctly abnormal.

PRINCIPLE 3 *The ECGs of well-trained endurance athletes may demonstrate AV block as well as atrial, nodal, and even ventricular escape rhythms; such "abnormalities" should disappear during exercise*

Ventricular preexcitation, such as the Wolff-Parkinson-White (W-P-W) syndrome, is due to the presence of an accessory AV conduction pathway that initiates early ventricular activation. Since this additional pathway is probably not under vagal control, endurance training may unmask the preexcitation pathway by impeding normal AV conduction. Consequently, ventricular preexcitation on the resting ECG may be slightly more frequent in athletes. However, W-P-W syndrome occurs in only 1 in 1000 in the general population[13]; this makes an accurate comparison of the incidence of preexcitation in athletes and with that in others impossible. It is important to note a short P-R interval on the resting electrocardiogram, however, because ventricular preexcitation may produce false-positive S-T segment responses to exercise, and because such athletes may face a slightly increased incidence of the cardiac complications discussed below.

In addition to the bradyarrhythmias and conduction disturbances related to enhanced vagal tone, a recent review[13] suggests that endurance athletes may experience an increased incidence of paroxysmal atrial fibrillation. The ventricular response to atrial fibrillation may be slower than in untreated patients of similar age, again, due to augmented vagal tone. The etiology of atrial fibrillation in athletes is rarely clear although alcohol use (the "holiday heart") is occasionally a factor. Most acute episodes of atrial fibrillation are transient and respond well to either patience, oral quinidine during telemetry monitoring, intravenous digoxin, or intravenous verapamil (Fig. 1–1).

Ventricular premature contractions (VPCs) reportedly occur with similar frequencies in athletes and sedentary subjects. Nevertheless, our clinical impression is that they are felt more frequently in athletes because bradycardia makes any cardiac disturbance more noticeable, because athletes are more attuned to such arrhythmias, or because VPCs are detected by pulse monitoring during training. VPCs should be judged by the cardiac company they keep, and in the company of an otherwise normal heart, they should be treated primarily with reassurance.

PRINCIPLE 4 *Ventricular premature contractions should be judged by the cardiac company they keep*

ST SEGMENT AND T-WAVE ABNORMALITIES AT REST

Increased vagal tone and reduced sympathetic stimulation may also be responsible for ST segment and T-wave abnormalities in athletes.[14] ST segment elevation characteristic of the "early repolarization" pattern is more common in young and old endurance athletes, but it is also common in other young subjects. Precordial T-wave inversions and biphasic T waves can be found in athletes. Both the ST segment and T-wave changes may resolve promptly when vagal tone is reduced by exercise or by atropine administration. Consequently, for the asymptomatic athlete with resting electrocardiographic abnormalities, the

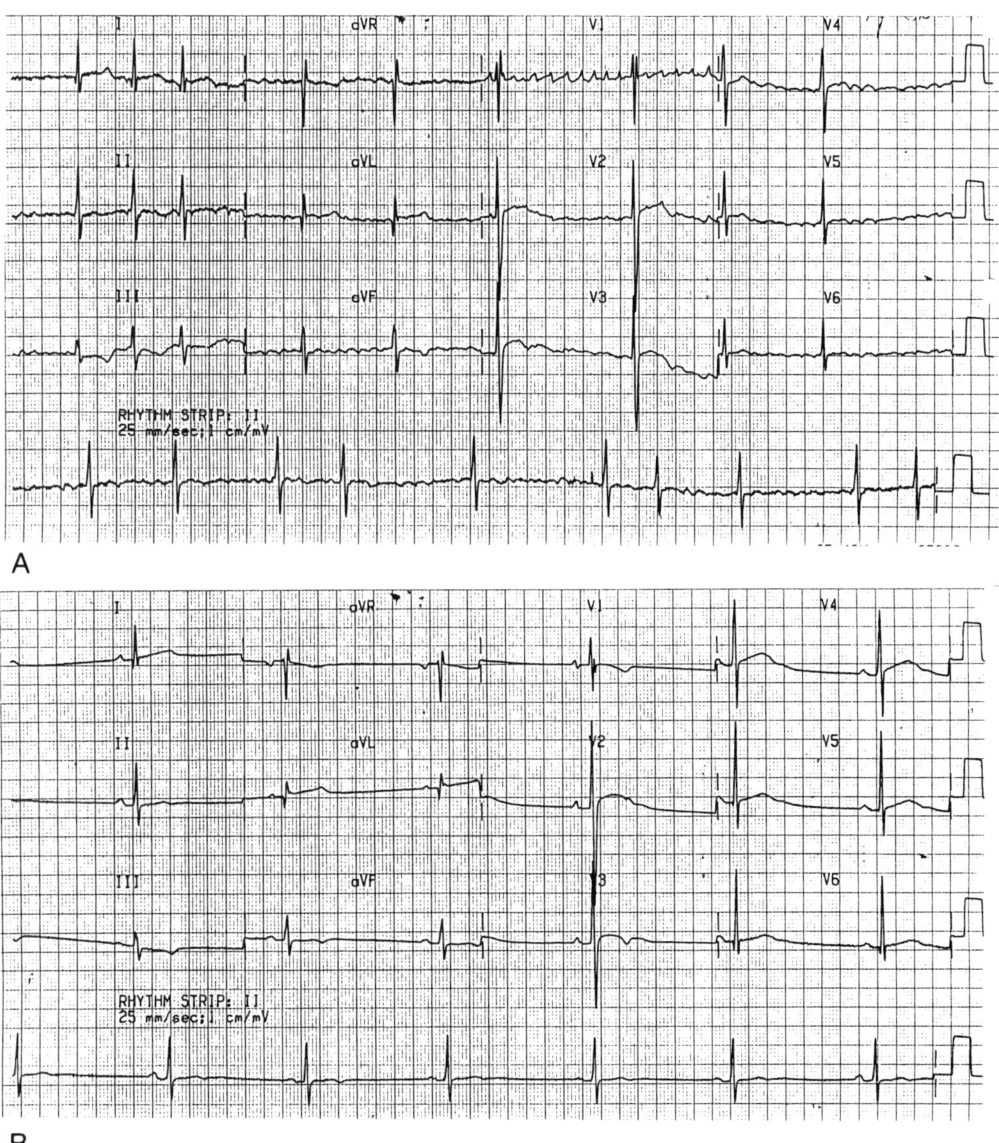

Figure 1–1. Case 2. ECG tracings during **(A)** and after **(B)** an episode of atrial fibrillation (AF) in a 42-year-old man who runs 35 miles per week. The ventricular response during AF is only 60 beats/min despite no medication. The patient was monitored and converted after oral quinidine. Postconversion heart rate was only 42 beats/min. Both tracings show the incomplete right bundle branch block, precordial ST elevation, and T-wave changes common in endurance athletes. This case illustrates that the ventricular response to AF is often slow in endurance athletes.

response of these abnormalities to exercise helps to differentiate physiologic from pathologic findings.

EVIDENCE OF CARDIAC HYPERTROPHY

Well-trained endurance athletes often have evidence of cardiac enlargement by electrocardiogram (ECG), chest radiograph, and echocardiogram. Such cardiac enlargement may include both ventricles, the left atrium, and even the right atrium.

Many endurance athletes meet voltage criteria for left ventricular hypertrophy (LVH) on ECG. The percentage of athletes with ECGs satisfying voltage criteria for LVH varies from 26% to 83%,[15,16] depending on the type of athletes studied and the LVH criteria used. It is uncommon, however, for athletes to have the ST segment depression of LVH even though they satisfy the voltage requirements. Raskoff and colleagues[17] reported that 26 (87%) of 30 runners satisfied at least one voltage criterion of LVH, but none of the athletes satisfied the more stringent Estes-Romhilt point criteria, which include ST segment depression.

Evidence of increased ECG voltage is also more common in endurance-trained athletes than in other types of athletes. Longhurst et al[18] obtained ECGs and echocardiograms in 12 runners, 17 competitive weightlifters, 10 lightweight controls, and 14 heavyweight controls. Both groups of athletes had a larger left ventricular mass than their controls. The QRS voltage on ECG was greatest in the runners, however, even though by echocardiography the left ventricular mass in the runners was equal to that in competitive weightlifters. This suggests that ECG voltage values observed in endurance athletes are due to both increased cardiac size and thin chest walls.

Athletes may also have ECG evidence of right ventricular hypertrophy (RVH). Roeske and colleagues[15] reported that 69% of professional basketball players had RVH on ECG. Ikaheimo and associates[16] compared the ECGs of distance runners, sprinters, and sedentary controls. Seven of 12 runners and 4 of 10 sprinters had partial right bundle branch block on ECG, presumably related to RVH (Fig. 1–2).

Abnormally tall P waves, suggesting right atrial enlargement, and P-wave notching have also been noted in endurance athletes.[13]

The ECG evidence of biventricular enlargement has been confirmed by both radiologic and echocardiographic studies of competitive athletes. Multiple studies have demonstrated that athletes' hearts on chest radiograph are larger than those of sedentary com-

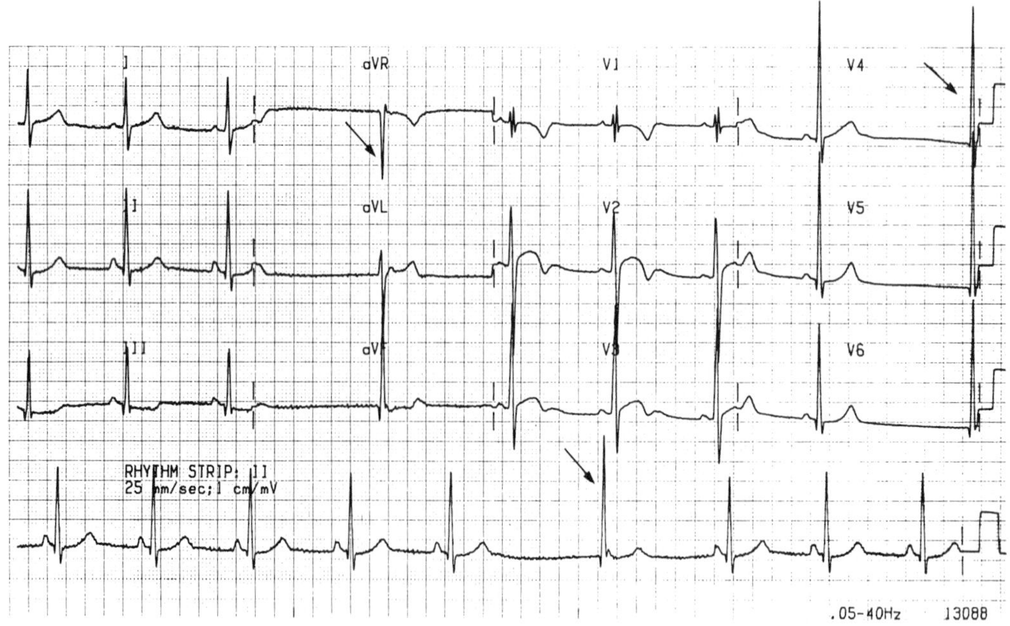

Figure 1–2. Case 3. ECG of a 28-year-old 2-hour, 17-minute marathoner evaluated for momentary chest discomfort. Cardiac examination was normal including splitting of S_2 with inspiration. The ECG tracing shows an axis of 110°, an incomplete right bundle branch block, sinus pauses with junctional escape beats *(arrows),* biphasic T waves in leads V_2 and V_3, and increased precordial voltage. The P wave is also slightly increased in lead II. These "abnormalities" are often normal in endurance athletes.

parison subjects.[16,17,19,20] The frequency of frank cardiomegaly, usually defined as a heart shadow of greater than half the width of the rib cage on posteroanterior view, varies. Parker and coworkers[20] reported that 3 of the 10 runners (30%) in their study had cardiomegaly on the chest radiograph, whereas only 10% of the distance runners studied by Raskoff et al[17] and 17% of the professional basketball players examined by Roeske et al[15] had radiologic cardiomegaly. Cardiomegaly on chest radiography is unusual in athletes participating in nonendurance sports and should prompt a search for other causes.

Echocardiographic studies of athletes confirm that their cardiac dimensions are larger than those of control subjects. The enlargement has been demonstrated to include the left ventricular internal diameter, the right ventricular internal diameter, the left atrium, and the left ventricular posterior wall.[13] Left ventricular function, as judged by wall motion and percent fractional shortening, is normal in the athletes.

The echocardiographic pattern of cardiac enlargement depends in general on the athlete's training activity. Endurance athletes have generalized cardiac enlargement. The walls of the left ventricle in endurance athletes may or may not be thickened.[16,18] Athletes involved in strength training tend to have an increased cardiac mass because of increased left ventricular wall thickness rather than because of chamber dilatation.

In the study of runners and weightlifters by Longhurst et al,[18] the calculated left ventricular mass in the athletes was increased over that in light–body weight and heavy–body weight control subjects, but the values for left ventricular mass were similar in the two groups of athletes. Posterior left ventricular wall thickness was greatest in the weightlifters, whereas left ventricular internal diameter was greatest in the distance runners. When left ventricular mass was normalized for body size, the left ventricular mass of the runners was greater than in all other groups. Furthermore, when the left ventricular mass of the weightlifters was corrected for lean body mass, the values for the weightlifters were not different from those of heavyweight controls. These results demonstrate that although left ventricular mass is increased in "strength" athletes, the increase is proportional to the increase in total body muscle mass. Endurance athletes, however, have an increase in left ventricular mass unrelated to changes in total body mass (Fig. 1–3).

The clinical implications of these findings are obvious: healthy athletes may have evidence of cardiac enlargement on ECG, radiograph, and echocardiography that may be interpreted as abnormal. In evaluating such findings, the physician must appreciate that the cardiac enlargement is not accompanied by evidence of diminished function.

PRINCIPLE 5 *Healthy endurance athletes may have evidence of atrial and ventricular enlargement on ECG, radiograph, and echocardiogram, but cardiac function is normal*

CAUSES OF EXERCISE-RELATED, NONTRAUMATIC DEATHS

Heat illness is dealt with elsewhere in this volume, and the cardiac causes of sudden death with exertion have been examined in several recent reviews.[21–23]

Congenital cardiovascular abnormalities are the most frequent cause of exercise-related deaths in young subjects. Commonly reported abnormalities include hypertrophic cardiomyopathy (Fig. 1–4), anomalous origin and course of the right or left coronary artery (Figs. 1–5 and 1–6), and Marfan's syndrome with aortic rupture. Valvular aortic stenosis was prevalent in early reports of exercise-related cardiac deaths, but has been largely absent from recent reviews either because it is no longer considered reportable or because screening has reduced the physical activity of potential victims. Other rare causes

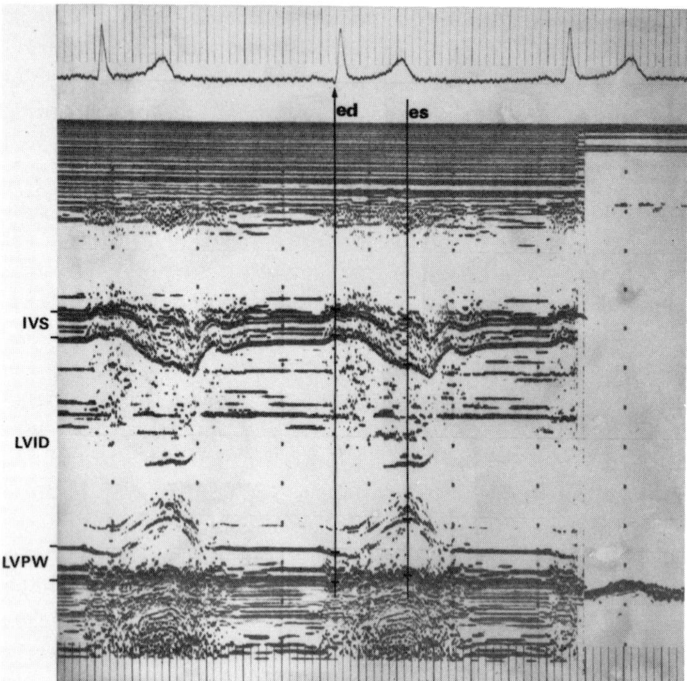

Figure 1–3. Case 4. The echocardiogram shows the septal (IVS) and posterior wall (LVPW) thickness and the left ventricular internal dimensions (LVID) at end diastole (ed) and end systole (es) in the author, formerly a 2-hour, 28-minute marathoner. The LVID ed is increased to 55 mm (normal is ≤55 mm), but wall thickness is normal, and the fractional shortening of the left ventricle is normal at 29%. The subject weighed 58 kg (128 lb) when this echocardiogram was performed.

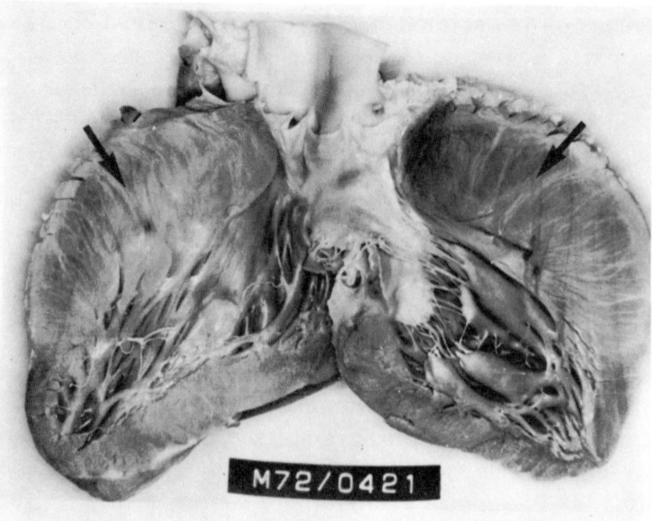

Figure 1–4. Case 5. The arrows point to the thickened left ventricular septum of a 15-year-old football player with hypertrophic cardiomyopathy who collapsed and died during warm-up exercises. (*From* Sturner WQ, Spruill FG: Asymmetrical hypertrophy of the heart: Two sudden deaths in adolescents. J Forensic Sci 19:566, 1974. Copyright ASTM. Reprinted with permission.)

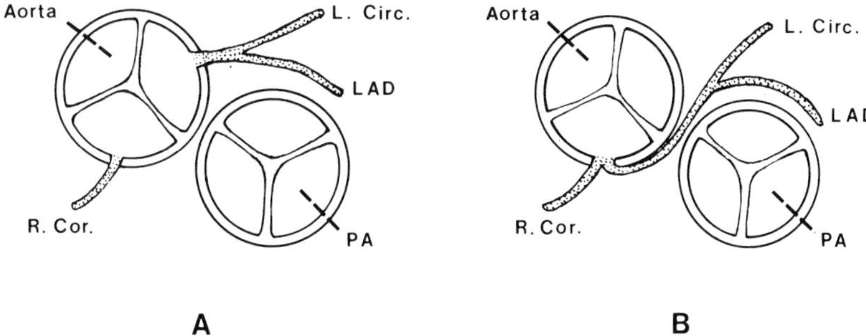

Figure 1–5. Anomalous origin of the left coronary artery. **A**: The normal origin of the right coronary artery is in the anterior sinus of Valsalva. The left coronary artery arises from the left sinus of Valsalva and divides into the left circumflex (L. Circ.) and left anterior descending (LAD) coronary arteries. The pulmonary artery (PA) is anterior to the aorta. **B**: Abnormal origin of the left coronary artery in the anterior sinus of Valsalva. In this picture, both the right and left coronary arteries arise from the same ostium. The left and right coronary arteries may also arise abnormally from separate ostia in the anterior sinus of Valsalva.

of sudden death during exercise include mitral valve prolapse, endomyocardial coronary arteries, and anomalous AV conduction, such as the Wolff-Parkinson-White syndrome. The rarity of these last three conditions as causes of exercise-related deaths is especially noteworthy because their prevalence in the general population is approximately 6%, 27%, and 0.1% respectively.[13,24,25] Unexplained left ventricular hypertrophy has been associated with death in young athletes[26] as well as probable myocarditis.[27] Some necropsies uncover no obvious culprit, implying that a primary arrhythmia with or without undetected conduction system disease was responsible. A recent report of sudden death in nonexercisers suggests that some of these unexplained exercise deaths may be related to an abnormally acute takeoff angle of the coronary arteries from the aorta or to the presence of coronary ostial ridges.[28] Both abnormalities can transiently occlude the coronary orifice when the stroke volume increases with exercise (Fig. 1–7).

In contrast, the most frequent cause of exercise-related death in adults is atherosclerotic coronary artery disease (CAD). Many of the victims have advanced CAD at autopsy with only half of the subjects showing an acute coronary lesion such as a recent thrombus, intramural hemorrhage, or recent myocardial infarction.[27] The absence of a recent infarction suggests that these deaths are arrhythmia-induced and occur without acute infarction or before pathologic evidence of an acute infarction has developed.

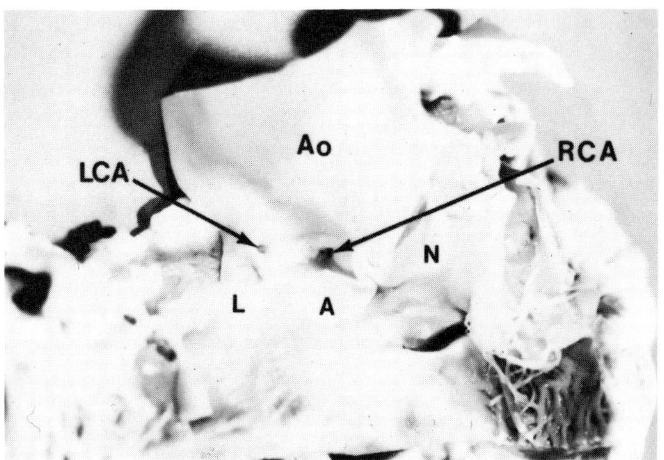

Figure 1–6. Case 6. The arrows indicate the origins of the left coronary artery (LCA) and the right coronary artery (RCA) in a 26-year-old man who collapsed and died while jogging. The LCA should originate from the left (L) coronary cusp, but here it originates between the left and right or anterior (A) cusps. N indicates the noncoronary cusp. Two ostia for the RCA are also visible. (Courtesy of Arthur C. Burns, MD, Providence, RI.)

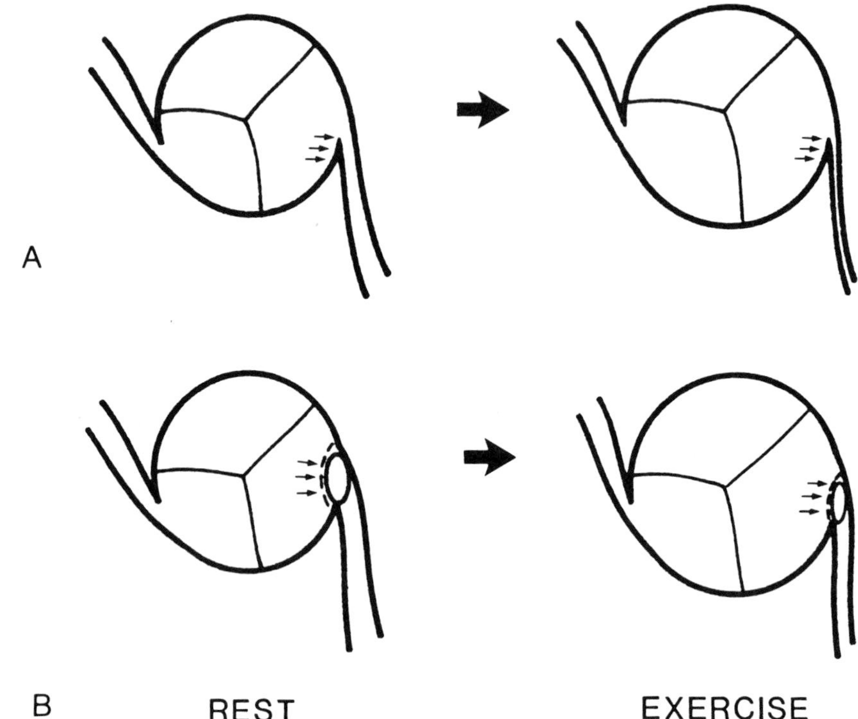

Figure 1–7. Illustrates possible occlusion of the coronary ostia when the aortic volume is increased during exercise in the presence of acute coronary artery takeoff angle (**A**) or ostial ridges (**B**).

INCIDENCE OF SUDDEN DEATH DURING EXERTION

Despite the widespread media attention given to sudden death in athletes, the incidence of death during exertion is extremely low. We collected all deaths occurring during jogging in Rhode Island over a 6-year period.[29] Twelve men died while jogging. All but two were aged 30 to 65 years and all but one died from coronary heart disease. The number of Rhode Island joggers was calculated using a random digit telephone survey and population statistics. We estimated that one jogging death occurred per year for every 7620 joggers aged 35 to 65 years. A premortem diagnosis of coronary heart disease was possible in five of the ten middle-aged men. If these men are eliminated and we assume that no surviving joggers had diagnosed heart disease, the incidence of death decreases to one death for every 15,240 healthy joggers. Siscovick et al[30] reported similar results in their study of cardiac arrests among previously healthy men in Seattle. Only one death per year occurred during exertion for every 18,000 healthy men. Nevertheless in both Rhode Island and Seattle, the hourly death rate during exercise exceeds that at other times. The absolute risk of death during exercise for asymptomatic individuals is extremely low, but exertion does transiently increase the risk for susceptible persons with known or occult disease.

PRINCIPLE 6 *The absolute risk of death during exercise for asymptomatic individuals is low, but exertion does transiently increase that risk for susceptible persons*

CARDIAC EXAMINATION OF THE ATHLETE

The cardiac examination is designed to detect pathologic conditions that may produce problems during exercise. The history should include inquiries about sudden death at a young age or congenital heart disease in family members as well as symptoms of exercise intolerance including exercise syncope, extreme dyspnea, chest discomfort, and palpitations in the patient.

The physical examination should exclude the possibility of hypertension, Marfan's syndrome, aortic stenosis, and hypertrophic cardiomyopathy. The possibility of Marfan's syndrome should be considered in all athletes but especially when evaluating athletes who participate in sports requiring increased height and arm length.

PRINCIPLE 7 *Marfan's syndrome should be considered in athletes who participate in sports requiring increased height and arm length*

Marfan's syndrome is an inherited defect of elastic tissue that affects the eyes, the cardiovascular system, and supporting structures.[31] Skeletal abnormalities include an increase in height compared with other family members, unusually long limbs, an increased lower body length, long slender fingers, and sternal deformities. Ocular problems include subluxation of the lens and increased globe length leading to myopia. Cardiac abnormalities include mitral valve prolapse and aortic root dilatation. Both dissecting aortic aneurysm and aortic rupture may occur during physical exertion. The ascending aorta is vulnerable owing to the force exerted by cardiac ejection and the high concentration of elastic fibers in the proximal aortic segment. Additional findings include a high, narrowly arched palate, inguinal hernias, cutaneous striae, lax joints, and a history of spontaneous pneumothorax. Despite obvious abnormalities in some, the diagnosis is often overlooked because contact lenses obscure otherwise obvious ocular abnormalities and because some patients have a paucity of structural abnormalities.

CASE 7

The patient was a champion high school cross-country runner. At age 28, he presented with chest pain, aortic root dilatation to 68 mm (normal is <40 mm), and aortic insufficiency. At this time, he was running 10 miles daily in preparation for the Newport Marathon. He underwent aortic root and valve replacement with reimplantation of the coronary arteries. He did well until age 36 when several hours after a free introductory workout at a health club, he developed a dissecting aneurysm of the descending aorta. This has been managed conservatively with antihypertensives and beta-adrenergic blockade. On examination, he is normal in appearance, in part because a sternal deformity was repaired during heart surgery. He is 5′8″ tall and weighs 77 kg. The wing span is not increased, the upper to lower body ratio is normal, and there is no joint laxity. The palate is highly arched, there are cutaneous striae on both buttocks, and the lens in the left eye is dislocated.

This case illustrates the importance of considering Marfan's syndrome in athletes and the risk of aortic damage with exercise in these patients. Proximal aortic dissections are more frequent than distal dissections, but distal dissections can occur.

Blood pressure should be measured with a cuff containing a bladder that covers two thirds of the arm circumference to avoid falsely elevated blood pressure readings in athletes with large arms. Mild increases in systolic blood pressure may occur in athletes because of their increased stroke volume. Widening of the pulse pressure to more than 60 mm Hg, however, may indicate aortic insufficiency from a bicuspid aortic valve, a condition that may occur in as many as 2% of the population.[32] A delay in carotid upstroke or the presence of audible or palpable murmurs over the carotids indicates aortic stenosis of significant degree. S_3 and S_4 gallops secondary to physiologic hypertrophy are common in athletes as are so-called innocent murmurs. Innocent or physiologically insignificant murmurs in young athletes are frequently related to pulmonic flow, whereas such murmurs in older subjects may be pulmonic or aortic in origin.[32] Both are more common when auscultation is performed in the supine position. The supine position augments venous return from the legs, which increases both stroke volume and the intensity of the murmur. Such murmurs should disappear or soften when the athlete is examined upright. Aortic flow murmurs are common in athletes more than 50 years old, but are often associated with mild early fibrosis and calcification of the aortic valve. In contrast to important aortic stenosis, the carotid upstroke is normal and innocent aortic murmurs rarely radiate to the carotids. The systolic murmur of hypertrophic cardiomyopathy may mimic either valvular aortic stenosis or mitral regurgitation. This murmur classically increases with the Valsalva maneuver because reduced venous return decreases left ventricular cavity size, allowing the septum to approach the free wall, which increases subvalvular obstruction.

WHY DO ATHLETIC HEARTS MURMUR?

Blood flow is laminar and without turbulence until a critical Reynolds number (Re) is exceeded. Re is equal to

$$\frac{\overline{V}d\rho}{\mu}$$

where $\overline{V}$ = average velocity, d = the diameter of the tube, ρ = fluid density, and μ = fluid viscosity.[33] Above an Re of 2000, laminar flow is disturbed, producing audible turbulence. Aortic and pulmonic valve orifice size (d) is not increased in athletes. Resting stroke volume can be greatly increased in endurance-trained athletes, however, and the athlete's more vigorous systolic function delivers much of this stroke volume in early systole. Velocity is consequently increased and the athletic flow murmur results.

We suggest that all screening examinations be done with the athletes standing or sitting. This position reduces or eliminates innocent murmurs, enhances the murmur of hypertrophic cardiomyopathy, and increases physiologic splitting of S_2. Absence of normal splitting of S_2 may indicate an atrial septal defect. In addition, all screening examinations should include the Valsalva maneuver. This decreases physiologic flow murmurs, but augments the murmur of hypertrophic cardiomyopathy.

PRINCIPLE 8 *Screening examinations should be done with subjects upright and should include the Valsalva maneuver*

CASE 8

A 20-year-old man was referred for evaluation of a heart murmur detected during a college blood drive. He plays racquetball 2 hours and practices karate 4 hours each week. Cardiac examination revealed a blood pressure of 122/74 mm

Hg in each arm and normal carotid upstrokes. No murmurs were audible with the patient sitting although a 2/6 early systolic ejection murmur was present with the patient supine and his legs elevated to increase venous return. No murmur was heard during Valsalva maneuver. The patient had been examined supine during the blood drive examination. Doppler echocardiography revealed normal cardiac dimensions and trace pulmonic and tricuspid regurgitation. The patient and his family were reassured that the murmur was an innocent flow murmur. Trace regurgitant lesions are common in normal Doppler echocardiographic studies.

We do not recommend any routine cardiac testing for healthy, asymptomatic, young or old athletes. Baseline ECGs may be useful for athletes in contact sports because such tracings may subsequently be useful in evaluating possible cardiac contusions. The rarity of occult structural abnormalities in athletes does not warrant baseline echocardiography. Similarly, we do not recommend routine exercise testing of adult athletes because of the rarity of exercise deaths,[29,30] the high frequency of false-positive ECG responses in healthy people,[34] and the observation that the largest absolute number of sudden cardiac deaths occurs in subjects with normal ST segment responses to exercise.[35] We do test any middle-aged athletes with symptoms suggestive of coronary disease.

Echocardiography is extremely useful in evaluating murmurs in athletes, and Doppler echocardiography is useful in quantifying the significance of valvular lesions. This latter technique is extremely sensitive, however, and may detect trivial regurgitation from all four cardiac valves in athletes.[36]

FURTHER EVALUATION AND RESTRICTION OF ACTIVITY

We prohibit patients with Marfan's syndrome, significant valvular aortic stenosis, or hypertrophic cardiomyopathy from vigorous exertion. Similarly, once the diagnosis of congenital or acquired coronary artery disease is seriously considered, we prohibit exercise until the diagnosis is excluded.

Subjects with asymptomatic valvular abnormalities other than aortic stenosis can exercise without restriction as long as the exercise does not provoke symptoms. All patients with valvular abnormalities require endocarditis prophylaxis and prompt attention to any skin infections. We permit patients with aortic insufficiency to participate in dynamic exercise but discourage isometric activities that may raise diastolic blood pressure and increase the regurgitant volume. Questions concerning children with congenital heart lesions are best handled in conjunction with a pediatric cardiologist. Furthermore, exercise syncope or possible exercise angina even in a young person requires complete cardiac evaluation by a cardiologist to exclude such rare abnormalities as anomalous coronary artery origin.

PRINCIPLE 9 *True exercise syncope or possible exercise angina even in a young person requires a complete cardiac evaluation*

Middle-aged athletes about to embark on a vigorous exercise program should know the nature of cardiac symptoms and their need for prompt medical attention.

PRINCIPLE 10 *Exercising adults should know the nature of cardiac prodromal symptoms*

Physicians should also be aware that some patients requesting permission to start an exercise program have experienced new symptoms and want to increase their activity to prove that their symptoms are not cardiac in origin. The physician should not overlook the possibility that new symptoms even in an active subject may indicate symptomatic coronary artery disease. We discourage adults with diagnosed coronary disease from competitive athletics, but we do encourage regular vigorous activity for this group.[37]

CASE 9

A 50-year-old man had bicycled 50 to 100 miles weekly most of his life and had run 30 miles per week for the last 7 years. He was evaluated for slight discomfort in his left arm that appeared 10 minutes into his 5-mile runs but would dissipate with continued exercise. During thallium stress testing, he exercised through the fifth stage of the Bruce protocol and achieved a peak heart rate of 182 beats per minute and a double product of 37,000. ST segment changes were abnormal (Fig. 1–8), and thallium imaging showed a reperfusing defect of the high anterior wall. Coronary angiography showed a high-grade stenosis of the first diagonal branch of the left anterior descending artery. He was treated with diltiazem and preexercise nitroglycerin, returned to noncompetitive running, and has been symptom-free during 18 months of follow-up. His highest serum lipid values are a total cholesterol of 227 mg/dL, triglycerides of 74 mg/dL, and an HDL cholesterol of 73 mg/dL. He never smoked, but he has had hypertension for many years treated with diuretics. This case illustrates the importance of suspecting occult coronary disease even in fit individuals at low risk for heart disease who present with atypical but exercise-induced symptoms.

COMMON CARDIAC PROBLEMS IN COMPETITIVE ATHLETES

Noncardiac Syncope

Cardiac syncope results in complete collapse, often with a short seizure and diaphoresis. Adolescent athletes, in contrast, may complain of "passing out" that is better described as a sense of weakness and disorientation. Frequently, these episodes are repetitive and happen at the end of a competitive event. Examinations, including echocardiography and exercise testing, are normal. Careful questioning often reveals a potential psychological factor in these episodes. Treatment consists of a full evaluation, attention to possible psychological factors, and reassurance for the parents and the athlete.

CASE 10

A 15-year-old female cross-country runner was evaluated for two episodes of exercise "syncope." Both episodes occurred near the finish line of 2- to 3-mile races in which she was running below her usual performance level. She was noted to stagger before collapsing. She denied loss of consciousness but was

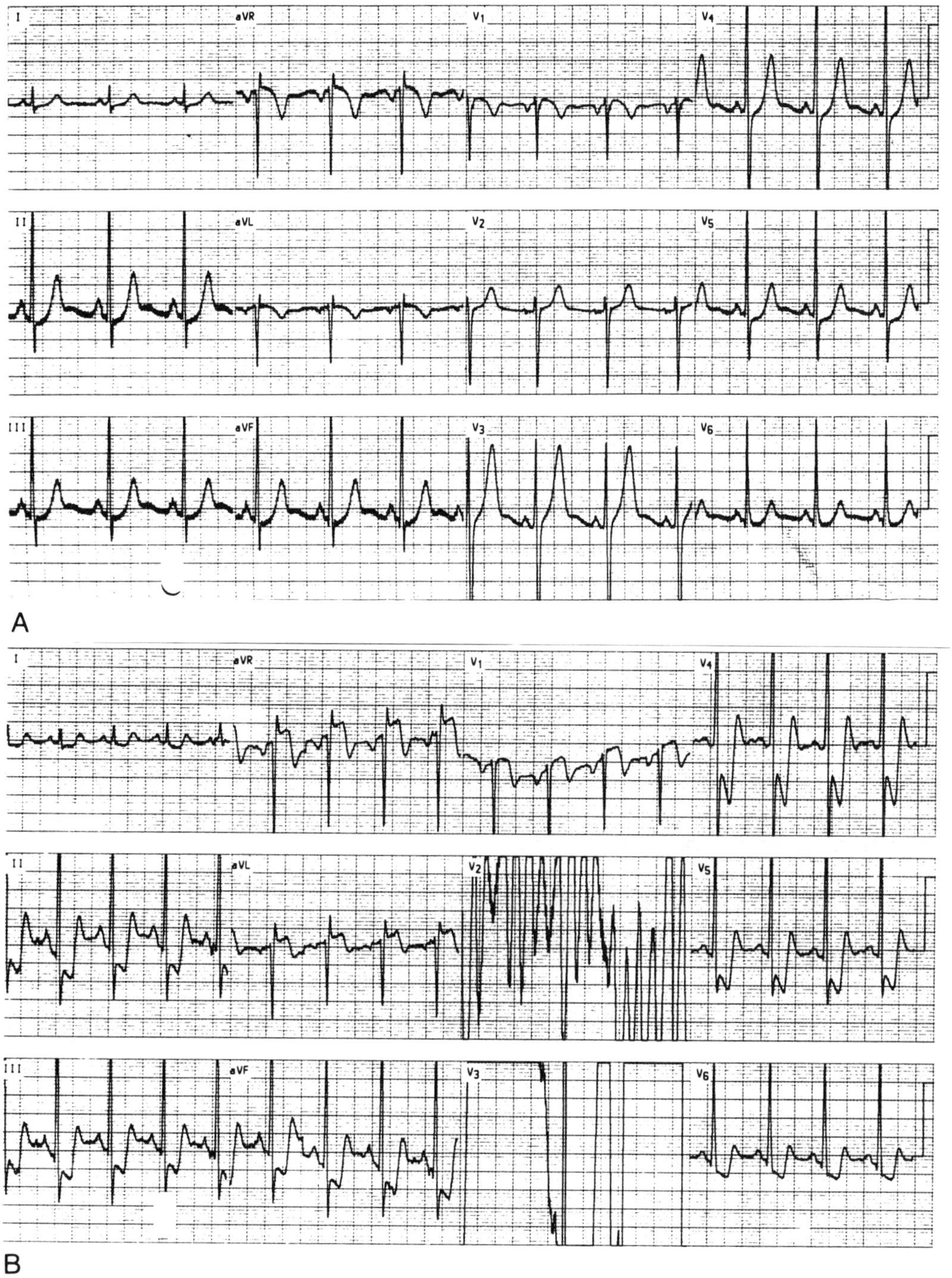

Figure 1–8. Rest **(A)** and postexercise **(B)** ECGs in case 9. Lead V_2 and V_3 tracings are obliterated by artifact in the postexercise tracing. The downsloping ST changes in the tracings from leads II, III, F, and V_1–V_6 and the persistence of ST depression after exercise suggest a true-positive ST response.

poorly responsive and felt "sleepy." Emergency room evaluation revealed a blood pressure of 94/60 mm Hg, a heart rate of 100 beats/min, and a blood glucose level of 90 mg/dL. Mitral valve prolapse was seen on the echocardiogram. An exercise test was normal. The patient and her family were reassured, and she has done well during 5 years of follow-up. The case illustrates that psychological exercise syncope often occurs in young athletes not performing up to expectations.

Elevation of Muscle Enzymes

The repetitive muscle trauma of endurance exercise can lead to the release of the muscle enzymes creatine phosphokinase (CPK), lactate dehydrogenase (LDH), and aspartate aminotransferase (AST). Because measurement of these enzymes is used clinically to diagnose myocardial infarction, their elevation may be erroneously interpreted as indicating myocardial injury. Furthermore, the myocardial band (MB) fraction of CPK has been used to distinguish CPK elevation of cardiac origin from other sources, but CPK-MB may also be elevated in athletes.[38] The cause of the MB fraction elevation is unknown, but it may be released from skeletal muscle cells involved in the muscle repair process. Consequently, elevations of "cardiac" enzymes in active endurance athletes should not be assumed to indicate myocardial infarction unless there is other supporting evidence. Because the athlete's ECG may appear abnormal, excluding disease may be difficult. Radionuclide cardiac imaging to detect myocardial perfusion defects or wall-motion abnormalities can be used to resolve the issue.

Exercise ST Segment Depression in the Athlete

Exercise stress testing is frequently performed prior to exercise training. Although we do not recommend such testing, the physician may be asked to advise appropriate treatment for an athlete whose routine exercise test revealed ST segment changes. "False-positive" exercise ECGs have been reported for competitive athletes. Five of 20 elite United States distance runners had such ECG changes, and in three instances, the ST displacement exceeded 2 mm.[39] Because such false-positive results can occur, the approach to these athletes depends on the probability that they have coronary disease if the exercise ECG is ignored. Athletes who have low coronary risk factors, especially those who are young nonsmokers with a low blood pressure and serum cholesterol level and who demonstrate excellent exercise tolerance, can be assumed to have a false-positive result. Older athletes frequently require additional testing, including myocardial imaging with thallium, and occasionally, coronary arteriography.

REFERENCES

1. Mitchell JH, Blomquist G: Maximal oxygen uptake. N Engl J Med 284:1018–1022, 1971.
2. Rowell LB: Human Circulation During Physical Stress. New York, Oxford University Press, 1986.
3. Amsterdam EA, Hughes JL, III, DeMaria AN, et al: Indirect assessment of myocardial oxygen consumption in the evaluation of mechanisms and therapy of angina pectoris. Am J Cardiol 33:737–743, 1974.
4. Clausen JP: Effect of physical training on cardiovascular adjustments to exercise in man. Physiol Rev 57:779–815, 1977.
5. Vatner SF, Pagani M: Cardiovascular adjustments to exercise: Hemodynamics and mechanisms. Prog Cardiovasc Dis 19:91–108, 1976.
6. Astrand P, Rodahl K: Textbook of Work Physiology: Physiological Basis of Exercise, ed 2. Philadelphia, McGraw-Hill, 1977, p 191.
7. Smith EE, Guyton AC, Manning RD, et al: Integrated mechanism of cardiovascular response and control during exercise in the normal man. Prog Cardiovasc Dis 18:421–444, 1976.
8. Gobel FL, Norstrom LA, Nelson RR, et al: The rate-pressure product as an index of myocardial oxygen consumption during exercise in patients with angina pectoris. Circulation 57:549–556, 1978.

9. Klocke FJ: Coronary blood flow in man. Prog Cardiovasc Dis 19:117–166, 1976.
10. Gordon JB, Ganz P, Nadel EG, et al: Atherosclerosis influences the vasomotor response of epicardial coronary arteries to exercise. J Clin Invest 83:1946–1952, 1989.
11. Smith ML, Hudson DL, Graitzer HM, et al: Exercise training bradycardia: The role of autonomic balance. Med Sci Sports Exerc 21:40–44, 1989.
12. Lewis SF, Nylander E, Gad P, et al: Non-autonomic component in bradycardia of endurance trained men at rest and during exercise. Acta Physiol Scand 109:297–305, 1980.
13. Huston TP, Puffer JC, Rodney WM: The athletic heart syndrome. N Engl J Med 313:24–32, 1985.
14. Lichtman J, O'Rourke RA, Klein A, et al: Electrocardiogram of the athlete: Alterations simulating those of organic heart disease. Arch Intern Med 132:763–770, 1973.
15. Roeske WR, O'Rourke RA, Klein A, et al: Noninvasive evaluation of ventricular hypertrophy in professional athletes. Circulation 53:286–291, 1976.
16. Ikaheimo MJ, Palatsi IJ, Takkunen JT: Noninvasive evaluation of the athletic heart: Sprinters versus endurance runners. Am J Cardiol 44:24–30, 1979.
17. Raskoff WJ, Goldman S, Cohn K: The "athletic heart": Prevalence and physiological significance of left ventricular enlargement in distance runners. JAMA 236:158–162, 1976.
18. Longhurst JC, Kelly AR, Gonyea WJ, et al: Echocardiographic left ventricular masses in distance runners and weight lifters. J Appl Physiol: Respirat Environ Exerc Physiol 48:154–162, 1980.
19. Gilbert CA, Nutter DO, Felner JM, et al: Echocardiographic study of cardiac dimensions and function in the endurance trained athlete. Am J Cardiol 40:528–533, 1977.
20. Parker BM, Londeree BR, Cupp GV, et al: The noninvasive cardiac evaluation of long distance runners. Chest 73:376–381, 1978.
21. Thompson PD: Cardiovascular hazards of physical activity. *In* Terjung RL (ed): Exercise and Sport Sciences Reviews, vol 10. Philadelphia, The Franklin Institute, 1982, pp 208–235.
22. Waller BF: Exercise-related sudden death in young (age $\leq$ 30 years) and old (age $>$ 30 years) conditioned subjects. Cardiovasc Clin 15:9–73, 1985.
23. Virmani R, Robinowitz M, McAllister HA Jr: Exercise and the heart: A review of cardiac pathology associated with physical activity. Pathol Annu 20 (part 2):431–462, 1985.
24. Procacci PM, Savran SV, Schreiter SL, et al: Prevalence of clinical mitral valve prolapse in 1,169 young women. N Engl J Med 294:1086–1088, 1976.
25. Case records of the Massachusetts General Hospital: Case 22–1989. N Engl J Med 320:1475–1483, 1989.
26. Maron BJ, Roberts WC, McAllister HA, et al: Sudden death in young athletes. Circulation 62:218–229, 1980.
27. Thompson PD, Stern MP, Williams P, et al: Death during jogging or running: A study of 18 cases. JAMA 242:1265–1267, 1979.
28. Virmani R, Chun PKC, Goldstein RE, et al: Acute takeoffs of the coronary arteries along the aortic wall and congenital coronary ostial valve-like ridges: Association with sudden death. J Am Coll Cardiol 3:766–771, 1984.
29. Thompson PD, Funk EJ, Carleton RA, et al: The incidence of death during jogging in Rhode Island joggers from 1975 through 1980. JAMA 247:2535–2538, 1982.
30. Siscovick DS, Weiss NS, Fletcher RH, et al: The incidence of primary cardiac arrest during vigorous exercise. N Engl J Med 311:874–877, 1984.
31. Prockop DJ: Marfan's syndrome. *In* Braunwald E (ed): Harrison's Principles of Internal Medicine, ed 11. New York, McGraw-Hill, 1987, pp 1687–1688.
32. Perloff JK: Innocent murmurs. *In* The Clinical Recognition of Congenital Heart Disease. Philadelphia, WB Saunders, 1970, pp 6–13.
33. Barry WH, Grossman W: Cardiac catheterization. *In* Braunwald E (ed): Heart Disease: A Textbook of Cardiovascular Medicine. Philadelphia, WB Saunders, 1980, p 295.
34. Spirito P, Maron BJ, Bonow RO, et al: Prevalence and significance of an abnormal ST segment response to exercise in a young athletic population. Am J Cardiol 51:1663–1666, 1983.
35. McHenry PL, O'Donnell J, Morris SN, et al: The abnormal exercise electrocardiogram in apparently healthy men: A predictor of angina pectoris as an initial coronary event during long-term follow-up. Circulation 70:547–551, 1984.
36. Douglas PS: Cardiac considerations in the triathlete. Med Sci Sports Exerc 21 (suppl):S214–S218, 1989.
37. Thompson PD: The benefits and risk of exercise training in patients with chronic coronary artery disease. JAMA 259:1537–1540, 1988.
38. Siegel AJ, Silverman LM, Holman BL: Elevated creatine kinase MB isoenzyme levels in marathon runners. JAMA 246:2049–2051, 1981.
39. Gibbons LW, Cooper KH, Martin RP, et al: Medical examination and electrocardiographic analysis of elite distance runners. Ann NY Acad Sci 301:283–296, 1977.

2

HYPERTENSION

Jeffrey L. Tanji, MD

HOW EXERCISE HELPS

Hypertension affects an estimated 23% of Americans,[1] and approximately 30% of Americans say they engage in a regular exercise program. It follows that many hypertensive patients may be interested in starting or maintaining an exercise program. Physicians who counsel these patients need to be familiar with the role of exercise in lowering blood pressure, guidelines for exercise prescription and safety, and recent research on exercise test results to predict hypertension.

How Effective Is Regular Exercise?

Although the final chapter has not yet been written, mounting evidence argues that regular exercise does lower blood pressure in hypertensive patients. A significant decrease in blood pressure in hypertensive subjects after repetitive periods of moderately intense aerobic exercise was documented by Nelson and associates in a controlled crossover study. The decreases in blood pressure were independent of changes in body weight and an associated decrease in total peripheral resistance.

Another study demonstrating that regular aerobic exercise lowers blood pressure was designed and conducted by Roman and colleagues.[3] They followed blood pressures longitudinally in a cohort of 30 hypertensive women, alternating exercise and sedentary phases. During the training phase, significant decreases in blood pressure occurred; higher blood pressures returned when the training ceased.

Exercise of moderate intensity has been shown in longitudinal cohort studies to be effective in decreasing blood pressure in hypertensive men[4] and in subjects with borderline hypertension.[5]

Recently, a well-designed longitudinal exercise/rest crossover study demonstrated that moderate-intensity, well-supervised aerobic training did not decrease blood pressure in subjects with mild hypertension.[6] In addition to standard blood pressures at rest, 24-hour ambulatory blood pressure was monitored to validate these standard measurements. Cardiac output was measured noninvasively during exercise testing to demonstrate that no alteration in cardiac output by measurement, or in total peripheral resistance by calculation, recurred during the study. These data need to be confirmed by further research because this study, although well designed, bucks the trend of other reports that strongly suggest the efficacy of exercise in the treatment of high blood pressure.

Mechanisms for Efficacy

A moderate-intensity exercise program can reduce high blood pressure, but the specific mechanisms for this benefit are not understood. One of these mechanisms is weight reduction.[7] Exercise has been demonstrated to decrease blood pressure in association with a decrease in body fat. In fact, one of the criticisms of research demonstrating the blood pressure–lowering effects of exercise is that the weight loss and decrease in obesity that follow an exercise program confound the issue; it is difficult to determine if the exercise itself lowers blood pressure, or if it is only weight loss facilitated through exercise that is responsible. This problem was first addressed by Hagberg and associates,[8–10] who demonstrated that regular aerobic exercise in teenagers lowered blood pressure independent of changes in body weight.

A second mechanism, although difficult to analyze, is the benefit of relaxation through exercise. The basis for a third mechanism is that some hypertensives have been noted to have a higher sympathetic resting tone, associated with a higher catecholamine output.[11] Regular physical exercise results in a decrease in resting heart rate and a decrease in the rate-pressure product at varying levels of work, which is hypothesized to have an effect similar to that of beta blockade on the sympathetic system, thus reducing blood pressure.[12] This phenomenon distinctly differs from beta blockade achieved with an antihypertensive agent. Both exercise and medication result in reducing the resting heart rate and left ventricular output at a given amount of work, but exercise does not place an upper limit on heart rate as does beta-blocker medication. This is particularly beneficial to exercising hypertensive patients who do not want their performance compromised by a limitation of maximal exercise capacity.

Establishing an Exercise Program

The American College of Sports Medicine (ACSM) recommends a screening exercise treadmill test for all patients over age 45 and all patients between the ages of 35 and 45 who have cardiovascular risk factors, even if they were asymptomatic before starting an exercise program.[13] There is considerable debate about these guidelines because of a high rate of false-positive tests among these age groups.[14] I recommend such testing for the hypertensive population, but not screening for coronary artery disease. Blood-pressure responses to exercise in hypertensive patients can be very high compared with normotensives at a given heart rate. It is useful to know the systolic and diastolic blood pressures at graded increases in heart rate so that hypertensive patients can be instructed not to exceed a particular heart rate and, consequently, a particular blood pressure.

In our laboratory, we are attempting to elucidate specific physiologic relationships among graded exercise, blood pressure, heart rate, total peripheral resistance, and catecholamines. We are examining the hypothesis that lower-intensity exercise (60% to 70% of maximal heart rate) as opposed to standard exercise (70% to 85% of maximal heart rate) or no exercise is the best way to control blood pressure among mild hypertensives (diastolic blood pressure 90 to 104 mm Hg). We have demonstrated and analyzed specific differences in blood pressure in normal, hypertensive, and borderline hypertensive populations at increasing degrees of exercise. We have identified a phenomenon termed the *point of maximal blood pressure depression*, a point during low intensities of exercise at which the diastolic blood pressure decreases before increasing in response to exercise.

We hypothesize that this is caused by a decrease in total peripheral resistance in conjunction with a cardiac output that has not yet started to increase. An intriguing question is whether hypertensive patients ought to exercise at an intensity where blood pressure is at this minimal point to best control blood pressure over a 24-hour period.

There is general consensus that standard aerobic exercise is beneficial for hypertensive patients. The ACSM recommends 20 to 30 minutes of aerobic exercise, three to four times a week, at 70% to 85% of maximum heart rate for normotensives.[13] As previously discussed, I am conducting studies analyzing the efficacy of lower-intensity training for hypertensives, but until the data are fully analyzed, I recommend the ACSM guidelines. Given the busy schedule of most patients, my preference is to let them choose the method of exercise. Walking, running, cycling, swimming, and high-repetition, low-resistance circuit training can be used to achieve fitness.

Hypertensive patients should avoid heavy-resistance training. MacDougall et al[15] have reported remarkable increases in blood pressure (355/281 mm Hg) with heavy-resistance training with maximal leg presses. Harris and Holly[16] demonstrated that high-repetition (20 to 30 repetitions), low-resistance weight training may effectively lower blood pressure in hypertensive patients. Thus, hypertensive patients should do light-resistance, not heavy-resistance, weight training.

Blair and associates demonstrated the benefit of physical fitness on all-cause mortality in both a normal[17] and hypertensive population (S. N. Blair, PED: personal communication, May 1990). Physical activity in excess of 2000 kcal per week has been associated with a decreased mortality in Harvard alumni.[18] The studies by Blair and colleagues[17] and Paffenbarger and Hale[18] demonstrate that the amount of exercise needed to achieve fitness levels that are associated with decreased mortality is within the grasp of the vast majority of the American population. It is particularly relevant that in the study by Blair and coworkers[17] of hypertensive patients, physical fitness almost negates the risk of mortality associated with hypertension.

There are no precise guidelines to determine whether an exercise program has been ineffective in treating a patient with hypertension and when to begin a medication regimen. I generally set a 3- to 6-month time frame to assess the impact of an exercise program; I monitor blood pressures every 1 to 2 months. If the diastolic pressure rises above 104 mm Hg, if there is any evidence of end-organ impact from hypertension, or if other cardiovascular risk factors worsen, I consider the use of medication.

Screening for Hypertension

Several studies[19–21] have suggested that the exercise test can be used to predict the development of hypertension. Wilson and Mayer[22] demonstrated that the relative risk for developing hypertension among normotensives with an exaggerated blood-pressure response to the Balke exercise protocol was 2.28. It may be that early in the course of hypertension, blood pressure at rest may not be a sensitive indicator of the presence of disease. Stress such as exercise might expose inadequate blood-pressure control mechanisms and unmask the latent tendency toward hypertension. Large-scale longitudinal studies are needed to validate the efficacy and cost-effectiveness of such tests before they can be broadly recommended.

THE ROLE OF MEDICATION

Nonpharmacologic therapy such as exercise may not be sufficient to control high blood pressure in some patients. Many patients enjoy exercise on a regular basis while being maintained on an antihypertensive medication regimen; however, the rules for prescribing antihypertensive medications for the sedentary adult do not necessarily hold true for the active exerciser.

The key issue facing physicians who prescribe medications for hypertensive patients who enjoy exercise is to find a medication that effectively controls blood pressure at rest and during exercise but does not compromise quality of life. Specifically, this means a medication that will not decrease exercise performance or increase the rate of perceived exertion for a given level of work. If the medication decreases exercise tolerance, the patient will either quit exercising or stop the medication in order to continue exercising. Clear communication and feedback between the patient and physician will probably result in adherence to both medication and exercise, thus helping to lower blood pressure at rest and during exercise.

I use a 3- to 6-month evaluation of nonpharmacologic therapy, such as exercise in the mildly hypertensive (90 to 104 mm Hg diastolic) patient. It is important not to simply use numbers in the management of hypertension. For instance, if a patient has no other cardiovascular risk factors, I may use a longer period to evaluate nonpharmacologic therapy. However, if a patient has any symptoms related to high blood pressure, evidence of end-organ damage, or rise in blood pressure to the moderate or severe range (>105 mm Hg diastolic), I strongly consider initiating pharmacologic management.

A discussion of current recommendations for the treatment of hypertension will help physicians choose the appropriate medication for hypertensive patients. The 1988 Report of the Joint National Committee on the Detection, Evaluation and Treatment of High Blood Pressure[23] broadened the step-care approach to the medical management of hypertension, thus allowing a more flexible approach to treating the exercising individual. The initial step is the use of nonpharmacologic therapy, such as diet, weight control, alcohol restriction, and exercise. This recommendation is a major advance in managing hypertension because it acknowledges the efficacy of nonpharmacologic therapy as the first step in treatment of mildly hypertensive patients.

If nonpharmacologic therapy is not effective, the committee recommends the use of a diuretic, beta-blocker, calcium antagonist, or angiotensin-converting enzyme (ACE) inhibitor (Fig. 2–1).

Diuretics

Diuretics, although a popular first-line agent for many hypertensive patients, may not be the best choice for exercising patients. The position paper on treatment of hypertension from the American Society of Hypertension (ASH) advocates that "a tailored, individualized approach should replace the rigid diuretic first-step-care approach now so com-

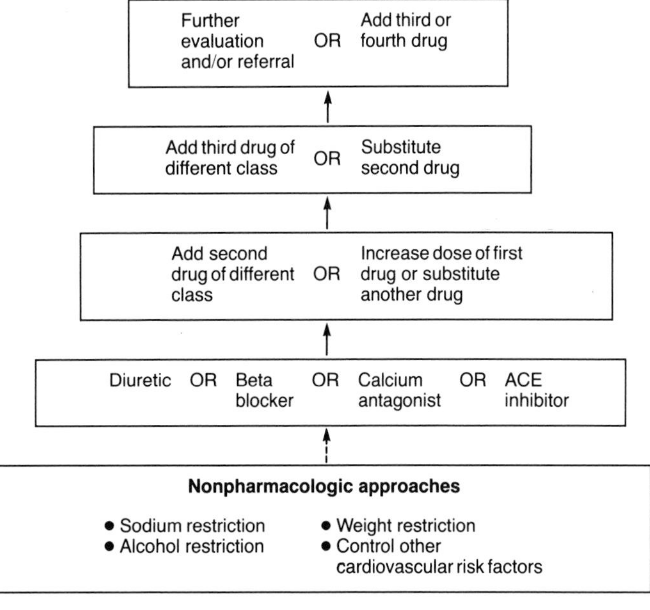

Figure 2–1. Individualized step-care therapy for hypertension. For some patients, nonpharmacologic therapy should be tried first. If the desired blood pressure is not achieved, add pharmacologic therapy. In patients who require pharmacologic therapy initially, nonpharmacologic treatment may be a helpful adjunct. (*Data from* The 1988 report of the Joint National Committee on Detection, Evaluation, and Treatment of High Blood Pressure. Arch Intern Med 148(5):1023–1038, 1988; with permission.)

monly followed."[24] Hypokalemia, a proven side effect of diuretic use, can be exacerbated during exercise, when high levels of catecholamines may be released. If a regularly exercising patient on a diuretic regimen is pleased with the medication, I advocate monitoring serum potassium levels as training levels increase or during seasonal variation in temperature (because increased fluid loss may occur). Although less well studied, dehydration may be exacerbated with exercise in conjunction with the use of diuretics. The use of aspirin or nonsteroidal anti-inflammatory agents is more common in athletes and exercising hypertensive patients and may antagonize the antihypertensive and natriuretic effectiveness of diuretics.

Beta-Blockers

No studies have conclusively demonstrated an antihypertensive therapeutic advantage of one beta-blocker over another for the treatment of hypertension. A key consideration, however, has been the search for a beta-blocking agent that minimizes the side effect of impairment of exercise performance. All beta-blocking agents, and specifically nonselective beta-blockers, reduce exercise tolerance significantly in patients with essential hypertension. Comparative studies have shown that in normal and hypertensive patients, β_1-selective agents impair exercise performance less than do nonselective agents. The ASH position paper advocates that those who wish to maintain a high level of exercise avoid nonselective beta-blockers.[24]

In contrast to diuretics, which can accentuate hypokalemia, the use of beta-blockers during exercise has been demonstrated to cause a transient increase in serum potassium.[25,26] This effect is present in both selective and nonselective beta blockade. The mechanism for this elevation in humans is not understood. Because increased serum potassium concentration during exercise has been associated with sudden death,[27] I recommend that potassium levels be monitored closely as training intensity is altered in subjects who use beta-blockers.

Nonselective beta-blockers, and to a lesser degree β_1-selective blockers, have been shown to impair heat dissipation during exercise,[28–30] either by diminishing blood flow to the skin or by indirect reflex vasoconstriction of peripheral arterioles as a result of decreased left ventricular pumping activity. These findings strongly suggest that hypertensive athletes who use beta-blockers should observe a strict fluid-replacement regimen, especially in endurance events. These athletes should be aware of the signs and symptoms of hyperthermia. Furthermore, because patients on beta-blockers tend to develop hyperkalemia during exercise, they should be careful if they use fluid-replacement drinks that contain potassium.

In summary, β_1-selective blockers are preferred for exercising patients with essential hypertension because they diminish exercise performance and impair thermoregulation to a lesser degree than do nonselective beta-blockers. It is important to realize that because limitation in exercise performance varies among individuals, it is not possible to predict who will or will not do well with beta-blockers.

Calcium Antagonists

Several studies[31–33] have documented that calcium-channel blockers have an antihypertensive effect without compromising exercise tolerance. These and other studies suggest that calcium-channel blockers may be excellent antihypertensive agents for exercising adults. These studies, however, were not performed on young, physically active adults.

A study by Myburgh and Gordon[34] comparing diltiazem (a calcium-channel blocker) and atenolol (a β_1-selective blocker) demonstrated equivalent decreases in blood pressure at rest, but a significant decrease in exercise blood pressure and heart rate with atenolol as compared with diltiazem. Maximal exercise performance was slightly but not significantly decreased with atenolol and not decreased at all with diltiazem. In this study, calcium-channel blockers were not definitively shown to be superior to β_1-selective blockers with regard to limiting exercise performance.

Calcium-channel blockers are an excellent choice for initial therapy in hypertensive patients who exercise. They are being widely used in this population without limiting exercise capacity, and to date no untoward side effects unique to exercise have been documented. Further studies are needed to compare their benefits with other antihypertensive agents.

ACE Inhibitors

ACE inhibitors are now considered first-line antihypertensive agents.[23] Because of their tolerance profile[35,36] and minimal side effects,[37,38] they are excellent agents for hypertensive patients who exercise. A study comparing captopril (an ACE inhibitor) with atenolol (a β_1-selective blocker) and nadolol (a nonselective blocker) demonstrated significantly greater maximal exercise performance with captopril as compared with nadolol, whereas performance was slightly but not significantly greater as compared with atenolol.

ACE inhibitors, like calcium-channel blockers, are an excellent initial agent for exercising hypertensive patients because they have minimal side effects and do not interfere with maximal exercise capacity. Like the calcium-channel blockers, however, it remains to be proved that a significant difference in limiting exercise capacity occurs as compared with β_1-selective blockers.

Aspirin and other nonsteroidal anti-inflammatory medications may magnify the potassium-retaining effects of ACE inhibitors,[23] so potassium levels should be monitored closely. Patients who use fluid-replacement drinks that contain potassium should be advised of this side effect as well.

Step-down Therapy

The Joint National Committee on the Detection, Evaluation, and Treatment of High Blood Pressure[23] in 1988 recommended that medications may be reduced in a stepwise fashion in patients whose mild hypertension has been satisfactorily controlled for at least 1 year. They noted that reducing medication may be particularly effective for patients who also follow nonpharmacologic therapeutic recommendations such as exercise. It is assumed that diet, exercise, and other life-style changes will be maintained as a foundation for the success of any attempt to step down from an antihypertensive regimen. In fact, most patients will require reinitiation of therapy if nonpharmacologic interventions are not continued.[39]

Few data exist regarding the interaction between exercise and multiple antihypertensive drug regimens, so this topic is not discussed here.

SUMMARY

A wide range of therapeutic options is available for the hypertensive patient who engages in regular exercise. The prudent physician individualizes therapy, with close follow-up of blood pressure, compliance, and side effects. No single agent is clearly superior. Physicians need to know the common and less well known side effects unique to the physically active patient to reach the goal of compliance with both medication and exercise.

REFERENCES

1. American Heart Association: Heart Facts. Dallas, 1988.
2. Nelson L, Jennings GL, Esler MD, et al: Effect of changing levels of physical activity on blood pressure and hemodynamics in essential hypertension. Lancet 2:473–476, 1986.
3. Roman O, Camuzzi AL, Villalon E, et al: Physical training program in arterial hypertension: A long-term prospective follow-up. Cardiology 67:230, 1981.
4. Boyer JL, Kasch FW: Exercise therapy in hypertensive men. JAMA 211:1168, 1970.
5. Choquette G, Ferguson RJ: Blood pressure reduction in "borderline" hypertensives following physical training. Can Med Assoc J 108:699, 1973.
6. Gilders RM, Voner C, Dudley GA: Endurance training and blood pressure in normotensive and hypertensive adults. Med Sci Sports Exerc 21(6):629–636, 1989.
7. Horton ES: The role of exercise in the treatment of hypertension in obesity. Int Obesity 5(suppl 1):165, 1981.
8. Hagberg JM, Goldring D, Ehsani A: Effect of exercise training on the blood pressure and hemodynamic features of hypertensive adolescents. Am J Cardiol 52:763–768, 1983.
9. Hagberg JM, Goldring D, Heath GW: Effect of exercise on plasma catecholamines and hemodynamics during rest, submaximal exercise and orthostatic stress. Clin Physiol 4:117–124, 1984.
10. Hagberg JM, Ehsani A, Goldring D: Effect of weight training on blood pressure and hemodynamics on hypertensive adolescents. J Pediatr 104:147–151, 1984.
11. Lorimer AR, MacFarlane PW, Provan G, et al: Blood pressure and catecholamine response to stress in normotensive and hypertensive subjects. Cardiovasc Res 5:161–173, 1971.
12. Duncan JJ, Hagan RD, Upton J, et al: The effects of an aerobic exercise program on sympathetic neural activity and blood pressure in mild hypertensive patients. Circulation 68:(suppl 3)285, 1983.
13. American College of Sports Medicine: Guidelines for graded exercise testing and exercise prescription. Philadelphia, Lea & Febiger, 1986.
14. Tanji JL: Exercise for hypertensives. Consultant 28(9):123–130, 1988.
15. MacDougall JD, Tuxen D, Sale DG, et al: Arterial blood pressure response to heavy resistance exercise. J Appl Physiol 58:785–790, 1985.
16. Harris KA, Holly RG: Physiological response to circuit weight training in borderline hypertensive subjects. Med Sci Sports Exerc 19:246–252, 1987.
17. Blair SN, Kohl HW, Paffenbarger RS, et al: Physical fitness to all-cause mortality. JAMA 262:2395–2401, 1989.
18. Paffenbarger RS, Hale WE: Work activity and coronary heart mortality. N Engl J Med 292:545–550, 1975.
19. Tanji JL, Champlin JJ, Wong GY, et al: Blood pressure recovery curves after submaximal exercise. Am J Hypertens 2:135–138, 1989.
20. Davidoff R, Schamroth CL, Goldman AP, et al: Postexercise blood pressure as a predictor of hypertension. Aviat Space Environ Med 53:591–594, 1982.
21. Dlin RA, Hanne N, Silverberg DS, et al: Follow-up of normotensive men with exaggerated blood pressure response to exercise. Am Heart J 106:316–320, 1983.
22. Wilson NV, Meyer BM: Early prediction of hypertension using exercise blood pressure. Prev Med 10:61–68, 1981.
23. The 1988 report of the Joint National Committee on Detection, Evaluation, and Treatment of High Blood Pressure. Arch Intern Med 148(5):1023–1038, 1988.
24. Kaplan NM, Alderman MH, Flamenbaum W, et al: Guidelines for the treatment of hypertension. Am J Hypertens 2(2 part 1):75–77, 1989.
25. Carlsson E, Fellenius E, Lungborg P, et al: Beta-adrenoceptor blockers, plasma-potassium, and exercise [letter]. Lancet 2(8086):424–425, 1978.
26. Lundborg P, Astrom H, Bengtsson C, et al: Effect of beta-adrenoceptor blockade on exercise performance and metabolism. Clin Sci 61(3):229–305, 1981.
27. Shephard RJ: Physiology and Biochemistry of Exercise. New York, Praeger, 1982, p 456.
28. Gordon NF: Effect of selective and nonselective beta-adrenoceptor blockade on thermoregulation during prolonged exercise in heat. Am J Cardiol 55(10):74D–78D, 1985.
29. Gordon NF, Kruger PE, Van Rensburg JP, et al: Effect of beta-adrenoceptor blockade on thermoregulation during prolonged exercise. J Appl Physiol 58(3):899–906, 1985.
30. Gordon NF, Van Rensburg JP, Russell HM, et al: Effect of beta-adrenoceptor blockade and calcium antag-

onism, alone and in combination on thermoregulation during prolonged exercise. Int J Sports Med 8(1):1–5, 1987.

31. Pool PE, Seagren SC, Salel AF: Effects of diltiazem on serum lipids, exercise performance and blood pressure: Randomized, double-blind, placebo-controlled evaluation for systemic hypertension. Am J Cardiol 56(16):86H–91H, 1985.
32. Szlachcic J, Hirsch AT, Tubau JF, et al: Diltiazem versus propranolol in essential hypertension: Responses of rest and exercise blood pressure and effects on exercise capacity. Am J Cardiol 59:(5)393–399, 1987.
33. Yamakado T, Oonishi N, Kondo S, et al: Effects of diltiazem on cardiovascular responses during exercise in systemic hypertension and comparison with propranolol. Am J Cardiol 52(8):1023–1027, 1983.
34. Myburgh DP, Gordon NF: Comparison of diltiazem and atenolol in young, physically active men with essential hypertension. Am J Cardiol 60(13):1092–1095, 1987.
35. Veterans Administration Cooperative Study Group on Antihypertensive Agents: Low-dose captopril for the treatment of mild to moderate hypertension: I. Results of a 14-week trial. Arch Intern Med 144(10): 1947–1953, 1984.
36. Croog SH, Levine S, Testa MA, et al. The effects of antihypertensive therapy on the quality of life. N Engl J Med 314(26):1657–1664, 1986.
37. Yodfat Y, Fidel J, Bloom DS: Captopril as a replacement for multiple therapy in hypertension: A controlled study. J Hypertens Suppl 3(2):S155–S158, 1985.
38. Hill JF, Bulpitt CJ, Fletcher AE: Angiotensin-converting enzyme inhibitors and the quality of life: The European trial. J Hypertens Suppl 3(2):S91–S94, 1985.
39. Stamler R, Stamler J, Grimm R, et al: Nutritional therapy for high blood pressure: Final report of a four-year randomized controlled trial—the Hypertension Control Program. JAMA 257(11):1484–1491, 1987.

3

CLINICAL EXERCISE TESTING

Steven P. Van Camp, MD

Clinical exercise testing now enjoys significant popularity because of the information it can provide, as well as its widespread application, safety, and ease of performance. During the past 50 years, exercise testing has evolved from its use in determining fitness and exercise capacity to the diagnosis of coronary artery disease. It is a test that provides clinical, hemodynamic, and electrocardiographic information in a safe, noninvasive, controlled manner.

EXERCISE PHYSIOLOGY

During acute, submaximal, and maximal exercise, multiple cardiovascular, respiratory, and metabolic changes occur.[1] These include increases in heart rate, blood pressure, stroke volume, A-V O_2 difference, arterial lactate concentration, respiratory rate, and respiratory quotient. The magnitude of these adjustments depends upon the intensity of exercise and the conditioning level of the test subject. In a multistage exercise test, many of these parameters can be monitored and recorded. Specifically, increases in heart rate and blood pressure are easily recorded. Using equipment to collect and analyze expired air, respiratory rate, respiratory quotient, and total body maximal oxygen consumption ($\dot{V}O_{2max}$) may be determined. The normal heart rate and blood pressure response to exercise in healthy men is shown in Figure 3–1.

Heart rate during exercise progressively increases as work load increases. Elevated heart rates during submaximal exercise or recovery may reflect poor physical conditioning, anemia, vasoregulatory asthenia with autonomic imbalance, conditions of decreased intravascular volume, or metabolic disorders. Relatively low heart rates may result from high levels of physical fitness or medications, including beta-adrenergic blocking agents and certain calcium-channel blockers (verapamil and diltiazem).

Maximal heart rate declines with age, apparently owing to the decreased responsiveness of cardiovascular tissue to beta-adrenergic stimulation.[3] Multiple formulas have been developed to estimate maximal heart rate (HR). One of the most commonly used formulas is

$$\text{maximal HR} = 220 - \text{age}$$

This approach generally underestimates the maximal heart rate, but is an acceptable one for clinical purposes. Additionally, it is necessary to appreciate that the standard deviation of maximal heart rate is approximately 10 beats/min.[4,5]

Systolic blood pressure rises with increases in work load, whereas diastolic blood pressure typically remains at the preexercise level or may decline slightly. An elevation of dia-

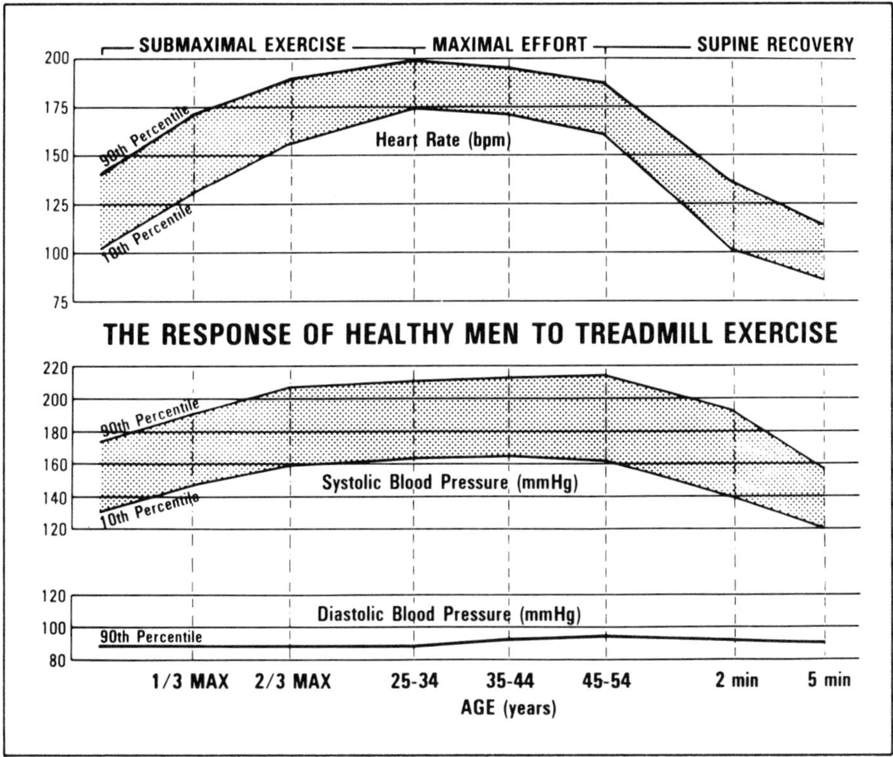

Figure 3–1. Physiologic response to submaximal and maximal treadmill exercise based on testing apparently healthy men 24 to 54 years of age. The bands represent the 10th and the 90th percentile limits. Therefore, 10% of normal individuals could have responses outside these limits without necessarily being abnormal. (*From* Froelicher VF: Exercise Testing and Training. New York, LeJacq Publishing, 1983, p 44; with permission.)

stolic blood pressure of 10 to 20 mm Hg may be seen in patients with either sustained or labile hypertension. Blood pressure typically declines to normal during the recovery period, and may decrease still further for a few hours after the test. The typically observed blood pressure response may be altered by medications. Beta-adrenergic blocking agents and calcium-channel blockers may result in lower blood pressures during both exercise and recovery.

During the exercise stimulus, myocardial contractility and myocardial wall tension also increase. These latter two phsyiologic changes, along with increases in heart rate, combine to increase myocardial oxygen consumption ($M\dot{V}O_2$).

CLINICAL USES OF EXERCISE TESTS

The heart rate, blood pressure, and electrocardiogram can be recorded with limited equipment during exercise in a controlled situation. The information available therefore extends beyond simply the presence or absence of electrocardiographic changes of ischemia (ie, ST segment changes) and includes (1) maximal exercise capacity, determined by work load performed or oxygen consumption measurement; (2) exercise-limiting and related symptoms; (3) maximal heart rate; (4) maximal blood pressure; (5) arrhythmias and conduction abnormalities; and (6) ST segment changes.

This information is especially important in its relationship to the amount of exercise that elicits the measured changes. This easily obtainable information makes exercise stress testing ideal for the following uses:

1. Determination of exercise capacity (functional capacity).
2. Assessment of exercise-related and limiting symptoms, especially those suggestive of myocardial ischemia.
3. Diagnosis of coronary artery disease.
4. Determination of prognosis in patients with coronary artery disease.
5. Evaluation of response to therapy (medical, revascularization—surgical or angioplasty, or exercise).
6. Screening prior to beginning an exercise program.
7. Assessment of arrhythmias.
8. Evaluation of patients with pulmonary or peripheral vascular disease.

Exercise tests can be performed on patients with a broad range of physiologic capacities and clinical states, including known or suspected cardiovascular or pulmonary disease. Healthy individuals and elite athletes are easily tested as well. The appropriateness of exercise testing in various clinical situations is discussed in detail in "Guidelines for Exercise Testing—A Report of the Joint American College of Cardiology/American Heart Association Task Force on Assessment of Cardiovascular Procedures (Subcommittee on Exercise Testing)."[6] The American College of Sports Medicine's *Guidelines for Exercise Testing and Prescription*[7] as well as several excellent textbooks[2,8] discuss exercise testing in greater detail. Clearly, exercise testing can provide important information in a variety of clinical circumstances.

TYPES OF EXERCISE TESTS

Various types of exercise tests may be performed depending on the type of exercise, the endpoint of the exercise test, the continuous or intermittent nature of exercise, and the exercise protocol used. The ideal stress test is not one with the same protocol for every subject, but one that is chosen to suit the individual. The specific type of test and protocol is one appropriate for the subject's clinical status, including symptoms, fitness level, and musculoskeletal limitations, and for the indication(s) for performance of the test. Generally, the appropriate exercise protocol will offer a progressive increase in work load with a type of exercise familiar to the test subject, lasting approximately 8 to 15 minutes before the achievement of maximal exercise capacity.

The type of exercise performed is usually a dynamic, rhythmic exercise using a large mass of muscle. A stationary bicycle or motor-driven treadmill is typically used. Arm ergometers may be used for individuals who are unable to perform leg exercise because of musculoskeletal or peripheral vascular disease limitations. Isometric exercises and step tests have been used in the past, but these have given way to the former two modes of exercise. Each apparatus has specific advantages and disadvantages. The stationary bicycle is less expensive and usually allows easier recording of blood pressure and an electrocardiogram freer of motion artifact. It may be, however, a mode of exercise unfamiliar to many people. It also requires somewhat greater motivation for the achievement of maximal exercise capacity than does the motor-driven treadmill. The treadmill is a more expensive piece of equipment; however, it does provide a type of exercise (walking) familiar to most people. It also is the mode of exercise used for most clinical research studies involving prognosis and angiographic correlations. With both types of equipment, the work load may be readily and individually adjusted.

The test may be terminated at a predetermined level of exercise work load, heart rate, or blood pressure (submaximal test), or it may be continued until the subject reaches his

TABLE 3–1. COMMONLY USED EXERCISE TEST PROTOCOLS

Bruce Protocol

Stage	*Duration (min)*	*Speed (mph)*	*Grade (%)*
1	3	1.7	10
2	3	2.5	12
3	3	3.4	14
4	3	4.2	16
5	3	5.0	18
6	3	5.5	20
7	3	6.0	22

Ellestad Protocol

Stage	*Duration (min)*	*Speed (mph)*	*Grade (%)*
1	3	1.7	10
2	2	3.0	10
3	2	4.0	10
4	2	5.0	10
5	2	5.0	15
6	2	6.0	15
7	2	7.0	15

Balke Protocol

Constant speed: 3.3 mph typically used
Grade: 1st min – 0%
2nd min –2%
Increased each minute by 1% until 25% grade reached at 25th min, then speed increased 0.2 mph each minute

or her level of maximal exercise capacity (maximal symptom-limited exercise test). Most clinicians favor maximal symptom-limited exercise tests, as they provide more complete symptomatic, hemodynamic, and electrocardiographic information.

The exercise may be performed in a continuous manner with increases in work load every few minutes, or in an intermittent, discontinuous manner. Continuous tests are usually performed for practical, rather than physiologic reasons. Multiple exercise protocols are available. The commonly used protocols of Bruce,[9] Ellestad,[8] and Balke[10] are presented in Table 3–1.

Bicycle test protocols also provide progressively increasing work loads. Work loads are calibrated in watts or kilogram-meters per minute (kg-m/min). (One kilogram-meter/minute equals 1 kg of resistance applied against a standard ergometer wheel at 50 rpm.) Initial work loads are generally 25 to 50 watts (150 to 300 kg-m/min) increasing by 25 watts (150 kg-m/min) every 2- or 3-minute stage.

EXERCISE TESTING

Evaluation Prior to Exercise Testing

Prior to the performance of an exercise stress test, the clinical indications and purpose(s) of the exercise test should be reviewed. A medical history and physical examination should be performed, along with appropriate laboratory work, to make certain no contraindications to exercise testing exist. Contraindications to exercise testing (Table 3–2) are con-

TABLE 3–2. CONTRAINDICATIONS TO EXERCISE TESTING

Absolute Contraindications
Acute myocardial infarction or any significant recent change in resting ECG
Unstable angina
Uncontrolled ventricular arrhythmias
Uncontrolled atrial arrhythmias that compromise cardiac function
Decompensated congestive heart failure
Severe aortic stenosis
Dissecting aortic aneurysm
Acute myocarditis or pericarditis
Deep venous thrombophlebitis
Recent systemic or pulmonary embolism
Acute infectious illness
Third-degree heart block (acquired)
Significant emotional distress (psychosis)

Relative Contraindications
Uncontrolled hypertension (resting diastolic blood pressure over 110 mm Hg or resting systolic blood pressure over 200 mm Hg)
Left main coronary artery disease or its equivalent
Significant valvular heart disease
Cyanotic congenital heart disease
Possible digitalis or other drug toxicity
Pulmonary hypertension
Electrolyte abnormalities, especially hypokalemia
Fixed-rate artificial pacemaker
Frequent or complex ventricular arrhythmias
Ventricular aneurysm
Cardiomyopathy, including hypertrophic cardiomyopathy
Uncontrolled metabolic disease (diabetes mellitus, thyrotoxicosis, myxedema)
Any serious systemic disorder (mononucleosis, hepatitis, etc)
Neuromuscular or skeletal disorders that would interfere with exercise
Congestive heart failure
Anemia
Marked obesity

ditions that carry a significant likelihood of risk with exercise. These are generally categorized as absolute or relative contraindications depending upon their severity and the risk they carry. Exercise testing should not be performed if any of the absolute contraindications are present. Relative contraindications may be considerd as conditions that require medical treatment and stabilization prior to the exercise test or which will require special attention during the test.

The preexercise clinical evaluation will also allow familiarization with the patient to determine the likelihood of development of cardiovascular symptoms or problems during the test. Particularly pertinent parts of the clinical evaluation include the patient's past medical history, especially cardiovascular problems; exercise-related symptoms; cardiovascular symptoms; coronary heart disease risk factors; and medications, especially those which may affect the exercise response or electrocardiographic response to exercise. The patient's activity status should also be determined to allow selection of the proper exercise protocol.

Patient Instructions

The patient should be instructed regarding what to expect during the exercise test. These instructions should (1) educate the patient as to the protocol to be used, (2) reassure the patient, and (3) encourage the patient to provide a maximal effort. Patients should be allowed to touch the treadmill handrails if necessary to maintain balance, but should be discouraged from gripping tightly or using them to prolong the exercise. Any patient questions should be answered at this time in a clear and reassuring manner. An informed consent should be obtained prior to the performance of the test. This document should include the nature of the test and the small, but finite, risk, and possible complications.

A resting 12-lead electrocardiogram (ECG) should be performed immediately before the exercise test to detect significant resting arrhythmias, heart block, or evidence of myocardial ischemia or infarction. This ECG should be a standard 12-lead ECG rather than the Mason-Likar modification, which is often used for exercise ECG recordings, as the latter does not provide an accurate resting 12-lead ECG.[11] The Mason-Likar modified ECG may result in patterns that falsely suggest lateral and apical myocardial infarctions. It may also falsely mask evidence of inferior, posterior, or apical infarctions.

Testing Preparations

The patient should fast for 2 to 3 hours, and avoid alcohol and tobacco for at least 3 hours before the test. Loose, comfortable clothing, and shoes appropriate for the exercise mode should be worn.

The decision to take medication before the exercise test depends on the indication for the medication, the purpose of the exercise test, and any potential problems that might occur if the medication is not taken. For example, use of a beta-adrenergic blocking agent prior to the test may (depending on the dosage and timing) limit the heart rate and blood pressure response to the extent that a nondiagnostic test for ischemia results. On the other hand, if the response to medical therapy needs to be assessed, the test should be performed without discontinuing the medication. Any medication that may have potential effects on the hemodynamic response to exercise or the exercise ECG should be documented, along with its time of administration relative to the test performance (eg, propranolol 40 mg q 6 hours, last dose taken 4 hours ago).

Prior to the performance of the test, it is important to have a well-practiced emergency plan along with adequate resuscitation equipment. A continuous electrocardiographic monitoring system should be used throughout the exercise and recovery periods. A defibrillator should be in the immediate area along with other resuscitation and ventilation equipment, including various airways, a laryngoscope, a ventilation bag, and a portable oxygen supply. Equipment for the establishment of an intravenous line is necessary including catheters, tubing, syringes, needles, and intravenous fluids (5% dextrose in water). Emergency drugs should also be immediately available including atropine, digoxin, dobutamine, dopamine, epinephrine, furosemide, isoproterenol, lidocaine, metaraminol, nitroglycerin, nifedipine, propranolol, procainamide, and verapamil.

Test Performance

Regardless of the protocol used, the initial work load should be a low-level one that allows adequate warm-up. The work load is then increased progressively, usually in 1- to 3-minute stages, to the patient's maximum capacity. Reasons for test termination vary with the type of exercise test performed. Submaximal exercise tests typically stop at a predetermined work load or heart rate. The more widely used maximal tests continue to a point of fatigue or the development of a sign or symptom indicating a need for test termination. The indications for test termination are listed in Table 3–3.

If the exercise test is negative for ischemia or shows no significant abnormalities, it

TABLE 3–3. INDICATIONS FOR TERMINATION OF EXERCISE TEST

Patient desires to stop
Excessive fatigue or dyspnea
Excessive chest discomfort or other exercise-induced symptom
Excessive ST segment deviation (2–4 mm)
Ventricular tachycardia
Frequent ventricular premature beats precipitated or aggravated by exercise (over 25% of beats)
Ectopic supraventricular tachycardia
Any intracardiac block precipitated by exercise (right bundle branch block, left bundle branch block, or intraventricular conduction delay)
Peripheral circulatory insufficiency (pallor, clammy skin, drop in blood pressure)
Failure of monitoring system
Significant drop in systolic blood pressure (greater than 10 mm Hg)
Lightheadedness, confusion, ataxia, locomotor difficulties

is generally not considered to be a diagnostic one unless the heart rate achieved is at least 85% of the maximal predicted heart rate (generally predicted as 220 − age).

Excessive blood pressure elevation also may be an indication to terminate the exercise test. Although there are no recorded instances of cerebrovascular accidents or other hypertensive complications during maximal exercise testing, it is usually considered appropriate to stop an exercise test with a systolic blood pressure above 280 mm Hg or a diastolic blood pressure above 115 mm Hg.

During the recovery stage of the test, the subject may be allowed to exercise for a few minutes at a low level that is consistent with adequate recovery. This approach will decrease the likelihood of postexercise hypotension. The subject is then allowed to sit for the remainder of the recovery period, which should last for at least 6 minutes, and certainly until all exercise-related abnormalities or symptoms have resolved.

The 12-lead ECG should be recorded before exercise as indicated previously. Single or multiple electrocardiographic leads are monitored during exercise tests. Because the standard placement of ECG electrodes on the limbs would result in unacceptable motion artifact during exercise, the Mason-Likar modified ECG lead system is generally used.[12] As indicated earlier, however, it should not be used as the preexercise ECG. This system brings the limb leads onto the more stable torso and maintains the position of the precordial electrodes. Figure 3–2 shows the Mason-Likar system for exercise electrocardiographic leads.

In general, single leads (V_5 or a comparable lead) may be adequate for testing young, apparently healthy subjects. In the testing of patients who are known to have, or to be at risk for, cardiovascular disease, multiple lead systems are advisable. These symptoms range from those with one or more inferior leads (II, III, or aVF) and a lateral precordial lead (V_5) to those with these leads plus additional precordial leads (V_1, V_4, or V_6). Full 12-lead ECGs are preferred by some. As one might expect, recording approaches that use multiple leads will increase test sensitivity (detection of subjects with disease), but decrease test specificity (proper identification of normals).[13]

During the exercise and recovery periods, the heart rate and rhythm should be monitored continuously. The blood pressure should be recorded at least once during every exercise stage and every 2 minutes during recovery. These readings should be performed every minute during exercise and recovery in patients with cardiovascular symptoms, disease, or abnormal ECGs or blood pressure readings. The ECG should be recorded at least once during every exercise stage, and preferably each minute during exercise and recovery. Additionally, careful clinical observation of the patient should be carried out to assure safety and the recording of any relevant exercise-related signs or symptoms.

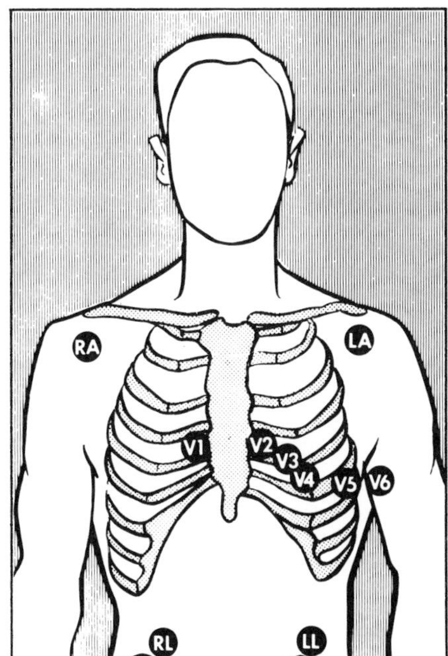

Figure 3–2. The Mason-Likar exercise electrocardiographic lead system is illustrated. The electrodes for the arms should be placed as far off the torso as possible so that the electrocardiogram most closely simulates the electrocardiogram obtained using standard wrist placement. (*From* Froelicher VF: Exercise Testing and Training. New York, LeJacq Publishing, 1983, p 17; with permission.)

Exercise Test Risks

The risk of death during exercise testing has been documented by Rochmis and Blackburn in a 1971 study as 1 fatality in 10,000 tests.[14] In a 1980 study, Stuart and Ellestad[15] compiled data from 1375 facilities that performed exercise stress tests during 1976. These centers reported complication rates of 3.6 myocardial infarctions per 10,000 tests and 1 fatality per 20,000 tests. However, less than 33% of centers responded to their questionnaire, raising the possibility that the facilities which provided data may have had better safety records than those which did not respond. Sheffield and associates[16] reported on tests performed on hyperlipidemic men in the Lipid Research Clinics' Prevalence Survey, finding no deaths, myocardial infarctions, or cardiac arrests in 9464 near-maximal graded exercise tests. A recent study from Gibbons and associates[17] reported on tests performed in patients with a low prevalence of known coronary heart disease. They reported only six major cardiac complications that occurred in relation to 71,914 maximal exercise tests. These complications consisted of two episodes of ventricular fibrillation and four myocardial infarctions. The infarctions occurred 10 minutes, 30 to 45 minutes, 12 hours, and 24 hours after the exercise tests. One of the subjects who experienced an infarction died of complications, but the others survived. These studies indicate that although finite risks do exist, when clinical safeguards are appropriately used, exercise stress testing may be performed with a high level of safety.

EXERCISE TEST INTERPRETATION

The pathophysiologic basis of exercise testing in the evaluation of coronary artery disease (CAD) is related to the fact that dynamic exercise produces an increase in myocardial oxygen consumption ($M\dot{V}O_2$) by increasing its primary components: heart rate, myocardial contractility, and intramyocardial wall tension. If $M\dot{V}O_2$ exceeds myocardial oxygen supply, myocardial ischemia occurs, and reportable or observable ischemic manifestations may occur. These manifestations are angina pectoris and electrocardiographic changes of ischemia (transient ST segment depression or elevation) or arrhythmias. Of these manifestations, only significant shifts of the ST segment are diagnostic for myocardial ischemia. Other data obtained with the stress test, however, enhance diagnostic accuracy and provide important clinical information.

The presently accepted criterion for myocardial ischemia is 1 mm or more of horizontal or downsloping ST segment depression for 0.08 second beyond the J-point (Fig. 3–3). Depressed and slowly upsloping ST segments are considered indicators of ischemia by some investigators if there is ≥1.5 mm of ST segment depression at 0.6 second beyond the J-point. Use of this criterion for ischemia will result in greater numbers of positive tests, thus enhancing sensitivity (more true positives). However, more false-positive tests will also occur, thus compromising the exercise test's specificity. (See section on sensitivity and specificity, below.) Contrary to common belief, ST depression helps to localize neither the area of myocardial ischemia nor the diseased coronary artery or arteries.[18] Inferior leads have more false positives with ST depression, possibly caused by atrial repolarization rather than myocardial ischemia.[13,19]

Exercise-induced ST segment elevation of ≥1 mm above the isoelectric line is also

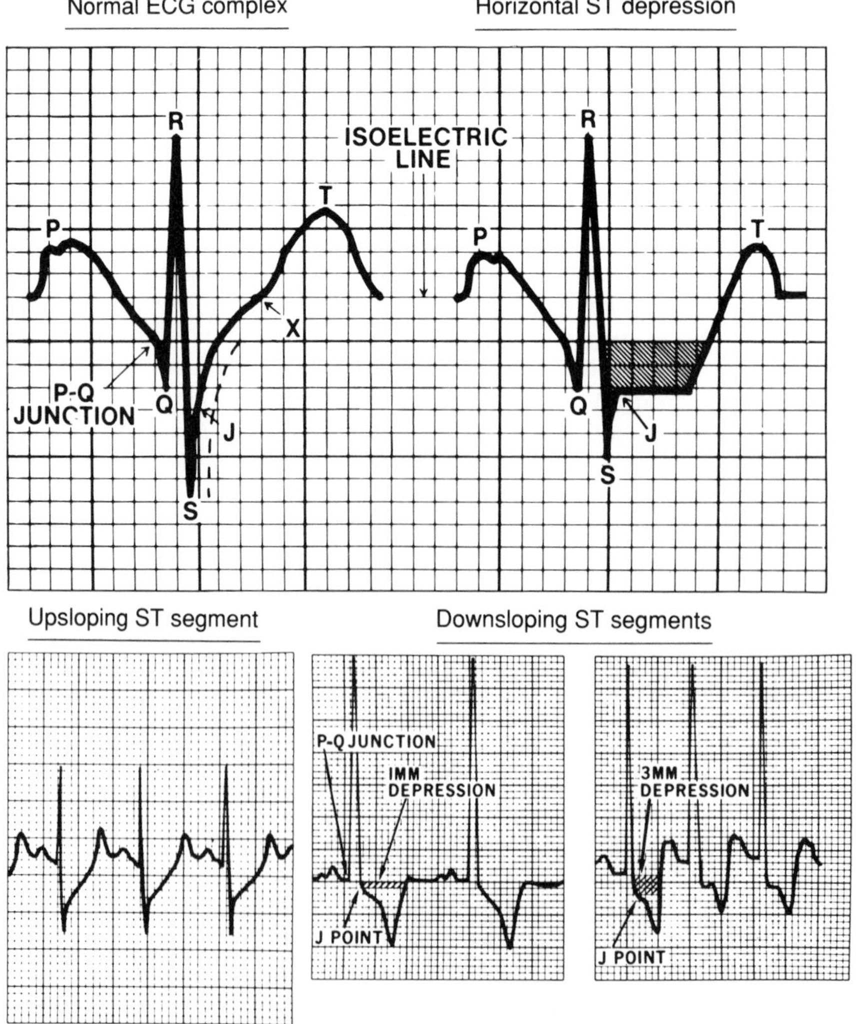

Figure 3–3. Deviation of ST segments associated with exercise. (*From* Ellerstad MH: Stress Testing: Principles and Practice, 3rd ed. Philadelphia, FA Davis, 1986, pp 225, 234, 238.)

accepted as a diagnostic criterion of myocardial (presumably transmural) ischemia, if it occurs in a lead without the Q wave of a previous myocardial infarction. Chahine and colleagues[20] reported its occurrence in 3.5% of 840 maximal exercise tests. In the majority of cases, it occurred in areas of previous myocardial infarction and abnormal Q waves. In these areas, the ST segment elevation is thought to simply reflect regional wall motion abnormalities rather than myocardial ischemia. Exercise-induced coronary artery spasm with transmural ischemia is also considered a cause of exercise-induced ST segment elevation. U-wave inversion occurring with exercise has also been reported as an indication of myocardial ischemia.[21] When right bundle branch block is present on the resting ECG, lead V_5 is the only lead that can be accurately interpreted.[22]

Conditions other than myocardial ischemia are also known to cause ST segment depression. A number of clinical conditions and electrocardiographic abnormalities may cause ST segment depression (hence "positive" tests) in the absence of myocardial ischemia. These conditions are therefore considered potential causes of "false-positive" tests (Table 3–4). Thus, ST segment shifts that would generally be accepted as indicative of ischemia occurring in patients with these conditions may be "falsely abnormal," resulting in false-positive tests. Exercise tests performed on patients with any of these conditions that show ST segment abnormalities should therefore be considered nondiagnostic for the presence of myocardial ischemia. Exercise tests, however, may provide other very useful information in these patients, in whom, with the exception of a patient who has hypokalemia, they may still be performed.

Conversely, exercise tests may show no diagnostic ST segment shifts in the presence of myocardial ischemia. These tests are usually considered "false-negative" tests. Such tests are more likely to occur in patients with mild (including single-vessel) CAD than in patients with more extensive CAD. The related concept is that an exercise stress test in a patient with CAD may be normal if no myocardial ischemia is present. Such a clinical situation would be found in a patient with CAD who has a healed myocardial infarction without areas of potentially ischemic myocardium. It must be remembered, of course, that the exercise ECG reflects the presence of myocardial ischemia rather than simply the presence of CAD. Therefore, the test would be expected to be normal in a patient with CAD who does not have myocardial ischemia with exercise. Additionally, it should be remembered that a test in which no ischemic ECG changes are present, but in which the maximal heart rate achieved is not at least 85% of the maximal predicted heart rate, should be considered nondiagnostic rather than negative (see section on test performance). Thus, medications that limit exercise heart rate response (eg, beta-blockers, verapamil, diltiazem), and situations that result in lower maximal heart rates (eg, inadequate work load, peripheral vascular disease, musculoskeletal limitations), should not be considered causes

TABLE 3–4. CAUSES OF FALSE-POSITIVE TESTS

Left bundle branch block
Left ventricular hypertrophy
Preexcitation electrocardiographic pattern (Wolff-Parkinson-White and Lown-Ganong-Levine syndromes)
Medications (digitalis, tricyclic antidepressants; possibly quinidine, procainamide, lithium, and phenothiazines)
Hypokalemia
Mitral valve prolapse
Hyperventilation syndrome
Resting ST-T wave changes
"Vasoregulatory asthenia"
Valvular heart disease
Congenital heart disease
Cardiomyopathies

of false-negative tests. Rather, they should be considered as potential causes of nondiagnostic tests.

SENSITIVITY, SPECIFICITY, AND PREDICTIVE VALUE

The accuracy of any test may be assessed by its sensitivity, specificity, and predictive value. The *sensitivity* of a test is the ability of the test to correctly identify abnormals or those with the condition or disease for which the test is performed. The *specificity* of a test is the ability of the test to correctly identify normals or those without the disease. The *predictive value* of a test is an indication of the likelihood that the test result obtained is an accurate one. The predictive value of a positive test is the likelihood that the positive test result obtained reflects a true-positive test. Conversely, the predictive value of a negative test is the likelihood that the negative test result obtained reflects a true-negative test. Thus, the predictive value of a test is the key issue once a test result is obtained.

The sensitivity of the exercise ECG for the detection of myocardial ischemia has been determined by comparison of exercise electrocardiographic results with coronary angiography (the accepted "gold standard"). However, CAD may be present in the absence of myocardial ischemia. An exercise test in a person with a healed myocardial infarction or functionally adequate collateral coronary vessels may be negative (and appropriately so) for ischemia but seemingly false-negative for CAD. Conversely, a test may be appropriately positive for myocardial ischemia in the presence of left ventricular hypertrophy or valvular heart disease but seemingly false-positive for CAD. The limitations of the correlations of the exercise ECG with coronary angiography therefore must be appreciated and accepted.

Correlations of the exercise ECG with coronary angiography have been performed in symptomatic patients (ie, those with known or suspected CAD). Tests in such patients have generally resulted in sensitivities of 54% to 80% and specificities of 88% to 97%.[23] In these patients, the predicted value of a positive test has been found to be high (87% to 96%). It must be accepted that the sensitivity, specificity, and predictive value of the exercise ECG are not fixed, but are dependent upon a number of factors related to the patients undergoing testing and the manner in which the tests are performed.

A critical factor determining the sensitivity of the exercise ECG is the severity of disease present. Not surprisingly, patients with more severe CAD are more likely to have abnormal tests than those with less severe disease. Bartel et al[24] found positive exercise stress tests in 39% of patients with single-vessel CAD, 66% with double-vessel CAD, 76% with triple-vessel CAD, and 87% with left main CAD. The sensitivity of the exercise ECG for all patients with CAD in their study was 65%. A patient with single-vessel CAD thus is more likely (61%) to have a normal test than to have a positive test (39%).

The sensitivity of the exercise ECG is increased by using multiple ECG leads; by recording the ECG during the exercise period as well as the recovery period; by using depressed, slowly upsloping ST segments as a criterion for test positivity; by performing maximal rather than submaximal exercise tests; and possibly by recording the ECG in the supine position during recovery.[13]

The specificity of the exercise ECG is increased by using strict ECG criteria for test positivity. Conversely, it is decreased in the testing of patients with abnormal resting ECGs.[13]

To study the possible causes of variations in reported sensitivity and specificity of exercise tests, Gianrossi and associates[25] applied meta-analysis to 147 published reports comparing exercise-induced ST depression with coronary angiography. These studies reported test sensitivities ranging from 23% to 100% (mean 68%) and specificities from

17% to 100% (mean 77%). Their analysis found that some, but not all, of the variation could be accounted for by patient population characteristics, technical factors, and methodologic factors. The factors significantly and independently influencing sensitivity were the treatment of equivocal test results; comparison with a "better" test, such as thallium scintigraphy; exclusion of patients on digitalis; and year of study publication. The factors affecting specificity were treatment of upsloping ST depression, exclusion of patients with prior infarction or left bundle branch block, and the use of hyperventilation before testing.

The predictive value of a test (the likelihood that a positive test result is a true positive) is dependent upon the likelihood of the disease's being present before the test is performed (ie, the prevalence of disease in the population being tested). This concept is Bayes' theorem, the statistical law of conditioned probability. If the population being tested (eg, middle-aged men with angina pectoris) has a high prevalence of disease or an individual has a high likelihood of disease, the predictive value of a positive test will be high. Conversely, in a population with a low prevalence of disease (eg, apparently healthy young women or any individual with a low likelihood of disease), the predictive value of a positive test may still be low. Weiner et al[26] correlated test results with CAD prevalence in the Coronary Artery Surgery Study. Their findings underscore two significant concepts. First, that the exercise test is an indicator of the likelihood of disease, and second, that the likelihood of disease after the test is performed is dependent upon the pretest likelihood of disease. Their analyses of descriptions of chest pain, results of exercise testing, and coronary arteriography findings are summarized in Table 3–5.

A man with definite angina in this study had a preexercise test likelihood of CAD of 89%. A positive exercise test increased his likelihood of disease to 96%, but even with a negative exercise test his likelihood of having CAD was still 65%. Similarly, because the prevalence of CAD in men with nonischemic pain in this study was 22%, such men had this pretest likelihood of CAD. A positive exercise test result increased this likelihood of CAD to 39%. This posttest likelihood was still less than that of a man with definite angina and a positive test (96%). Furthermore, it is even lower than that of a man with definite angina and a negative exercise test (65%). A negative exercise test in a man with nonischemic pain decreased his likelihood of CAD from 22% to 14%. Women in this study had a lower prevalence of CAD and hence a lower pretest likelihood of CAD, but their results paralleled those of the men.

TABLE 3–5. CORRELATIONS AMONG HISTORY OF ANGINA, EXERCISE TEST RESULTS, AND PREVALENCE OF CORONARY ARTERY DISEASE

	Prevalence of CAD (%)	Prevalence of CAD if ET + (%)	Prevalence of CAD if ET − (%)
Men			
Definite angina	89	96	65
Probable angina	70	87	44
Nonischemic pain	22	39	14
Women			
Definite angina	62	73	33
Probable angina	40	54	22
Nonischemic pain	5	6	5

Abbreviations: CAD = coronary artery disease, ET = exercise test.

Adapted from information in N Engl J Med, Weiner DA, Ryan TJ, McCabe CH, et al: Exercise stress testing: Correlations among history of angina, ST segment response and prevalence of coronary-artery disease in the Coronary Artery Surgery Study (CASS). N Engl J Med 301:230–235, 1979; with permission.

DIAGNOSTIC AND PROGNOSTIC INFORMATION AVAILABLE FOR EXERCISE TESTS

Although the ST-segment shifts are the basis for the diagnosis of myocardial ischemia and, hence, usually CAD, other information obtained from the exercise test can be used diagnostically and prognostically. Additionally, the proper interpretation of an exercise test requires the assessment of the interrelation of the electrocardiographic changes with hemodynamic and clinical parameters.

Patients with CAD exhibit a wide spectrum of disease severity with a resultant great range of clinical outcomes (ie, prognosis). Exercise test results are related to extent of CAD and left ventricular dysfunction. They therefore logically provide prognostic information in patients with CAD. The exercise ECG may, in fact, be a more accurate indicator of prognosis than coronary and left ventricular angiography alone.[27]

Configuration of ST Segment Shifts

Goldschlager and associates[28] correlated types of ST segment shifts with coronary angiography in patients with suspected CAD. They demonstrated that significant diagnostic information can be obtained from the assessment of the configuration of the ST segment shifts.

Their study included 269 patients with angiographic evidence of CAD and 141 patients without significant CAD. Downsloping ST segments were found in 123 patients. Only one of the 123 did not have significant CAD (one false positive). Of the 123, 91% had double- or triple-vessel CAD and 56% had either left main or triple-vessel disease.

Horizontal ST segment depression was present in 60 patients in their study. Of the 60 patients, nine (15%) did not have significant CAD (ie, the results were false-positive), 58% had double- or triple-vessel CAD, and 38% had left main or triple-vessel disease.

Depressed but slowly upsloping ST segments were present in 47 patients, 15 (32%) of whom did not have significant CAD. Of patients with this ST segment configuration, 55% had double- or triple-vessel CAD, and 34% had left main or triple-vessel disease.

Thus, downsloping ST segment depression was found to be highly predictive of CAD (99%) and multivessel disease (91%). Horizontal ST segment depression is less predictive (85%) of CAD, but more predictive than slowly upsloping ST segment depression (68%). Inclusion of slowly upsloping ST depression to horizontal and downsloping ST depression raised sensitivity (ability to detect those with CAD) from 64% to 76%, but decreased specificity (ability to detect those without CAD) from 93% to 82%. They concluded that "the slowly upsloping ST segment is best considered an 'equivocal' response—neither diagnostic of ischemia nor necessarily normal."[28]

Maximal Work Load and Heart Rate Achieved

The time of appearance of ischemia has been shown by McNeer and associates[29] to have diagnostic importance, correlated with the likelihood and severity of CAD. Of patients with positive tests in stages I and II of the Bruce protocol, 98% and 97%, respectively, had significant CAD. Seventy-three percent and 51% of patients with these results had triple-vessel disease, and 27% and 24% had significant left main disease. Conversely, triple-vessel disease was infrequent in patients with negative tests for ischemia who reached stage III (11%) or greater (9%).

Both the heart rate and work load at the onset of ischemia have been shown to also correlate with prognosis. McNeer and associates[29] demonstrated that ischemia occurring at a heart rate less than 120/minute carries a worse prognosis than ischemia occurring at higher heart rates. The pathophysiologic basis for this observation is that because heart rate correlates linearly with myocardial oxygen consumption, ischemia occurring at relatively low heart rates occurs at relatively low levels of myocardial oxygen consumption. It is likely, therefore, to be due to severe CAD. Similarly, ischemia occurring at low work loads, such as stage I of the Bruce protocol, carries a worse prognosis than does ischemia occurring at higher work loads. The relationship of prognosis and maximal exercise capacity persists in patients with CAD even if the exercise test does not show ST segment changes of ischemia.

Goldschlager and associates also found that early appearance of ischemic ST responses was highly predictive of multivessel CAD.[28] Of the 59 patients with positive tests in stage I of the Bruce protocol, 51 (87%) had double-vessel, triple-vessel, or left main CAD. However, in their study a significant number (14 of 23, 61%) of patients who exercised more than 6 minutes before developing positive tests also had multivessel disease.

Persistence of ECG Abnormalities

The persistence of ischemic changes in recovery was also found by Goldschlager and associates to be related to severe CAD.[28] Ninety percent (34 of 38) of patients with ST segment depression for more than 8 minutes of recovery had double- or triple-vessel disease, with 63% (24 of 38) having the latter. As would be expected, though, multivessel and even left main disease was also found in patients with early resolution of ST changes (within the first minute of recovery).

Degree of ST Segment Changes

The magnitude of ST segment depression also correlates with extent of CAD. Goldman and colleagues found the prevalence of triple-vessel CAD to be 33% in patients with 1 to 2.9 mm of ST segment depression and 69% in patients with ≥3 mm of ST segment depression. It should be remembered, however, that the magnitude of ST segment depression is dependent upon the manner in which the test is performed. For example, patients will manifest more ST segment depression if allowed to continue exercising once angina has developed than if they are stopped at the onset of angina.

Blood Pressure Changes

Blood pressure responses also provide important information. The normal blood pressure response to exercise is shown in Figure 3–1. This type of blood pressure response is not seen in patients with impaired left ventricular function due to myocardial ischemia or other conditions. The typically observed blood pressure response may also be altered by medications. Beta-adrenergic blocking agents and calcium-channel blockers may result in lower blood pressure during exercise and recovery. Both the failure to normally increase blood pressure and the drop in systolic blood pressure during exercise (exertional hypotension) are abnormal and prognostically important blood pressure responses.

Data from the Seattle Heart Watch correlated maximal exercise blood pressure with subsequent clinical course.[31] The maximal systolic blood pressure was inversely correlated with the annual mortality for sudden and nonsudden cardiac deaths. Subjects with maximal systolic blood pressures of greater than 200 mm Hg had an annual rate of cardiac death of 8.3 per 1000 men. These rates rose to 32.7 and 114.2 per 1000 men for maximal systolic pressures of 140 to 199 mm Hg and less than 140 mm Hg, respectively.

Exertional hypotension, defined as a greater than 10 mm Hg decrease in systolic blood pressure during exercise, has been demonstrated to be a highly specific although insensitive sign of multivessel disease. It occurred in 23 of 460 exercise tests performed on patients with known or suspected CAD.[32] Coronary angiography in these test subjects revealed seven with double-vessel disease and 15 with triple-vessel disease. Thus, its presence indicates a strong likelihood of multivessel disease, but its absence does not preclude severe disease.

Multiple Exercise Test Findings

A combination of factors was studied by Weiner and colleagues.[33] They found that ≥2 mm of downsloping ST segment depression in stage I of the Bruce protocol in five or more ECG leads persisting for ≥6 minutes in recovery was a highly predictive (74%) but only moderately sensitive indicator of the presence of left main or triple-vessel CAD.[33]

Exercise-Induced Arrhythmias

Ventricular arrhythmias have many causes other than CAD. Thus, as indicated earlier, their occurrence during an exercise test is not diagnostic of myocardial ischemia or CAD. They are present in approximately one third of asymptomatic men performing a maximal exercise test, with prevalence increasing slightly with age.[34] They are most likely to occur at maximal exercise levels, but generally are poorly reproducible on subsequent tests. Reproducibility with regard to presence or absence of exercise-induced ventricular arrhythmias, though generally low, appears to be greater in subjects with definite or suspected cardiovascular disease than in normal subjects.[34] The exercise-induced ventricular arrhythmias have also not been found to be highly reproducible by type or complexity both in normal subjects and in those with definite or suspected cardiovascular disease.[34]

Ventricular arrhythmias, however, are found more frequently in patients with CAD than in those without CAD.[35,36] Additionally, paired premature ventricular contractions (PVCs) and ventricular tachycardia are more likely, though not invariably, to be found in patients with extensive CAD and abnormal left ventricular function. Udall and Ellestad[37] found the presence of ventricular arrhythmias in patients with ST segment depression to be associated with a more adverse prognosis than in patients with ST depression and no ventricular arrhythmias. Other studies, however, have not found exercise-induced ventricular arrhythmias to provide independent prognostic information in patients with known CAD.[36,38] Findings from the Baltimore Longitudinal Study of Aging address the issue of prognostic importance of ventricular arrhythmias in asymptomatic subjects over a broad age range (21 to 96 years). Even frequent (greater than 10% of beats in any 1 minute) or repetitive (greater than three in a row) PVCs on a maximal treadmill exercise test were not found to predict increased cardiac morbidity or mortality. The suppression of PVCs with exercise does not exclude the diagnosis of CAD, nor does it imply a "benign" prognosis.[39] Supraventricular arrhythmias occurring during exercise testing have not been found to be related to myocardial ischemia or CAD.

Chest Pain

The presence of chest discomfort during the exercise or early recovery period may be an indicator of myocardial ischemia even without diagnostic ST segment shifts. Cole and

Ellestad[40] found an increase in test sensitivity from 64% to 85% when chest discomfort "characteristic of angina" was used as a criterion for a positive test. The use of this criterion, of course, will decrease the test specificity, because patients without myocardial ischemia may report such symptoms with exercise. Cole and Ellestad did not report its effect on test specificity in their study. Conversely, myocardial ischemia can occur without symptoms of chest discomfort (ie, "silent ischemia"). The reproduction of a patient's typical exertional chest discomfort during an exercise test, however, strengthens the likelihood that the patient's symptom is angina, that the patient has CAD, and that any ST segment shifts that occur are due to myocardial ischemia.

R-wave Amplitude

The failure of the R-wave amplitude to decrease during exercise has been proposed as a criterion for myocardial ischemia.[41] However, further studies have not been in agreement with the original proposition, and thus this finding is not believed to be diagnostic of myocardial ischemia.[42,43]

EXERCISE TESTING OF ATHLETES

When testing persons who are physically active, the athletic heart syndrome[44] must be remembered. This syndrome is defined as findings on the physical examination, chest radiograph, ECG, and echocardiogram that do not reflect disease but rather are physiologic adaptations to training. These findings should be regarded as normal in athletes and persons who participate in cardiovascular and endurance training programs. Physical examination findings may include sinus bradycardia, third and fourth heart sounds, and functional heart murmurs. The chest radiograph or echocardiogram may identify four-chamber cardiac enlargement. The ECG may show multiple changes including sinus bradycardia with or without sinus arrhythmia, prolongation of the PR interval (first-degree atrioventricular block) and second-degree atrioventricular block, typically the Wenckebach type. These changes are related to increased vagal tone and decreased sympathetic tone. Typically, they will disappear with exercise. Other changes on the ECG include P-wave changes suggestive of right and/or left atrial enlargement and increased QRS voltage at times accompanied by intraventricular conduction delays. ST-T wave changes of early repolarization and the so called juvenile T-wave inversion of leads V_1 through V_4 may be seen as well as U waves.

Resting ECGs of athletes show many "abnormalities" in the absence of any apparent organic heart disease.[45,46] Additionally, when an abnormal ST segment response to exercise occurs in an athlete, it is very likely also to occur in the absence of organic heart disease.[47] This concept is in keeping with the application of Bayes' theorem to a population with a low prevalence (likelihood) of CAD. It may also reflect a unique physiologic aspect of the athlete—physiologic cardiac hypertrophy. Whatever the cause, it is very important to cautiously interpret apparently abnormal electrocardiographic findings in athletes.

EXERCISE TESTING IN WOMEN

Using Coronary Artery Surgery Study (CASS) data, Weiner and associates[26] compared the false-positive and false-negative results in the men and women with differing types of chest pain. They found that women were 4.5 times more likely to have false-positive results than men, and that for both groups the percentage of false-positive responses increased as the pattern of chest pain was less characteristic of angina. Conversely, men were 2.8 times more likely than women to have a false-negative response.

These results (more false-positive tests in women) have been found by most investigators. However, when men and women with comparable ages and extents of CAD were compared in the study by Weiner and co-workers,[26] there was no statistically significant difference between men and women in false-positive responses (44% versus 51%) or false-negative responses (12% versus 14%).

Thus, exercise tests may provide less diagnostic information in women, but this appears to simply be in keeping with Bayes' theorem and the decreased prevalence of CAD in women compared with men. However, if these concepts are appreciated, exercise testing can be properly interpreted in women and in subjects with low likelihood of CAD.

EXERCISE TESTING IN ASYMPTOMATIC INDIVIDUALS

Less diagnostic information is available from exercise testing performed in asymptomatic individuals than in those who are symptomatic, because the former have a lower risk (prevalence) of CAD. Multiple studies have indicated a greater risk of subsequent cardiac events in asymptomatic individuals with an abnormal exercise test.[48,49] However, as pointed out by Detrano and Froelicher[50] in their review of the current status of exercise testing, most of these studies included angina pectoris as a cardiac event, and this diagnosis may have been more likely to be made in a patient with an abnormal exercise test. Also, most of the patients identified as abnormal by the exercise test did not develop cardiac events in the follow-up period (usually 3 to 8 years). Thus, the predictive value of an abnormal test in such a population with a low prevalence of disease is, in keeping with Bayes' theorem, low.

These tests can be valuable if appropriately applied and interpreted. Asymptomatic subjects suitable for exercise testing fall into one of three categories: (1) men over age 40 and women over age 50 who have two or more strongly abnormal risk factors for CAD or a family history of premature cardiovascular disease; (2) men over age 40 and, possibly, women over age 50 who will be engaging in vigorous exercise programs, especially if they have significant risk factors for CAD; and (3) individuals over age 40 who are involved in work that may affect public safety, such as airline pilots, truck or bus drivers, police, or firemen. These categories are minor modifications of the ones from a Joint American College of Cardiology/American Heart Association Task Force.[6]

It is critically important to interpret a positive test as an indicator of the likelihood rather than an absolute indicator of disease. Furthermore, interpretation should include assessment of maximal heart rate, blood pressure, and work load achieved, along with evaluation of symptoms and degree and configuration of ST segment changes.

EXERCISE TESTING FOLLOWING MYOCARDIAL INFARCTION

Exercise tests may be performed following myocardial infarction to assess prognosis and functional capacity, and to aid in therapeutic decisions.[6] They may also provide patients with reassurance relative to their physical capabilities. These tests are typically performed at the time of discharge or at 3 or more weeks following the myocardial infarction. They are performed in selected patients in whom the clinical course either was uncomplicated or has been stabilized following initial complications. The tests selected are usually begun at low levels of exercise and are slowly progressive. Submaximal tests, stopping at a specific heart rate or work load, are used by some investigators, while others use symptom-limited tests. These tests have been found to be predictive of subsequent events and useful in identifying high- and low-risk groups of patients.[51–53]

EXERCISE TESTING IN CONJUNCTION WITH RADIONUCLIDE IMAGING

Radionuclide imaging tests using thallium 201 for myocardial perfusion studies or technetium 99m for radionuclide angiography may be performed in conjunction with exercise. These tests have been found to have increased diagnostic power compared with standard exercise tests.[54] Sensitivities of 80% to 90% are reported for properly performed thallium exercise tests compared with a general sensitivity of 65% for the exercise ECG. Additionally, thallium scans provide information regarding the amount of myocardium jeopardized by ischemia. Thallium 201 studies are performed by injecting the radionuclide at near-peak exercise and continuing the exercise for an additional 30 to 60 seconds. Myocardial perfusion imaging is then performed within 5 to 10 minutes of exercise completion and again 2 to 4 hours later. The homogeneous distribution of the thallium 201 isotope occurs in normal subjects. In the presence of myocardial ischemia, a perfusion defect is present with immediate imaging but not on the later (redistribution) image. A perfusion defect that does not resolve with later imaging is indicative of myocardial scarring. Tomographic thallium scintigraphic images and quantitative analysis of the thallium images can be produced with computer-assisted processing.[55] These techniques add to the diagnostic accuracy of the test.

The use of radionuclide angiography with exercise is based on the principle that transient myocardial ischemia results in ventricular wall motion abnormalities. Left ventricular ejection fraction increases of at least 5% normally occur with maximal exercise. An abnormal response to exercise is either the failure of the left ventricular ejection fraction to increase normally (at least 5%) or the presence of an exercise-induced wall motion abnormality. The sensitivity of radionuclide angiography for the detection of myocardial ischemia is very good (greater than 90%).[56] Its specificity, however, is variable and highly dependent upon the patients being evaluated, as abnormal responses may occur with other conditions producing left ventricular dysfunction.

These tests have found their greatest usefulness in the evaluation of patients with nondiagnostic exercise ECGs (eg, those with left ventricular hypertrophy, ECG patterns of Wolff-Parkinson-White syndrome, left bundle branch block, and resting ST-T changes) and of asymptomatic patients with positive exercise tests. They are also used in the assessment of patient prognosis and significance of borderline hemodynamically significant CAD lesions.

CONCLUSION

Exercise testing in clinical situations can be performed with relative ease and a high degree of safety. Very significant data can be obtained from properly performed and interpreted exercise tests. These tests are very likely to continue to have a high level of clinical utility in this era of sophisticated medical technology and financial accountability. It will, of course, be vitally important to appropriately apply the exercise test, to critically assess the information it generates, and to continually reassess its role in the fields of cardiology and sports medicine.

REFERENCES

1. Clausen JP: Circulatory adjustments to dynamic exercise and the effect of physical training in normal subjects and patients with coronary heart disease. Prog Cardiovasc Dis 18:459–495, 1976.
2. Froelicher VF: Exercise Testing and Training. New York, LeJacq Publishing, 1983 p. 44.
3. Weisfeldt ML, Gerstenblith G: Cardiovascular aging and adaptation to disease. *In* Hurst JW (ed): The Heart, ed 6. New York, McGraw-Hill, 1986, pp 1403–1411.
4. Lester FM, Sheffield LT, Reeves TJ: Electrocardiographic changes in clinically normal older men following near maximal and maximal exercise. Circulation 36:5, 1967.
5. Sheffield LT, Maloof JA, Sawyer JA, et al: Maximal heart rate and treadmill performance of healthy women in relation to age. Circulation 57:79–84, 1978.
6. Guidelines for exercise testing: A report of the Joint American College of Cardiology/American Heart Association Task Force on Assessment of Cardiovascular Procedures (Subcommittee on Exercise Testing). Circulation 74:653A–667A, 1986.
7. American College of Sports Medicine: Guidelines for Exercise Testing and Prescription. Philadelphia, Lea & Febiger, 1986.
8. Ellestad MH: Stress Testing: Principles and Practice, ed 3. Philadelphia, FA Davis, 1986.
9. Bruce RA, Blackman JR, Jones JW, et al: Exercise testing in adult normal subjects and cardiac patients. Pediatrics 32(suppl):742–745, 1963.
10. Balke B, Ware RW: An experimental study of physical fitness of Air Force personnel. US Armed Forces Med J 10:675, 1959.
11. Sevilla DC, Dohrmann ML, Somelofski CA, et al: Invalidation of the resting electrocardiogram obtained via exercise electrode sites as a standard 12-lead recording. Am J Cardiol 63:35–39, 1989.
12. Mason RE, Likar I: A new system of multiple lead exercise electrocardiography. Am Heart J 71:196–198, 1966.
13. Chaitman BR, Hanson JS: Comparative sensitivity and specificity of exercise electrocardiographic lead systems. Am J Cardiol 47:1335–1349, 1981.
14. Rochmis P, Blackburn H: Exercise tests: A survey of procedures, safety and litigation experience in approximately 170,000 tests. JAMA 217:1061–1066, 1971.
15. Stuart RJ Jr, Ellestad MH: National survey of exercise stress testing facilities. Chest 77:94–97, 1980.
16. Sheffield LT, Haskell W, Heiss G, et al: Safety of exercise-testing volunteer subjects: The Lipid Research Clinics' Prevalence Study Experience. J Cardiol Rehabil 2:395, 1982.
17. Gibbons L, Blair SN, Kohn HW, et al: The safety of maximal exercise testing. Circulation 80:846–852, 1989.
18. Karnegis JN, Matts J, Tuna N, et al: Directional ST-segment deviation in graded exercise tests correlated with motion of the individual segments of the left ventricular wall. Am J Cardiol 52:449–454, 1983.
19. Riff DP, Carleton RA: Effect of exercise on the atrial recovery wave. Am Heart J 82:759–763, 1971.
20. Chahine RA, Raizner AE, Ishimori T: The clinical significance of exercise-induced ST segment elevation. Circulation 54:209–213, 1976.
21. Gerson MC, Phillips JF, Morris SN, et al: Exercise induced U-wave inversion as a marker of stenosis of the left anterior descending coronary artery. Circulation 60:1014–1020, 1979.
22. Tanaka T, Friedman MS, Okada RD, et al: Diagnostic value of exercise-induced ST segment depression in patients with right bundle branch block. Am J Cardiol 41:670–673, 1978.
23. Fortuin NJ, Weiss JL: Exercise stress testing. Circulation 56:699–712, 1977.
24. Bartel AG, Behar VS, Peter RH, et al: Graded exercise stress tests in angiographically documented coronary artery disease. Circulation 49:348–356, 1974.
25. Gianrossi R, Detrano R, Mulvihill D, et al: Exercise-induced ST depression in the diagnosis of coronary artery disease: A meta-analysis. Circulation 80:87–98, 1989.
26. Weiner DA, Ryan TJ, McCabe CH, et al: Exercise stress testing: Correlations among history of angina, ST-segment response and prevalence of coronary-artery disease in the Coronary Artery Surgery Study (CASS). N Engl J Med 301:230–235, 1979.
27. Bonow RO, Kent KM, Rosing DR, et al: Exercise-induced ischemia in mildly symptomatic patients with coronary-artery disease and preserved left ventricular function: Identification of subgroups at risk of death during medical therapy. N Engl J Med 311:1339–1345, 1984.
28. Goldschlager N, Selger A, Cohn K: Treadmill stress tests as indicators of presence and severity of coronary artery disease. Ann Intern Med 85:277–286, 1976.
29. McNeer JF, Margolis JR, Lee KL, et al: The role of the exercise test in the evaluation of patients for ischemic heart disease. Circulation 57:64–70, 1978.
30. Goldman S, Tselos S, Cohn K: Marked depth of ST-segment depression during treadmill exercise testing: Indicator of severe coronary artery disease. Chest 69:729–733, 1976.
31. Irving JB, Bruce RA, DeRouen TA: Variations in and significance of systolic pressure during maximal exercise (treadmill) testing. Am J Cardiol 39:841–848, 1977.

32. Morris SN, Phillips JF, Jordan JW, et al: Incidence and significance of decreases in systolic blood pressure during graded treadmill exercise testing. Am J Cardiol 41:221–226, 1978.
33. Weiner DA, McCabe CH, Ryan TJ: Identification of patients with left main and three vessel coronary disease with clinical and exercise test variables. Am J Cardiol 46:21–27, 1980.
34. Faris JV, McHenry PL, Jordan JW, et al: The prevalence and reproducibility of exercise-induced ventricular arrhythmias during maximal exercise testing in normal men. Am J Cardiol 37:617–622, 1976.
35. McHenry PL, Morris SN, Kavalier M, et al: Comparative study of exercise-induced ventricular arrhythmias in normal subjects and patients with documented coronary artery disease. Am J Cardiol 37:609–616, 1976.
36. Califf RM, McKinnis RA, McNeer JF, et al: Prognostic value of ventricular arrhythmias associated with treadmill exercise testing in patients studied with cardiac catheterization for suspected ischemic heart disease. J Am Coll Cardiol 2:1060–1064, 1983.
37. Udall JA, Ellestad MH: Predictive implications of ventricular premature contractions associated with treadmill stress testing. Circulation 56:985–989, 1977.
38. Sami M, Chaitman B, Fisher L, et al: Significance of exercise-induced ventricular arrhythmias in stable coronary artery disease: A coronary artery surgery study project. Am J Cardiol 54:1182–1185, 1984.
39. Jelinek MV, Lown B: Exercise stress testing for exposure of cardiac arrhythmias. Prog Cardiovasc Dis 16:497–506, 1974.
40. Cole JP, Ellestad MH: Significance of chest pain during treadmill exercise: Correlation with coronary events. Am J Cardiol 41:227–232, 1978.
41. Bonoris PE, Greenberg PS, Castellanet MJ, et al: Significance of changes in R wave amplitude during treadmill stress testing: Angiographic correlation. Am J Cardiol 41:846–851, 1978.
42. Fox K, England D, Jonathan A, et al: Inability of exercise-induced R wave changes to predict coronary artery disease. Am J Cardiol 49:674–679, 1982.
43. Alijarde-Guimera M, Evangelista A, Galve E, et al: Useless diagnostic value of exercise-induced R wave changes in coronary artery disease. Eur Heart J 4:614–621, 1983.
44. Huston TP, Puffer JC, Rodney WM: The athletic heart syndrome. N Engl J Med 313:24–32, 1985.
45. Oakley DG, Oakley CM: Significance of abnormal electrocardiograms in highly trained athletes. Am J Cardiol 50:985–989, 1982.
46. Balady GJ, Cadigan JB, Ryan TJ: Electrocardiogram of the athlete: An analysis of 289 professional football players. Am J Cardiol 53:1339–1343, 1984.
47. Spirito P, Maron BJ, Bonow RO, et al: Prevalence and significance of an abnormal S-T segment response to exercise in a young athletic population. Am J Cardiol 51:1663–1666, 1983.
48. Froelicher VF, Thomas MM, Pillow C, et al: Epidemiologic study of asymptomatic men screened by maximal treadmill testing for latent coronary artery disease. Am J Cardiol 34:770–776, 1974.
49. Allen WH, Aronow WS, Goodman P, et al: Five-year follow-up of maximal treadmill stress test in asymptomatic men and women. 62:522–527, 1980.
50. Detrano R, Froelicher VF: Exercise testing: Uses and limitations considering recent studies. Prog Cardiovasc Dis 331:173–204, 1988.
51. Theroux P, Waters DD, Halphen C, et al: Prognostic value of exercise testing soon after myocardial infarction. N Engl J Med 301:341–345, 1979.
52. Davidson DM, DeBusk RF: Prognostic value of a single exercise test three weeks after uncomplicated myocardial infarction. Circulation 61:236–242, 1980.
53. Weld FM, Chu KL, Bigger JT Jr, et al: Risk stratification with low level exercise testing two weeks after acute myocardial infarction. Circulation 64:306–314, 1981.
54. Beller G: Nuclear cardiology: Current indications and clinical usefulness. Curr Probl Cardiol 10(10):1–76, 1985.
55. Holman BL: Nuclear cardiology. *In* Braunwald E (ed): Heart Disease: A Textbook of Cardiovascular Medicine, ed 3. Philadelphia, WB Saunders, 1988, pp 311–355.
56. Okada RD, Boucher CA, Strauss HW, et al: Exercise radionuclide imaging approaches to coronary artery diseases. Am J Cardiol 46:1188–1204, 1980.

4

EXERCISE PRESCRIPTION

Barry A. Franklin, PhD
Michael Buchal, MS
Victoria Hollingsworth, MA
Seymour Gordon, MD
Gerald C. Timmis, MD

Exercise training is widely advocated in the prevention and treatment of several "chronic" health problems. Appropriately prescribed endurance exercise training, when maintained on a regular basis, has a favorable effect on cardiorespiratory function, increasing the anaerobic threshold and maximal oxygen consumption ($\dot{V}O_{2max}$).[1] Aerobic exercise training programs can result in moderate losses in body weight, moderate-to-large losses in body fat, and small-to-moderate increases in lean body weight.[2] Regular endurance exercise can also promote decreases in blood pressure (particularly among hypertensives),[3] serum triglycerides, and low-density lipoprotein cholesterol, and increases in the "protective" high-density lipoprotein cholesterol subfraction.[4] The physician who prescribes exercise for such purposes must consider the patient's age, sex, clinical status, related medical problems, habitual physical activity, orthopedic and musculoskeletal integrity, and, most importantly, the information derived from a multistage exercise tolerance test.

This chapter reviews the physiologic and clinical bases for the prescription of exercise in the healthy adult, with specific reference to the appropriate intensity, frequency, duration, and types of training activities. Similar principles for physical conditioning apply equally well to patients with coronary heart disease, including those with residual left ventricular dysfunction or exercise-induced ischemia, and patients who have undergone coronary artery bypass graft surgery or angioplasty.[5]

COMPONENTS OF THE EXERCISE SESSION

Exercise training sessions should include three phases: a preliminary warm-up, a stimulus (endurance) phase, and a cool-down.[6] Recreational activities can also be employed after the endurance phase, before the cool-down. A brief review of the rationale and components for each phase is provided below.

Warm-up

The warm-up period, generally lasting 5 to 10 minutes, prepares the body for the transition from rest to the endurance phase, stretching postural muscles and increasing blood flow. More importantly, a preliminary warm-up serves to decrease the susceptibility to orthopedic injury and the potential for adverse responses such as ischemic ST segment

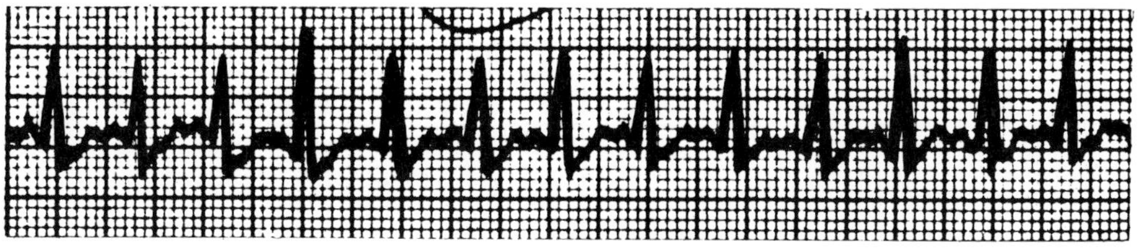

A

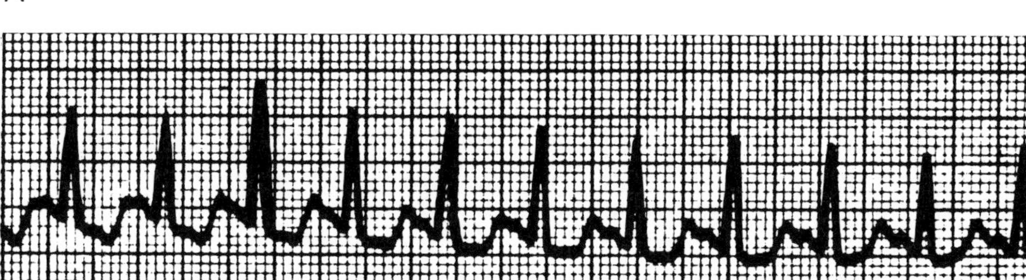

B

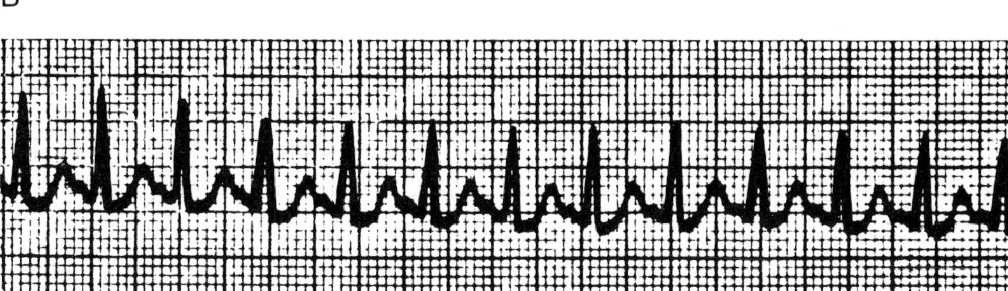

C

Figure 4–1. ECG recordings obtained from a 35-year-old man. **A**: At maximal exercise during multistage treadmill testing. **B**: Immediately after 10-second run at 9 mph, 30% grade, with no prior warm-up. Significant horizontal to downsloping ST segment depression is apparent. **C**: Immediately after 10-second run at 9 mph, 30% grade, preceded by a 2-minute warm-up of jogging in place. ST segment abnormalities were reduced in severity. (*From* Barnard RJ, Gardner GW, Diaco NV, et al: Cardiovascular responses to sudden strenuous exercise: Heart rate, blood pressure, and ECG. J Appl Physiol 34:833–837, 1973; with permission.)

depression (Fig. 4–1), ventricular ectopy, decreased left ventricular ejection fraction, and diffusely hypokinetic wall motion—abnormalities that may be provoked by sudden strenuous exertion.[7–10] Thus, warm-up has musculoskeletal and cardiovascular preventive value.

Warm-up exercises should include calisthenics and cardiorespiratory activities that involve rhythmic body movement (eg, alternate walking-jogging, swimming, mild-to-moderate resistance cycle ergometry) sufficient to evoke a heart rate response within 20 beats/min of the heart rate recommended for endurance training.

Our experience suggests that the ideal warm-up for any endurance activity is the same activity only at a lower intensity.[11] Hence, participants who use jogging during the endurance phase should conclude the warm-up period with brisk walking (ie, 3.5 to 4.5 mph); for participants who use the stationary cycle ergometer, "zero" load or mild tension cycling serves as an ideal warm-up. Cardiorespiratory warm-up exercises can also be modified to incorporate playground balls, and individual, partner, or group activities or relays.[12] However, with partner or small-group activities, participants should ideally be grouped with individuals who have similar aerobic capacities ($\dot{V}O_{2max}$).

TABLE 4–1. EXERCISE PRESCRIPTION FORM

M.D. ______________________

EXERCISE PRESCRIPTION

Name ______________________ Age ________ Starting Date ____________

Clinical Status:

Arrhythmia	Angina	CABG	CAD	HTN	MI	PTCA	VR

NOTE: This prescription is valid only if you remain on the same medications (type and dose), and you are in the same clinical status as on the day your exercise test was conducted.

CONTRAINDICATIONS: *Angina at rest *Fever *Illness
*Temperature and Weather Extremes (below 30 degrees or over 80 degrees with high humidity)

ACTIVITIES TO AVOID: *Sudden strenuous lifting or carrying
*Exertion that leads to holding your breath

EXERCISE TYPE: Aerobic types of exercise that are continuous, dynamic, and repetitive in nature
FREQUENCY: ____________ times/day ____________ days/week
DURATION: Total duration of exercise session: ____________ minutes
TO BE DIVIDED AS FOLLOWS:
WARM-UP: (light flexibility/stretching routine) ____________ minutes
AEROBIC TRAINING ACTIVITY: ____________ to ____________ minutes
COOL-DOWN: (slow walking and stretching): ____________ minutes

INTENSITY:
TARGET HEART RATE ____________ to ____________ beats/minute
____________ to ____________ beats/10 seconds
PERCEIVED EXERTION SHOULD NOT EXCEED "SOMEWHAT HARD"

RE-EVALUATION

Your next graded exercise test is due: ______________________
Call our office to schedule an appointment.
Exercise Physiologist ______________________

CABG, Coronary artery bypass graft; CAD, coronary artery disease; HTN, hypertension; MI, Myocardial infarction; PTCA, percutaneous transluminal coronary angioplasty; VR, valve replacement.

Endurance Phase

The endurance phase (at least 20 to 30 minutes) serves to directly stimulate the oxygen transport system and to maximize caloric expenditure. This phase should be prescribed in specific terms of intensity (how strenuously a person exercises), frequency (how often a person exercises), duration (how long is each exercise session), and mode (the type of exercise that is best). An "exercise prescription form" (Table 4–1) serves as an ideal way of providing your recommendations to the patient. It should be emphasized, however, that interrelationships among the training intensity, frequency, and duration may permit a decrease in the intensity to be partially or totally compensated for by increases in the exercise duration or frequency, or both.[13]

Recreational Games

The inclusion of enjoyable recreational games after the endurance phase often enhances compliance. However, 6 to 10 weeks of preliminary conditioning with achievement of a minimal exercise capacity of 5 metabolic equivalents [METs; 1 MET = 3.5 mL of oxygen per kilogram of body weight per minute ($mL \cdot kg^{-1} \cdot min^{-1}$)] is recommended before participation in games.[14] To accommodate even the most deconditioned participant, game rules should be modified to decrease the energy cost and heart rate response to play. Modifications that serve to minimize skill and competition and maximize participant success are particularly important in adult fitness and cardiac exercise programs. For example, volleyball played allowing one or more bounces of the ball per side, facilitates longer rallies and provides additional fun, while minimizing the skill level required to play the game. Through such modifications, the participant is better able to appreciate the primary objective of the activity: enjoyment of the game itself.[15]

Cool-down

Cool-down activities such as slow walking or low-tension pedaling permit a gradual recovery from the endurance phase and recreational games. Exercises of a muscle-stretching or muscle-lengthening nature are encouraged. Special attention should be paid to the extensor muscles of the back, lower legs, and upper extremities. Such activities encourage a return of the heart rate and blood pressure to near resting values; enhance venous return, thereby reducing the potential for postexercise hypotension and dizziness; facilitate heat dissipation; promote the removal of lactic acid[16]; and combat the potentially deleterious effects of the postexercise rise in plasma catecholamines.[17]

During exercise, vasodilation in the active muscles accommodates the blood flow necessary for increased metabolic demands. The potential for "pooling" of blood in the lower extremities is countered by a "milking action" of the muscles on the veins and one-way valves that prohibit retrograde flow. Abrupt cessation of exercise may result in a transient decrease in venous return, reducing coronary blood flow when heart rate and myocardial oxygen demands are still high. This scenario, in persons with a compromised coronary circulation, may lead to angina pectoris, ischemic ST segment depression, or threatening ventricular dysrhythmias. Of 61 cardiovascular complications reported (by survey questionnaire) during the exercise training of cardiac patients, at least 44 (72%) occurred during either the warm-up or cool-down phase.[18]

INTENSITY

Exercise intensity may be regulated by several methods: a prescribed training heart rate range; assigned pace for walking or jogging; recommended work load for the cycle ergometer; and the Borg category or category-ratio scales for rating of perceived exertion.[19] This latter method, particularly when used in conjunction with other clinical, psychological, and physiologic information (eg, pulse rate), provides a reliable method for regulating exercise intensity within safe and effective limits.

The prescribed exercise intensity should be above a minimal level required to induce a "training effect," yet below the metabolic load that evokes significant symptoms, or ECG or blood pressure abnormalities. For most deconditioned adults and cardiac patients, the threshold intensity for exercise training probably lies between 40% and 60% $\dot{V}O_{2max}$[14]; moreover, considerable evidence suggests that it increases in direct proportion to the pretraining $\dot{V}O_{2max}$ or the level of habitual activity.[20]

The optimal intensity for aerobic exercise training probably occurs between 60% and 80% $\dot{V}O_{2max}$, as indicated by two physiologic variables that signify increasing reliance on anaerobic metabolism: the respiratory exchange ratio ($\dot{V}CO_2/\dot{V}O_2$) as it approaches unity, and blood lactate when it increases abruptly—acute responses that are associated with favorable long-term adaptation and improvement in oxygen transport capacity.[5]

Improvement in $\dot{V}O_{2max}$ increases curvilinearly with increasing intensities of exercise to a peak of about 80% $\dot{V}O_{2max}$, with little additional cardiorespiratory benefit thereafter. Although higher intensity training (ie, up to 90% $\dot{V}O_{2max}$) may provide "direct" cardiac

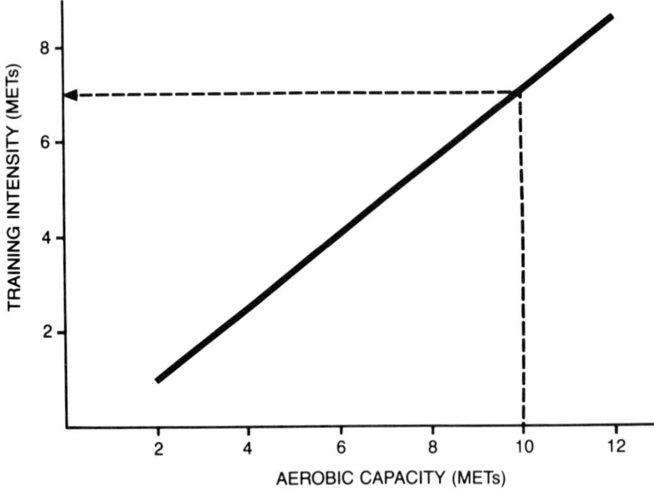

Figure 4–2. Sliding scale method for estimating relative exercise-training intensity (METs) from the peak or symptom-limited aerobic capacity (METs). For example, a cardiac patient with an aerobic capacity of 10 METs would use a training intensity of 7 METs.

benefits such as an improvement in stroke volume and left ventricular ejection fraction,[21–22] such regimens are generally considered inadvisable because of the increased risk of orthopedic and cardiovascular complications (ie, significant dysrhythmias, ischemic ST segment depression, myocardial infarction, and cardiac arrest).[23–26]

The "sliding scale" method, as recommended by the American College of Sports Medicine,[14] empirically estimates a relative exercise training intensity that increases in direct proportion to the initial peak or symptom-limited aerobic capacity ($\dot{V}O_{2max}$). The baseline intensity, set at 60% $\dot{V}O_{2max}$, is added to the $\dot{V}O_{2max}$, expressed as METs, to obtain the percentage of $\dot{V}O_{2max}$ that should be used for physical conditioning. For example, an individual with a 10-MET capacity would train at 70% of his or her $\dot{V}O_{2max}$ (60 + 10), corresponding to an average training intensity of 7 METs. Accordingly, Figure 4–2 shows the prescribed training intensity (METs) for persons with aerobic capacities ranging from 2 to 12 METs. For physical conditioning intensities of 3 METs or more, it is recommended that the initial exercise intensity be set at about 1 MET lower than suggested, until the participant has become accustomed to exercise.[14]

Heart Rate Monitoring

To attain a desired metabolic load for exercise training, one must either measure the oxygen uptake directly or have an equivalent index. Since heart rate (HR) and oxygen uptake are linearly related during dynamic exercise involving large-muscle groups, a predetermined training or target heart rate (THR) has become widely adopted as an indicator of exercise intensity. Heart rate monitoring offers several advantages in regulating the intensity of exercise[20]: (1) it can be used to assess the relative strenuousness of occupational or recreational activities; (2) it provides a built-in regulator for changes in fitness; (3) it adjusts for extremes in environmental conditions, so that the cardiac work (myocardial oxygen consumption) remains unchanged[27]; and (4) it allows for the detection of dysrhythmias.

The limitations of age-predicted maximal heart rates as indices of $\dot{V}O_{2max}$ and of training intensity are well documented.[28] Although maximal heart rates (HR_{max}) in normal healthy men and women may be estimated from equations such as 220 minus age, the predicted HR_{max} may differ from the actual HR_{max} by 20 beats/min (standard deviation is approximately ±10 beats/min). THRs for aerobic conditioning can be more accurately determined by one of four methods from data obtained during graded exercise testing (GXT): (1) the HR versus $\dot{V}O_2$ regression method, (2) the Karvonen method, (3) the percentage HR_{max} method, and (4) the HR slightly below the anaerobic or ventilatory threshold.

The first method involves identifying the HR that occurred at a given $\dot{V}O_2$ during GXT, using a plot of the HR versus $\dot{V}O_2$ or METs.[29] The THR is equal to the HR that occurred at 60% to 80% aerobic capacity or $\dot{V}O_{2max}$. This method is most accurate when steady-state HR and $\dot{V}O_2$ are determined during at least two, and ideally three, progressive submaximal work loads.

Another method of establishing the THR is the maximal heart rate reserve method of Karvonen and associates,[30] in which THR equals (HR_{max} minus resting HR) times 60% to 80%, plus resting HR. This method, which requires reliable measurements of resting (standing) and maximal HR, closely approximates the percentage of aerobic capacity in healthy young men.[31] On the other hand, it may overestimate the desired aerobic training intensity in cardiac patients, particularly during the initial stages of rehabilitation.[32]

The third method that is widely used to compute the THR is to calculate a fixed percentage (eg, 70% to 85%) of the measured maximal HR (HR_{max}).[33,34] This method has the advantage of requiring only the measurement of HR_{max}. Moreover, it has been shown to yield remarkably similar regressions of $\%\dot{V}O_{2max}$ on $\%HR_{max}$ (ie, 60% to 80% $\dot{V}O_{2max} \sim$ 70% to 85% HR_{max}), regardless of the subject's age or sex, the presence or absence of coronary artery disease, $\dot{V}O_{2max}$, body weight, relative body fat, muscle groups involved, exercise testing mode, or cardiac medications.[35,36] However, limitations of the method include the underestimation of the THR for a given MET level (corrected by adding 15% to the calculated THR)[14]; and considerable individual variability in the relationship between $\%HR_{max}$ and $\%\dot{V}O_{2max}$.[37]

The final method of intensity prescription involves determining the gas exchange anaerobic threshold (AT) and establishing the THR at the work rate or oxygen consumption just below the point of increase in minute ventilation ($\dot{V}E$)/$\dot{V}O_2$ during exercise without a change in $\dot{V}E/CO_2$ production ($\dot{V}CO_2$) (Fig. 4–3).[38] Coplan and associates[39] compared

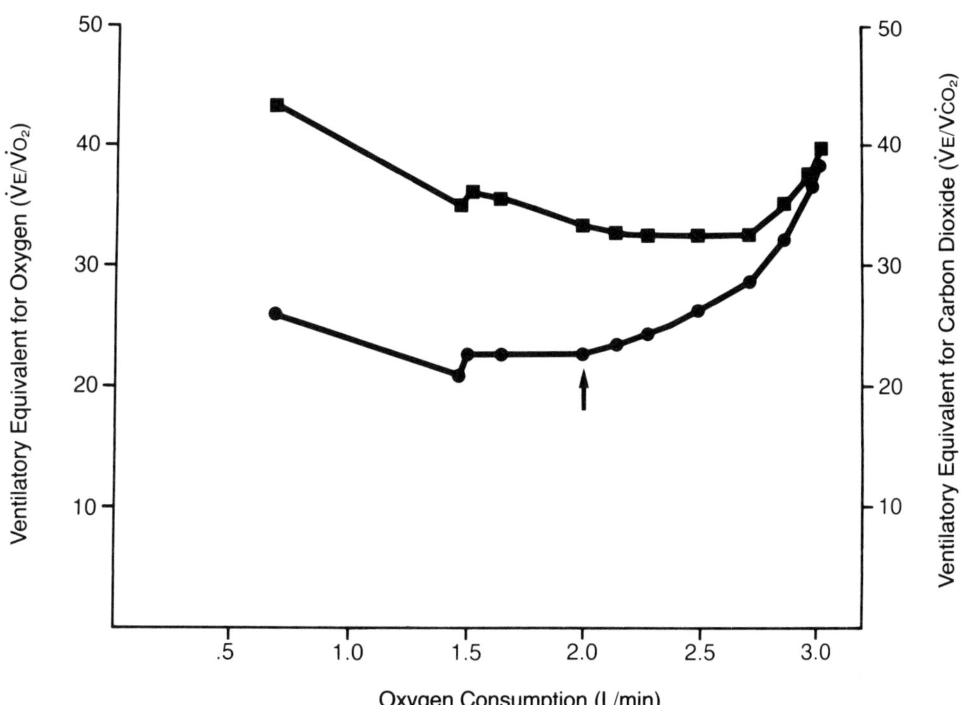

Figure 4–3. Ventilatory equivalent for oxygen (●) and carbon dioxide (■) as a function of oxygen consumption for one subject. Arrow indicates gas exchange anaerobic threshold, which occurred at 67% of the $\dot{V}O_{2max}$.

several methods for determining exercise intensity, using heart rate at the AT and at 50% $\dot{V}O_{2max}$ as the recommended upper and lower limits for training. Exercise prescription based on either 80% HR_{max} or the heart rate corresponding to 70% $\dot{V}O_{2max}$ yielded the greatest number of subjects falling within this range. Nevertheless, even these methods yielded an exercise intensity that exceeded the anaerobic threshold 15% to 20% of the time. It was concluded that exercise prescriptions should be based on direct assessment of the AT. The preferred method to use when respiratory measurements are not available is an exercise intensity based on 80% HR_{max}.

In summary, HR provides a safe and reliable monitor of the exercise intensity. Once a THR is established, participants should be taught to correctly count their pulse. HR can be estimated most reliably by counting the pulse using palpation of the radial artery for 10 seconds immediately after cessation of activity and then multiplying the resulting number by six.[40] Excessive pressure when monitoring heart rate via the carotid can produce

PERCEIVED EXERTION

Category scale

6	
7	VERY, VERY LIGHT
8	
9	VERY LIGHT
10	
11	FAIRLY LIGHT
12	
13	SOMEWHAT HARD
14	
15	HARD
16	
17	VERY HARD
18	
19	VERY, VERY, HARD
20	

Category–ratio scale

0	NOTHING AT ALL	
0.5	VERY, VERY WEAK	[just noticeable]
1	VERY WEAK	
2	WEAK	[light]
3	MODERATE	
4	SOMEWHAT STRONG	
5	STRONG	[heavy]
6		
7	VERY STRONG	
8		
9		
10	VERY, VERY STRONG	[almost max]
	MAXIMAL	

Figure 4–4. Perceived exertion scales with descriptive "effort ratings." (*Data from* Borg G: Psychophysical bases of perceived exertion. Med Sci Sports Exerc 14:377–381, 1982.)

bradycardia, yielding an underestimation of the relative exercise intensity. However, this problem can be eliminated when adult exercisers are taught how to palpate the carotid artery correctly.[41]

Rating of Perceived Exertion

The rating of perceived exertion (RPE) is a useful and important adjunct to heart rate as an intensity guide for exercise training. It must, however, be interpreted in the proper context to insure valid responses. Accordingly, the use of explicit preliminary instructions is important.

The RPE scale, first introduced by Borg,[19] consists of 15 grades from 6 to 20 or 10 grades from 0 to 10 (Fig. 4–4). The ratings, based on one's overall feeling of exertion and physical fatigue, correlate highly with metabolic changes (eg, heart rate, oxygen consumption) experienced during exercise, particularly when these variables are expressed as percentages of their respective maximums. Participants are advised not to overemphasize any one factor, such as leg pain or dyspnea, but to try to assess their total feelings of somatic exertion. Among healthy young persons, the effort rating on the 6 to 20 scale generally approximates one tenth of the heart rate response.

Exercise rated as 11 to 13 (6 to 20 scale) or 3 to 4 (0 to 10 scale), between "fairly light" and "somewhat hard" (6 to 20 scale), or between "moderate" and "somewhat strong" (0 to 10 scale), is generally appropriate for weight reduction programs, corresponding to 60% to 70% of the maximal HR, which is equivalent to 45% to 60% $\dot{V}O_{2max}$. During this relative intensity, blood lactate levels generally remain low, allowing the individual to exercise for sustained periods, and free fatty acids are used preferentially as a fuel source.[42,43] In contrast, exercise rated 13 to 16 (6 to 20 scale), between "somewhat hard" and "hard," or 4 to 6 (0 to 10 scale), between "somewhat strong" and "very strong," is generally considered more appropriate for cardiorespiratory conditioning, corresponding to 70% to 85% of maximal HR, which is equivalent to 60% to 80% $\dot{V}O_{2max}$. This relative intensity is associated with decreased fat and increased carbohydrate utilization (Fig. 4–5).[44]

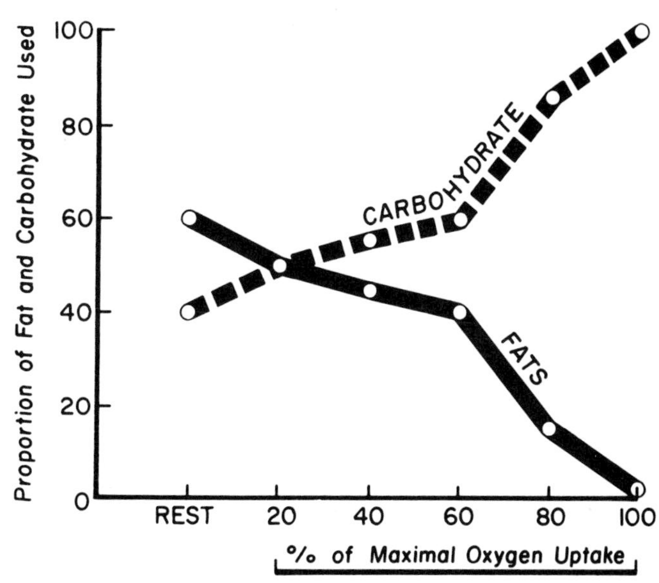

Figure 4–5. Relative contributions from fat and carbohydrate as a function of exercise intensity, expressed as a percentage of the maximal oxygen uptake ($\dot{V}O_{2max}$). During mild intensity exercise (ie, below 60% $\dot{V}O_{2max}$), fat serves as an important energy substrate. However, at higher intensities, there is decreased fat and increased carbohydrate utilization. (*Data from* Åstrand PO, Rodahl K: Textbook of Work Physiology. New York, McGraw-Hill, 1970, p 460.)

The concept of perceived exertion appears to be valid even for patients whose heart rates are attenuated by propranolol, since similar RPEs are obtained at a given percentage of maximum HR reserve, regardless of the beta-blocker dosage or peak HR.[45] However, there are limitations in using RPE alone to gauge exercise intensity. Although the subjective rating correlates well with HR, oxygen uptake, and work load, ischemic ST segment depression and threatening ventricular dysrhythmias can occur without symptoms (silent ischemia) at low ratings of perceived exertion.[46]

DURATION

The duration of exercise required to elicit a significant training effect varies inversely with the intensity; the greater the intensity, the shorter the duration of exercise necessary to achieve favorable adaptation and improvement in cardiorespiratory fitness. Significant increases in aerobic capacity have been reported with high-intensity (>85%–90% $\dot{V}O_{2max}$) exercise sessions of only 5 to 10 minutes duration.[14] However, such regimens are not generally recommended for sedentary adults and cardiac patients because of potential complications and compliance problems. Fortunately, exercise programs of low intensity but long duration can yield results similar to those of higher intensity and shorter duration when the caloric expenditure is equalized.[13]

Generally, the duration of continuous or discontinuous aerobic exercise varies from 15 to 60 minutes; however, there appears to be little additional cardiovascular benefit beyond 30-minute sessions, excluding the warm-up and cool-down.[47] Even longer training sessions (≥45 minutes) are associated with a disproportionate incidence of orthopedic injury (Fig. 4–6).[48]

The initial exercise prescription should include sessions of moderate duration and intensity, such as 20 to 30 minutes and 40% to 70% of aerobic capacity ($\dot{V}O_{2max}$). If the participant experiences no musculoskeletal complications and does not have persistent fatigue, the duration and/or intensity may be gradually increased over a period of weeks.[14]

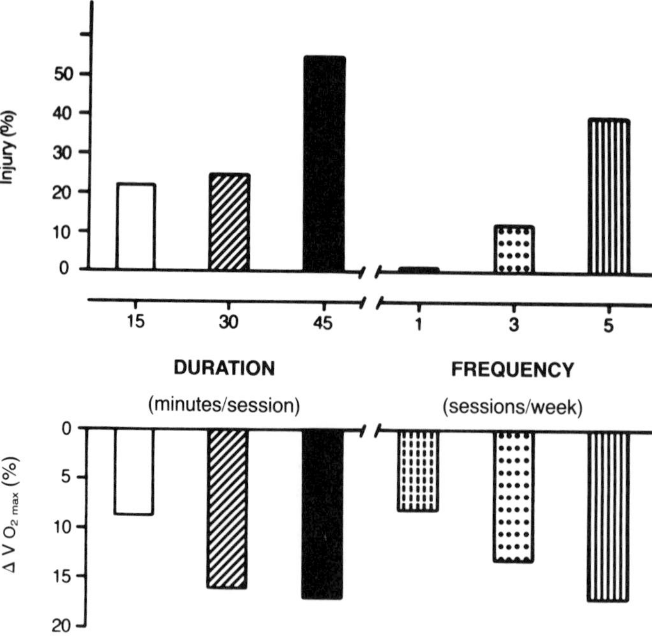

Figure 4–6. Relationships among exercise frequency and duration, improvement in maximal oxygen consumption ($\Delta\dot{V}O_{2max}$), and the incidence of orthopedic injury. Above an exercise duration of 30 minutes/session or a frequency of 3 sessions/week, additional improvement in $\dot{V}O_{2max}$ is small, and the injury rate increases disproportionately. (*Data from* Pollock ML, Gettman LR, Milesis CA, et al: Effects of frequency and duration of training on attrition and incidence of injury. Med Sci Sports 9:31–36, 1977.)

FREQUENCY

The optimal training frequency for persons with or without heart disease appears to be three or four evenly spaced workouts per week.[11,47] Additional cardiorespiratory benefits of five or more training sessions per week appear to be minimal, whereas the incidence of lower-extremity injuries increases abruptly (Fig. 4–6).[48] Although improvements in cardiorespiratory fitness can occur in deconditioned subjects exercising only one to two times per week, such regimens evoke little or no reduction in body weight and fat stores.[49,50] For adults initiating a jogging program, exercise every other day is recommended; however, if weight reduction is the primary objective, lower impact activities such as walking may be performed more frequently in order to augment caloric expenditure.

TYPES OF TRAINING ACTIVITIES

The most effective exercises for the endurance phase employ large-muscle groups, are maintained continuously, and are rhythmic and aerobic in nature. Examples include walking, jogging (in place or moving), running, stationary or outdoor cycling, swimming, skipping rope, rowing, climbing stairs, and stepping on and off a bench. Because of the relative consistency of energy expenditure in walking, jogging, and cycling, these activities lend themselves particularly well to exercise prescription, offering comparable cardiorespiratory improvements when the exercise frequency, intensity, and duration are equated.[51] Other training activities commonly used in conditioning programs for sedentary adults include calisthenics, particularly those involving sustained total body movement, arm exercise, and weight training. The latter is a particularly important option, since traditional aerobic conditioning regimens often fail to accommodate participants who have an interest in improving muscular strength and endurance.

Walking and Jogging

Walking and jogging on level ground are the most facile and easily regulated exercises for cardiorespiratory conditioning. Moreover, inherent neuromuscular limitations to the speed of walking have established it as the most appropriate activity in early cardiac rehabilitation, offering an exercise intensity of 2 METs or more, even at the slowest walking speeds ($\leq$2 mph) (Fig. 4–7).[52]

Fitness walking programs can elicit significant increases in aerobic capacity and/or decreases in body weight and fat stores, if three or more 30- to 60-minute exercise sessions are performed each week.[53,54] Advantages of such regimens include a low dropout rate, an easily tolerable work intensity, and fewer musculoskeletal and orthopedic problems of the legs, knees, and feet. Swimming-pool walking in shallow water and walking with a backpack offer additional options for those who wish to lose weight and improve fitness.[55,56]

The gross caloric cost of walking approximates 1.15 kilocalories (kcal) per kilogram of body weight per mile.[57] Furthermore, unless the individual walks at an extremely slow or fast pace (ie, less than 1.9 mph or greater than 3.7 mph), the caloric cost per mile is relatively independent of speed, increasing linearly as a function of body weight. Although many sedentary adults may be unable to maintain a jog or run, they can expend considerable energy by moving their body weights over considerable distances. Tables 4–2 and

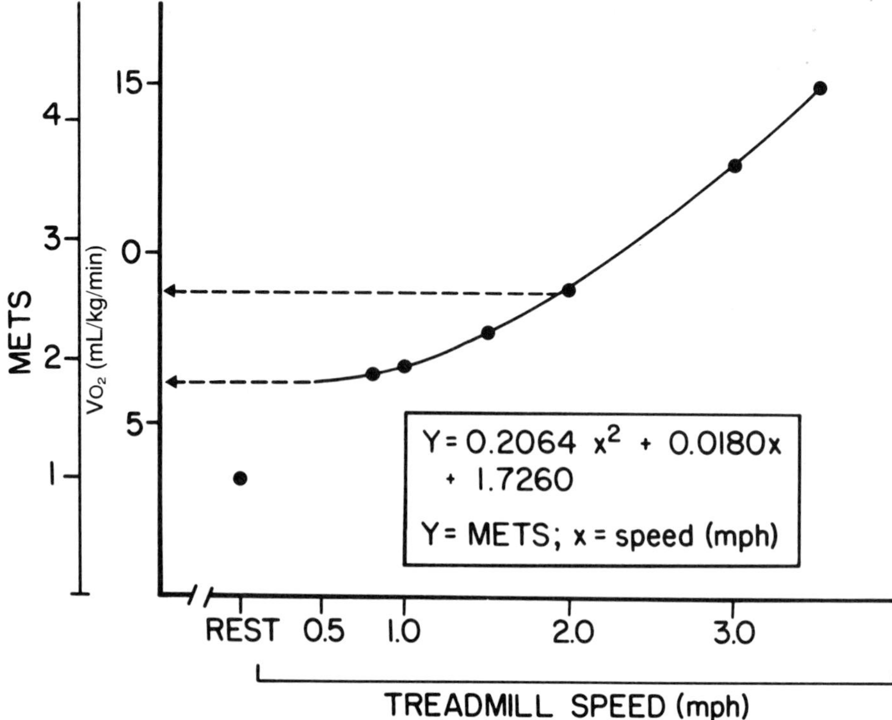

Figure 4–7. Relationship between $\dot{V}O_2$ and treadmill walking speed. The energy cost of walking at ≤2.0 mph, indicated by broken lines, approximates 2 METs. (*From* Franklin BA, Pamatmat A, Johnson S, et al: Metabolic cost of extremely slow walking in cardiac patients: Implications for exercise testing and training. Arch Phys Med Rehabil 64:564–565, 1983; with permission.)

4–3 provide progressive walking programs for individuals with low and average fitness levels, with specific reference to the recommended exercise frequency, intensity, duration, pace, and distance over 20 weeks.[58]

Rebounding

Walking or running-in-place on units that resemble minitrampolines constitutes rebound exercise. Among sedentary adults, average HR and oxygen consumption responses to rebound running were 116 beats/min and 17 $mL \cdot kg^{-1} \cdot min^{-1}$, respectively, equivalent to the aerobic cost of walking at a 4.0 mph pace.[59] However, the maximal energy expenditure that may be attained on these units is relatively low, because the subject's vertical displacement decreases as the stepping rate increases. Thus, few individuals are able to attain high exercise HRs and levels of oxygen consumption.

In summary, rebound exercise may be an appropriate training modality for many deconditioned adults and cardiac patients, particularly during the initial weeks of conditioning. Intensity limitations, however, may preclude its effectiveness in highly fit or trained subjects.

Swimming

Although lap swimming is an excellent exercise for cardiorespiratory conditioning, incorporating both the upper and lower extremities, it is difficult to prescribe for three reasons:

TABLE 4–2. 20-WEEK WALKING PROGRAM FOR INDIVIDUALS WITH FUNCTIONAL CAPACITIES LESS THAN 25 mL·kg^{-1}·min^{-1}

Week*	Distance (miles)	Pace† (min/mile)	Intensity (%HR_{max})	Duration (min)	Frequency (days/wk)
1	1.5	20	60–65	30	5
2	1.5	20	60–65	30	5
4	1.75	20	60–65	35	5
6	2.0	20	60–65	40	5
8	2.25	17	65–70	38	5
10	2.50	17	65–70	43	5
12	2.50	17	65–70	43	5
14	2.75	17	65–70	47	5
16	3.0	15	70–80	45	5
18	3.0	15	70–80	45	5
20	3.0	15	70–80	45	5

*Training recommendations for the odd-numbered weeks can be those listed for the even-numbered week immediately before or after, depending on progression.

†The pace listed is only an approximation. The actual pace should be the one that keeps the heart rate at the indicated intensity, provided that the perceived exertion is less than or equal to "somewhat hard."

Data from Rippe JM, Southmayd W: The Sports Performance Factors. New York, Putnam, 1986, p 64; with permission.

(1) energy expenditure for a given stroke or pace is extremely variable and is highly dependent on skill and mechanical efficiency; (2) THRs extrapolated from maximal treadmill or cycle ergometer testing may be too high, typically by 5 to 10 beats/min[60]; and (3) swimming pool facilities are often inaccessible. Additional drawbacks to swimming, even at slow speeds, include a relatively high aerobic cost, 6.5 and 8.6 METs for untrained and trained swimmers, respectively,[61] camouflaged anginal symptoms,[62] and sudden HR and blood pressure fluctuations with exposure to cold water.

TABLE 4–3. 20-WEEK WALKING PROGRAM FOR INDIVIDUALS WITH FUNCTIONAL CAPACITIES OF 25 TO 35 mL·kg^{-1}·min^{-1}

Week*	Distance (miles)	Pace† (min/mile)	Intensity (%HR_{max})	Duration (min)	Frequency (days/wk)
1	2.00	20	65–70	40	5
2	2.25	20	65–70	45	5
4	2.50	20	65–70	50	5
6	2.75	17	70–75	47	5
8	2.75	17	70–75	47	5
10	3.00	17	70–75	51	4–5
12	3.00	15	75–80	45	4–5
14	3.25	15	75–80	49	4–5
16	3.50	14	75–80	49	3–5
18	3.50	14	75–80	49	3–5
20	3.50	14	75–80	49	3–5

*Training recommendations for the odd-numbered weeks can be those listed for the even-numbered week immediately before or after, depending on progression.

†The pace listed is only an approximation. The actual pace should be the one that keeps the heart rate at the indicated intensity, provided that the perceived exertion is less than or equal to "somewhat hard."

Data from Rippe JM, Southmayd W: The Sports Performance Factors. New York, Putnam, 1986, p 65; with permission.

TABLE 4–4. ENERGY EXPENDITURE IN METs DURING BICYCLE ERGOMETRY AT PROGRESSIVE WORK RATES FOR PERSONS OF DIFFERENT BODY WEIGHT

Body Weight		Work Rate ($kg \cdot m \cdot min^{-1}$)						
kg	*lb*	*300*	*450*	*600*	*750*	*900*	*1050*	*1200*
50	110	4.4	6.1	7.9	9.6	11.3	13.0	14.7
60	132	3.9	5.3	6.7	8.1	9.6	11.0	12.4
70	154	3.4	4.7	5.9	7.1	8.3	9.6	10.8
80	176	3.1	4.2	5.3	6.4	7.4	8.5	9.6
90	198	2.9	3.9	4.8	5.8	6.7	7.7	8.6
100	220	2.7	3.6	4.4	5.3	6.1	7.0	7.9

Data from American College of Sports Medicine: Guidelines for Graded Exercise Testing and Exercise Prescription, ed 3. Philadelphia, Lea & Febiger, 1986, p 168; with permission.

Bicycling

Bicycling programs offer the potential for outdoor or indoor training, using a mobile bicycle or stationary-cycle ergometer, respectively. However, with the latter, care should be taken to insure that the seat height provides a slight bend in the knee when the pedal is in the down position,[6] and sustained tight gripping of the handlebars should be avoided.

The relative oxygen consumption ($\dot{V}O_2$) for outdoor bicycle riding (on the level) can be reasonably estimated for speeds from 9.3 to 19.9 mph, equivalent to 250 to 531 meters per minute (m/min), using the following regression equation[63,64]: $\dot{V}O_2$ ($mL \cdot kg^{-1} \cdot min^{-1}$) = 0.1 (m/min) − 12. Accordingly, the $\dot{V}O_2$ for a cycling speed of 9.3 mph (250 m/min) would be 13 $mL \cdot kg^{-1} \cdot min^{-1}$ or 3.7 METs. This value, however, may vary with the type of bicycle, cycling skill of the individual, terrain, and air (wind) resistance.

The power output (and oxygen consumption) associated with stationary leg ergometry is determined by the weight applied (kg), the distance (m) this weight moves per revolution, and the number of revolutions per minute (rpm), or $kg \cdot m \cdot min^{-1}$. Since the work rate is independent of body weight, the absolute $\dot{V}O_2$ (expressed as mL/min) at any power output is comparable among individuals of different size.[14] However, a lighter individual would have a greater relative $\dot{V}O_2$ (ie, in METs or $mL \cdot kg^{-1} \cdot min^{-1}$) than a heavier person when exercising at the same work rate (Table 4–4).

Calisthenics

Although stretching of isolated muscle groups is generally thought to be ineffective in raising HR and total body oxygen demands to the levels needed to obtain a training effect, rhythmic total-body calisthenics involving large-muscle groups (eg, straddle hops or jumping jacks) have been shown to elicit cardiorespiratory responses that are of sufficient intensity to promote favorable adaptation and improvement in oxygen transport capacity. The key lies in alternating rapidly from one exercise to another so as to maintain the HR at or near the prescribed training level. Hellerstein[65] reported a mean HR response of 120 beats/min during sustained calisthenic exercise in men with coronary artery disease, which corresponded to approximately 60% of their $\dot{V}O_{2max}$. For these subjects, peak HR responses during running sequences averaged 140 beats/min.

Rope Skipping

Rope skipping is an easily accessible and enjoyable endurance activity that has been suggested as a superior method (over running) for improving cardiovascular efficiency.[66]

However, recent studies suggest that rope skipping is no more effective than other training modalities, including running.[67] At a given HR, running evokes a greater somatic oxygen cost than does skipping rope, which suggests that the former may better promote cardiorespiratory conditioning. Furthermore, the relatively high aerobic requirements of rope skipping preclude it as an appropriate training activity for many sedentary adults and cardiac patients. Skipping at 60 to 70 skips/min requires approximately 31.5 $mL \cdot kg^{-1} \cdot min^{-1}$, or 9 METs. Doubling the rate of skipping to 120 to 140 skips/min increases the aerobic requirement only slightly, to 11 to 12 METs.[14,68] This relatively flat relationship of energy expenditure to skipping rate presents an additional problem when prescribing rope skipping, since the cardiorespiratory stress placed on the subject will be nearly the same, regardless of the skipping rate.

Aerobic Dance

Although some authorities have denigrated the cardiovascular training value of aerobic dance, studies of the acute cardiorespiratory responses to this enjoyable activity in men and women have demonstrated relatively high values for HR and oxygen uptake, particularly for medium- and high-intensity dance routines.[69] Moreover, aerobic-dance training has been shown to increase cardiovascular fitness in young and middle-aged women, as substantiated by a decreased resting HR and improved walk-run performance on a 12-minute field test for distance.[70] Thus, aerobic dance, appropriately adjusted for intensity, should provide effective cardiovascular conditioning in previously sedentary adults, and the potential for enhanced compliance.

Bench Stepping/Stair Climbing

The impetus for stair climbing as a fitness activity probably originated from early research studies that popularized stepping up and down on a 17-inch bench for cardiovascular conditioning.[71] Subsequently, fitness enthusiasts realized that bench stepping was not that different from climbing stairs. However, to maximize effectiveness, authorities recommended that the climbing be limited to the same set of three steps. Because the energy cost of stepping down (negative work) is only about one third the work done stepping up (positive work), it was reasoned that the shorter descent would allow less time for recovery.[72]

Today, bench stepping is still widely used in many adult fitness and cardiac rehabilitation programs. The energy requirement for bench stepping varies with the height of the step and the stepping rate,[73] generally regulated by a metronome (Table 4–5).[14] In addition, several manufacturers have now developed simulated stair-climbing devices, which are widely employed in health clubs and rehabilitation centers. Such units provide progressive, computerized workout routines, along with estimated feedback on caloric expenditure and the HR response.

The cardiovascular benefits of stair climbing appear to be comparable to those of conventional training modalities such as walking, running, and stationary-cycle ergometry. One investigation involved 15 women between the ages of 25 and 48 years who climbed a stair-treadmill ergometer at 75% of their $\dot{V}O_{2max}$ for 30-minute sessions, three times a week, for 12 weeks. The women demonstrated a 36% improvement in $\dot{V}O_{2max}$ after the training program.[74] A study of an at-work stair-climbing program in healthy men also showed that a work load of 5500 kg/day (approximately 25 flights for a 70-kg man) resulted in a significant increase in aerobic capacity.[75] Similar or greater improvements may occur at a reduced total work load in cardiac patients with low baseline fitness levels.

TABLE 4–5. ENERGY EXPENDITURE IN METs DURING STEPPING AT DIFFERENT RATES ON STEPS OF DIFFERENT HEIGHTS

Step Height		Steps/Minute (Metronome Setting)*			
cm	in	12 (48)	18 (72)	24 (96)	30 (120)
0	0	1.2	1.8	2.4	3.0
8	3.2	1.9	2.8	3.7	4.6
16	6.3	2.5	3.8	5.0	6.3
24	9.4	3.2	4.8	6.3	7.9
32	12.6	3.8	5.7	7.7	9.6
40	15.8	4.5	6.7	9.0	11.2

*Metronome setting (ie, clicks per minute) for a given stepping rate is determined by the desired steps/minute, times four. Thus, one complete ascent and descent is equal to four metronome clicks (ie, up-up, down-down).

Data from American College of Sports Medicine: Guidelines for Graded Exercise Testing and Exercise Prescription, ed 3. Philadelphia, Lea & Febiger, 1986, p. 169; with permission.

Cross-country Skiing

Cross-country skiing is widely recognized as an excellent activity for improving aerobic capacity and is apparently even more effective than running.[76] The somatic and myocardial oxygen demands of level cross-country skiing are considerably greater than those of level walking, jogging, or running at similar speeds.[14,77,78] This is generally attributed to the increased weight of the ski clothing and equipment, arm work, snow surface, and cold temperatures. Thus, caution should be used when prescribing cross-country skiing for cardiac patients, since physiologic responses are often inordinately high and do not correspond with ratings of perceived exertion.[79] The availability of simulated cross-country skiing devices should help to alleviate this problem; however, such exercise may be difficult to prescribe, since HR and oxygen uptake responses are extremely variable and highly dependent on skill and mechanical efficiency.[11]

Arm Exercise

The limited degree of crossover of training benefits from the lower to the upper extremities appears to discredit the general practice of pursuing cardiovascular exercise programs that involve leg work exclusively.[80] Because many occupational and leisure-time activities require more arm work than leg work,[81] it appears reasonable to encourage individuals to train the arms as well as the legs, with the expectation of attenuated cardiorespiratory, hemodynamic, and perceived exertion responses to both forms of effort.

Guidelines for upper extremity conditioning should include recommendations regarding three variables[82]: (1) the prescribed exercise HR; (2) the power output ($kg \cdot m \cdot min^{-1}$) that will elicit a sufficient metabolic load for training; and (3) the proper training equipment or modalities.

Although the prescribed HR for arm training should ideally be derived from arm ergometer testing, this may not always be practical. Mean peak (or maximal) HRs obtained during arm ergometry are equivalent to 88% to 98% of the maximal HRs elicited during leg ergometry, with a mean value of 93%.[80] This applies to men and women, with or without heart disease. Consequently, an arm exercise prescription that is based on the maximal HR response to lower extremity testing may result in an inappropriately high THR for upper extremity training. As a general guideline, we have reduced the prescribed HR for leg training by approximately 12 beats/min for arm training, using perceived exertion as a complementary method for regulating the exercise intensity.

In establishing the work load for arm training, it is important to emphasize that, at a given submaximal work load, arm exercise is performed at a greater HR, blood pressure, and oxygen uptake than is leg exercise; however, maximal responses are generally lower during arm exercise.[83,84] Consequently, a work load suitable for leg training will generally be too high for arm training. In our experience, work loads approximating 50% to 60% of those used for leg training are appropriate for arm training. Accordingly, a subject using 300 $kg \cdot m \cdot min^{-1}$ for leg training would use 150 to 180 $kg \cdot m \cdot min^{-1}$ for arm training, demonstrating similar HRs and perceived exertion ratings at these work loads.

Equipment suitable for dynamic upper extremity training includes arm ergometers, rowing machines, wall pulleys, vertical climbing devices, and cross-country skiing simulators. Walking while swinging 0.45- to 2.27-kg handheld weights or wrist weights can, with exaggerated arm movements, significantly increase the energy expenditure at any given pace, promoting simultaneous conditioning of the upper and lower extremities.[85–87] However, careful assessment of the individual systolic blood pressure responses to exercise with and without hand weights should be conducted before recommending this form of exercise, particularly in patients in whom an increased cardiac afterload is contraindicated.[88] Finally, combined arm-leg exercise may be more readily tolerated than arm or leg training alone, presumably because the work load can be apportioned over a greater muscle mass.[89–91]

Weight Training

Blomqvist[92] reviewed the exercise literature on strength training and upper extremity conditioning. He concluded that

> . . . in a general sense the physiologic data support the concept that therapeutic exercise programs should not be limited to dynamic leg exercise but should include upper body activities. Exercise specifically designed to improve muscle strength may be beneficial, and the exclusion of all activities requiring predominantly static efforts is not warranted.

Several lines of evidence seem to support weight training as an adjunct to an aerobic exercise program, especially in persons whose occupational or leisure-time activities require lifting, pushing, or carrying moderate-to-heavy loads. Sustained isometric exertion is characterized by a pressor response, which is proportionate to the relative intensity [percentage of maximal voluntary contraction (MVC)],[93] duration, and muscle mass involved.[94] Consequently, increased muscular strength should result in an attenuated blood pressure response to any given load, since the load now represents a lower percentage of the MVC.

Although previous studies have reported that weight training programs do not benefit cardiovascular function, these studies generally evaluated training effectiveness with dynamic treadmill or cycle ergometer testing. When comparing hemodynamic responses to a standardized lifting or isometric test before and after isometric strength training, improvement has been noted.[95] There are also intriguing data to suggest that strength training can increase endurance time to exhaustion without an accompanying increase in $\dot{V}O_{2max}$.[96] Moreover, regular progressive resistance exercise training may have a favorable effect on resting blood pressure,[3] and lipid and lipoprotein levels.[97]

TABLE 4–6. WEIGHT TRAINING GUIDELINES* FOR HEALTHY ADULTS AND "LOW-RISK"† CARDIAC PATIENTS

1. To prevent soreness and injury, initially choose a weight that will allow the performance of 10 to 12 repetitions comfortably, corresponding to approximately 50% to 60% of the maximal weight load that can be lifted in one repetition. Adults with major coronary risk factors and "low-risk" cardiac patients should select an initial weight load that can be lifted for 12 to 15 repetitions.
2. Generally, two to three sets of each exercise is recommended.
3. Don't strain! Ratings of perceived exertion (6–20 scale) should not exceed "fairly light" to "somewhat hard" during lifting.
4. Avoid breath-holding. Exhale (blow out) on the most strenuous part of an exercise. For example, exhale when lifting a weight stack overhead and inhale when lowering it.
5. Increase weight loads by 5 to 10 lb when 10 to 12 repetitions can be comfortably accomplished; for high-risk adults and cardiac patients, weight may be added when 12 to 15 repetitions can be managed easily.
6. Raise the weight to a count of two and lower the weight gradually to a count of four; emphasize complete extension of the limbs when lifting.
7. Exercise large-muscle groups before small-muscle groups. Include devices (exercises) for both the upper and lower body.
8. Weight train three times per week.
9. Avoid sustained handgripping when possible because this may evoke an excessive blood pressure response to lifting.
10. Stop exercise in the event of warning signs or symptoms, especially dizziness, abnormal heart rhythm, unusual shortness of breath, or chest pain.
11. Stay moving from one device to another; in other words, don't rest for extended periods between sets.

*The modes of exercise most frequently prescribed are the use of free weights, Universal, Nautilus, and Cybex Eagle equipment.

†Arbitrarily defined as individuals with good left ventricular function (ie, ejection fraction ≥50%) and reasonable cardiorespiratory fitness (ie, completion of Stage III, Bruce's protocol) without ischemic ST segment depression, significant blood pressure abnormalities, or serious ventricular arrhythmias or symptoms.

Weight training guidelines for healthy adults and selected cardiac patients are shown in Table 4–6, with specific reference to the appropriate number of sets and repetitions, progression, proper breathing technique, and safety concerns.

SPECIAL CONSIDERATIONS IN EXERCISE PRESCRIPTION

Variables potentially affecting the exercise prescription include concomitant drug therapy and environmental factors such as extreme heat or cold.

Drug Therapy

Exercise guidelines should be appropriately modified to accommodate the increasing number of cardiac and hypertensive patients who are taking a variety of cardiovascular medications.[98,99] Pharmacologic treatment in physically active subjects may include the following: (1) diuretics, (2) beta-blockers, (3) vasodilators, (4) angiotensin-converting enzyme (ACE) inhibitors, (5) calcium-channel blockers, (6) central nervous system (CNS)–active drugs, and (7) alpha-receptor blockers. Special considerations for exercise prescription are extensively reviewed elsewhere,[14,99] and are briefly summarized below.

Diuretics. Under normal circumstances, diuretics do not alter chronotropic reserve or aerobic capacity. Thus, prescribed HRs for exercise training can be determined in the standard fashion.[14]

Beta-Blockers. Beta-blocker therapy acts to decrease submaximal and maximal HR, cardiac output, muscle blood flow and, frequently, exercise capacity. The reduction in functional capacity and/or ability to exercise may be even greater with nonselective than cardioselective agents,[100,101] perhaps because the utilization of carbohydrates is impaired by the former.[102]

Although it has been previously suggested that beta-blockade may attenuate desired training benefits,[103] several studies have shown that patients may derive considerable physiologic benefit from a physical conditioning program in the presence of both cardioselective and nonselective beta-blocking drugs, despite therapeutic doses and a reduced THR.[104–107] This premise was verified in a report showing comparable cardiorespiratory and hemodynamic effects of exercise training in two groups of cardiac patients, one with and one without beta-blocker treatment.[108]

Because beta-blockers do not alter the remarkably consistent relationship between oxygen consumption ($\dot{V}O_2$) and HR (expressed as percentages of their respective maximal values[109]), it appears that the generally accepted metabolic load for training (60% to 80% $\dot{V}O_{2max}$), associated with favorable adaptation and improvement, may be achieved by patients on beta-blockade at the conventional relative HR recommendation for training (70% to 85% HR_{max}). However, patients on "long-acting" beta-blockers should have their prescribed THR based on the results of an exercise test that is conducted at a time similar to that at which the subject will be exercising, as the significant reduction in HR response may dissipate over time.[110]

Vasodilators. Because vasodilators do not generally modify the HR response to submaximal and maximal work loads, exercise intensity can be based on conventional prescription methods.[14] It should be emphasized, however, that patients on vasodilators may be subject to hypotensive episodes in the postexercise period, unless an adequate cool-down is performed.

Angiotensin-Converting Enzyme Inhibitors. Because ACE inhibitors do not generally affect the HR response to exercise,[111] training intensity may be prescribed in the usual manner.[14] However, in view of the potential for reduced afterload and preload, an adequate cool-down is advised to prevent hypotension in the postexercise recovery period.

Calcium-Channel Blockers. In contrast to beta-blocker therapy, these drugs do not generally impair cardiac output, muscle blood flow, functional capacity, or exercise trainability.[112–115] However, certain calcium-channel blockers may alter the HR response to exercise. Verapamil, for example, tends to have a negative chronotropic effect.[99] Consequently, the prescribed THR should be based on the medicated patient's individual response to an exercise test.[14]

Central Nervous System–Active Drugs. These agents, including clonidine, guanfacine, and guanabenz, can have varying effects on the HR and blood pressure during exercise.[116] Accordingly, the exercise prescription should be formulated with caution, and the potential for hypotension, dizziness, and syncope should be carefully monitored in patients taking several of the central antagonists, especially in conjunction with beta-blockers.[14]

Alpha-Receptor Blockers. Although alpha-receptor blockers effectively lower systolic and diastolic blood pressure, they appear to have minimal effects on HR, cardiac output, and metabolic responses to exercise. Therefore, training may be prescribed in the usual manner, using HR as an indicator of exercise intensity.[14]

Warm Weather

Vigorous exercise when the temperature or humidity is high can lead to heat stress. Hyperthermic conditions can place excessive demands on the circulation and temperature regulation mechanisms designed to dissipate the heat generated by the environment and the increased metabolism of exercise. Moreover, excessive sweating may alter serum and intracellular sodium and potassium levels, increasing the potential for dysrhythmias.

To prevent dramatic increases in body temperature during exercise, a substantial portion of the cardiac output is shunted from the core to the periphery (skin) where it is more easily cooled. This process is complemented by the evaporation of perspiration, which serves as a powerful mechanism to cool the body.

Malfunctions in the temperature regulation mechanism can result from excessive body water losses, high humidity, or both, decreasing the effectiveness of the sweating response. Dehydration reduces the magnitude of sweating response, whereas high humidity impairs the evaporation of sweat. As a result, core temperature rises abruptly, increasing the potential for heat stroke and related complications.

Several suggestions are offered to help reduce heat stress when exercising in hot and/or humid environments:

- Maintain salt and water balance by drinking cool fluids (either water or a weak electrolyte solution) before, during, and after physical activity.
- Exercise during the cooler parts of the day, preferably when the sun's radiation is minimal (early morning or early evening).
- Decrease exercise intensity and duration at high temperatures and/or relative humidity. Under such conditions, a reduced walking or jogging speed or work rate will achieve the prescribed THR.[27]
- Wear minimal amounts of clothing to facilitate cooling by evaporation. Porous, light-colored, loose-fitting clothing is ideal (eg, a T-shirt and running shorts). Rubberized sweat suits, often worn to "enhance weight loss," block the evaporation of sweat, depriving the body of its normal mechanism for cooling.
- Allow the body to partially adapt to heat through incremental daily exposures. An increase in the somatic circulatory and cooling efficiency (called acclimatization) generally occurs within 2 weeks.[117]

Cold Weather

Outdoor exercise during the winter months usually presents fewer problems than expected. Adequate clothing promotes heat conservation while exercise actually serves to offset the effects of cold by increasing body heat production.

Physiologically, the body acts to maintain core temperature by reducing blood flow to the skin. If this first line of defense is inadequate, shivering occurs, which adds to the metabolic heat production.

A few extra precautions will help prevent excessive exposure to cold[118]:

- Monitor the "wind chill factor." Temperature alone is not a valid index of cold stress. The wind serves to remove the thin layer of warm air surrounding the body. The wind chill factor measures the effective decrease in temperature resulting from moving air. For example, at 20°F in a 20-mph wind, the cooling effect is equivalent to calm air at −10°F.[50]
- Change wet clothing. Because water is an excellent conductor, damp clothing extracts heat from the body much faster than dry clothing. Consequently, adults should be encouraged to change wet clothing, particularly socks and gloves. In contrast to most other materials, wool, when wet, will still keep the body warm.
- Dress appropriately. Overdressing for exercise in the cold may result in overheating and excessive sweating. **A general guideline for dressing for exercise in the cold is to wear several layers of light clothing that can be shed or replaced separately as body heat changes.** Between each layer, there is trapped air which, when heated by the body, acts as an excellent insulator.

- Stay moving. Because of the potential increase in metabolic rate during strenuous exercise, body temperature can be easily maintained even in subzero conditions, as long as one continues to exercise.
- Protect certain body areas. Body heat is most easily lost from parts that have a large surface area to mass ratio—for example, the hands and feet. Because of a poor vasoconstriction response, a tremendous loss of body heat can occur from an uncovered head.[117] This can, of course, be avoided by wearing a hat or cap when exercising in the cold. An anecdotal complication of winter jogging has also been reported—penile frostbite.[119]

CONCLUSION

The prescription of medications and exercise should, in many ways, be managed similarly. Both have a dose-response relationship with therapeutic levels, a potential for overdose, indications and contraindications, side effects, and special precautions. The salutary effects of each are relatively short-lived. Moreover, both types of therapy are associated with poor long-term compliance.

To simply tell a patient to "get more exercise" is tantamount to saying "take more medicine" without providing specific instructions. If exercise guidelines were approached with the same precision and caution as when any pharmacologic agent is prescribed, fewer complications and greater benefits would undoubtedly occur.[47]

ACKNOWLEDGMENT

The authors thank Brenda White for typing this manuscript.

REFERENCES

1. Davis J, Frank M, Whipp B, et al: Anaerobic threshold alterations caused by endurance training in middle-aged men. J Appl Physiol 46:1039–1046, 1979.
2. Wilmore J: Body composition in sport and exercise: Directions for future research. Med Sci Sports 15:21–31, 1983.
3. Seals DR, Hagberg JM: The effect of exercise training on human hypertension: A review. Med Sci Sports Exerc 16:207–215, 1984.
4. Streja D, Mymin D: Moderate exercise and high-density lipoprotein cholesterol: Observations during a cardiac rehabilitation program. JAMA 242:2190–2192, 1979.
5. Franklin BA, Hellerstein HK, Gordon S, et al: Cardiac patients. *In* Franklin BA, Gordon S, Timmis GC (eds): Exercise in Modern Medicine. Baltimore, Williams & Wilkins, 1989, pp 44–80.
6. Zohman LR: Beyond Diet. . . . Exercise Your Way to Fitness and Heart Health. Englewood Cliffs, NJ, CPC International, 1974, p 16.
7. Barnard RJ, Gardner GW, Diaco NV, et al: Cardiovascular responses to sudden strenuous exercise: Heart rate, blood pressure, and ECG. J Appl Physiol 34:833–837, 1973.
8. Barnard RJ, MacAlpin R, Kattus AA, et al: Ischemic response to sudden strenuous exercise in healthy men. Circulation 48:936–942, 1973.
9. Foster C, Anholm JD, Hellman CK, et al: Left ventricular function during sudden strenuous exercise. Circulation 63:592–596, 1981.
10. Foster C, Dymond DS, Carpenter J, et al: Effect of warm-up on left ventricular response to sudden strenuous exercise. J Appl Physiol 53:380–383, 1982.
11. Franklin BA, Hellerstein HK, Gordon S, et al: Exercise prescription for the myocardial infarction patient. J Cardiopulmonary Rehabil 6:62–79, 1986.
12. Franklin BA, Oldridge NB, Stoedefalke KG, et al: On the Ball: Innovative Activities for Adult Fitness and Cardiac Rehabilitation Programs. Indianapolis, Benchmark Press, 1990, pp 62–187.
13. Pollock ML: Quantification of endurance training programs. *In* Wilmore JH (ed): Exercise and Sport Sciences Reviews, vol 1. New York, Academic Press, 1973, pp 155–188.
14. American College of Sports Medicine: Guidelines for Graded Exercise Testing and Exercise Prescription, ed 3. Philadelphia, Lea & Febiger, 1986.

15. Stoedefalke KG: Physical fitness programs for adults. Am J Cardiol 33:787–790, 1974.
16. Belcastro AN, Bonen A: Lactic acid removal rates during controlled and uncontrolled recovery exercise. J Appl Physiol 39:932–936, 1975.
17. Dimsdale JE, Hartley H, Guiney T, et al: Postexercise peril: Plasma catecholamines and exercise. JAMA 251:630–632, 1984.
18. Haskell WL: Cardiovascular complications during exercise training of cardiac patients. Circulation 57:920–924, 1978.
19. Borg G: Psychophysical bases of perceived exertion. Med Sci Sports Exerc 14:377–381, 1982.
20. Wilmore JH: Exercise prescription: Role of the physiatrist and allied health professional. Arch Phys Med Rehabil 57:15–19, 1976.
21. Hagberg JM, Ehsani AA, Holloszy J: Effect of 12 months of intense exercise training on stroke volume in patients with coronary artery disease. Circulation 67:1194–1199, 1983.
22. Ehsani AA, Martin WH III, Heath GW, et al: Cardiac effects of prolonged and intense exercise training in patients with coronary artery disease. Am J Cardiol 50:246–254, 1982.
23. Mann GV, Garrett HL, Farhi A, et al: Exercise to prevent coronary heart disease: An experimental study of the effects of training on risk factors for coronary disease in man. Am J Med 46:12–27, 1969.
24. Kibom A, Hartley LH, Saltin B, et al: Physical training in sedentary middle-aged older men: I. Medical evaluation. Scand J Clin Lab Invest 24:315–322, 1969.
25. Mead WF, Pyfer HR, Trombold JC, et al: Successful resuscitation of two near simultaneous cases of cardiac arrest with a review of fifteen cases occurring during supervised exercise. Circulation 53:187–189, 1976.
26. Hossack KF, Hartwig R: Cardiac arrest associated with supervised cardiac rehabilitation. J Cardiac Rehabil 2:402–408, 1982.
27. Pandolf KB, Cafarelli E, Noble BJ, et al: Hyperthermia: Effect on exercise prescription. Arch Phys Med Rehabil 56:524–526, 1975.
28. Ward A, Malloy P, Rippe J: Exercise prescription guidelines for normal and cardiac populations. Cardiol Clin 5:197–210, 1987.
29. Wilmore JH, Haskell W: Use of the heart rate–energy expenditure relationship in the individual prescription of exercise. Am J Clin Nutr 24:1186–1192, 1971.
30. Karvonen M, Kentala K, Mustala O: The effects of training on heart rate: A longitudinal study. Ann Med Exp Biol 35:307–315, 1957.
31. Davis JA, Convertino VA: A comparison of heart rate methods for predicting endurance training intensity. Med Sci Sports 7:295–298, 1975.
32. Dressendorfer RH, Smith JL: Predictive accuracy of the maximum heart rate reserve method for estimating aerobic training intensity in early cardiac rehabilitation. J Cardiac Rehabil 4:484–489, 1984.
33. American Heart Association: Exercise Testing and Training of Individuals with Heart Disease or at High Risk for Its Development: A Handbook for Physicians. Dallas, American Heart Association, 1975, p 25.
34. Hellerstein HK, Hirsch EZ, Ader R, et al: Principles of exercise prescription for normals and cardiac subjects. *In* Naughton JP, Hellerstein HK (eds): Exercise Testing and Exercise Training in Coronary Heart Disease. New York, Academic Press, 1973, pp 129–167.
35. Taylor HL, Haskell W, Fox SM III, et al: Exercise tests: A summary of procedures and concepts of stress testing for cardiovascular diagnosis and function evaluation. *In* Blackburn H (ed): Measurement in Exercise Electrocardiography (The Ernst Simonson Conference). Springfield, IL, Charles C Thomas, 1969, pp 259–305.
36. Hossack KF, Bruce RA, Clark LJ: Influence of propranolol on exercise prescription of training heart rates. Cardiology 65:47–58, 1980.
37. Franklin B, Hodgson J, Buskirk ER: Relationship between percent maximal O_2 uptake and percent maximal heart rate in women. Res Q Exerc Sport 51:616–624, 1980.
38. Caiozzo VJ, Davis JA, Ellis JF, et al: Comparison of gas exchange indices used to detect anaerobic threshold. J Appl Physiol 53:1184–1189, 1982.
39. Coplan NL, Gleim GW, Nicholas JA: Using exercise respiratory measurements to compare methods of exercise prescription. Am J Cardiol 58:832–836, 1986.
40. Pollock ML, Broida J, Kendrick Z: Validity of the palpation technique of heart rate determination and its estimation of training heart rate. Res Q 43:77–81, 1972.
41. Oldridge NB, Haskell WL, Single P: Carotid palpation, coronary heart disease and exercise rehabilitation. Med Sci Sports Exerc 13:6–8, 1981.
42. Girandola RN: Body composition changes in women: Effects of high and low exercise intensity. Arch Phys Med Rehabil 57:297–300, 1976.
43. Sharkey BJ: Physiology of Fitness. Champaign, IL, Human Kinetics, 1979, p 132.
44. Åstrand PO, Rodahl K: Textbook of Work Physiology. New York, McGraw-Hill, 1970, p 460.
45. Pollock ML, Foster C: Exercise prescription for participants on propranolol [abstract]. J Am Coll Cardiol 1:624, 1983.

46. Williams MA, Fardy PS: Limitations in prescribing exercise. J Cardiovasc Pulm Technique 8:36–38, 1980.
47. Dehn MM, Mullins CB: Physiologic effects and importance of exercise in patients with coronary artery disease. Cardiovasc Med 2:365–387, 1977.
48. Pollock ML, Gettman LR, Milesis CA, et al: Effects of frequency and duration of training on attrition and incidence of injury. Med Sci Sports 9:31–36, 1977.
49. The recommended quantity and quality of exercise for developing and maintaining fitness in healthy adults. American College of Sports Medicine Position Statement. Med Sci Sports 10:7–9, 1979.
50. Pollock ML, Wilmore J, Fox SM: Health and Fitness Through Physical Activity. New York, John Wiley & Sons, 1978, p 113.
51. Pollock ML, Dimmick J, Miller HS, et al: Effects of mode of training on cardiovascular function and body composition of adult men. Med Sci Sports 7:139–145, 1975.
52. Franklin BA, Pamatmat A, Johnson S, et al: Metabolic cost of extremely slow walking in cardiac patients: Implications for exercise testing and training. Arch Phys Med Rehabil 64:564–565, 1983.
53. Pollock ML, Miller HS, Janeway R, et al: Effects of walking on body composition and cardiovascular function of middle-aged men. J Appl Physiol 30:126–130, 1971.
54. Gwinup G: Effect of exercise alone on the weight of obese women. Arch Intern Med 135:676–680, 1975.
55. Evans BW, Cureton KJ, Purvis JW: Metabolic and circulatory responses to walking and jogging in water. Res Q Exerc Sport 49:442–449, 1978.
56. Shoenfeld Y, Keren G, Shimoni T, et al: Walking: A method for rapid improvement of physical fitness. JAMA 243:2062–2063, 1980.
57. Franklin BA, Rubenfire M: Losing weight through exercise. JAMA 244:377–379, 1980.
58. Rippe JM, Southmayd W: The Sports Performance Factors. New York, Putnam, 1986, pp 64–65.
59. Katch VL, Villanacci JF, Sady SP: Energy cost of rebound-running. Res Q 52:269–272, 1981.
60. Thompson DL, Boone TW, Miller HS: Comparison of treadmill exercise and tethered swimming to determine validity of exercise prescription. J Cardiac Rehabil 2:363–370, 1982.
61. Fletcher GF, Cantwell JD, Watt EW: Oxygen consumption and hemodynamic response of exercises used in training of patients with recent myocardial infarction. Circulation 60:140–144, 1979.
62. Magder S, Linnarsson D, Gullstrand L: The effect of swimming on patients with ischemic heart disease. Circulation 63:979–986, 1981.
63. Adams WC: Influence of age, sex, and body weight on the energy expenditure of bicycle riding. J Appl Physiol 22:539–545, 1967.
64. Pugh LGCE: The relation of oxygen intake and speed in competition cycling and comparative observations on the bicycle ergometer. J Physiol 241:795–808, 1974.
65. Hellerstein HK: Exercise therapy in coronary disease. Bull NY Acad Med 44:1028–1047, 1968.
66. Baker JA: Comparison of rope skipping and jogging as methods of improving cardiovascular efficiency of college men. Res Q Exerc Sport 39:240–243, 1968.
67. Getchell B, Cleary P: The caloric costs of rope skipping and running. Phys Sportsmed 8:56–60, 1980.
68. Town GP, Sol N, Sinning WE: The effect of rope skipping rate on energy expenditure of males and females. Med Sci Sports Exerc 12:295–298, 1980.
69. Weber H: The energy cost of aerobic dancing. Med Sci Sports 5:65–66, 1973.
70. Watterson VV: The effects of aerobic dance on cardiovascular fitness. Phys Sportsmed 12:138–145, 1984.
71. Benzaquin P: Stairway to fitness. Runner's World, March:66–67, 1981.
72. Koszuta LE: Can fitness be found at the top of the stairs? Phys Sportsmed 15:165–169, 1987.
73. Nagle FJ, Balke B, Naughton JP: Gradational step tests for assessing work capacity. J Appl Physiol 20:745–748, 1965.
74. Verstraete D, Rosentswieg J, Bassett G: Stairclimbing as a training modality for women [abstract]. Med Sci Sports Exerc 18(April suppl):S28, 1986.
75. Fardy PS, Ilmarinen J: Evaluating the effects and feasibility of an at-work stairclimbing intervention program for men. Med Sci Sports 7:91–93, 1975.
76. Oja P, Vuori I, Nieminen R, et al: Effects of running and cross-country skiing on cardiorespiratory response to exercise [abstract]. Med Sci Sports Exerc 17:270, 1985.
77. Oldridge NB, MacDougall JD: Cross-country skiing: Precautions for cardiac patients. Phys Sportsmed 9:64–70, 1981.
78. MacDougall JD, Hughson R, Sutton JR, et al: The energy cost of cross-country skiing among elite competitors. Med Sci Sports 11:270–273, 1979.
79. Oldridge NB, Connolly C: Oxygen uptake and heart rate during cross-country skiing and track walking after myocardial infarction. Am Heart J 117:495–497, 1989.
80. Franklin BA: Aerobic exercise training programs for the upper body. Med Sci Sports Exerc 21:S141–148, 1989.
81. Hellerstein HK: Prescription of vocational and leisure activities: Practical aspects. Adv Cardiol 24:105–115, 1978.
82. Franklin BA: Exercise testing, training and arm ergometry. Sports Med 2:100–119, 1985.

83. Bergh U, Kanstrup IL, Ekblom B: Maximal oxygen uptake during exercise with various combinations of arm and leg work. J Appl Physiol 41:191–196, 1976.
84. Gleim GW, Coplan NL, Scandura M, et al: Rate pressure product at equivalent oxygen consumption on four different exercise modalities. J Cardiopulmonary Rehabil 8:270–275, 1988.
85. Auble TE, Schwartz L, Robertson RJ: Aerobic requirements for moving handweights through various ranges of motion while walking. Phys Sportsmed 15:133–140, 1987.
86. Graves JE, Pollock ML, Montain SJ, et al: The effect of handheld weights on the physiological responses to walking exercise. Med Sci Sports Exerc 19:260–265, 1987.
87. Zarandona JE, Nelson AG, Conlee RK, et al: Physiological responses to handcarried weights. Phys Sportsmed 14:113–120, 1986.
88. Graves JE, Sagiv M, Pollock ML, et al: Effect of hand-held weights and wrist weights on the metabolic and hemodynamic responses to submaximal exercise in hypertensive responders. J Cardiopulmonary Rehabil 8:134–140, 1988.
89. Mostardi RA, Gandee RN, Norris WA: Exercise training using arms and legs versus legs alone. Arch Phys Med Rehabil; 62:332–336, 1981.
90. Stenberg J, Åstrand PO, Ekblom B, et al: Hemodynamic response to work with different muscle groups, sitting and supine. J Appl Physiol 22:61–79, 1967.
91. Gutin B, Ang KE, Torrey K: Cardiorespiratory and subjective responses to incremental and constant load ergometry with arms and legs. Arch Phys Med Rehabil 69:510–513, 1988.
92. Blomqvist CG: Upper extremity exercise testing and training. *In* Wenger NK (ed): Exercise and the Heart, ed 2. Philadelphia, FA Davis, 1985, pp 175–183.
93. Lind AR, McNichol GW: Muscular factors which determine the cardiovascular responses to sustained and rhythmic exercise. Can Med Assoc J 96:706–715, 1967.
94. Mitchell JH, Payne FC, Saltin B, et al: The role of muscle mass in the cardiovascular response to static contractions. J Physiol 309:45–54, 1980.
95. Lewis S, Nygaard E, Sanchez J, et al: Static contraction of the quadriceps muscle in man: Cardiovascular control and responses to one-legged strength training. Acta Physiol Scand 122:341–353, 1984.
96. Hickson RC, Rosenkoetter MA, Brown MM: Strength training effects on aerobic power and short-term endurance. Med Sci Sports Exerc 12:336–339, 1980.
97. Goldberg L, Elliot DL, Schutz RW, et al: Changes in lipid and lipoprotein levels after weight training. JAMA 252:504–506, 1984.
98. Rost R: Physical exercise and antihypertensive drugs. Nephron 47 (suppl 1):27–29, 1987.
99. Lund-Johansen P: Exercise and antihypertensive therapy. Am J Cardiol 59:98A–107A, 1987.
100. Kaiser P, Hylander B, Eliasson K, et al: Effect of $beta_1$-selective and nonselective beta blockade on blood pressure relative to physical performance in men with systemic hypertension. Am J Cardiol 55:79D–84D, 1985.
101. Wilmore JH, Freund BJ, Joyner MJ, et al: Acute response to submaximal and maximal exercise consequent to beta-adrenergic blockade: Implications for the prescription of exercise. Am J Cardiol 55:135D–141D, 1985.
102. Hossack KF, Bruce RA, Kusumi F: Altered exercise ventilatory responses by apparent propranolol-diminished glucose metabolism: Implications concerning impaired physical training benefit in coronary patients. Am Heart J 102:378–382, 1981.
103. Zohman LR: Exercise stress test interpretation for cardiac diagnosis and functional evaluation. Arch Phys Med Rehabil 58:235–240, 1977.
104. Pratt CM, Welton DE, Squires WG, et al: Demonstration of training effect during chronic beta-adrenergic blockage in patients with coronary artery disease. Circulation 64:1125–1129, 1981.
105. Stuart RJ, Koyal SN, Lundstrom R, et al: Does exercise training alter maximal oxygen uptake in coronary artery disease during long-term beta-adrenergic blockade? J Cardiopulmonary Rehabil 5:410–414, 1985.
106. Froelicher V, Sullivan M, Myers J, et al: Can patients with coronary artery disease receiving beta blockers obtain a training effect? Am J Cardiol 55:155D–161D, 1985.
107. Fletcher GF: Exercise training during chronic beta blockade in cardiovascular disease. Am J Cardiol 55:110D–113D, 1985.
108. Vanhees L, Fagard R, Amery A: Influence of beta-adrenergic blockade on the hemodynamic effects of physical training in patients with ischemic heart disease. Am Heart J 108:270–275, 1984.
109. Hossack KF, Bruce RA, Clark LJ: Influence of propranolol on exercise prescription of training heart rates. Cardiology 65:47–58, 1980.
110. Timmis GC, Franklin BA, Borysyk L, et al: Failure of once-daily atenolol to prevent an ischemic response to exercise late in the afternoon. Chest 92:S71, 1987.
111. Fagard R, Bulpitt C, Lijnen P, et al: Response of the systemic and pulmonary circulation to converting-enzyme inhibition (captopril) at rest and during exercise in hypertensive patients. Circulation 65:33–39, 1982.

112. Mooy J, van Baak M, Bohm R, et al: The effects of verapamil and propranolol on exercise tolerance in hypertensive patients. Clin Pharmacol Ther 41:490–495, 1987.
113. Myburgh DP, Gordon NF: Comparison of diltiazem and atenolol in young, physically active men with essential hypertension. Am J Cardiol 60:1092–1095, 1987.
114. Szlachcic J, Hirsch AT, Tubau JF, et al: Diltiazem versus propranolol in essential hypertension: Responses of rest and exercise blood pressure and effects on exercise capacity. Am J Cardiol 59:393–399, 1987.
115. Chang K, Hossack KF: Effect of diltiazem on heart rate responses and respiratory variables during exercise: Implications for exercise prescription and cardiac rehabilitation. J Cardiac Rehabil 2:326–332, 1982.
116. Timmis GC, Westveer DC, Hauser AM, et al: Cardiovascular Review, ed 8. New York, Pergamon Press, 1987, pp 378–380.
117. Lamb DR: Physiology of Exercise: Responses and Adaptations. New York, MacMillan, 1978, p 282.
118. Franklin BA: Take care in the cold. Heartline 18:1–2, 1988.
119. Hershkowitz M: Penile frostbite, an unforeseen hazard of jogging [letter to the editor]. N Engl J Med 296:178, 1977.

5

CARDIOVASCULAR BENEFITS AND RISKS OF EXERCISE: THE SCIENTIFIC EVIDENCE

William L. Haskell, PhD

The concept that regular exercise provides some protection against the clinical manifestations of coronary artery atherosclerosis, especially myocardial infarction and sudden death, has become generally accepted by the public and health professionals during the past several decades. This belief has been promoted by individual scientists, clinicians, and educators as well as by major health organizations. Most often, the idea has been expressed that regular exercise, in conjunction with other risk-reducing behaviors, will help protect against an initial cardiac episode *(primary prevention);* will aid in the recovery of patients following myocardial infarction, coronary artery bypass surgery, or angioplasty *(cardiac rehabilitation);* and will reduce the risk of recurrent cardiac events *(secondary prevention).*

As is the case for other regimens promoted for the prevention or treatment of coronary heart disease (CHD), definitive evidence in support of an increase in exercise significantly decreasing morbidity and mortality is still lacking. However, substantial data exist that demonstrate improvements in clinical status and functional capacity as a result of exercise training. There are also strong indications that regular exercise leads to a reduced risk of myocardial ischemia and sudden death.

Information relating level of habitual physical activity to CHD risk has been derived from a variety of sources including animal studies, clinical impressions, observational surveys of the general population or special groups, and experimental studies in which the exercise of treatment subjects was significantly increased in relation to sedentary, control subjects. None of these studies provides irrefutable evidence of a cause-and-effect relationship between exercise status and CHD pathology, even though many sources of information do generally support such a contention. Until the basic biologic process of atherosclerosis at the cellular or molecular level has been established, it is highly unlikely that any exercise training study will definitively demonstrate a cause-and-effect relationship.

This situation is not unique to the preventive role of exercise as it relates to CHD because it very likely applies to all other generally accepted risk factors. Additional observational studies will provide only more data on association or will demonstrate the predictive value of an active lifestyle. No plans presently exist to initiate a randomized control trial to determine the effect of habitual exercise on the progression of coronary atherosclerosis or on the rate of initial or subsequent CHD clinical events. Thus, it appears that decisions regarding the application of exercise as a therapeutic modality for CHD prevention and rehabilitation will have to be based on presently available information.

The presentation of information in this chapter is designed to provide the scientific basis for making decisions regarding the potential use of exercise in the primary and secondary prevention of CHD and the rehabilitation of patients following myocardial infarction or coronary artery bypass surgery. Available data on the relationship of exercise to CHD morbidity and mortality are reviewed, and the possible biologic mechanisms by which beneficial effects may occur are presented. The issue of a dose-response relationship between exercise amount and CHD risk is discussed, as are the program and participant characteristics associated with the development of cardiac complications during exercise.

DOES EXERCISE DECREASE CARDIOVASCULAR MORBIDITY AND MORTALITY?

Primary Prevention of Coronary Heart Disease

During the past 40 years, as many as 50 studies have been published that report the association between habitual level of physical activity and the prevalence or incidence of initial clinical manifestations of CHD, especially myocardial infarction and sudden cardiac death. These studies have included the determination of on-the-job or leisure-time activity in free-living populations of men with activity classifications based on job category, self-report questionnaires, or interviewer determinations. Manifestations of CHD were established by examination of death certificates, hospital or physician records, questionnaires completed by the subjects or physicians, and medical evaluations conducted by the investigators. Reported activity levels range from daily caloric expenditures exceeding 6000 kilocalories (kcal) per day in Finnish lumberjacks at one extreme, to very sedentary civil servant managers and postal clerks at the other. Studies have been conducted in major industrial environments as well as rural or primitive living areas, with data from North and South America, Europe, Asia, Africa, and the Middle East.

As a result of the diverse protocols used in the various studies, including sample selection procedures, physical activity classification methods, clinical event determination criteria, and statistical treatment of the data, it is not possible to collate the results into a single summary statement or interpretation. However, certain findings, although not universally obtained, occur with sufficient frequency to warrant the formulation of preliminary conclusions to use as a basis for clinical recommendations and the planning of future research.

MORE ACTIVE PERSONS APPEAR TO BE AT LOWER RISK

The general impression obtained from a comprehensive review of scientific reports containing data on the primary preventive effect of physical activity is that more active people develop less CHD than their inactive counterparts, and when they do develop CHD, it occurs at a later age and tends to be less severe.[1] The results of the numerous reports are quite variable, with some studies demonstrating a highly significant beneficial effect of exercise,[2–4] others showing a favorable but nonsignificant trend in favor of the more acitve,[5,6] and some showing no difference in CHD rates.[7,8] Of major importance is the consistent finding that being physically active *does not increase* an individual's risk of CHD.

No specific study characteristics can be identified that explain the differences in results among the various studies, but in some cases, the physical activity measure is not very accurate or reliable, and the activity gradient among the population is quite small.[2] Also, with populations in which CHD mortality is exceptionally high and in which major risk factors such as hypercholesterolemia, hypertension, and cigarette smoking are prevalent, even very high levels of physical activity do not appear to exert a major protective effect. Finnish lumberjacks are an example of physically active individuals in whom CHD risk remains high.[9] These results argue strongly for a multifactor approach to CHD prevention.

A major criticism of the observational studies that demonstrate a protective effect of exercise is that the differences in CHD rates between active and inactive individuals may be due to less healthy people selecting a less active lifestyle—not to increased activity preventing disease. Such self-selection may account for some of the differences reported; but in several reports, the investigators considered this problem in their data analyses and still found that being physically active was of significant benefit.[3,10]

MODERATE AMOUNTS OF EXERCISE MAY BE PROTECTIVE

A striking feature of many studies demonstrating a reduced CHD risk for more active individuals is that the greatest difference in risk is achieved between those people who do almost nothing and those who do a moderate amount of exercise on a regular basis. Much smaller differentials in risk are observed when moderately active individuals are compared with the most active participants.[1,2,11]

The amount of activity, in both intensity and duration, that is associated with a decrease in CHD clinical manifestations varies substantially among different reports. Several studies have observed significant differences in CHD indicators with quite small increases in habitual activity level at a relatively low intensity,[2,10] whereas other authors interpret their data to indicate that a "threshold" of higher intensity or amount of activity is needed to obtain benefit.[3,12] The types of activity performed by the more active groups include brisk walking on level ground or up stairs, lifting and carrying light objects, lifting heavy objects, operating machinery or appliances, light and heavy gardening and doing home maintenance or repairs, and participating in active games and sports. Participation in "physical fitness" or "athletic conditioning" programs contributes very little to the active classification in most observational studies so far reported.

Most of the initial observations establishing an association between physical activity status and CHD manifestations used on-the-job activity. It is much easier to classify individuals as inactive or active according to their job title or description than it is to obtain accurate self-assessments by interview, questionnaire, or direct observation of job-related or leisure-time activity. The early studies that obtained a difference in CHD rates between inactive and active classifications, such as the reports by Morris and associates[13] on London busmen and postal workers, Kahn's observation on Washington, DC, postal workers,[10] or Taylor and Parlin's studies on U.S. railroad workers,[14] included job situations in which the major exercise of the more active groups was walking on flat ground, up stairs, or up and down hills. If the more physically active status is responsible for the lower CHD rates in these populations, then the threshold for an activity-related benefit is not high. More recent results from on-the-job studies, however, have not found any protective association with activity level until a classification of "heavy work" was obtained.[12,15]

Examples of studies that demonstrate a benefit associated with quite small differences in reported activity levels include the earlier studies by Zukel and colleagues,[16] and the project of the Health Insurance Plan (HIP) of Greater New York.[2] The Zukel study observed a striking difference in CHD rates between individuals who had active and sedentary occupations in a six-county area of North Dakota. A more detailed analysis of these data shows that persons reporting from 1 to 2 hours of "heavy physical work" per day had 18% of the CHD incidence of those individuals reporting less than 1 hour of heavy physical activity per day. There appears to be very little added protection associated with an additional increase in the number of reported hours of heavy physical activity up to 6 hours a day. Data from the HIP study also indicate that the greatest difference in fatal myocardial infarction rates by on-the-job activity classification is obtained in moving from a least active to a first intermediate category. Here again, some small additional benefit appears to be associated with being classified as second intermediate or most active.

Prevalence data collected during the original survey in Evans County, Georgia,[17] indicated a substantial difference in CHD rates according to classification by occupational physical activity. The intensity and amount of activity associated with significant differences in CHD rates were quite low. The difference in the average occupational activity intensity between the low- and high-activity groups was less than 1 kcal/min. It was estimated that during the entire workday, this difference consisted of 400 to 600 kcal.

In a later report regarding the Evans County population,[12] in which CHD incidence data between 1960 and 1962 and between 1967 and 1969 were analyzed, the investigators concluded that an activity threshold existed and that CHD rates did not become lower until "higher" levels of activity were performed. Also, when job-related and non–job-related activity status categories were analyzed together, a "protective effect" was not observed systematically until at least a classification of moderate activity was reached for both categories.

The longshoremen studies reported by Paffenbarger and colleagues[15] have been cited the most frequently as evidence of a needed "threshold" of intensity and amount of activity in order to obtain a significant CHD benefit. At least for longshoremen between the ages of 35 and 54, intermediate intensity of occupational activity does not carry with it the CHD-protective effect that the heavy activities of cargo handling provide. The rates of calorie expenditure are reported to range from 5.2 to 7.5, 2.4 to 5.0 and 1.5 to 2.0 kcal/min for the heavy, moderate, and light job classifications, respectively. These rates of energy expenditure result in a total workday expenditure above a basal metabolic rate of 856 kcal for light workers, 1473 kcal for moderate workers, and 1876 kcal for heavy workers.

Other observational studies relating on-the-job activity to CHD prevalence or incidence have included job classifications that have energy requirements somewhere between the extremes reported here. For example, the estimated difference in daily work-related calorie expenditure between U.S. railroad clerks and switchmen range from 200 to 700 kcal.[14] Similar values would be expected for Italian railroad workers,[18] postal employees (clerks versus carriers),[10] or London busmen (drivers versus conductors).[13]

The estimated net energy expenditure (above the inactive group energy expenditure) associated with a decrease in CHD mortality in the various occupational studies ranges from 300 to 800 kcal/day. The intensity of the activity contributing to this increased energy expenditure includes walking, lifting and carrying objects, farming, and laboring-type jobs. In most cases, the higher-intensity activities (ie, heavy lifting or carrying) are performed in reasonably short bursts throughout the workday with the lower-intensity activities (ie, walking) being carried out for longer durations.

From the limited data available, these types of activities, at least those requiring 400 to 500 kcal/day more than inactive occupations, do not substantially increase physical fitness levels. Skinner and colleagues[19] conducted multistage treadmill exercise tests on samples of men in Evans County (Georgia) whose daily physical activity varied as determined by their occupation and answers to a detailed physical activity questionnaire. The prevalence of CHD was significantly less in the more active groups, but no differences were observed between their work capacity and that of the less active groups. In the railroad study by Taylor and Parlin,[14] the more active switchmen had a heart rate response to a standard submaximal exercise test (treadmill walk at 3 mph with a 5% grade for 3 minutes) that was approximately nine beats slower than the response for the less active clerks. About a third of this difference, however, can probably be attributed to the poorer mechanical efficiency of the clerks, and the remainder, to actual differences in exercise tolerance.

Accurate quantitative assessments of leisure-time or nonjob activity status are very difficult to obtain on samples of the size needed to evaluate the relationship of habitual activity status and CHD events. Various diary and recall techniques have been attempted, and they all present significant validation and scoring difficulties. However, in the few studies that have attempted to quantitate various aspects of nonjob activities, several have identified an association between activity status and CHD similar to the relationship reported for occupation-based studies.

Evidence of some protection possibly being provided by nonjob, low-intensity activity on a regular basis was reported by Rose.[20] He observed that the prevalence of "ischemic-type" resting electrocardiographic abnormalities was inversely associated with duration of walking to work among 8948 executive-grade civil service workers in London. Those employees who walked 20 or more minutes to work on a regular basis had one third fewer electrocardiographic abnormalities than their counterparts who rode to work. This association could be accounted for as a result of differences in age, grade of employment, smoking habits, serum cholesterol, or glucose tolerance. Those who walked regularly, however, tended to be a little less overweight.

The relationship of leisure-time activity to CHD mortality among middle-aged male civil servant workers in Britain has been studied by a 2-day activity recall procedure.[4] Morris and co-workers reported that nonjob activity, as assessed by a self-administered, 48-hour recall questionnaire completed on a Monday for the preceding Friday and Saturday, was significantly associated with CHD mortality only when activities requiring a peak energy expenditure of 7.5 kcal/min for 30 minutes or longer each day were performed ("vigorous activity"). Lesser amounts of activity appeared to carry no protective benefit. This conclusion was based on a survey of 1138 first clinic episodes of CHD in 17,994 men during 8.5 years of follow-up. In the men reporting vigorous activity, there was a CHD rate of 3.1% versus 6.9% for those men not reporting any vigorous activity ($P < 0.01$). The more active men had fewer fatal (1.1% versus 2.9 %; $P < 0.01$) and nonfatal (2.0% versus 4.0%; $P < 0.01$) events than inactive men. Examples of vigorous activity included brisk walking, running, stair climbing (500 or more stairs), cycling, heavy gardening, heavy home repairs or construction, swimming, sailing as crew, and morning exercises (Canadian 5BX). To meet the vigorous exercise criteria, a calorie expenditure during the activity could be as low as 225 kcal/day (30 min × 7.5 kcal/min). This apparent protective action of "vigorous activity" was not related to plasma total cholesterol level, blood pressure, cigarette smoking, or adiposity, and it occurred at all ages from 40 to 69 years.

The association of physical activity level with the risk of death was analyzed for a cohort of 636 healthy Finnish men, aged 45 to 64 years, followed up for 20 years. Thirty-nine percent of the cohort were classed as highly active at baseline in 1964.[21] Up to 1984, there were 287 deaths, 106 of them due to CHD. During the first two thirds of the follow-up, men with high physical activity had a lower risk of death than did men with low physical activity. During the last one third of follow-up, the survival curves of the men with high and low physical activity gradually converged. Of the men who died, those with high physical activity lived 1 to 2 years longer ($P = 0.002$) than those with low physical activity, after adjustment for age, smoking, blood pressure, serum cholesterol level, and body mass index. This difference was due mainly to fewer CHD deaths among the highly active group. High physical activity may thus independently prevent premature death among middle-aged men, but it probably does not prolong the maximum achievable life span.

The relation of self-selected leisure-time physical activity (LTPA) to first major CHD events and overall mortality was studied in 12,138 middle-aged men participating in the Multiple Risk Factor Intervention Trial.[11] Total LTPA over the preceding year was quantitated (in mean minutes per day) at baseline by questionnaire, with subjects classified into tertiles (low, moderate, and high) based on LTPA distribution. During 7 years of follow-up, moderate LTPA was associated with 63% as many fatal CHD events and sudden

TABLE 5–1. DEATH RATES (RISK RATIO) BY TERTILE OF LEISURE-TIME PHYSICAL ACTIVITY IN THE MULTIPLE RISK FACTOR INTERVENTION STUDY

	Tertile of Physical Activity		
	Low	*Middle*	*High*
CHD death	1.0	0.64†	0.67*
Sudden death	1.0	0.64†	0.67*
All-cause death	1.0	0.73*	0.87
	Mean Values for Each Tertile of Activity		
Minutes/day	15	47	134
Light	5	18	53
Moderate	6	17	41
Heavy	3	9	28
Other	1	3	12
Cal/day	74	224	638

*$P < 0.05$.

†$P < 0.01$ compared to low tertile.

Data from Leon AS, Cornett J, Jacobs DR, et al: Leisure-time physical activity levels and risk of coronary heart disease and death: The Multiple Risk Factor Intervention Trial. JAMA 258:2388, 1987.

deaths, and 70% as many total deaths as low LTPA ($P < 0.01$)(Table 5–1). Mortality rates for those with high LTPA were similar to those with moderate LTPA; however, combined fatal and nonfatal major CHD events were 20% lower with high as compared with low LTPA ($P < 0.05$). These risk differentials persisted after statistical adjustments for possible confounding variables, including other baseline risk factors. The authors concluded that LTPA has a modest inverse relation to CHD and overall mortality in middle-aged men at high risk for CHD.

The relationship of non–job-related activity and CHD mortality in the HIP study[2] is quite similar to that reported for job-related activity: a substantial reduction in rapidly fatal and all fatal cardiac events is associated with only modest increases in reported activity, with even further benefits achieved with a more active status. The amount of activity needed to be considered first intermediate instead of least active appears to be quite small—probably not more than several hundred kilocalories daily or every other day. The activities include levels ranging from walking (4 kcal/min), up to running, singles tennis, or handball (12 kcal/min). The differences in total daily caloric expenditure between inactive and active categories, however, as one would expect, are consistently less than that reported for on-the-job activity classifications.

PHYSICAL FITNESS AND PRIMARY PREVENTION

Only in the last few years have studies been published that have adequately measured cardiovascular functional capacity or physical fitness in a sample of sufficient size and then followed clinical status long enough to be able to effectively evaluate the relationship of physical fitness to future CHD or total mortality. If a higher level of habitual activity causes a reduction in cardiovascular morbidity and/or mortality, then a similar association should be observed with accurate, reliable measure of fitness.

This issue was examined in a study of 4276 men, 30 to 69 years of age, who were screened as part of the Lipid Research Clinic's prevalence survey and followed for an average of 8.5 years.[22] Examination at baseline included assessment of conventional coronary risk factors and treadmill exercise testing. The heart rate during submaximal exer-

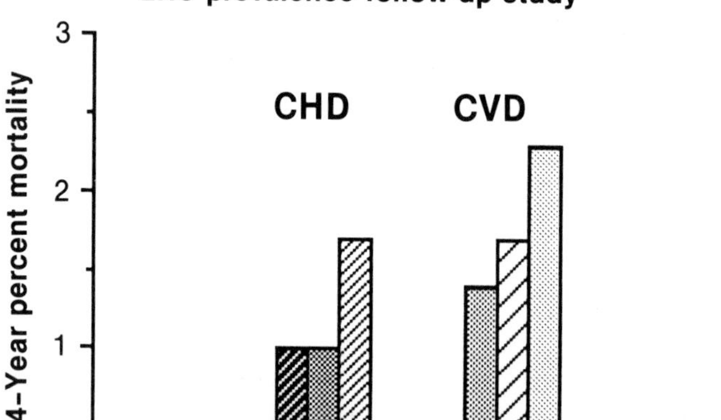

Figure 5–1. The relationship of treadmill performance to the development of coronary heart disease (CHD) and cardiovascular disease (CVD) mortality in men: Lipid Research Clinic (LRC) Follow-up Study. (*Data from* Ekelund LG, Haskell WL, Johnson JL, et al: Physical fitness as a prevention of cardiovascular mortality in asymptomatic North American men. N Engl J Med 319:1379, 1988.)

cise (stage 2 of the exercise test) and the duration of exercise were used as measures of physical fitness. Men with incomplete data (n = 308) or men who were using cardiovascular drugs (n = 213) were excluded from the analysis. Men who had clinical evidence of cardiovascular disease at baseline (n = 649) were analyzed separately. Forty-five deaths from cardiovascular causes occurred among the remaining 3106 men.

A lower level of physical fitness was associated with a higher risk of death from cardiovascular and coronary heart disease, after adjustment for age and cardiovascular risk factors. The relative risk of death from cardiovascular causes was 2.7 (95% confidence interval, 1.4 to 5.1; $P = 0.003$) for healthy men with an increment of 35 beats/min in the heart rate during stage 2, and 3.0 (95% confidence interval, 1.6 to 5.5; $P = 0.0004$) for those with a decrement of 4.4 minutes in the exercise time spent on the treadmill. The corresponding values for death from CHD were 3.2 (95% confidence interval, 1.5 to 6.7; $P = 0.003$) and 2.8 (95% confidence interval, 1.3 to 6.1; $P = 0.007$), respectively (Fig. 5–1). Thus, a low level of physical fitness is associated with a higher risk of death from CHD and cardiovascular disease in healthy men, independent of conventional coronary risk factors.

The relationship of physical fitness as measured by maximal treadmill performance and all-cause and cause-specific mortality rates was evaluated in 10,224 men and 3,120 women who had comprehensive medical examinations at the Cooper Clinic.[23] Average follow-up was slightly more than 8 years, for a total of 110,482 person-years of observation. There were 240 deaths in men and 43 deaths in women. Age-adjusted all-cause mortality rates declined across physical fitness quintiles from 64.0 per 10,000 person-years in the least-fit men to 18.6 per 10,000 person-years in the most-fit men. Corresponding values for women were 39.5 per 10,000 person-years to 8.5 per 10,000 person-years. These trends remained after statistical adjustments for age, smoking habit, cholesterol level, systolic blood pressure, fasting blood glucose level, parental history of CHD, and follow-up interval. Lower mortality rates in higher fitness categories also were seen for cardiovascular disease and cancer of combined sites. Attributable risk estimates for all-cause mortality rates indicated that low physical fitness was an important risk factor in both men and women. Higher levels of physical fitness appear to delay all-cause mortality, primarily due to lowered rates of cardiovascular disease and cancer.

The results of these two physical fitness studies are highly consistent with the observational data on physical activity and cardiovascular mortality: the least fit and least active have the highest rate of disease—moderate increases in fitness and activity are associated with a significant reduction in risk. There is a small dose-response relationship at higher levels of activity and fitness, but the magnitude of the benefit declines rapidly as fitness levels increase. This is especially true for the data from the Institute for Aerobics Research.[23]

Secondary Prevention of Coronary Heart Disease

As with primary prevention, there is no definitive study demonstrating a significant reduction in new cardiac events as a result of exercise training in patients with established CHD. However, in addition to studies that have simply compared morbidity or mortality for active versus inactive cardiac patients, controlled experimental trials have been conducted in which postmyocardial infarction patients have been randomly assigned to exercise and control groups.

Here again, the trend in morbidity and mortality favors the more physically active patients, with benefits apparently derived from an increase in caloric expenditure of no more than 300 to 400 kcal per session, three to four times per week, at a moderate intensity (66% to 75% of $\dot{V}O_{2max}$). All of the studies published, which show either no differences or lower mortality in the active population, have either design or implementation flaws that prohibit definitive conclusions regarding the hypothesis: "Does an increase in exercise reduce the future likelihood of recurrent myocardial infarction, cardiac arrest, or sudden cardiac death?"

Overall, patients who participated in a program of active rehabilitation after myocardial infarction had a much more favorable prognosis than those with similar clinical characteristics who did not participate in any formal program. In many of the earlier studies, the CHD mortality rate of exercise program participants was reported to be only one half or even one third that of patients in nonparticipant comparison groups.[24–26] It is very likely that these large differences in mortality were due, at least in part, to patient selection criteria, with lower-risk patients being recruited for participation in the exercise programs. In addition, lower mortality may have occurred in the program participants because of the modification of other risk factors, especially cigarette smoking and hypertension, and better medical management, leading to fewer sudden deaths.

Randomized Clinical Trials

Randomized clinical trials of cardiac rehabilitation following hospitalization for myocardial infarction usually have demonstrated lower mortality in treated patients, but a statistically significant reduction occurred in only one trial.[27–30] To overcome the problem of the inadequate power of any one study to detect small but clinically important benefits for mortality in randomized trials of exercise and risk factors rehabilitation, a meta-analysis was performed on the combined results of ten clinical trials.[31] All of the trials were required to have good documentation of myocardial infarction, randomization of patients, a rehabilitation program lasting at least 6 weeks, follow-up for 24 months or longer, and comprehensive documentation of outcome. Data on a total of 4347 patients were analyzed. The pooled ratios of 0.76 (95% confidence interval, 0.63 to 0.92) for all-cause deaths and 0.75 (95% confidence intervals, 0.62 to 0.93) for cardiovascular death were significantly lower for the rehabilitation group than for the control group, with no significant difference for recurrent myocardial infarction (Fig. 5–2). A similar review, which evaluated a total of 22 randomized trials of rehabilitation after myocardial infarction, reached a similar conclusion.[32]

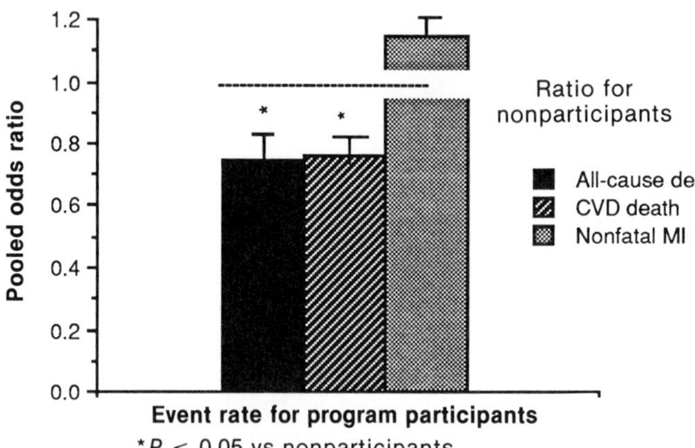

Figure 5–2. Pooled results for cardiovascular events in ten clinical trials of cardiac rehabilitation. Pooled odds ratio for nonparticipants expressed as 1.0. (*Data from* Oldridge NB, Guyatt GH, Fisher ME, et al: Cardiac rehabilitation after myocardial infarction: Combined exercise of randomized clinical trials. JAMA 266:945, 1988.)

Probably the best designed and best executed trial of the exercise benefits in secondary prevention of CHD has been the National Exercise and Heart Disease Project (NEHDP) conducted at five clinical centers in the United States from 1974 to 1979.[30] This study enrolled 651 men with myocardial infarction in a randomized 3-year clinical trial of the effects of prescribed supervised exercise. The subjects, aged 30 to 64 years, were screened for eligibility 2 to 36 months after their qualifying myocardial infarction. The men in the exercise group pursued supervised exercise training in the laboratory for 8 weeks and then in a gymnasium for 34 months.

The experience of the exercise group was more favorable than that of the control group in most of the comparisons made. The cumulative 3-year total mortality was 7.3% for the control group and 4.6% for the exercise group. The 3-year rate for recurrent myocardial infarction was 7.0% and 5.3%, respectively. Mortality rates in the two groups did not differ significantly, but the data were consistent with an assumption of substantial benefit from exercise. Compliance to treatment assignment was better in this project than that reported previously. By the end of 2 years, 23% of the exercise group were not attending the supervised exercise sessions and were not exercising elsewhere, whereas 31% of the control subjects reported exercising regularly.

In all of these clinical trials, as well as in others investigating different risk modification procedures, a major design problem has been the surprisingly low mortality in the control group, thus significantly reducing the statistical power of the study. For example, in the NEHDP, the total mortality in the control group, expected to be approximately 15% over the 3 years of follow-up, was only 7.3%. Such low rates may be due to exclusion of higher-risk patients from the trial, improved medical treatment as a participant in the trial (even when assigned to a control group), or an increase in risk-reducing behaviors by the control subjects during the course of the trial. However, even with these limitations, the NEHDP investigators estimate that in a study approximately twice the size of theirs (1400 versus 651 patients), the 37% reduction in mortality they achieved would be judged statistically significant.[30]

BIOLOGIC MECHANISMS PROTECTING AGAINST CORONARY HEART DISEASE

A variety of biologic changes or mechanisms have been proposed to explain how physical activity might decrease the development of CHD clinical manifestations or improve the clinical status of CHD patients (Table 5–2). Most of these mechanisms act in some way to

TABLE 5–2. BIOLOGIC MECHANISMS BY WHICH EXERCISE MAY CONTRIBUTE TO THE PRIMARY OR SECONDARY PREVENTION OF CORONARY HEART DISEASE*

Maintain or Increase Myocardial Oxygen Supply
- Delay progression of coronary atherosclerosis (possible)
  - Improve lipoprotein profile (increase HDL-C/LDL-C ratio) (probable)
  - Improve carbohydrate metabolism (increase insulin sensitivity) (probable)
  - Decrease platelet aggregation and increase fibrinolysis (probable)
  - Decrease adiposity (usually)
- Increase coronary collateral vascularization (unlikely)
- Increase epicardial artery diameter (possible)
- Increase coronary blood flow (myocardial perfusion) or distribution (unlikely)

Decrease Myocardial Work and Oxygen Demand
- Decrease heart rate at rest and during submaximal exercise (usually)
- Decrease systolic and mean systemic arterial pressure during submaximal exercise (usually) and at rest (possible)
- Decrease cardiac output during submaximal exercise (probable)
- Decrease circulating plasma catecholamine levels (decrease sympathetic tone) at rest (probable) and during submaximal exercise (usually)

Increase Myocardial Function
- Increase stroke volume at rest and during submaximal and maximal exercise (likely)
- Increase ejection fraction at rest and during exercise (possible)
- Increase intrinsic myocardial contractility (unlikely)
- Increase myocardial function resulting from decreased "afterload" (probable)
- Increase myocardial hypertrophy (probable); but this may not reduce CHD risk

Increase Electrical Stability of Myocardium
- Decrease regional ischemia at rest or during submaximal exercise (possible)
- Decrease catecholamines in myocardium at rest (possible) and during submaximal exercise (probable)
- Increase ventricular fibrillation threshold due to reduction of cyclic AMP (possible)

*Expression of likelihood that effect will occur for an individual participating in endurance-type training program for 16 weeks or longer at 65% to 80% of functional capacity for 25 minutes or longer per session (300 kcal) for 3 or more sessions per week ranges from unlikely, possible, likely, probable, to usually.

Abbreviations: HDL-C = high-density lipoprotein cholesterol; LDL-C = low-density lipoprotein cholesterol; CHD = coronary heart disease; AMP = adenosine monophosphate.

decrease the likelihood that the oxygen demands of the myocardium will exceed the oxygen delivery capacity of the coronary arteries and to prevent the development of myocardial ischemia. Thus, mechanisms can be classified as either those that contribute to the maintenance or increase of oxygen supply to the myocardium, or those that contribute to a decrease in myocardial work and oxygen demands. It is these very same mechanisms through which all preventive and therapeutic measures for reducing clinical manifestations of CHD work.

Maintenance of Myocardial Oxygen Supply

Because the primary cause of symptoms resulting from coronary atherosclerosis is myocardial ischemia, the most direct beneficial effect of physical training is an increase in myocardial oxygen supply. Enhanced oxygen delivery to the myocardium can be achieved (1) by the regression or delayed progression of coronary atherosclerosis, (2) by an increase in the lumen diameter of major coronary arteries, or (3) by coronary collateral vascularization. Also, it has been speculated that exercise training might reduce ischemia by redistributing myocardial regional blood flow, thus increasing the volume of blood flowing to the previously ischemic area. A major factor limiting our ability to directly collect information about these possibilities is the difficulty in obtaining the necessary invasive measurements before and after training in both an exercise-training group and a comparable control group.

DELAY OF ATHEROSCLEROSIS

One way in which exercise training could maintain or enhance myocardial oxygen supply would be by halting or delaying the progression of coronary atherosclerosis or even by stimulating regression of existing plaques. The concept of coronary atherosclerosis prevention or reversibility as observed in primates[33] is very attractive, but only limited human experimental data are available to support the isolated animal and epidemiologic observations that lend support to such a possibility.

No study has been reported in which the progression of coronary atherosclerosis in relation to exercise status has been measured in asymptomatic individuals, and only a few studies have reported any such data in cardiac patients.[34–37] A few investigators have attempted to study myocardial perfusion changes using thallium 201 radionuclide imaging, but reproducibility and precision problems with the measurement technique have contributed to inconclusive results.[38,39]

The preliminary report by Selvester and colleagues[34] using repeat coronary arteriograms obtained from 104 cardiac patients at a mean interval of 20 months has been the only study so far to observe an association between exercise and rate of atherosclerosis. During the period between the two arteriograms, all patients were enrolled in a CHD risk–reduction program consisting of exercise training, diet modifications (calories, saturated fat, and cholesterol), cigarette smoking abatement, and blood pressure control. All cineangiogram films were reviewed independently by two experienced angiographers, with each obstructive coronary lesion graded as to the percentage of narrowing of cross-sectional area present. A lesion was considered to have progressed between the first and second study if lumen narrowing of at least 30% or progression to total occlusion was observed. Patients in the more physically active groups, especially when they showed an increase in their levels of fitness, experienced a decreased incidence of atherosclerotic progression in their coronary arteries; progression occurred in 21 of 47 (45%) possible arteries in the inactive patients and in 3 of 16 (19%) possible arteries in the high-level training subjects ($P = 0.06$).

The design of this study creates several serious problems in data interpretation and generalizability:

1. The participants were not randomly allocated to treatments.
2. There was no control group.
3. The results are confounded by the various degrees of change in risk behaviors other than exercise.

In three other studies in which coronary cineangiography was performed before and after training, no changes in coronary artery lesions were noted.[35–37] The time between arteriograms in one study was 11 to 15 weeks, and no change in lesions, either regression or progression, should be expected in such a short time.[35] In the other two studies, approximately 1 year elapsed between evaluations, in which case one might have expected significant progression to have occurred in some patients.[36,37] Because none of these studies included a control or comparison group, it is not possible to determine whether a lack of progression of atherosclerosis in the exercising subjects is itself a favorable response. The only study that has included repeat coronary arteriograms on a nonexercising control group, as well as patients who participated in a standard exercise training program for 7 months, did not find any difference in the progression of atherosclerosis between the two groups.[40]

Indirect evidence that vigorous exercise might beneficially influence the rate of atherosclerosis is suggested by the relationship of exercise to several established CHD risk factors. In both healthy adults and cardiac patients, exercise training has been shown to alter the blood lipoprotein profile in a direction thought to be less atherogenic: high-density lipoprotein cholesterol (HDL-C) level is increased; and low-density lipoprotein cholesterol (LDL-C), very-low-density lipoprotein cholesterol (VLDL-C), total cholesterol, and triglyceride levels are sometimes lower.[41,42] Of particular interest is the apparent antiatherogenic effect of increased HDL-C levels and the demonstration that HDL-C levels increase more systematically with exercise than with dietary change or weight loss.[43] In addition to improving lipid metabolism, exercise training also tends to normalize the carbohydrate metabolism of hyperglycemic and diabetic individuals and may favorably influence the accelerated atherosclerosis frequently seen in these patients.[44]

If occlusion of narrowed coronary arteries resulting from blood clots significantly contributes to the increased incidence of infarction or cardiac arrest, exercise might exert a beneficial influence by delaying clotting[45] or by increasing fibrinolysis.[46] Moderate-intensity exercise (70% of functional capacity for 30 minutes), which is well within the capability of many CHD patients, significantly increases fibrinolytic activity.[46] This enhanced fibrinolysis, which appears to be independent of any delayed blood clotting resulting from exercise, is caused by an increased concentration of a plasminogen activator and may last for up to 60 minutes following exercise. As a result of the complexity of the blood-clotting mechanism, a dose-response relationship between exercise and this phenomenon has not yet been defined.

CORONARY COLLATERAL VASCULARIZATION

The intriguing hypothesis that exercise training might be an adequate stimulus for the development of coronary collateral vessels was supported by some early animal studies.[47] Such encouraging results, however, have not been obtained systematically in any human study using coronary arteriography. The necessary stimulus for enhancing coronary collateral vascularization appears to be myocardial hypoxia induced by the atherosclerotic disease process itself; increases in myocardial work, coronary blood flow, or coronary perfusion pressure produced during exercise do not appear to significantly alter the size of the functional vascular bed.

Ferguson and colleagues[37] performed coronary arteriograms on 14 cardiac patients before and after 13 months of exercise training consisting of three hourly sessions per week of walking and low-intensity games (average attendance, 68%). The average total distance walked per patient in 13 months was 219 ± 63 miles. As a result of this training, functional capacity increased in all patients. Maximal oxygen uptake increased an average of 25%, and the seven patients with angina on entry were asymptomatic at the final evaluation. In spite of these changes in functional capacity and clinical status, new collaterals were visualized in only 2 of the 21 coronary arteries with 50% to 95% obstruction before training. Thus, an increase in functional capacity and relief of angina at rest and during exercise associated with exercise training can occur without coronary collateral development as visualized by cineangiograms.

These results are consistent with those of at least five other studies in which no significant increase in coronary collaterals was observed with exercise training lasting from 11 weeks to 12 months.[35,36,40,48,49] Thus, human studies using coronary arteriography to detect coronary collaterals have not supported the exercise-induced collateralization hypothesis derived from animal studies. This discrepancy is probably due to a species difference, although the insensitivity of the measurement technique in detecting small changes in coronary anatomy and coronary flow should not be overlooked. Also, it would be of interest to observe subjects before and after exercise training of greater intensity than that used in the studies just described.[50]

CORONARY BLOOD FLOW

Exercise training, even when increasing the work load at the onset of angina, does not necessarily enhance coronary blood flow (CBF) at peak exercise. It does, however, usually decrease CBF both at rest and at submaximal work loads.

Ferguson and co-workers[51] measured coronary sinus blood flow (CSBF) by thermodilution in ten cardiac patients before and after 6 months of exercise training (30 minutes of stationary bicycle riding and 20 minutes of volleyball 2.6 times per week for 16 to 22 weeks). Symptom-limited exercise capacity increased 38% (560 to 770 kg-m/min), and patients could perform 18% more work at the same heart rate (114 beats/min). At rest, CSBF decreased slightly (95 to 90 mL/min), as did resting heart rate and blood pressure. At a preanginal standard work load of 400 kg-m/min, CSBF decreased from 163 to 135 mL/min, primarily as a result of decreases in heart rate from 120 to 103 beats/min, and in systolic blood pressure from 180 to 168 mm Hg. At the onset of angina, work load increased from 493 to 703 kg-m/min (43%), but the increase in mean CSBF was not significant (200 to 214 mL/min).

That the intensity of exercise training usually performed by cardiac patients probably does not increase peak CBF or the oxidative capacity of the myocardium in humans is supported by the data of Sim and Neill,[35] who observed no improvement in CBF or myocardial lactate extraction at the anginal threshold during pacing following 11 to 15 weeks of conditioning. Detry and Bruce,[52] who reported that the posttraining increase in pressure-rate product (RPP) at the onset of angina was accompanied by an increase in the magnitude of ST segment depression, demonstrated that onset of angina may not be as good an indicator as needed to study this question. Thus, patients who have an increase in CSBF or RPP at the onset of angina or at angina-limited maximal exercise may have an altered pain threshold following training.

Longer and more vigorous exercise training may improve myocardial oxygen delivery, as indicated by the study results of Ehsani and colleagues.[50] For 12 months, they trained ten patients who had developed ischemic-type ST segment depression during exercise testing. Patients usually trained at 70% to 80% of $\dot{V}O_{2max}$ with 2- to 5-minute intervals of training requiring 80% to 90% of $\dot{V}O_{2max}$ included in the sessions after the first 3 months. Average attendance at training sessions was 4.5 times per week. The heart rate–systolic blood pressure product threshold for ST segment depression increased an average of 22% after the 12 months of training and there was a decrease in the extent of ST segment depression at the same RPP. No such change was seen in eight control subjects. These findings suggest that myocardial ischemia is reduced at the same or higher myocardial work load. This may be due to an increase in CBF following long-term, high-volume, vigorous endurance training.

Decreases in Myocardial Oxygen Demand

A reduction in the frequency or severity of the clinical manifestations of CHD may occur with physical training as a result of decreases in myocardial oxygen requirements at rest and during exercise. Following exercise training, a substantial percentage of angina patients increase the exercise intensity necessary to provoke ischemia, and in some patients, exertional angina is eliminated altogether.[53]

The primary reason for this increase in ischemia-free working capacity is a decrease in myocardial oxygen demand attributable to systematic decreases in exercise heart rate with less of a reduction in systolic blood pressure. The decrease in heart rate at a given work load or oxygen uptake appears to be the key to improving the clinical status of many CHD patients with angina pectoris, because it is the major factor in the exercise-related decrease in indexes of myocardial work.

The precise mechanism by which training produces exercise bradycardia is still not fully understood. The training-induced decrease in exercise heart rate appears to be due to changes in the skeletal muscle used for training (usually leg muscles in cardiac patients) and to some other more central change, such as increased blood volume, myocardial hypertrophy, increased myocardial contractility, or altered central nervous system regulation.[54] A number of studies have been conducted in which one set of limbs (arms or legs) was trained and the training response was determined at rest and during exercise in both the trained and untrained limbs. These studies consistently demonstrate that the greatest reduction in submaximal exercise heart rate occurs with trained limbs,[55] and that in training studies of shorter duration, little if any reduction in heart rate occurs during exercise of the nontrained limbs.[56] These data indicate that much of the decrease in heart rate observed during the early stages of exercise training, especially when the training is performed at lower intensities, is due to changes taking place in the trained skeletal muscle. Changes in heart rate at rest and during exercise using untrained limbs may occur only if training is conducted for a longer duration or at a higher intensity.

At maximal or peak exercise, indirect indexes of myocardial oxygen demand tend to increase somewhat, again primarily because patients are willing or able to exercise to a higher heart rate. The main question precipitated by these data is whether or not this apparent increase tolerated by cardiac patients following training is met by an increase in myocardial oxygen supply. Most of the data presented in the previous section suggest that this increased myocardial oxygen demand is tolerated with greater ischemia rather than with an increase in CBF.

Reduction in Myocardial Irritability

Any significant antidysrhythmic effect that exercise training might have could contribute to the reduction in sudden deaths frequently seen in epidemiologic studies reporting lower mortality for active individuals. But this idea is still highly speculative, because very little information on which to evaluate this question has been published. The concept is plausible because of the known effects of training on the nervous system regulation of the heart, on the reduction of myocardial oxygen demand, and in the lowering of circulating plasma catecholamines.[57] Because of the rather low test-retest reproducibility of cardiac dysrhythmias during 24-hour ambulatory monitoring and exercise testing, the measurement problems associated with answering this question are substantial.

Blackburn and associates[58] have reported the only controlled trial so far in asymptomatic men who were at high risk for CHD. They randomly assigned half of a group of 196 middle-aged men to an 18-month exercise training program (three 45- to 60-minute sessions a week) and the other half to a control group. Following the program, repeat exercise testing did not result in any significant difference between the two groups in terms of the incidence or frequency of premature ventricular complexes (PVCs). When only those subjects who were classified as compliers to the program (greater than 75% attendance) were compared with the controls, the number of PVCs per man in those subjects displaying ventricular ectopic activity was significantly less in the conditioned group ($P = 0.04$), but the percentage of subjects manifesting PVCs was not different. Although inconclusive, these data do suggest that exercise training may have an antidysrhythmic potential for some individuals.

CARDIOVASCULAR RISKS DURING EXERCISE

Risks in the General Public

At least in the United States, whenever someone dies suddenly during participation in recreational or sporting activities, the event receives much more publicity than if the same individual had died while at home or work. Because of this publicity, the percentage of all sudden cardiac deaths (SCDs) that occur during sporting activities in the general population is probably lower than it would seem to be, based on casual observation. However, if an individual has underlying cardiac disease that significantly reduces myocardial perfusion, the increased myocardial oxygen demand—imposed by either static or dynamic exercise—can precipitate sudden cardiac arrest or sudden death.[59] It appears that most instantaneous deaths do not result from new anatomic lesions, but from an electrical event taking place in an already chronically and severely damaged heart.

Adults in the general population who participate in vigorous sporting activities such as long-distance running, cross-country skiing, cycling, or vigorous sports may be at greater risk of SCD during exercise than when not exercising.[60,61] Based on the circumstances surrounding 2606 sudden deaths in Finland during 1 year, Vuori and colleagues[60] concluded that SCD in connection with sporting activities in the general population is quite rare; instantaneous deaths were even rarer (<1% of all incidences of SCD) and occurred only with coexisting activity. Of the deaths associated with exercise, 73% were caused by acute or chronic ischemic heart disease and most of the subjects had serious cardiovascular risk factors that were known in advance or could have been identified easily.

Thompson and colleagues[62] investigated the circumstances of death and the medical and activity histories of 18 individuals who died during or immediately after jogging in the United States. Thirteen men died of CHD, and four men and one woman died of other causes. Six SCD subjects experienced prodromal symptoms but continued vigorous exercise programs, and ten had seen their physician in the past year, a significantly higher rate than would be expected of healthy adults in the United States. Two subjects had exercised regularly for not more than a month, but most had trained regularly for years. This study supports the ideas that most SCDs during exercise in adults over 35 are due to coronary artery disease (CAD), that CAD can occur in habitually active and reasonably well-conditioned individuals, and that many of the victims have significant risk factors for heart disease.

In adults who have had a recent medical evaluation, the risk for SCD during exercise is extremely small. Gibbons and colleagues[63] documented only two nonfatal cardiac arrests and no deaths in 374,798 person-hours of vigorous exercise. In a very large experience obtained by Vander and associates[64] from 40 exercise facilities over 5 years, the fatality rate associated with exercise in the general population was quite low. In 33,726,000 participant-hours of exercise, only 38 fatal cardiovascular complications occurred for a fatality rate of one death every 887,526 hours of participation. This means one could expect one death per year if 3400 adults were exercising 5 hours per week each. Also, the mortality rate while exercising in this group is about 1% per year, nearly the same as the annual CHD mortality rate in the United States. Most of the fatalities reported in this study occurred during court games, jogging, and swimming.

Risks In Cardiac Patients

As a result of the increase in myocardial oxygen demand imposed by vigorous physical activity, caution has been recommended to individuals thought to be at increased risk or

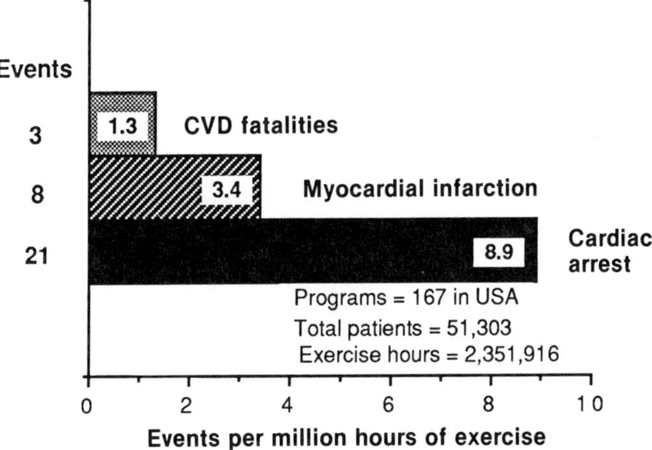

Figure 5–3. Cardiovascular events occurring in conjunction with exercise training by patients with ischemic heart disease. (CVD = cardiovascular disease.) (*Data from* Van Camp SP, Peterson RA: Cardiovascular complications of cardiac rehabilitation programs. JAMA 256:1160, 1986.)

to patients with known cardiovascular disease. Of particular concern are those patients with symptomatic CAD or left ventricular outflow tract obstruction (such as produced by aortic stenosis or idiopathic hypertrophic subaortic stenosis). Numerous instances have been cited in which SCD has occurred during vigorous exercise in such patients. However, increasing experience suggests that properly monitored exercise can be relatively safe for patients with CAD.

Haskell[65] determined by questionnaire the occurrence of major cardiovascular complications during exercise training of CAD patients in 30 cardiac rehabilitation programs in North America. These programs conducted medically supervised cardiac exercise classes in 103 locations and reported information on 13,570 participants who accumulated a total of 1,629,624 patient-hours of supervised exercise. A total of 50 cardiac arrests were experienced during exercise, 42 of which were successfully resuscitated, and eight of which were fatal. Seven myocardial infarctions were reported; two were fatal, and five were nonfatal. Four other deaths occurred, all from acute cardiopulmonary disorders. The average complication rate was one nonfatal and one fatal event every 34,673 and 116,040 patient-hours of participation, respectively.

The results of a more recent survey of 167 randomly selected cardiac rehabilitation programs in the USA were even more favorable relative to risk of cardiac death during medically supervised exercise.[66] These 167 programs reported that 51,303 patients exercised 2,361,916 hours from January 1980 through December 1984. During this time, 21 cardiac arrests (18 in which the patient was successfully resuscitated) and eight nonfatal myocardial infarctions were reported. The incidences per million patient hours of exercise were 8.9 for cardiac arrests (one per 111,996 patient-hours), 3.4 for myocardial infarction (one per 293,990 patient-hours) and 1.3 for fatalities (one per 783,972 patient-hours) (Fig. 5–3). There was no statistically significant difference in frequency of these events among programs of varying size on extent of electrocardiographic monitoring. These data support the safety of cardiac exercise programs as they are now conducted in the United States. Similar experiences have been reported from Finland, Austria, West Germany, and Australia.

The safety of exercise for cardiac patients can be increased by proper medical evaluation including symptom-limited exercise testing, effective patient counseling and education, and proper monitoring of exercise performance. However, techniques have not been developed to identify all of those ambulatory patients with such a high risk of sudden death that they should not exercise. Those patients at greatest risk may be characterized by one or more of the following:

1. Poor left ventricular function (ejection fraction <30%).
2. Exercise hypotension.
3. Multivessel disease (>70% narrowing).
4. Very low exercise capacity.
5. Frequent complex PVCs.
6. Multiple myocardial infarctions.
7. Angina pectoris at rest or low-level exercise.

PREVENTION OF CARDIOVASCULAR COMPLICATIONS DURING EXERCISE

The prevention of all SCDs during exercise cannot be achieved because some victims are asymptomatic until the fatal event, or because the anomaly could only have been detected by costly and, in some cases, potentially dangerous invasive evaluation procedures. Even if it were able to be detected, there has been a general tendency to misdiagnose or disregard selected cardiac anomalies in the younger population. In some cases, the dangers of the anomaly are downplayed in order to avoid restricting the individual inappropriately.

The causes of SCD in young people are reasonably well established, and when the causes are identified, proper precautions should be taken. The generally recognized causes include:

1. Congenital coronary anomalies, such as anomalous origin of the left coronary artery from the pulmonary artery, and origin of the left coronary artery from the anterior sinus of Valsalva.
2. Hypertrophic cardiomyopathy.
3. Aortic stenosis.
4. Atherosclerotic coronary artery disease.

Rarer causes of SCD include:

1. Prolapsed mitral valve.
2. Dissection of the aorta with rupture into the pericardium.
3. Coronary emboli from atrial myxoma.
4. Occlusion of the coronary ostium by vegetation.
5. Benign papillary fibroelastoma of the aortic valve.

Electrophysiologic problems include accelerated atrioventricular conduction with atrial fibrillation; this causes ventricular fibrillation and prolonged QT interval syndrome. In the United States, more than 90% of all incidences of SCD with coexisting exercise in both men and women over age 40 appears to be due to progressive CAD. Structural myocardial anomalies, especially hypertrophic cardiomyopathies and atrioventricular conduction defects, account for many of the remaining nonaccidental deaths during moderate-to-vigorous exercise.

In individuals at all ages, but especially after age 30, those with established risk factors of CHD should be considered at increased risk for SCD. Routine screening for hypertension, hyperlipidemia, glucose intolerance, and cigarette smoking should be performed on those individuals participating in high-level, competitive activities. Such screening should be followed up by aggressive therapy when indicated. Of particular concern should be genetic-based hyperlipidemias in which the low-density fraction of cholesterol is elevated. Up to a third of the current events could be prevented by (1) more aggressive medical intervention when patients at high risk for SCD are identified; and (2) more extensive use of cardiovascular evaluation procedures. Such procedures include resting and exercise electrocardiograms, echocardiography, magnetic resonance imaging, and radionuclide imaging during exercise to determine myocardial perfusion and ventricular function abnormalities.

SUMMARY

Results of animal, experimental, clinical, and observational research support the hypothesis that more physically active individuals have greater resistance to the development of coronary atherosclerosis and its clinical manifestations. Large-muscle dynamic exercise that requires a substantial increase in calorie expenditure and places a greater volume than pressure load on the myocardium appears to be most useful in providing protection. Both job-related and leisure-time activity seem to provide benefit with only recent activity making a contribution: No credits or advantages appear to be gained from being more active earlier in life.

At average rates of energy expenditure of less than 7 kcal/min, a daily expenditure of 300 to 500 kcal above that expended by inactive peers is associated with a decreased risk of CHD; above 7 kcal/min, it seems that less activity needs to be performed, probably no more than 200 to 300 kcal at least every other day. The benefits of exercise in terms of reducing CHD risk occur at all ages for men over 40, but the advantages have not been studied adequately for younger men or women.

The biologic pathways through which exercise exerts any protective effect have not been fully elucidated. Even though the evidence on whether or not exercise directly influences the rate of progression of atherosclerosis is as much negative as it is positive, recent data on the favorable lipid and carbohydrate metabolic changes produced by exercise provide a potential mechanism. Myocardial hypertrophy and possibly increased contractility and capillarization as well as coronary blood flow, are produced by long-term vigorous exercise training. However, such changes usually are not seen at the low levels of exercise that seem to provide some protection against CHD.

It is very unlikely that exercise is an adequate stimulus for systematically producing collateral coronary vessels in humans. Most of the risk-reducing benefit of exercise may be due to its oxygen-sparing effects as evidenced by lower heart rates, blood pressure, and general sympathetic tone. Such changes are of particular importance to individuals with hemodynamically significant coronary atherosclerosis and may be major contributors to the reduction in sudden death observed in some studies.

REFERENCES

1. Powell KE, Thompson PD, Cospersen CJ, et al: Physical activity and incidence of coronary heart disease. Annu Rev Public Health 8:253, 1987.
2. Shapiro S, Weinblatt E, Frank CW, et al: Incidence of coronary heart disease in a population insured for medical care (HIP). Am J Public Health 59 (suppl):1, 1969.
3. Paffenbarger RS, Wing AL, Hyde RT: Physical activity as an index of heart attack in college alumni. Am J Epidemiol 108:161, 1978.
4. Morris JN, Pollard R, Everitt MG, et al: Vigorous exercise in leisure time: Protection against coronary heart disease. Lancet ii:1207, 1980.
5. Costas R, Garcia-Palmieri MR, Nazario E, et al: Relation of lipids, weight and physical activity to incidence of coronary heart disease: The Puerto Rico Heart Study. Am J Cardiol 42:653, 1978.
6. Salonen JT, Puska P, Tuomilehto J: Physical activity and risk of myocardial infarction, cerebral stroke and death: A longitudinal study in Eastern Finland. Am J Epidemiol 115:526, 1982.
7. Chapman JM, Massey FJ: The interrelationship of serum cholesterol, hypertension, body weight and risk of coronary disease. J Chronic Dis 17:933, 1964.
8. Paul O: Physical activity and coronary heart disease (part II). Am J Cardiol 23:303, 1969.

9. Karvonen MJ, Rautaharju PM, Orma E, et al: Heart disease and employment: Cardiovascular studies on lumberjacks. J Occup Med 3:49, 1961.
10. Kahn HA: The relationship of reported coronary heart disease mortality to physical activity of work. Am J Public Health 53:1058, 1963.
11. Leon AS, Cornett J, Jacobs DR, et al: Leisure-time physical activity levels and risk of coronary heart disease and death: The Multiple Risk Factor Intervention Trial. JAMA 258:2388, 1987.
12. Cassel J, Heyden S, Bartel AG, et al: Occupation and physical activity and coronary heart disease. Arch Intern Med 128:920, 1971.
13. Morris JN, Heady JA, Raffle PAB, et al: Coronary heart disease and physical activity of work. Lancet ii:1053–1057, 1111–1120, 1953.
14. Taylor HL, Parlin RW: The physical activity of railroad clerks and switchmen: Estimation of on-the-job calorie expenditure by time and task measurements and classification of recreational activity by a questionnaire. Written Presentation at "Three Days of Cardiology." Seattle, June 25, 1966.
15. Paffenbarger RS, Hale WE, Brand RJ, et al: Work-energy level, personal characteristics, and fatal heart attack: A birth-cohort study. Am J Epidemiol 105:200, 1977.
16. Zukel WJ, Lewis RH, Enterline PE, et al: A short-term community study of the epidemiology of coronary heart disease. Am J Public Health 49:1630, 1959.
17. McDonough JR, Hames CG, Stulb SC, et al: Coronary heart disease among negroes and whites in Evans County, Georgia. J Chronic Dis 18:443, 1965.
18. Menotti A, Puddu V, Monti M, et al: Habitual physical activity and myocardial infarction. Cardiologia 54:119, 1969.
19. Skinner JS, Benson H, McDonough HR, et al: Social status, physical activity and coronary proneness. J Chronic Dis 19:773, 1966.
20. Rose G: Physical activity and coronary heart disease. Proc R Soc Med 62:1183, 1969.
21. Pekkanan J, Marti B, Nissinen A, et al: Reduction of premature mortality by high physical activity: A 20-year follow-up of middle-aged Finnish men. Lancet i:1473, 1987.
22. Ekelund LG, Haskell WL, Johnson JL, et al: Physical fitness as a prevention of cardiovascular mortality in asymptomatic North American men. N Engl J Med 319:1379, 1988.
23. Blair SN, Kohl HW, Paffenbarger RS, et al: Physical fitness and all-cause mortality: A prospective study in healthy men and women. JAMA 262:2395, 1989.
24. Hellerstein HK: Exercise therapy in coronary disease. Bull NY Acad Med 44:1028, 1968.
25. Kellerman JJ: Physical conditioning in patients after myocardial infarction. Schweiz Med Wochenschr 103:79, 1973.
26. Kavanagh T, Shephard RJ, Chisholm AW, et al: Prognostic indexes for patients with ischemic heart disease enrolled in an exercise-centered rehabilitation program. Am J Cardiol 44:1230, 1979.
27. Kentala E: Physical fitness and feasibility of physical rehabilitation after myocardial infarction in men of working age. Ann Clin Res 91 (suppl):1, 1972.
28. Wilhelmsen L, Sanne H, Elmfeldt D, et al: A controlled trial of physical training after myocardial infarction: Effects on risk factors, nonfatal reinfarction and death. Prev Med 4:491, 1975.
29. Rechnitzer PA, Cunningham DA, Andre GM, et al: Relation of exercise to the recurrence rate of myocardial infarction in men. Am J Cardiol 51:65, 1983.
30. Shaw L: Effects of a prescribed supervised exercise program on mortality and cardiovascular morbidity in patients after myocardial infarction. Am J Cardiol 48:39, 1981.
31. Oldridge NB, Guyatt GH, Fisher ME, et al: Cardiac rehabilitation after myocardial infarction: Combined exercise of randomized clinical trials. JAMA 260:945, 1988.
32. O'Conner GT, Boving JE, Yusuf S, et al: An overview of randomized trials of rehabilitation with exercise after myocardial infarction. Circulation 80:234, 1989.
33. Kramsch DM, Aspen A, Abramowitz B, et al: Reduction of coronary atherosclerosis by moderate conditioning exercise in monkeys on an atherogenic diet. N Engl J Med 305:1483, 1981.
34. Selvester R, Camp J, Sanmarco M: Effects of exercise training on progression of documented coronary atherosclerosis in men. *In* Milvey P (ed): The Marathon: Physiological, Medical, Epidemiological, and Psychological Studies. New York, New York Academy of Sciences, 1977, p 495.
35. Sim DN, Neill WA: Investigation of the physiological basis for increased exercise threshold for angina pectoris after physical conditioning. J Clin Invest 54:763, 1974.
36. Kennedy CC, Spiegerman RE, Lindsay MI, et al: One-year graduated exercise program for men with angina pectoris. Mayo Clin Proc 51:231, 1976.
37. Ferguson RJ, Petitclerc R, Choquette G, et al: Effect of physical training on treadmill exercise capacity, collateral circulation and progression of coronary disease. Am J Cardiol 34:764, 1974.
38. Verani M, Hartung H, Hoepfel-Harris J, et al: Effects of exercise training on left ventricular performance and myocardial perfusion in patients with coronary artery disease. Am J Cardiol 47:797, 1981.
39. Atwood E, Jensen D, Froelicher V, et al: Radionuclide perfusion images before and after cardiac rehabilitation. Aviat Space Environ Med 51:892, 1980.

40. Nolewjka AJ, Kostuk WJ, Rechnitzer PA, et al: Exercise and human collateralization: An angiographic and scintigraphic assessment. Circulation 60:114, 1979.
41. Wood PD, Haskell WL, Blair S, et al: Increased exercise level and plasma lipoprotein concentrations: A one-year randomized, controlled study in sedentary, middle-aged men. Metabolism 32:31, 1983.
42. Ballantyne FC, Clark RS, Simpson HS, et al: The effect of moderate physical exercise on the plasma lipoprotein subfractions in male survivors of myocardial infarction. Circulation 65:913, 1982.
43. Wood PD, Haskell WL: The effect of exercise on plasma high-density lipoproteins. Lipids 14:417, 1979.
44. Saltin B, Lindgarde F, Houston M, et al: Physical training and glucose tolerance in middle-aged men with chemical diabetes. Diabetes 28 (suppl):30, 1979.
45. Rouramaa R, Salonen J, Kukkonon-Harjula K, et al: Effects of mild physical exercise on serum lipoproteins and metabolites of arachidonic acid: A controlled randomized trial in middle-aged men. Br Med J 288:603, 1984.
46. Astrup T: The effects of physical activity on blood coagulation and fibrinolysis. *In* Naughton JP, Hellerstein HR (eds): Exercise Testing and Training in Coronary Heart Disease. New York, Academic Press, 1973, pp 169–192.
47. Eckstein RW: Effect of exercise and coronary artery narrowing on coronary collateral circulation. Circ Res 5:230, 1957.
48. Conner JF, La Camera F, Swanick EF, et al: Effects of exercise on coronary collateralization—angiographic studies of six patients in a supervised exercise program. Med Sci Sports 8:145, 1976.
49. Kattus AA, Grollman J: Patterns of coronary collateral circulation in angina pectoris: Relation to exercise training. *In* Russek H, Zohman B (eds): Changing Concepts in Cardiovascular Disease. Baltimore, Williams & Wilkins, 1972, p 352.
50. Ehsani A, Heath G, Hagberg J, et al: Effects of 12 months of intense exercise training on ischemic ST-segment depression in patients with coronary artery disease. Circulation 64:1116, 1981.
51. Ferguson RJ, Cote P, Gauthier P, et al: Changes in exercise coronary sinus blood flow with training in patients with angina pectoris. Circulation 58:41, 1978.
52. Detry JM, Bruce RA: Effects of physical training on exertional ST-segment depression in coronary heart disease. Circulation 45:390, 1971.
53. Redwood DR, Rosing DR, Epstein SE: Circulatory and symptomatic effects of physical training in patients with coronary-artery disease and angina pectoris. N Engl J Med 286:959, 1972.
54. Varnauskas E, Björntorp P, Fahlen M, et al: Effects of physical training on exercise blood flow and enzymatic activity in skeletal muscle. Cardiovasc Res 4:418, 1970.
55. Thompson P, Cullinane E, Lazarus B, et al: Effect of exercise training on the untrained limb exercise performance of men with angina pectoris. Am J Cardiol 48:844, 1981.
56. Clausen JP, Klausen K, Rasmussen B, et al: Central and peripheral circulatory changes after training of the arms or legs. Am J Physiol 225:675, 1973.
57. Cousineau D, Ferguson R, de Champlain J, et al: Catecholamines in coronary sinus during exercise in man before and after training. J Appl Physiol 43:801, 1977.
58. Blackburn H, Taylor H, Hamrell B, et al: Premature ventricular complexes induced by stress testing: Their frequency and response to physical conditioning. Am J Cardiol 31:441, 1973.
59. Dawson A, Leon A, Taylor H: Effect of submaximal exercise on vulnerability to fibrillation in the canine ventricle. Circulation 60:798, 1979.
60. Vuori I, Makarainen M, Jaaselainen A: Sudden death and physical activity. Cardiology 63:287, 1978.
61. Thompson P, Funk E, Carleton R, et al: Incidence of death during jogging in Rhode Island from 1975 through 1980. JAMA 247:2535, 1982.
62. Thompson P, Stern M, Williams P, et al: Death during jogging or running: A study case of 18 cases. JAMA 242:1265, 1979.
63. Gibbons LW, Cooper KH, Myer B, et al: The acute cardiac risk of strenuous exercise. JAMA 244:1799, 1980.
64. Vander L, Franklin B, Rubenfire M: Cardiovascular complications of recreational physical activity. Physician Sports Med 10:89, 1982.
65. Haskell WL: Cardiovascular complications during exercise training of cardiac patients. Circulation 57:920, 1978.
66. Van Camp SP, Peterson RA: Cardiovascular complications of cardiac rehabilitation programs. JAMA 256:1160, 1986.

SECTION II

DISORDERS OF VARIOUS ORGAN SYSTEMS

6

IMMUNE MECHANISMS AND INFECTIOUS DISEASES IN EXERCISE AND SPORTS

Harvey B. Simon, MD

Exercise places unique demands on the human body; patients who exercise place unique demands on their physicians.

The physiologic responses to habitual exercise are generally adaptive and beneficial, thus, athletes tend to be healthy patients. But because of their commitment to exercise, athletes with intercurrent illnesses pose special challenges for their physicians. This is particularly true with regard to infectious diseases. Standard medical practice is to prescribe rest in the management of almost all infections. Because compliance with this advice is very difficult for many athletes, patients who exercise require more precise guidelines. Although data is still limited, these guidelines should be based on current understanding of the interactions between physical exertion, the immune system, and infectious agents. And insofar as the athlete forces us to reevaluate older empiric recommendations, this reappraisal of exercise and infection may improve medical management of infectious illness in sedentary people as well.

The study of exercise and immunity begins with the work of Larrabee who observed a brisk leukocytosis in four men at the conclusion of the 1901 Boston Marathon.[1] Unfortunately, interest in this subject has not been sustained throughout this century; indeed most of our current understanding of exercise, infection, and immunity is based on in vitro studies performed within the past decade. Although information is still incomplete in this rapidly evolving field, an overall picture is beginning to emerge.

In this review, I will discuss first the effects of exercise on the immune system. Next, I will summarize the much smaller body of epidemiologic data dealing with the incidence and severity of infections in people who exercise. I will also review the effects of exercise on established infections and the effects of infection on athletic performance. Finally, I will propose guidelines for the prevention and management of certain common infections in people who exercise.

EXERCISE AND HUMAN IMMUNE FUNCTION

The immune system is a complex network composed of bone marrow and lymphoid tissues, circulating leukocytes, and soluble mediators including antibody, complement, and numerous cytokines and interferons. These elements function together to recognize, entrap, and destroy invading microbes and tumor cells. In addition to these immunologically specific mechanisms, resistance to infection depends on a series of nonimmunologic anatomic and physiologic barriers designed chiefly to prevent penetration of microorganisms from the body's cutaneous and mucosal surfaces and from the environment.

Exercise can affect each element of the immune system. Although there is little data on the effects of exercise on the immune system as a whole, a substantial amount of information on how exercise affects individual components of the immune network is now available. Hence, I will consider each aspect of the immune system individually in this chapter, returning at the end to an evaluation of the overall significance of the changes that have been observed.

Even omitting animal data, there are certain difficulties in comparing studies of exercise and immunity. In almost all the studies, healthy adult volunteers served as subjects; a great majority of the subjects were men. However, the fitness level of the study subjects varies widely, ranging from unconditioned people to elite athletes. To further compound the difficulties in interpreting these studies, most rely on only a small number of subjects.

The exercise protocols also vary greatly, ranging from 5 minutes of stair climbing, to much more carefully controlled treadmill running or bicycle ergometry, to marathon running and a 24-hour march covering 120 km. In a few studies, immune parameters were investigated only at rest, and conditioned athletes were compared with sedentary control subjects. In most studies, however, the subjects in each investigation served as their own controls, as various immunologic parameters were measured before and after exercise. In most cases, only the acute effects of exercise were studied, with blood samples drawn for in vitro immunologic assays within minutes to hours after the termination of exercise.

The host defense parameters that were measured in these studies are also very disparate, ranging from simple determinations of leukocyte counts to sophisticated evaluations of lymphocyte subsets and functions. Since these studies were performed between 1902 and 1990, it is not surprising that the immunologic assays used also vary greatly.

In view of these many disparities, it is not surprising that the results of these investigations also display considerable variability; in some cases, the findings are even contradictory. Clearly, further studies will be needed to resolve these ambiguities and to extend our understanding in this newest area of exercise physiology.

Lymphocytes

Lymphocytes are the primary cells in the immune response. Originally derived from pleuripotential stem cells in the bone marrow, lymphocytes differentiate during embryogenesis into T cells, B cells, and non-T non-B cells. In recent years, the development of monoclonal antibodies capable of recognizing surface antigens on these cells has produced an explosive growth in knowledge about lymphocyte subtype.

T lymphocytes develop in the thymus, and populate germinal centers in lymph nodes and the spleen; about 80% of circulating lymphocytes are T cells. T cells have many important functions: they regulate the immune response, produce many lymphokines, are responsible for cell-mediated immunity (such as resistance to intracellular pathogens including certain bacteria, mycobacteria, fungi, viruses, and some parasites), and induce B cells to produce antibody. There are two major subclasses of T cells, each with two subsets. CD4+ cells (formerly called helper or T4 cells) comprise 50% to 65% of circulating T cells; they include helper/inducer T cells, which stimulate the immune response, and helper/suppressor T cells, which downregulate antibody production. CD8+ cells (formerly called suppressor or T8 cells) include suppressor T cells, which inhibit antibody production, and cytotoxic T cells, which lyse antigen-bearing target cells.

B lymphocytes develop in the bone marrow and comprise 5% to 15% of circulating lymphocytes. B lymphocytes undergo a second cycle of differentiation and proliferation when exposed to antigen, becoming nondividing plasma cells which secrete immunoglobulins.

A final group of lymphocytes do not bear the surface markers of T or B cells. These null cells include at least two important subtypes. Natural killer (NK) cells are capable of killing a wide variety of targets without the presence of antibody or prior sensitization; various tumor cells and infectious agents are susceptible to NK cells. Finally, K cells are lymphocytes that can kill targets that have been sensitized by antibody in the antibody-dependent cellular cytotoxicity (ADCC) system.

Current studies of exercise and human immune function have focused the greatest attention on lymphocytes. Because of the complexity of lymphocyte subtypes, it is not surprising that a unified picture has not yet emerged. In addition, immunologic techniques are evolving with particular speed in this area. Changes in technique may explain some of the contradictory results which have been reported over the past two decades. For example, early studies identified B lymphocytes on the basis of surface immunoglobulins or Fc receptors. NK cells can be misidentified as B cells by these criteria, but this would not occur in newer studies, which use monoclonal antibodies to specific surface markers to discriminate among lymphocyte types. Finally, it must be remembered in interpreting these studies that the human investigations examine only changes in peripheral blood lymphocytes, which comprise no more than 10% of man's total lymphocyte pool.

Total lymphocyte counts and lymphocyte subsets at rest are no different in trained athletes than in sedentary control subjects.[2] However, exercise does produce significant changes in lymphocyte trafficking. A lymphocytosis is consistently observed following exercise; the rise in peripheral blood lymphocyte counts is prompt,[3] beginning as early as 3 minutes after exercise is initiated.[4] Whereas strenuous exercise can produce a substantial lymphocytosis, with peak counts often reaching three times control values, the lymphocytosis of exercise is brief. When lymphocyte kinetics have been monitored following the cessation of exercise, baseline levels have been restored in as little as 15 minutes,[5] and counts are almost always normal within 2 hours.

The mechanism of exercise-induced lymphocytosis is unknown. Human studies involving hepatic vein catheterization suggest that splenic and splanchnic lymphoid tissues are not the source.[6] Canine studies suggest that exercise stimulates lymph flow from skeletal muscle, and that this "tissue pump" effect can deliver large numbers of lymphocytes to the circulation very promptly.[7] Increased perfusion of lung may also serve to deliver lymphocytes from tissue sites to the circulation.[8]

In addition to the effects of altered blood flow, hormonal influences may contribute to the lymphocytosis of exercise. Catecholamine and cortisol levels rise with exercise; both hormones can affect lymphocyte trafficking, probably in opposite directions. Beta(β)-adrenergic receptors are present on the lymphocyte cell surface. The level of postexercise lymphocyte counts correlates with serum epinephrine levels, and the effects of exercise are mimicked by adrenergic activity.[9] Physically fit individuals secrete less epinephrine during exercise than do unconditioned people; exercise training appears to blunt the lymphocytes of exercise,[10] perhaps because of adrenergic changes. β-blockade inhibits the acute leukocyte response to exercise,[11] further supporting a role for adrenergic mechanisms. However, β-blockade does not alter the effects of long-term conditioning programs on lymphocyte function,[12] suggesting that other mechanisms contribute as well.

In contrast to epinephrine, cortisone probably acts to limit exercise-induced lymphocytosis. Postexercise lymphocyte counts are not correlated with plasma cortisol levels,[13] and exogenous corticosteroid administration blocks exercise-induced lymphocytosis.[14] Whereas circulating epinephrine and cortisone appear to act in opposite directions on peripheral blood lymphocyte counts, both hormones contribute to the granulocytosis of exercise.[3]

Although exercise can increase all lymphocyte subtypes, not all lymphocyte populations increase to the same degree. B-cell counts are elevated by exercise.[3,15] T-cell counts also increase as a result of exercise. The effect of exercise on T-cell subsets, however, is controversial. Some studies report no important changes in the distribution of T-lymphocyte subsets[16] or in the helper-suppressor ratio.[17] A recent study recorded an elevation in the helper-suppressor ratio due to a decline in suppressor T cells.[3] However, many studies note a decline in the helper-suppressor ratio, generally because exercise produces a greater rise in suppressor T cells than in helper T cells.[2,4,18–20] A fall in the helper-suppressor ratio could have immunosuppressive effects; however, ratios are normalized within 2 hours after the cessation of exercise.[2,4]

Exercise can also affect lymphocyte functions, but here too, the impact is unclear. One study found enhanced blastogenesis[3] whereas another study found blastogenesis to be unchanged following exercise.[21] In contrast, several investigations have reported that lymphocyte blastogenesis in response to mitogens and antigens is suppressed immediately after exercise.[2,13,22] However, suppressed lymphocyte transformation returns to normal levels within 24 hours after the cessation of exercise.[2] In addition, antibody synthesis in athletes is normal, even if the antigenic stimulus is given immediately following the stress of marathon running.[13]

Exercise has important, if transient, effects on non-B non-T lymphocytes.[23] NK-cell counts and NK-cell activity are both increased in highly trained athletes who were tested at rest.[24] Lymphocytes bearing surface markers of NK cells increase in the circulation immediately after exercise;[25,26] in addition to an increase in numbers, enhanced NK-cell activity following exercise has also been observed.[27,28] NK cells appear to have a role in antiviral and antitumor immunity, and this enhanced activity could be protective. However, the exercise-induced changes in NK-cell activity are short-lived: counts of NK cells return to baseline 1 hour after the cessation of exercise.[29] NK activity, which is enhanced immediately after exercise, is depressed below baseline levels 2 hours later, but returns to normal within 24 hours.[30] MacKinnon and co-workers[31] have also reported suppressed NK activity 1 hour after exercise, with recovery by 24 hours.

K-cell activity, as measured by antibody-dependent cellular cytotoxicity, is acutely enhanced by exercise.[6,22,32] The kinetics of K-cell stimulation have been evaluated in only one study; Hanson and Flaherty[32] found that antibody-dependent cellular cytotoxicity remains elevated 24 hours after an 8-mile run, making this the most enduring exercise-induced lymphocyte alteration.

The effects of exercise on lymphocytes are complex, and more studies will be needed to elucidate the details. At present, we can say that alterations in blood and lymph flow and adrenergic stimulation account for the significant, but short-lived lymphocytosis produced by exercise. All lymphocyte classes participate, but suppressor T cells increase more than helper T cells. Lymphocyte mitogenesis is depressed by exercise, but this suppression is brief and long-term lymphocyte function is normal in athletes. Exercise produces a particularly striking increase in null lymphocytes; NK-cell enhancement is brief, but K-cell enhancement may be more durable.

Immunoglobulins

B lymphocytes and their mature derivatives, plasma cells, secrete five classes of immunoglobulins. Three of the five are important in host defense against microbial agents. IgM, the largest immunoglobulin, is produced earliest in response to antigenic challenge. Although IgM antibodies are short-lived, they can help fight infection by agglutinating and lysing gram-negative bacilli and other bacteria. IgG is the principal serum immunoglobulin and is crucial for resistance to bacterial infections. IgG can opsonize bacteria, preparing them for phagocytosis and killing by leukocytes. IgG can also neutralize bacterial toxins and viruses. IgG antibodies are long-lasting. IgA is also present in serum, but it is most important as the predominant immunoglobulin in the body's external secretions, including tears, saliva, and secretions of the respiratory and gastrointestinal tracts. IgA antibodies can block the adherence of organisms to mucosal surfaces, neutralize viruses, and opsonize bacteria.

There have been relatively few studies of the effects of exercise on human serum immunoglobulin levels and antibody formation. Exhaustive physical exercise does not alter serum immunoglobulin concentrations.[19,33–35] The stress of marathon running does not affect the ability to form antibody, even when the antigenic stimulus is administered immediately after exercise.[13] In mice, however, exercise may enhance antibody synthesis.[36] In highly trained human athletes, immunoglobulin levels are normal,[32,34,37] arguing against a long-term adaptation of antibody function in response to repetitive exercise. Strength-trained athletes also have normal serum immunoglobulin levels, but anabolic steroid abuse appears to depress IgA and IgM levels in bodybuilders.[38]

Secretory immunoglobulin levels are affected by exercise. Highly trained Nordic skiers have reduced salivary IgA levels, and these levels decline further after strenuous competition.[15] Highly trained bicyclists, however, have normal levels of secretory IgA as well as normal levels of salivary IgM and IgG.[31] After intense exercise, salivary IgA and IgM concentrations of these athletes fall, but this decline is transient; levels rise within 1 hour after exercise ceases, and normal values are restored within 24 hours.

Lower secretory antibody levels could predispose athletes to infections with organisms that colonize the respiratory tract. However, the decline in salivary antibody levels is transient, except in skiers, whose low levels may be due to cold exposure rather than exercise per se. Interestingly, psychological stress also reduces salivary IgA levels.[39] Moreover, approximately 1 in 650 adults are entirely deficient in IgA; the majority of these individuals are healthy and do not experience an increased incidence of infection. Hence, I believe that exercise-induced alterations in secretory antibody levels are not likely to be functionally significant. There is no evidence that exercise alters serum immunoglobulin concentrations or antibody function.

Complement

At least 20 proteins produced by the liver and by macrophages interact together in the complement system. Present in the circulation as inactive precursor proteins, the complement sequence can be activated by various stimuli, including antigen-antibody complexes and bacterial cell wall components. The activated complement cascade serves many roles in host defense, including bacterial opsonization, bacterial cell wall damage, and leukocyte chemotaxis. Complement is also an important mediator in producing tissue inflammation.

Two investigations have reported that complement levels at rest are normal in highly conditioned athletes.[32,37] In contrast, Nieman and associates[34] observed that 11 marathon runners had lower levels of C3 and C4 than did nine sedentary control subjects, both before and after the acute stress of exercise. However, two studies[32,35] found that post-exercise complement levels are normal, and two others[40,41] reported that intense exertion produced elevations in C3 and C4 levels.

Although studies of exercise and serum complement levels are limited, it seems unlikely that exercise produces clinically important alterations in the complement system.

Polymorphonuclear Leukocytes

Originally derived from pleuripotential stem cells, polymorphonuclear leukocytes differentiate subsequently from myeloid stem cells in the bone marrow. Polymorphonuclear leukocytes are short-lived cells, but they are present in huge numbers in the bone marrow, peripheral blood, and the marginal pool (a reserve of polymorphonuclear leukocytes adherent to the walls of postcapillary venules). Polymorphonuclear leukocytes are crucial to the host defense against bacterial infection.

Perhaps the best-documented effect of exercise on the host-defense network of man is the acute leukocytosis induced by exertion. Larrabee[1] documented a three to five fold increase in blood leukocyte counts in four runners who completed the 1901 Boston Marathon. The leukocytosis was due chiefly to a rise in neutrophils, although lymphocytes also increased. In addition, exertion-induced eosinopenia was documented in these athletes. During the past nine decades, the observations of this early study have been confirmed many times, but we have made relatively little progress in understanding the significance of exertional leukocytosis.

Exercise-induced granulocytosis is an acute response to exertion.[42] Primitive circulating hematopoietic progenitor cells appear in the blood shortly after intense exertion, but their counts return to baseline levels within 15 minutes.[43] The great majority of the leukocytosis of exercise is accounted for by mature granulocytes.[11,13,22,43] Leukocyte counts increase promptly with exercise; granulocyte counts often peak at levels four times above baseline values, and are accompanied by a 30% rise in platelet counts.[44]

Exercise-induced leukocytosis has been observed in both conditioned and unconditioned subjects. Some investigators have reported that training blunts the leukocytosis of exercise,[43] which could be explained by lower postexercise cortisol and catecholamine levels in conditioned athletes. However, many other groups have observed a brisk leukocyte response even in highly conditioned athletes.[13,21,44–46] Indeed, Soppi and colleagues[10] found that exercise produced a leukocytosis both before and after a 6-week physical conditioning program.

The leukocytosis induced by exercise is transient. Immature precursor cells return to baseline levels within 15 minutes,[43] and granulocyte counts are significantly reduced within 45 minutes[5] to 2 hours.[45,46] The return to normal counts continues over the next 12 hours,[44] and counts are fully normal within 24 hours.[47] In fact, during extreme endurance events, granulocyte counts return to baseline values even before exercise is terminated.[45] The resting baseline leukocyte counts in highly conditioned athletes are no different from those of sedentary control subjects.[37] An intense 20-month training program, which converted 78 sedentary men and women into marathon runners, did not change their resting leukocyte counts.[48]

Leukocyte function has been studied less extensively. Exercise has been reported to produce a decrease in neutrophil adherence and bactericidal capacity in conditioned athletes, but not in untrained subjects; exercise increased phagocytic activity of the neutrophils of untrained men, but not of athletes.[46] However, the clinical significance of these changes is unclear, because neutrophil function returned to baseline levels within 2 hours of the cessation of exercise. Indeed, resting neutrophil function is normal in highly trained athletes.[37]

The mechanisms responsible for exercise-induced leukocytosis have not been fully clarified, but five factors probably contribute to this phenomenon. Strenuous exercise rapidly causes significant shifts in extracellular fluids, producing hemoconcentration, which can elevate the concentration of formed elements in the blood.[44] Exercise produces an increase in blood flow to lung and other tissues, which may deliver additional leukocytes to the circulation.[8] Exercise elevates catecholamine levels, and epinephrine in turn mobilizes granulocytes from the marginal pool. Indeed, Ahlborg and Ahlborg[11] found that propranolol blunts the leukocytosis of exercise, suggesting that adrenergic mechanisms do play an important role. Cortisol levels are also increased by exercise; cortisol mobilizes granulocytes from the marrow pool and also slows their egress from the circulation. Finally, exercise increases interleukin-1 (IL-1) levels (see later), and IL-1 can in turn stimulate granulocytosis.

Polymorphonuclear leukocytes are crucial in the host defense against bacterial infection. Within minutes of bacterial invasion, polymorphonuclear leukocytes are mobilized from the circulation to the inflammatory site in a process called chemotaxis. Polymorphonuclear leukocytes ingest bacteria, especially those which have been opsonized by antibody and complement; once phagocytized, many bacteria are promptly killed.

It might be tempting to speculate that the leukocytosis of exercise could help protect athletes from bacterial infection. There is no direct data to answer this question, but I doubt that this is the case. The leukocytosis of exercise is an acute response to physical stress, but it is transient; there is no evidence that regular exercise produces long-term adaptation in polymorphonuclear leukocyte numbers, mobilization, or function.

Mononuclear Phagocytes

Mononuclear phagocytes are of crucial importance in initiating, modulating, and effecting the immune response. Myeloid precursor cells in the bone marrow differentiate into monocytes, which travel through the circulation to the tissues, where they mature into macrophages. The body's 200 billion mononuclear phagocytes have three important immunologic roles: (1) they process antigens and present the essential epitopes to lymphocytes to facilitate the induction of immunity; (2) they are very active secretory cells, producing many biologically important substances such as the cytokines, which modulate the immune response (see IL-1 later), complement components, prostaglandins, and various enzymes; and (3) they are effector cells, which migrate to sites of inflammation and infection less rapidly than polymorphonuclear leukocytes, but nevertheless, they ingest and kill microorganisms. Macrophages can be activated by helper T lymphocytes to enhance their bactericidal capacity, and they are particularly important in defending against intracellular parasites including mycobacteria, fungi, viruses, and certain bacteria and parasites.

The influence of exercise on the mononuclear phagocyte system has been studied only recently, and data is still relatively scant. In murine models, exercise appears to activate peritoneal macrophages, increasing enzyme content and phagocytic activity.[49,50] In man, exercise produces an increase in circulating monocyte counts; counts may rise as much as 87%,[51] but the monocytosis of exercise is transient, lasting less than 2 hours.[46] Exercise also increases monocyte phagocytic activity[52] and metabolic rate,[51] but decreases monocyte adherence in conditioned men.[46] Strenuous exertion increases the sensitivity of circulating human monocytes to in vitro stimulation by lipopolysaccharide.[53] Athletes in training who lose weight due to caloric restriction experience a decrease in monocyte phagocytic activity.[54] However, strenuous exertion increases both phagocytic activity and enzyme content of human tissue macrophages.[54]

The duration of these exercise-induced changes in monocyte function has not been studied. Exercise-induced increases in mononuclear cell secretory activity are transient (see cytokines, next). In contrast, serum concentrations of neopterine (a metabolite of guanosine triphosphate), which reflects macrophage activity, remain elevated for 24 hours after intense exertion.[55]

The clinical impact of exercise-induced changes in monocyte numbers and function is unclear.

Cytokines, Fever, and Hyperthermia

Mononuclear phagocytes are active secretory cells. Among their most important products are cytokines, proteins which travel in the circulation to modulate the activity of leukocytes and other cells. Interleukin-1 (IL-1) is one of the most important of these cytokines. IL-1, a protein of 17,000 daltons, is produced by mononuclear cells (and, in lesser quantities, by many other cells) in response to endotoxin, immune complexes, phagocytosis, and other stimuli (including exercise; see later). IL-1 has three major actions: (1) IL-1 is an immunostimulator, increasing both T-lymphocyte activity and the production of antibody by B lymphocytes; (2) IL-1 mediates the acute phase response that characterizes so many infectious and inflammatory states, including leukocytosis, hepatic synthesis of fibrinogen and other acute phase proteins, fibroblast proliferation and collagen production, and muscle catabolism; and (3) IL-1 produces fever by traveling in the circulation to the thermal control center in the anterior hypothalamus, where it increases prostaglandin levels, thereby resetting the "thermostat" upwards. At least three other cytokines produced by macrophages (tumor necrosis factor, interleukin-6, and interferon γ) are pyrogenic; the inflammatory activities of tumor necrosis factor (TNF) are also very similar to those of IL-1.[56]

IL-1 and TNF produce immunostimulation and inflammation as well as fever. The immunostimulatory activity of IL-1 is in fact increased at elevated temperatures. Although it is tempting to speculate that these events help fight infection, there is still no direct proof that fever is beneficial in fighting infection in man. Quite apart from the immunostimulatory activity of IL-1 and TNF, fever per se may also provide benefit by directly injuring thermolabile microorganisms and by lowering serum iron levels. Whereas fever can enhance recovery from infection in certain experimental animals, the importance of fever in clinical infection in man is uncertain.

Exercise increases IL-1 levels in man. Cannon and Kluger[57] demonstrated that 1 hour of exercise increased serum endogenous pyrogen activity in 14 men. These increased levels were documented immediately after exercise and they persisted for 3 hours. In addition, circulating blood monocytes harvested from five of these subjects immediately after exercise also released endogenous pyrogen after incubation in vitro, whereas monocytes obtained from these men prior to exercise did not. It is now clear that "endogenous pyrogen" is IL-1; indeed elevated IL-1 levels can be demonstrated following exercise.[58] The mechanism by which physical exercise stimulates IL-1 production and release is not known, but it does not appear to depend on mononuclear cell phagocytic activity or on stress-induced increases in epinephrine or cortisone levels.[59] The exercise-induced increase in IL-1 levels is relatively brief; increased levels persist in the circulation for 2 to 6 hours, but are returned to baseline by 9 hours.[4,56]

Exercise also increases circulating TNF levels, but only 8 subjects have been studied, and the elevations were significant only 1 hour after the conclusion of strenuous exercise.[55] The effect of exercise on other cytokines has been studied in even less detail. Exercise has been reported to increase interleukin-2 levels,[60] but other investigators have observed that exercise decreases interleukin-2 levels.[4]

Although the observations of exercised-induced increases in IL-1 and TNF are based on small studies, they provide a potentially important link between exercise and host-defense mechanisms. First, these cytokines are immunostimulators, increasing the activity of both T and B lymphocytes; hence exercise-induced production of IL-1 and TNF might account for the lymphocyte activation reported in other studies (see earlier), and could potentially enhance host-defense mechanisms in athletes. Second, IL-1 and TNF mediate the acute phase response to infection and inflammation; in this capacity, they produce leukocytosis and could therefore be a contributing factor in the leukocytosis of exercise. Finally, these cytokines are pyrogenic; fever can enhance recovery from infection in some experimental animals, but the effects of fever per se on clinical host defense in man remains uncertain. Body temperatures are regularly elevated as a result of intense exercise and sports.[61] However, the hyperthermia of exercise has been regarded as entirely different from the fever of infection in terms of its pathogenesis.[56] In infections and other inflammatory states, IL-1, TNF, and other pyrogenic cytokines act on the anterior hypothalamus to elevate the set-point of the body's "thermostat." Neural control mechanisms then produce vasoconstriction, cessation of sweating, and increased heat production by skeletal muscle until body temperature rises to the new set-point. In contrast, the hypothalamic set-point is unchanged in exercise hyperthermia; body temperature is elevated simply because intense exercise generates heat faster than it can be dissipated by thermal control mechanisms.

Clearly the studies of exercise and pyrogenic cytokine production should lead to a reexamination of this hypothesis. It should be noted that only a modest number of subjects have been studied and that body temperatures were not reported. Hence, I believe that these fascinating observations should be confirmed before we conclude that exercise hyperthermia involves the production of cytokines, much less immunologic enhancement. Indeed, it seems likely that exercise hyperthermia may depend on both excessive heat production by metabolically active skeletal muscle and on pyrogenic cytokine production. The relative importance of these two mechanisms, as well as the possible contribution of each to host-defense mechanisms, will require further study.

Interferons

The interferons are a group of proteins produced by host cells in response to viral infections and other stimuli. In man, interferon α is produced by blood leukocytes and lymphoid cells, interferon β is derived from fibroblasts, and interferon γ is produced by immunologically stimulated helper T lymphocytes. Interferons exert antiviral effects against a broad spectrum of viruses, and also act on tumor cells and various immunologic functions. Indeed, interferon α is now being used therapeutically for certain viral and neoplastic disorders.

Exercise has been reported to increase circulating levels of interferon α.[62] However, only eight men were studied; more importantly, levels rose only from three to seven units, and were restored to baseline values within 3 hours. Because interferon α is produced by leukocytes, this transient increase may simply reflect the leukocytosis of exercise. Unfortunately, Viti and co-workers[62] did not report leukocyte counts in their subjects.

Although these exercise-induced increases in interferon levels are statistically significant, I doubt that they are biologically significant because the magnitude is small and the duration brief. Indeed, viral infections in man produce interferon levels that are 10 to 20 fold higher, and which are sustained for much longer periods.

NONIMMUNOLOGIC HOST-DEFENSE MECHANISMS

Anatomic and Physiologic Barriers

The first line of defense against infection is a series of anatomic and physiologic barriers, which prevent penetration of microorganisms from the environment and from the body's cutaneous and mucosal surfaces into vulnerable body tissues. These are nonimmunologic mechanisms, which do not depend on the recognition of foreign antigens. The intact skin and mucous membranes constitute one such important barrier to infection. The mucus that lines the respiratory epithelium serves to entrap bacteria; enzymes and other substances present in secretions limit bacterial growth; and ciliary action helps expel bacteria and other particulate material. Other examples of nonspecific host-defense mechanisms include the cough and gag reflexes, gastric acidity, intestinal motility, free drainage of body cavities ranging from the paranasal sinuses to the bladder, and intact lymphatic and circulatory networks.

The stress of exercise has only modest effects on certain nonspecific defense mechanisms. Exercise does promote bronchial clearance in man,[63] which could help prevent bronchopulmonary infections; on the other hand, nasal mucus transport is depressed by exercise.[64] Exercise increases intestinal motility;[65] this could help prevent gastroenteritis, but studies to evaluate this possibility have not been performed. Strenuous exercise and sports can result in trauma, which may disrupt the integrity of the cutaneous barrier to infection. This does not seem to be a clinically important problem, but the maceration caused by exercise-induced perspiration can predispose one to annoying superficial fungal infections ("athlete's foot," "jock itch").

Neuroendocrine Factors

Exercise produces many changes in neuroendocrine function. Interestingly, the changes produced by the physical stress of exercise are strikingly similar to the changes produced by psychosocial stress or adversive physiologic stimuli. Aerobic exercise acutely elevates plasma levels of β-endorphins,[66] and endurance training increases this effect.[67] Like other forms of stress, exercise increases plasma catecholamine and glucocorticoid levels. These exercise-induced changes are acute and transient. It is tempting to speculate that changes in neuroendocrine hormones mediate bidirectional interactions between the central nervous system and the immune system[68]; additional study in this area is needed.

EXERCISE, FITNESS, AND SUSCEPTIBILITY TO INFECTION

Exercise produces many alterations in the immune system of humans. Some of these changes tend to enhance immune function, whereas others tend to depress host-defense mechanisms. Most of the immunologic effects of exercise, whether immunoenhancing or immunosuppressive, are relatively modest in magnitude and very brief in duration. Do these changes produce clinically important results?

Unfortunately, relatively little data is available in this important area. Investigations of the immunology of infection are numerous and depend on sophisticated in vitro assays. In contrast, investigation of clinical infections in people who exercise are few in number and depend on relatively crude epidemiologic observations.

Four small studies suggest that athletes may be more vulnerable to infection of the respiratory tract. In an abstract published in 1978, Douglas and Hanson[69] reported that upper respiratory tract infection symptoms were more common in members of a college crew team than in their unconditioned classmates; however, there was no difference in fever or in overall absenteeism. An abstract published in 1988 reported more "infectious" symptoms in subjects in heavy training for the Los Angeles Marathon[70]; however, there were no control subjects, and the symptoms were retrospectively self-reported without criteria to separate bona fide infections from fatigue and overtraining. However, Peters and Bateman[71] did find an increased incidence of upper respiratory tract symptoms in ultramarathoners who were compared with age-matched sedentary household contacts. The upper respiratory tract symptoms were mild and were confined to the 2 weeks following a 56-km road race. Finally, Linde[72] reported more self-diagnosed upper respiratory symptoms in 44 elite Danish orienteers who were compared with age-matched sedentary control subjects over a 1-year period. But here too, the differences were slight.

The athletes experienced 2.5 infections per year, whereas the controls reported 1.7 episodes, and there were no differences in the duration or severity of the infections.

Whereas these four investigations suggest an increased risk of respiratory infections in people who exercise, two other studies do not support these conclusions. Osterback and Ovarnberg[73] prospectively studied 62 adolescent athletes and 75 age-matched control subjects. Over the course of 1 year, there was no difference in respiratory infections or school absences. Most recently, a retrospective study of 199 young adults in Finland found no correlation between respiratory infections and physical activity or maximal aerobic power.[74]

Many athletes insist that exercise has promoted their "resistance" to infections. Other anecdotes blame exercise for an enhanced vulnerability to infection. Unfortunately, objective data on this question are limited, and they are also divided. Even granting the small sizes and methodologic limitations of these studies, however, I think it is quite unlikely that habitual physical activity exerts a clinically important influence in the incidence or severity of clinical infections.

EXERCISE AND CANCER: DOES THE IMMUNE SYSTEM PLAY A ROLE?

One of the major roles of the immune system of humans is to identify and contain invading infectious agents; the other major role is the detection and destruction of tumor cells. Do the immunologic effects of exercise affect neoplastic diseases?

Habitual exercise enhances longevity; the major reason for this is the decreased incidence of cardiovascular disease in people who exercise. However, a recent study documents that people of both sexes who exercise also have a significant decrease in mortality due to cancer.[75] Women who are former college athletes have a lower risk of developing cancer of all noncutaneous sites than do sedentary women.[76] It is far from clear, however, that these exercise-related benefits depend on immunologic mechanisms.

Four independent studies in five different population groups have reported a reduced risk of colon cancer in physically active people. The earliest American study[77] evaluated 2950 cases of colon cancer in California men. Physical activity was assessed by occupation. Men with sedentary jobs were found to have a colon cancer risk 1.6 times greater than men with physically active jobs; moreover, the cancer risk increased in a stepwise manner as activity level decreased. A second study[78] examined the risk for colon cancer in 1.1 million Swedish men during a 19-year follow-up. Sedentary work increased the risk of colon cancer 1.3 times. A third study[79] evaluated 430,000 men and 25,000 women in Washington state; the risk of colon cancer increased progressively with decreased physical activity as measured by occupation. These same investigators also performed a case-control investigation of men treated for colon cancer in Buffalo, New York. Again, the most active people had the lowest risk of colon cancer. A smaller European case-control study[80] reported similar findings.

Although these studies are impressive, we should note that they are all limited by their reliance on job description as an index of physical activity. This technique has been validated in studies of exercise and cardiovascular disease and should be valid for cancer studies as well. Even so, studies evaluating leisure-time exercise and colon cancer risk will be of interest. In addition, although these studies were well controlled for race, age, and socioeconomic class, careful controls for diet and family history are lacking. Finally, excellent studies of exercise and mortality in college alumni and longshoremen did not report a decreased colon cancer risk in physically active people.[81] Clearly, more studies will be required to resolve these disparities.

Although fewer studies have examined the relationship between exercise and female breast and reproductive tract cancers, the magnitude of protection conferred by exercise is even more impressive. Frisch and associates[82] evaluated the lifetime risk of these cancers in 5398 college alumnae as a function of college athleticism. Women who were sedentary during their college years experienced a 2.5 times greater risk of reproductive cancers and a 1.8 times greater risk of breast cancer when compared with college athletes. The Washington State study[79] also reported a decreased risk of breast cancer in women with physically active jobs, but did not evaluate reproductive tract cancers. Once again, however, another study[81] did not note a protective effect of exercise on breast and reproductive cancers, emphasizing the need for further study.

Even if we accept that exercise helps protect against colon, breast, and reproductive cancers, does this protection depend on immunologic mechanisms? Probably not. These cancers are not among the neoplasia that are dramatically increased in immunosuppressed individuals. Exercise may protect against colon cancer by decreasing intestinal transit time.[81] In the case of female breast and reproductive cancers, the mechanism of protection may be hormonal, depending on decreased estrogenic stimulation of these end organs. Clearly, additional studies will be required to evaluate the mechanisms by which exercise protects against neoplasia; at present, I believe that this protection is nonimmunologic.

EXERCISE AND SPORTS IN PATIENTS WITH INFECTIONS

Exercise affects many components of the human immune system, but the alterations which result are modest in magnitude, variable in direction, and brief in duration. Not surprisingly, the few epidemiologic studies that are currently available fail to demonstrate a consistent effect of exercise on the risk of acquiring an infectious illness. Although the in vitro immunologic data is not yet directly applicable to clinical situations, and the epidemiologic data is scant and inconclusive, the clinician is still faced with the need to provide practical advice for athletes who acquire infectious illnesses.

Rest is a time-honored part of the treatment regimen for patients who are infected. Indeed, traditional bedside observation suggests that physical activity can worsen certain infections; polio, now rare in the United States, is a classic example.[83] For other infections, unfortunately, controlled data to support standard clinical practice is lacking. Whereas rest would seem the prudent recommendation for most serious acute infections, unnecessarily prolonged rest can produce deconditioning, resulting in adverse physiologic and functional consequences.[61] Moreover, people who exercise habitually are characteristically reluctant to accept blanket admonitions against exercise. Hence, we should strive to individualize our recommendations, prescribing rest when necessary and exercise when possible. Such recommendations should be based on controlled trials when available, or on animal models and clinical observations when more precise data are lacking.

To aid in the practical management of athletes with infections, we can subdivide these infections into acute and chronic processes, which may be localized or systemic in extent, and viral or bacterial in etiology.

Acute Infections

Localized viral infections are the most common infections encountered in clinical sports medicine. By far, the most common of these is the viral *upper respiratory tract infection* (URI). These infections are frequent because they can be caused by so many viral strains that immunity does not develop. For example, more than 110 serotypes of rhinovirus can cause URIs. Person-to-person transmission by aerosol route or direct contact, and the close living conditions which prevail during the winter months in temperate climates also contribute to the frequency of these events. Athletes who belong to teams, particularly when they are housed in the same living quarters, are particularly likely to pass respiratory viruses back and forth to each other. However, despite numerous admonitions by the mothers of America, exposure to cold temperature, damp environments, or drafts does not seem to enhance vulnerability to the URI[84]; hence, athletes who participate in winter sports are not at increased risk.

The symptoms of the URI are familiar to all physicians, and are no different in athletes than in sedentary people. The overwhelming majority of those processes are brief and self-limited, although more serious bacterial infections may sometimes supervene. Management is strictly symptomatic. However, a word of caution regarding the use of cold remedies by athletes may be in order. Many of these over-the-counter preparations contain sympathomimetic amines that can cause tachycardia and might disqualify athletes from certain high-level competitive events. On occasion, mycoplasmal or chlamydial species can produce illnesses similar to the viral URI. These organisms respond to erythromycin or tetracyclines, but specific diagnosis is very difficult in the clinical setting, and antibiotics are rarely indicated in patients with URI symptoms.

Mild-to-moderate URIs do not ordinarily require interruption of exercise schedules. In fact, some athletes report an amelioration of symptoms with exercise, possibly because of the increased mucus flow that results from physical activity.

Viruses can also cause acute *lower respiratory tract infections*. In clinical terms, cough and possibly dyspnea will be present instead of, or in addition to, the coryza and congestion that characterize the URI. Lower respiratory tract infections may produce bronchospasm, which can be further exacerbated by exercise, especially in cold, dry ambient air. Hence, it would seem prudent to advise athletes with lower respiratory tract symptoms to avoid strenuous exercise until they have recovered.

Gastroenteritis is another localized acute viral infection that produces similar manifestations in athlete and nonathlete alike. Mild-to-moderate cases call for symptomatic treatment only, and exercise can be continued as symptoms permit. But in more severe cases, dehydration and electrolyte imbalance can impair athletic performance; more importantly, exercise might precipitate cardiovascular abnormalities in such patients. Hence, exercise should be restricted until gastrointestinal motility is normal and fluids and electrolytes have been replaced.

Whereas localized viral infections of the upper and lower respiratory tracts and gastrointestinal tract are not characteristically related to exercise, a final localized viral infection is linked to sports participation: herpes gladiatorum.[85] Because this infection involves direct skin-to-skin transmission of herpes simplex virus 1, it is most common in wrestlers, occurring in about 3% of all high-school wrestlers. Vesicular lesions of the head and neck are most common, but autoinoculation can spread the virus to other cutaneous sites as well. Ocular involvement may be manifested as conjunctivitis, keratitis, or blepharitis. Initial infection in nonimmune individuals commonly results in lymphadenopathy, fever, and malaise as well as vesicular skin lesions. Recurrences usually appear as vesicles or "cold sores" without systemic manifestations. Oral acyclovir, 200 mg 5 times daily, appears to shorten the course of the episode, although controlled observations are lacking. Athletes should be prohibited from participation in contact sports until their lesions have dried and crusted. Herpes gladiatorum can be prevented by screening athletes for suspicious skin lesions and preventing participation when lesions are identified.

Systemic acute viral infections are less common in athletes than are localized infections, but they are potentially more hazardous. Animal data suggest that exercise during experimental systemic infections with cardiotoxic viruses may increase the risk of acute myocarditis and late myocardiopathy. Weanling mice that are forced to swim vigorously in heated water during the acute phase of infection with virulent coxsackievirus B3 develop myocardial inflammation, dilatation, and necrosis.[86] Viral titers are 500 times higher than in sedentary control animals. Half the exercised animals die in pulmonary edema, and survivors have an increased risk of dilated cardiomyopathy. In a similar murine model, treadmill running increased the severity of myocarditis in adult mice infected with coxsackievirus B3, but exercise did not increase mortality in these animals.[87] Even during infection with less virulent coxsackievirus A9, swimming produced reversible myocarditis in adult mice.[88]

The relevance of this murine model to human exercise is unclear. Myocarditis is uncommon as a cause of sudden death in athletes. However, myocarditis is a recognized cause of sudden death in physically active military recruits.[89] In addition, a recent prospective study of 32 young adults with various systemic viral infections revealed subtle electrocardiographic and echocardiographic abnormalities in some patients despite normal physical examinations and the absence of cardiac symptoms.[90]

Additional observations of exercise and systemic infections in humans would be scientifically desirable. However, the limited experimental and clinical data that are available can justify practical guidelines for athletes with systemic infections. Athletes should avoid strenuous exercise in the presence of fever, myalgias, and other systemic symptoms. Rest should be the rule during the acute phases of influenza and other systemic viral infections, but if symptoms permit, gentle stretching exercises would seem safe substitute activities for the committed athlete who is reluctant to eschew all exercise. After acute systemic symptoms abate, training can resume in a gradual, graded fashion. As a rule of thumb, I generally ask the convalescing athlete to build up slowly, allowing 2 days of reduced intensity exercise for each day of rest during the preceding acute illness.

If data on exercise during viral infections are scant, data on exercise during *bacterial infections* are nearly nonexistent. In an experimental model, exercise promoted the recovery of mice infected with *Salmonella typhimurium*.[91] Nevertheless, it seems prudent to use the same guidelines for bacterial infections as for viral processes. In mild, localized infections, such as pharyngitis or cystitis, modest exercise schedules can be maintained. Even so, athletes with mild or localized infections should be instructed to "listen to their bodies," and to rest when fatigue or other warning symptoms appear. In cases of more severe bacterial infections, such as pneumonitis or pyelonephritis, rest should be the rule until recovery is well underway.

The only bacterial infections that can be directly linked to exercise are *skin infections*. Trauma is the major offender: abrasions or puncture wounds occurring during sports allow the direct inoculation of microorganisms. Mild, localized skin and soft tissue infections can be managed by elevation of the affected limb, warm soaks, and orally administered antibotics; abscesses require surgical drainage rather than antibiotics. Deeper infections, such as cellulitis and lymphangitis, require parenteral antibiotics, rest, and elevation; clearly, exercise is not possible until healing occurs.

Even in the absence of trauma, moisture and maceration produced by perspiration can predispose the individual to infections with bacteria or fungi. The latter are more common; the organisms responsible are superficial dermatophytes. Because these molds do not live free in nature but are spread from person to person, shared locker-room facilities play an epidemiologic role in the spread of these infections. Although these processes can be unsightly and uncomfortable, they are confined to the superficial layers of the epidermis and are rarely serious. However, they can be a focus for secondary bacterial infection and should therefore be treated promptly.

Because infection with superficial dermatophytes is so common in athletes, several varieties pay tribute to the athlete in their common names. Tinea cruris is an infection of the inguinal region which is also known as "jock itch." Tinea pedis involves the interdigital areas of the foot and is called "athlete's foot." Both of these processes respond promptly to topical antimycotic agents such as tolnaftate, miconazole, or clotrimazole. Rarely, refractory cases may require oral therapy with ketoconazole. Meticulous drying is very important in preventing and treating these processes as well.

Subacute and Chronic Infections

Whereas modified exercise schedules can generally be permitted in localized or mild acute infections, systemic acute infection should generally be managed with rest. In certain subacute or chronic systemic infections, however, the situation is a bit different. The major infections in this category are viral hepatitis and infectious mononucleosis. Bed rest is the classic treatment for both; whereas rest is surely appropriate during the acute phases of both illnesses, the available data do not support the traditional approach of prolonged rest even during the convalescent stages of these processes.

In the case of *viral hepatitis,* Chalmers and co-workers[92] demonstrated in 1955 that bed rest does not enhance recovery. In their careful study, soldiers who were allowed free activity recovered as quickly as did men who were confined to bed. More recent studies have gone one step further. In small European trials of exercise conditioning,[93,94] it has been shown that aerobic training does not impair recovery from hepatitis. Even in chronic active hepatitis, exercise training does not adversely affect liver function tests; work capacity improves, as does the patient's subjective well-being.[95]

Infectious mononucleosis is a more common problem facing the sports medicine practitioner. In 1964, Dalrymple[96] studied Harvard college students with infectious mononucleosis. One hundred thirty-one consecutive patients were randomly assigned to strict bed rest or to unrestricted activity schedules, limited only by symptoms. The results fly in the face of traditional management: the students randomized to activity actually recovered more rapidly than did the students treated with bed rest.

Infectious mononucleosis is very common in high-school and college athletes. Even the most committed athlete will not feel like exercising strenuously when fever, pharyngitis, lymphadenopathy, and fatigue are present. Indeed, it seems prudent to caution against such exercise when mononucleosis is acute or severe. However, in my practice, I permit ordinary daily activities to the limits of tolerance even in the early stages of mononucleosis.

As patients recover from mononucleosis, fever and pharyngitis resolve, but fatigue often persists. Lingering fatigue is often treated with additional bed rest. In my view, this is counterproductive; rest produces cardiovascular deconditioning, which in turn contributes to fatigue. A self-perpetuating cycle can persist, which can even lead to rather prolonged invalidism. Indeed, I suspect that "chronic mononucleosis" is not due to persistent active infection with Epstein-Barr virus, but is due to functional derangements, including deconditioning. In my experience, gradual exercise training (sometimes in conjunction with small doses of amitriptyline) has been helpful for these patients.

How soon can the athlete with mononucleosis return to sports? Exercise should be postponed until fever and other acute symptoms have resolved. Although the guidelines for return to sports must be individualized, training can be resumed in about 3 weeks in many cases. But exercise should begin at a modest level and should progress only in a graded fashion, allowing perhaps 2 days of rehabilitation for each day of rest during the acute illness.

Because many patients with mononucleosis develop splenomegaly, contact sports represent a special problem. To minimize the risk of splenic rupture, contact sports should be prohibited until splenomegaly has resolved. This is true also for noncontact sports, which may nevertheless produce abdominal trauma; diving is an example. Abdominal ultrasonography can be used to monitor spleen size.

The Effects of Infection on Athletic Performance

Thus far I have considered only the ways in which exercise affects recovery from infections. But for the athlete, the converse of this question is also important: how does infection affect athletic performance?

Despite the paucity of detailed data here, I see no reason to doubt the widespread anecdotal observations of athletes, coaches, and team physicians: infections do indeed impair performance. In fact, the experimental and clinical studies that are available support clinical lore.[97,98] In general, more serious infections will produce more deleterious effects on performance, but athletes participating at high levels often note impairment with mild or moderate infections. Clearly, athletes with constitutional symptoms should not be allowed to participate in competition. Even strenuous training should be discouraged because optimal form cannot be expected. In addition, impaired concentration, coordination, endurance, and strength could lead to musculoskeletal injuries in these circumstances.

IMMUNIZATIONS FOR ATHLETES

It is a truism that prevention is always the best form of medical treatment. Fortunately, many infectious diseases can be prevented by immunization. Although the guidelines for immunizations in athletes are basically similar to the guidelines for sedentary people,[99] a few specifics deserve emphasis.

Tetanus immunizations should be kept up to date in all adults. Because of the risk of trauma, this is particularly important for athletes. A Td booster every 10 years will maintain immunity following a primary series. Traumatic wounds that occur in athletes who are not fully immunized should be managed according to the guidelines in Table 6–1.

Influenza immunizations are not ordinarily indicated in healthy athletes. However, athletes can be offered influenza vaccination if supplies are adequate to meet first the needs of people who are elderly, chronically ill, or providers of medical and essential community services. This immunization may be particularly helpful for athletes who play fall and winter sports because close contact among team members can result in rapid spread of influenza, which can disrupt an entire season. Influenza vaccine should not be administered to people who are allergic to eggs.

Measles vaccination is of unique importance for young athletes. Despite the availability of an excellent attenuated vaccine, the incidence of measles is increasing rapidly in the United States. Although still a far cry from the 500,000 cases that occurred annually in the prevaccine era, it is worrisome that the incidence of measles has increased from a low of 1497 reported cases in 1983 to more than 17,000 cases in 1989. The majority of these cases are in young patients, either in children who have not received their recommended immunization or in college-age individuals whose immunity has waned.

Quite apart from the medical consequences for the individuals involved, measles outbreaks can have a deleterious effect on team sports. For example, the University of Maine hockey team was forced to abandon participation in the 1990 Hockeyfest Tournament at the Boston Garden because of an outbreak of measles in students at the University.

Individuals born before 1957 can be considered immune to measles by virtue of natural infection. Younger individuals should receive live attenuated measles vaccine if (1)

TABLE 6–1. SUMMARY GUIDE TO TETANUS PROPHYLAXIS IN ROUTINE WOUND MANAGEMENT—UNITED STATES

History of Adsorbed Tetanus Toxoid (Doses)	Clean, Minor Wounds		All Other Wounds*	
	Td†	*TIG*	*Td†*	*TIG*
Unknown or <3	Yes	No	Yes	Yes
≥3‡	No§	No	No‖	No

*Such as, but not limited to, wounds contaminated with dirt, feces, soil, saliva, etc; puncture wounds; avulsions; and wounds resulting from missiles, crushing, burns, and frostbite.

†For children under 7 years old, DTP (DT, if pertussis vaccine is contraindicated) is preferred to tetanus toxoid alone. For persons 7 years old and older, Td is preferred to tetanus toxoid alone.

‡If only three doses of *fluid* toxoid have been received, a fourth dose of toxoid, preferably an adsorbed toxoid, should be given.

§Yes, if more than 10 years since last dose.

‖Yes, if more than 5 years since last dose. (More frequent boosters are not needed and can accentuate side effects.)

Abbreviations: Td = tetanus-diphtheria toxoid, adult type; TIG = tetanus immune globulin; DT = diphtheria-tetanus; DTP = diphtheria-tetanus-pertussis.

From Morbidity and Mortality Weekly Reports 34:405, 1986; with permission.

they received only the older, less potent inactivated vaccine which was in use between 1963 and 1967; (2) they received measles vaccine before 15 months of age; or (3) they received measles vaccine before 1980.

SUMMARY

Exercise produces direct effects on the immune network of humans. These effects have been documented by in vitro studies of leukocytes and serum proteins in blood samples from people who exercise.

The response of human lymphocytes to the stress of exercise has been studied in detail. Exercise produces a substantial rise in blood lymphocyte counts, but this lymphocytosis is transient, with the return of normal counts within 2 hours after the conclusion of exercise. Counts of all lymphocyte types increase due to exercise, but T cells and non-B non-T cells increase more than B cells. Among T cells, suppressor cells rise more than helper cells; however, the depressed helper-suppressor ratio that results is rapidly restored to normal after exercise ceases. Similarly, although exercise produces a depression in lymphocyte transformation, this too is transient. Exercise increases NK cell and K counts and activity. The exercise-induced changes in NK cells are brief, but K-cell stimulation after exercise may persist for 24 hours or longer.

Serum immunoglobulin levels are not altered by exercise, nor is antibody synthesis. However, secretory immunoglobulin levels are altered by physical exertion. After intense exercise, salivary IgA and IgM levels fall. However, this decline is transient, except that secretory IgA levels remain depressed in highly trained athletes who exercise in cold weather.

Although studies of serum complement and exercise are limited, there is at present no evidence that complement levels or function are significantly altered by exercise.

Exercise produces an acute polymorphonuclear leukocytosis in humans. Exercise-induced leukocytosis was first documented in 1902, and has been confirmed many times in subsequent years. Polymorphonuclear leukocyte counts may rise three times or more above baseline values, but they return to normal promptly after exercise is terminated. Polymorphonuclear cell function is not affected by exercise.

Studies of mononuclear phagocytes and exercise are much more limited. In murine models, exercise appears to activate macrophages. In humans, exercise produces a transient rise in blood monocyte counts. Monocyte phagocytic activity and metabolic rate are also elevated, but monocyte adherence is depressed. Mononuclear cell secretory activity, as measured by IL-1 and TNF production, is increased following exercise.

Exercise increases serum IL-1 levels in humans; this elevation persists for less than 9 hours. TNF levels are also elevated, but for only 1 hour after the cessation of exercise. Other cytokines have been studied in even less detail. IL-2 levels have been reported to increase or to decrease.

Although exercise appears to increase serum interferon α levels, this increase is small in magnitude and brief in duration.

Exercise produces acute elevations in blood levels of neuroendocrine hormones, including β-endorphins, catecholamines, and glucocorticoids. These changes resemble the effects of psychosocial stress; in both situations, changes in neuropeptides, endorphins, and corticosteroids may affect the immune system.

The effects of exercise on immune function can perhaps be understood best in the context of the feedback loops that modulate human immune mechanisms. The immune network is regulated by an elegant series of homeostatic controls that are designed to balance immune function, avoiding both immunologic deficiencies and hyperactivity. The stress of exercise disturbs the status quo, and produces many alterations in immune function. Eventually, however, counterregulatory control mechanisms prevail; within minutes to hours after exercise ceases, most immune functions are back to normal. In this respect, the immune mechanisms of humans respond to exercise as do lung, kidney, and intestinal organs, with short-term responses but not long-term adaptations. We know that repeated exercise produces both short-term responses and long-term adaptation in other human systems, including cardiac and skeletal muscle, bone, and certain metabolic and endocrine functions. Further study will be required to learn if the transient immunologic responses to the stress of exercise can summate and result in biologically important phenomena.

Although exercise has many effects on immune mechanisms, the functional importance of these changes is uncertain. Whereas significant exercise-induced immune alterations can be demonstrated by in vitro assay systems, there are persently no in vivo studies which demonstrate that these changes are biologically meaningful. Preliminary epidemiologic studies suggest that exercise reduces the risk of bowel cancer in men and of breast and reproductive tract cancer in women, but this protection probably depends on nonimmunologic mechanisms. Similarly, there is no evidence that physical activity substantially alters susceptibility to infections.

Exercise may produce adverse effects in patients with certain systemic viral infections, such as polio and possibly infections with viruses that have cardiotoxic potential. Hence, rest should be advised in the management of acute systemic infections. However, symptom-limited modified exercise schedules can be permitted in athletes with infections that are mild and localized. In contrast, traditional concerns that physical activity may harm patients with mononucleosis or hepatitis do not appear warranted. A gradual return to activity should be encouraged after the acute phase of these infections has subsided.

Immunizations should be administered to athletes just as they are to other people. Tetanus and measles immunizations warrant special attention.

Professor J. N. Morris, a pioneer in the study of exercise and health, has concluded that "vigorous exercise is a natural defense of the body, with a protective effect on the aging heart against ischemia and its consequences."[100] Until further studies become available, we are unable to conclude that exercise has a similar protective effect on the body's natural defense against infection.

REFERENCES

1. Larrabee RC: Leucocytosis after violent exercise. J Med Res 7:76–82, 1902.
2. Oshida Y, Yamanouchi K, Hayamizu S, et al: Effect of acute physical exercise on lymphocyte subpopulations in trained and untrained subjects. Int J Sports Med 9:137–140, 1988.
3. Nieman DC, Berk LS, Simpson-Westerberg K, et al: Effects of long-endurance running on immune system parameters and lymphocyte function in experienced marathoners. Int J Sports Med 10:317–323, 1989.
4. Lewicki R, Tchorzewski H, Majewska E, et al: Effect of maximal physical exercise on T-lymphocyte subpopulations and on interleukin 1 (IL-1) and interleukin 2 (IL-2) production in vitro. Int J Sports Med 9:114–117, 1988.
5. Robertson AJ, Ramesar KCRB, Potts RC, et al: The effect of strenuous physical exercise on circulating blood lymphocytes and serum cortisol levels. J Clin Lab Immunol 5:53–57, 1981.
6. Hedfors E, Biberfeld P, Wahren J: Mobilization of the blood of human non-T and K lymphocytes during physical exercise. J Clin Lab Immunol 1:159–162, 1978.
7. Lindena J, Kupper W, Trautschold I: Enzyme activities in thoracic duct lymph and plasma of anaesthetized, conscious resting and exercising dogs. Eur J Applied Physiol 52:188–195, 1984.
8. Muir AL, Cruz M, Martin BA, et al: Leukocyte kinetics in the human lung: Role of exercise and catecholamines. J Applied Physiol 57:711–718, 1984.
9. Landmann MA, Muller FB, Perini CH, et al: Changes of immunoregulatory cells induced by psychological and physical stress: Relationship to plasma catecholamines. Clin Exp Immunol 58:127–135, 1984.
10. Soppi E, Varjo P, Eskola J, et al: Effect of strenuous physical stress on circulating lymphocyte number and function before and after training. J Clin Lab Immunol 8:43–46, 1982.
11. Ahlborg B, Ahlborg G: Exercise leukocytosis with and without beta-adrenergic blockade. Acta Med Scand 187:241–246, 1970.
12. Watson RR, Moriguchi S, Jackson JC, et al: Modification of cellular immune functions in humans by endurance exercise training during β-adrenergic blockade with atenolol or propranolol. Med Sci Sports Exerc 18:95–100, 1986.
13. Eskola J, Ruuskanen AO, Soppi MK, et al: Effect of sport stress on lymphocyte transformation and antibody formation. Clin Exp Immunol 32:339–345, 1978.
14. Yu DTY, Clements PJ, Pearson CM: Effect of corticosteroids on exercise-induced lymphocytosis. Clin Exp Immunol 28:326–331, 1977.
15. Tomasi TB, Trudeau FB, Czerwinski D, et al: Immune parameters in athletes before and after strenuous exercise. J Clin Immunol 2:173–178, 1982.
16. Gmunder FK, Lorenzi G, Bechler B, et al: Effect of long-term physical exercise on lymphocyte reactivity: Similarity to spaceflight reactions. Aviat Space Environ Med 59:146–151, 1988.
17. Kanonchoff AD, Cavanaugh DJ, Mehl VL, et al: Changes in lymphocyte subpopulations during acute exercise [abstract]. Med Sci Sports Exerc 16:175, 1984.
18. Berk LS, Tan SA, Nieman DC, et al: The suppressive effect of stress from acute exhaustive exercise on T-lymphocyte helper 1 suppressor cell ratio in athletes and non-athletes [abstract]. Med Sci Sports Exerc 17:492, 1985.
19. Berk LS, Nieman DC, Tan SA, et al: Complement and immunoglobulin levels in athletes vs sedentary controls [abstract]. Med Sci Sports Exerc 20:519, 1988.
20. Tchorzewski H, Lewicki R, Majewska E: Changes in the helper and suppressor lymphocytes in human peripheral blood following maximal physical exercise. Arch Immunol Ther Exp 35:307–312, 1987.
21. Moorthy AV, Zimmerman SW: Human leukocyte response to an endurance race. Eur J Applied Physiol 38:271–276, 1978.
22. Hedfors E, Holm G, Ohnell B: Variations of blood lymphocytes during work studied by cell surface markers, DNA synthesis and cytotoxicity. Clin Exp Immunol 24:328–335, 1976.
23. MacKinnon LT: Exercise and natural killer cells: What is the relationship? Sports Med 7:141–149, 1989.
24. Pedersen BK, Tvede N, Christensen LD, et al: Natural killer cell activity in peripheral blood of highly trained and untrained persons. Int J Sports Med 10:129–131, 1989.
25. Berk LS, Nieman D, Tan SA, et al: Lymphocyte subset changes during acute maximal exercise [abstract]. Med Sci Sports Exerc 18:706, 1986.
26. Fiatarone MA, Morley JE, Bloom ET, et al: The effect of exercise on natural killer cell activity in young and old subjects. J Gerontol 44:M37–45, 1989.
27. Targan S, Britvan L, Dorey F: Activation of human NKCC by moderate exercise: Increased frequency of

NK cells with enhanced capability of effector-target lytic interactions. Clin Exp Immunol 45:352–360, 1981.

28. Edwards AJ, Bacon TH, Elms CA, et al: Changes in the populations of lymphoid cells in human peripheral blood following physical exercise. Clin Exp Immunol 58:420–427, 1984.
29. Deuster PA, Curiale AM, Cowan ML, et al: Exercise-induced changes in populations of peripheral blood mononuclear cells. Med Sci Sports Exerc 20:276–280, 1988.
30. Pederson BK, Tvede N, Hansen FR, et al: Modulation of natural killer cell activity in peripheral blood by physical exercise. Scand J Immunol 27:673–678, 1988.
31. MacKinnon LT, Chick TW, van As A, et al: The effect of exercise on secretory and natural immunity. Adv Exp Med Biol 216A:869–876, 1987.
32. Hanson PG, Flaherty DK: Immunological responses to training in conditioned runners. Clin Sci 60:225–228, 1981.
33. Poortmans JR: Serum protein determination during short exhaustive physical activity. J Appl Physiol 30:190–192, 1971.
34. Nieman DC, Tan SA, Lee W, et al: Complement and immunoglobulin levels in athletes and sedentary controls. Int J Sports Med 10:124–128, 1989.
35. Sawka MN, Young AJ, Dennis RC, et al: Human intravascular immunoglobulin responses to exercise-heat and hypohydration. Aviat Space Environ Med 60:634–638, 1989.
36. Liu YG, Wang SY: The enhancing effect of exercise on the production of antibody to *Salmonella typhi* in mice. Immunol Lett 14:117–120, 1986–1987.
37. Green RL, Kaplan SS, Rabin BS, et al: Immune function in marathon runners. Ann Allergy 47:73–75, 1981.
38. Calabrese LH, Kleiner SM, Barna BP, et al: The effects of anabolic steroids and strength training on the human immune response. Med Sci Sports Exerc 21:386–392, 1989.
39. Jemmott JB III, Borysenko M, Chapman R, et al: Academic stress, power motivation, and decrease in secretion rate of salivary secretory immunoglobulin A. Lancet 1:1400–1402, 1983.
40. Dufaux B, Hoffken K, Hollman W: Acute phase proteins and immune complexes during several days at severe physical exercise. *In* Knultgen HG (ed): Biochemistry of Exercise. Champaign, I1, Human Kinetics, 1983, pp 356–362.
41. Dufaux B, Order U: Complement activation after prolonged exercise. Clin Chim Acta 179:45–50, 1989.
42. McCarthy DA, Dale MM: The leucocytosis of exercise: A review and model. Sports Med 6:333–363, 1988.
43. Busse WW, Anderson CL, Hanson PG, et al: The effect of exercise on the granulocyte response to isoproterenol in the trained athlete and unconditioned individual. J Allergy Clin Immunol 65:358–364, 1980.
44. Davidson RJL, Robertson JD, Galea G, et al: Hematological changes associated with marathon running. Int J Sports Med 8:19–25, 1987.
45. Galun E, Burnstein R, Assia E, et al: Changes of white blood cell count during prolonged exercise. Int J Sports Med 8:253–255, 1987.
46. Lewicki R, Tchorzewski H, Denys A, et al: Effect of physical exercise on some parameters of immunity in conditioned sportsmen. Int J Sports Med 8:309–314, 1987.
47. Wells CL, Stern JR, Hecht LH: Hematological changes following a marathon race in male and female runners. Eur J Applied Physiol 48:1–49, 1982.
48. Janssen GME, van Wersch JWJ, Does RJMM: White cell system changes associated with a training period of 18–20 months: A transverse and a longitudinal approach. Int J Sports Med 10:S176–S180, 1989.
49. Fehr HG, Lotzerich H, Michna H: The influence of physical exercise on peritoneal macrophage functions: Histochemical and phagocytic studies. Int J Sports Med 9:77–81, 1988.
50. Voronina NP, Maianskiĭ DN: Functional rearrangements in macrophages following intensive physical exercise. Biull Eksp Biol Med 104:207–209, 1987.
51. Bieger WP, Weiss M, Michel G, et al: Exercise-induced monocytosis and modulation of monocyte function. Int J Sports Med 1:30–36, 1980.
52. Koliada TI, Abzaeva LN, Baboshko IuA: Effect of exposure to physical loading, hypoxia, and hyperthermia on the cellular and anti-infection resistance factors of the body. Zh Mikrobiol Epidemiol Immunobiol 2:76–79, 1988.
53. Osterud B, Olsen JO, Wilsgard L: Effect of strenuous exercise on blood monocytes and their relation to coagulation. Med Sci Sports Exerc 21:374–378, 1989.
54. Kono I, Kitao H, Matsuda M, et al: Weight reduction in athletes may adversely affect the phagocytic function of monocytes. Physician Sports Med 16:56–65, 1988.
55. Fehr HG, Lotzerich H, Michna H: Human function and physical exercise: Phagocytic and histochemical studies. Eur J Applied Physiol 58:613–617, 1989.
56. Simon HB, Swartz MN: Pathophysiology of fever and fever of unknown origin. *In* Rubenstein E, Federman D (eds): Scientific American Medicine. New York, Scientific American, 1989.

57. Cannon JG, Kluger MJ: Endogenous pyrogen activity in human plasma after exercise. Science 220:617–618, 1983.
58. Cannon J, Dinarello C: Interleukin-1 activity in human plasma [abstract]. Fed Proc 43:462, 1984.
59. Cannon J, Evans WJ, Hughes VA, et al: Physiological mechanisms contributing to increased interleukin-1 secretion. J Appl Physiol 61:1859–1874, 1986.
60. Schechtman O, Elizondo R, Taylor M: Exercise augments interleukin-2 induction [abstract]. Med Sci Sports Exerc S18:108, 1988.
61. Simon HB: Exercise, health and sports medicine. *In* Rubenstein E, Federman D (eds): Scientific American Medicine. New York, Scientific American, 1988.
62. Viti A, Muscettola M, Paulesu L, et al: Effect of exercise on plasma interferon levels. J Appl Physiol 59:426–428, 1985.
63. Wolff RK, Dolovich MB, Obminski G, et al: Effects of exercise and eucapnic hyperventilation on bronchial clearance in man. J Appl Physiol 43:46–50, 1977.
64. Cederlund A, Camner P, Svartengren M: Nasal mucociliary transport before and after jogging. Physician Sports Med 15:93–98, 1987.
65. Holdstock DJ, Misiewicz JJ, Smith T, et al: Propulsion (mass movements) in the human colon and its relationship to meals and somatic activity. Gut 11:91–99, 1970.
66. Howlett TA, Tomlin S, Ngahfoong L, et al: Release of β-endorphin and met-enkephalin during exercise in normal women: Response to training. Br Med J 288:1950–1952, 1984.
67. Carr DB, Bullen BA, Skrinar GS, et al: Physical conditioning facilitates the exercise-induced secretion of β-endorphin and β-lipotropin in women. N Engl J Med 305:560–563, 1981.
68. Simon HB: Exercise and human immune function. *In* Ader R, Felten DL, Cohen N (eds): Psychoneuroimmunology II. Orlando, FL, Academic Press, 1991.
69. Douglas DJ, Hanson PG: Upper respiratory infections in the conditioned athlete [abstract]. Med Sci Sports Exerc 10:55, 1978.
70. Nieman DC, Johansen LM, Lee JW: Infectious episodes in runners before and after the Los Angeles Marathon [abstract]. Med Sci Sports Exerc S18, 1988.
71. Peters EM, Bateman ED: Ultramarathon running and upper respiratory tract infections. S Afr Med J 64:582–584, 1983.
72. Linde F: Running and upper respiratory tract infections. Scand J Sports Sci 9:21–23, 1987.
73. Osterback L, Ovarnberg Y: A prospective study of respiratory infections in 12-year-old children actively engaged in sports. Acta Paediatr Scand 76:944–949, 1987.
74. Schouten WJ, Verschuur R, Kemper HCG: Physical activity and upper respiratory tract infections in a normal population of young men and women: The Amsterdam growth and health study. Int J Sports Med 9:451–455, 1988.
75. Blair SN, Kohl HW III, Paffenbarger RS, et al: Physical fitness and all-cause mortality: A prospective study of healthy men and women. JAMA 262:2395–2401, 1989.
76. Frisch RE, Wyshak G, Albright NL, et al: Lower prevalence of non-reproductive system cancers among female former college athletes. Med Sci Sports Exerc 21:250–253, 1989.
77. Garabrant DH, Peters JM, Mack TM, et al: Job activity and colon cancer risk. Am J Epidemiol 119:1005–1114, 1984.
78. Gerhardsson M, Norell SE, Kiviranta H, et al: Sedentary jobs and colon cancer. Am J Epidemiol 123:775–780, 1986.
79. Vena JE, Graham S, Zielezny M, et al: Occupational exercise and risk of cancer. Am J Clin Nutr 45:318–327, 1987.
80. Husemann B, Neubauer MG, Duhme C: Sitzende tatigkeit und rektum-sigma-karzinom. Onkologie 4:168–171, 1980.
81. Paffenbarger RS, Hyde RT, Wing AL: Physical activity and incidence of cancer in diverse populations: A preliminary report. Am J Clin Nutr 415:312–317, 1987.
82. Frisch RE, Wyshak G, Albright NL, et al: Lower prevalence of breast cancer and cancers of the reproductive system among former college athletes compared to non-athletes. Br J Cancer 52:885–891, 1985.
83. Horstmann DM: Acute poliomyelitis. JAMA 135:11, 1956.
84. Douglas GR, Lindgren KM, Couch RB: Exposure to cold environment and rhinovirus common cold. N Engl J Med 279:742–747, 1968.
85. Herpes gladiatorum at a high school wrestling camp—Minnesota. MMWR 39(5):69–71, 1990.
86. Gatmaitan BG, Chason JL, Lerner AM: Augmentation of the virulence of coxsackie virus B-3 myocardiopathy by exercise. J Exp Med 131:1121–1136, 1970.
87. Ilback N-G, Fohlman J, Friman G: Exercise in coxsackie B3 myocarditis: Effects on heart lymphocyte subpopulations and the inflammatory reaction. Am Heart J 117:1298–1302, 1989.
88. Tillis IG, Elson SH, Shaka JA, et al: Effects of exercise on coxsackie A-9 myocarditis in adult mice. Proc Soc Exp Biol Med 117:777–782, 1964.

89. Phillips M, Robinowitz M, Higgins JR, et al: Sudden cardiac death in Air Force recruits: A 20-year review. JAMA 256:2696–2699, 1986.
90. Montague TJ, Marrie TJ, Bewick DJ, et al: Cardiac effects of common viral illnesses. Chest 94:919–925, 1988.
91. Cannon JG, Kluger MG: Exercise enhances survival rate in mice infected with *Salmonella typhimurium.* Proc Soc Exp Biol Med 175:518–521, 1984.
92. Chalmers TC, Eckhardt RD, Reynolds WE, et al: The treatment of acute infectious hepatitis: Controlled studies of the effects of diet, rest and physical reconditioning in the acute course of the disease and the incidence of relapses and residual abnormalities. J Clin Invest 34:1163–1235, 1955.
93. Edlund A: The effect of defined physical exercise in the early convalescence of viral hepatitis. Scand J Infect Dis 3:189–196, 1971.
94. Graubaum HJ, Metzner C, Ziesenhenn K: Korperliche belastung and hepatitisverlauf. Dtsch Med Wochenschr 112:47–49, 1987.
95. Ritland S, Petlund CF, Knudsen T, et al: Improvement of physical capacity after long-term training in patients with chronic active hepatitis. Scand J Gastroenterol 18:1083–1087, 1983.
96. Dalrymple W: Infectious mononucleosis. Postgrad Med 35:345–349, 1964.
97. Daniels WL, Vogel JA, Sharp DS, et al: Effects of virus infection on physical performance in man. Milit Med 150:8–14, 1985.
98. Friman G, Wright JE, Ilback NG, et al: Does fever or myalgia indicate reduced physical performance capacity in viral infections? Acta Med Scand 217:353–361, 1985.
99. Simon HB: Immunization and chemotherapy for viral infections. *In* Rubenstein E, Federman D (eds): Scientific American Medicine. New York, Scientific American, 1990.
100. Morris JN, Pollard R, Everitt MG, et al: Vigorous exercise in leisure-time: Protection against coronary heart disease. Lancet 2:1207–1210, 1980.

7

THE SKIN

Wilma Fowler Bergfeld, MD, FACP
Thomas N. Helm, MD

Skin disorders in athletes are similar to those of the general population. Because athletes spend many long hours in training, however, the skin is often subjected to unusual stresses. Certain processes are seen more frequently as the protective effects of the skin are overcome. The intimate contact and strenuous exercise in some sports predispose the athlete to certain infectious diseases. This chapter discusses the clinical presentation and treatment of commonly encountered skin conditions in athletes resulting from mechanical irritation, physical factors, infections, and contact allergy. Miscellaneous skin disorders that may have a modified course in the athlete as well as rare disorders unique to the athlete will also be discussed.

MECHANICAL IRRITATION

Friction blisters are perhaps the most common skin disorder of athletes. They can be a major problem, especially in running and team activities. Blisters occur most commonly on the feet as a result of friction between the shoe and the foot. Blisters can, however, occur anywhere and are especially prominent over the joints, at the ends of fingers or toes, or on the heel of the foot (Fig. 7–1 [see color plates for all figures in this chapter]). Shearing forces on the skin may lead to cleavage in the spinous layer of the epidermis. This is especially likely to occur in those athletes who have not trained regularly and who have not undergone epidermal hyperplasia in areas of maximal pressure. Excessive or abrupt friction can induce an immediate blister, and blisters may even occur under a callus if frictional forces are great enough. Hyperhidrosis may contribute to the formation of blisters by allowing the skin surface to slide within the shoe, enhancing shearing forces.

Blisters can be treated in several different ways. A friction blister has sterile contents, and the blister roof provides a natural occlusive dressing, which promotes healing. Often, however, it may not be feasible to leave a blister in place because it will most certainly rupture if left alone. This is especially true for blisters on the feet. A sterile needle may be used to drain the blister fluid and an occlusive pressure dressing should then be placed over the wound. Occlusive dressings can increase the speed of epithelialization and should be used whenever possible. Some commonly used occlusive dressings include various pads (Telfa, Curad, and Band-Aids), hydrocolloid dressings (Duoderm and Actiderm), hydrogel dressings (Geliperm, Second Skin, and Vigilon), polyurethane films (Bio-occlusive, Op-site, and Tegaderm), and simple ointment dressings (petrolatum, bacitracin, Polysporin, and Bactroban). Transparent film dressings appear to give superior results when compared with standard antibiotic ointment and gauze dressings. Unfortunately, the recently developed occlusive dressings cost considerably more than a simple dressing of antibiotic ointment and gauze. Blisters should be watched for secondary infection. Should infection occur, antiseptic soaks with agents such as chlorhexidine (Hibiclens) and iodine prove highly effective. Antibiotic ointments also hasten resolution when infection occurs.

Calluses are another common change in the skin seen in athletes. Astute observers have been able to deduce what sport an athlete engages in simply by observing his or her calluses. The calluses represent epidermal hyperplasia, which protects underlying structures from trauma. Calluses occur commonly over pressure points such as bony prominences. Other reactive changes may occur as well. Activities like rowing may produce lichenified plaques on the buttocks. The repetitive trauma to the toes in ballet commonly induces changes in the nailplate (Fig. 7–2). If a callus becomes cosmetically objectionable, soaking of the affected area followed by gentle debridement with a pumice stone can be most helpful. Keratolytics with salicylic acid (Saligel, Ureacin, Keralyt Gel, Whitfield's Ointment, and Hydrisalic Gel) can also be helpful. Nail changes are difficult to treat as long as the causative trauma continues. Corns (clavi) often need to be debrided with a scalpel. Once the firm center of the corn is removed, discomfort is relieved. Protective pads are helpful in preventing corns, but sometimes osteotomies are necessary to treat persistent areas of callus or corn formation.

Certain areas on the body do not form calluses. The inability to form calluses can often be more troubling than their presence. The nipples of runners become sensitive after prolonged friction; this is known as "jogger's nipples." Placing bandages over the nipples, avoiding nylon athletic jerseys, or applying petrolatum helps prevent this problem.

The black heel (also known as talon noir, and hyperkeratosis haemorrhagica) has a similar pathogenesis to that of friction blisters but is especially common in sports that involve quick stops and starts, such as tennis, soccer, track, and basketball. Areas where blood vessels are relatively susceptible to injury, such as at the edge of the heel, are particularly prone to this form of injury. Treatment involves reassurance. When it is difficult to differentiate black heel from a nevus or melanoma, gentle paring of the stratum corneum should be undertaken. The black heel lesion can be painlessly removed with the stratum corneum whereas pigmented growths are at the level of the epidermis or below and cannot be removed by this technique. Well-fitting athletic shoes may help cushion the feet and prevent this form of injury.

Subungual bleeding gives rise to the subungual hematoma. This lesion is painful and results from blunt external trauma, most commonly involving the great toe. Treatment consists of evacuation of the hematoma by incision. One effective and easy technique involves heating a metal wire and applying it to the nailplate. The trapped blood is under pressure if the hematoma is of recent onset, and will squirt forth from the opening with immediate relief of pain. Proper foot protection, such as shoes with reinforced toe sections, is helpful for prevention. If there is any doubt that the lesion is a subungual hematoma, a nail biopsy should be performed to rule out a dysplastic nevus or melanoma.

Other types of athletic injury may give characteristic patterns. Ping-pong patches are erythematous or purpuric lesions with an annular appearance that occur where high velocity ping-pong balls hit the skin. Tennis players appear particularly likely to develop splinter hemorrhages of the halluces known as tennis toes. Bicyclists who rest their volar forearms on their racing bike handlebars are predisposed to developing characteristic purpura. Surfers develop nodules in areas of repetitive injury from contact with their surf boards. A careful history usually clarifies the etiology of these otherwise perplexing dermatoses.

Piezogenic papules are herniations of fat through the connective tissue. These papules are found in the non–weight-bearing areas of the foot and are usually tender. They may only be apparent upon weight bearing. Women are affected more frequently than men. Treatment is most often unsuccessful.

Intertrigo is another common condition in athletes, which develops in bodyfold areas of friction. The groin, axillae, and inframammary folds are most often involved. The lesions are symmetric and well demarcated. Obesity is important in enhancing the friction that exacerbates this disorder. Bacterial and fungal superinfection is common, especially during the warm summer months. Potassium hydroxide examination of scales for fungi is usually negative. Immediate treatment involves soothing compresses with Burow's 1:40 solution (Domeboro) and combination anti-inflammatory antibacterial agents (Vytone 1% Cream). Weight loss is most helpful for prevention.

ENVIRONMENTAL FACTORS

Although more and more sports are played indoors, athletes are frequently forced to brave the elements. Frostbite, cold-induced urticaria (Fig. 7–3), cold-induced purpura, and immersion foot (Fig. 7–4) may all affect the outdoor athlete. Women who horseback ride in the cold may develop cold panniculitis on their thighs. Warm clothing can help to prevent these problems. In the case of cold urticaria, antihistamines may be helpful. Frostbite should be treated by immediate rewarming of affected areas, preferably with water of 40.0 to 40.5°C.

Sunburn

Sunburn is a frequently encountered problem of all athletes engaging in outdoor activities. This is especially true when unusually intense sunlight is encountered during sports like mountaineering or skiing. Exposure to ultraviolet B (UVB) light (290 to 320 nm) is usually the cause. This radiating energy meets the earth's surface with its greatest intensity between 10 AM and 3 PM in the northern hemisphere. Increasing cloud cover and humidity reduce the incident ultraviolet radiation to the earth's surface, but it is a common misconception that one cannot become sunburned on a cloudy or hazy day. An individual's response to light will depend upon the skin type, time of day, duration of exposure, use of photosensitizing medications, protective clothing, and use of sunscreens. Erythema may be noted a few hours after exposure to excessive UVB light, but peak effects are not seen until almost a day later. Clinically, sunburn reactions have been classified as (1) first-degree burn: consists of a mild erythema; (2) second-degree burn: consists of erythema and blister formation; and (3) third-degree burn: consists of blisters and skin ulceration (Fig. 7–5).

Ultraviolet B light exposure has been linked to skin cancer and acute blistering sunburns have been associated with melanoma development. Sun exposure may also trigger a wide variety of disorders such as herpes simplex, lupus erythematosus, porphyria cutanea tarda, solar urticaria, polymorphous light disorder, erythema multiforme, telangiectasia, photoaging, and sunstroke. Other diseases, such as vitiligo, may become more apparent after sun exposure.

Sunscreens (Table 7–1), protective clothing, and short exposures to the sun, which promote tanning, should all be part of the first line of defense against sunburn. Most dermatologists recommend sunscreens with sun protective factor (SPF) of 15 or greater (if someone usually burns within 1 hour of sun exposure, a sunscreen with SPF 15 will theoretically prevent sunburn until 15 hours after application). Much attention has recently been focused on the role of ultraviolet A light (320 to 400 nm) exposure in skin cancer formation, photoaging, and triggering of photosensitive disease such as lupus ery-

TABLE 7–1. SOME COMMONLY USED SUNSCREENS

Agent	Protective Range	Brand Names
PABA	UVB	Hawaiian Tropic Gel, Presun Gel, Pabanol, Sunbrella
Paba ester	UVB	Aztec, Block Out, Eclipse Original, Sundown, Sea and Ski
Padimate-O and Parsol 1789	UVA, UVB	Photoplex
PABA ester/benzophenone	UVA, UVB	Chapstick Sunblock 15, Presun 39, Solbar Plus, Sundown 24, Supershade 15, Coppertone 4 Body Mousse
Opaque agents	UVA, UVB, and beyond	UVB Covermark, Clinique Continuous Coverage, Reflecta, RVPaque, Shadow

thematosus. Newer broad spectrum sunscreens with padimate-O and parsol 1789 (Photoplex) have been developed with these factors in mind.

In very sensitive individuals, sunscreens can be used in conjunction with other agents, such as antimalarials or psoralens (Trisoralen), to help increase tolerance of the sun. Aspirin at a dose of 300 to 600 mg 1 to 2 hours before sun exposure may minimize the intensity of a sunburn reaction by inhibiting the production of inflammatory mediators.

When acute sunburn occurs, treatment should be directed at reducing skin inflammation and heat. Cold compresses should be frequently applied to the affected area. Compresses of water and milk are simple to use and may prevent excessive drying of the sunburned area. Mid potency corticosteroid creams (Westcort Cream, Aclovate Cream) may be applied three times daily for 1 or 2 days to hasten resolution. Corticosteroid creams of high potency should not be applied around the eyes as they may increase intraocular pressure. Oral corticosteroids, aspirin at a dose of 600 mg three times daily, or indomethacin (Indocin) at a dosage of 25 mg three times daily have all been reported to hasten resolution.

BACTERIAL INFECTIONS

Impetigo

Impetigo is an infectious, contagious disorder that may present as honey-colored, crusted lesions or as bullae (Fig. 7–6). The crusted form of impetigo is typically due to β-hemolytic streptococci and occurs in preschool children and adults. Certain strains may cause acute nephritis, but this is usually limited to infants. Epidemic infection by nephritogenic streptococci on a rugby team has, however, been reported. If streptococcal impetigo is suspected, a urinalysis should be performed. The bullous form of impetigo occurs most commonly in newborns and older children and is typically due to *Staphylococcus aureus* of phage group 2 (Fig. 7–7).

Treatment consists of erythromycin 250 mg four times daily for 10 days in adults, or approximately 125 mg four times daily in most children. An intramuscular injection of 1.2 million units penicillin G can be given to adults as an alternative to erythromycin therapy. Other effective treatments include a 10- to 14-day course of antibiotics, such as clindamycin (Cleocin), first-generation cephalosporins (Keflex), or amoxicillin–clavulanic acid (Augmentin). If lesions fail to clear with penicillin therapy, the etiologic agent is likely to be penicillinase-producing *Staphylococcus aureus*. These patients should be treated with penicillinase-resistant antibiotics, such as dicloxacillin, oxacillin, or nafcillin. Compresses with Burow's solution (Domeboro powder/tabs), gentle soap and water cleansing, and topical antibiotics all hasten resolution. The new topical antibiotic, mupirocin (Bactroban), has a mode of action different from that of other antibiotics. Cross-resistance is, therefore, unlikely to occur and when used three times daily on affected areas, mupirocin has been found to be as effective as oral antibiotics in the treatment of impetigo. The cost of this agent is its major drawback.

Folliculitis and Furunculosis

Folliculitis and furunculosis are inflammatory disorders characterized by papular, pustular, and nodular lesions. Tender fluctuant abscesses may develop. Staphylococci and streptococci are the primary causative organisms. Topical treatment with warm compresses, benzoyl peroxide in concentrations ranging from 5% to 10%, or antibiotic solutions (erythromycin 2% solution or clindamycin 1% solution) is helpful in controlling folliculitis. Furuncles should be cultured so that the sensitivity of the causative organism(s) can be determined. The appropriate oral antibiotic should then be given for periods of up to 3 months or longer. If they are treated early, incision and drainage of these lesions may not be needed. Rifampin may sometimes be needed in resistant cases. The anterior nares should be cultured for causative organisms in not only the affected athlete but also in other family members. Team members may also need careful evaluation. If nasal carriage of staphylococci with the same sensitivity pattern as the lesional organisms is found, topical agents such as mupirocin may be applied to the anterior nares three times daily to eradicate colonization. All affected family members should be treated. Fluctuant abscesses should be incised and drained. An athlete with active furunculosis should be disqualified from a contact or swimming sport.

Erythrasma

Erythrasma is an infection most often found in the groin folds or axillae, but it may occur in webs of the feet. Lesions typically have a dull red-brown appearance. The infection is caused by *Corynebacterium minutissimum* but frequently may mimic tinea cruris or intertrigo. Potassium hydroxide examination will, however, be negative for fungi. Wood's light (long-wave ultraviolet light) examination will reveal a characteristic coral red fluorescence, which helps establish the diagnosis. A porphyrin produced by the metabolism of the organism is responsible for this striking color. Gram's stain reveals gram-positive rods.

Eradication of the infection is usually easily achieved by topical antibiotics, soap and water washing, or a regimen of either tetracycline or erythromycin at a dosage of 1 g daily given for 10 to 21 days.

Pitted Keratolysis

Pitted keratolysis is a bacterial infection of the plantar skin with *Corynebacterium* and other bacterial species. Profuse sweating and a warm environment are thought to be important in its development. Careful inspection of the soles reveals many tiny pits in the stratum corneum. The lesions are asymptomatic.

Treatment includes agents that promote drying, such as 20% aluminum chloride (Drysol), erythromycin 2% solution, or benzoyl peroxide preparations. Absorbent cotton socks should always be worn and changed frequently.

VIRAL INFECTIONS

Herpes Simplex

Herpes simplex is a common cutaneous viral infection of the skin and mucous membranes. Both physical and emotional stress may precipitate lesions. The clinical course is characterized by three stages: a primary infection, a latent phase, and recurrence at the initial site of infection.

Two types of herpes simplex are recognized. Type 1 is usually localized above the waist (Fig. 7–8); type 2 usually affects the genital areas (Fig. 7–9). This classic distribution is now less useful clinically than it was in the past, presumably due to changing sexual practices. Lesions consist of grouped vesicles on an erythematous base. Athletes with moist lesions may infect other athletes during contact sports. The spread of herpes infection during wrestling is well recognized and known as "herpes gladiatorum." Injury from abrasive clothing may facilitate this type of infection. Infection can be severe and may even lead to a monoarticular arthritis. Other sports, such as rugby, have also been associated with the spread of herpes simplex virus 1. Diagnosis is established by Tzanck test, Papanicolaou smear, or culture. The Tzanck test can be immediately performed on a suspicious vesicular lesion and is, therefore, the diagnostic method of choice. Culture allows for differentiation of herpes simplex viruses 1 and 2. Serologic testing is rarely useful.

Treatment was once solely directed at drying lesions to hasten resolution and minimize infectivity. Many drying agents, such as compresses, benzoyl peroxide (Persa-Gel 5%, Panoxyl Aq, Oxy-10), astringent lotions (Sea-breeze), sulfacetamide (Sulfacet R), and tretinoin (Retin-A Gel), are useful in this regard. Mild combination antibacterial and anti-inflammatory medications such as Vytone or Vioform-HC may also prove useful. The most effective therapy is probably oral acyclovir (Zovirax) given at a dosage of 200 mg five times daily for 7 to 10 days. Acyclovir 2% ointment (Zovirax ung) may also hasten resolution of lesions, but convincing evidence of this is lacking. Those athletes who can recognize a characteristic prodrome before cutaneous lesions appear may be able to abort reactivation with a 1-week course of oral acyclovir at the previously mentioned dosage. Sunburn can precipitate labial herpes (Fig. 7–10), and lip balm with sunscreen should be used by athletes prone to labial recurrences. Zovirax has also been reported to prevent reactivation of herpes labialis in skiers.

Molluscum Contagiosum

Molluscum contagiosum is a common viral disease caused by the pox virus. Multiple flesh-colored papules are usually encountered, although solitary lesions can also be seen. The classic central umbilication of lesions may not always be readily apparent. The surrounding skin is usually devoid of an inflammatory response (Fig. 7–11). The trunk, axillae, perineum, thighs, and face are common sites. The cheeselike material found within the lesions contains active pox virus and accounts for the infectivity of lesions.

Not only contact sports, but also sports like cross-country running, orienteering, and swimming have been associated with transmission of molluscum contagiosum. Lesions may have an unusual distribution and appearance and are often misdiagnosed. Minor breaks in the skin may predispose to infection.

Diagnosis is established by skin biopsy or smear. Treatment methods include a light application of liquid nitrogen (−196°C), cantharidin, electrodesiccation, salicylic acid/lactic acid (Duofilm), curettage, and topical retinoic acid (Retin-A) applied to affected areas twice daily.

Common Warts and Condyloma Acuminata

Warts are epithelial tumors caused by the many types of human papillomavirus. Any site on the skin can be involved and lesions may also appear on the mucous membranes. The size of these tumors may vary from 1 millimeter to many centimeters. Lesions can appear flat or dome-shaped and usually have an irregular surface (Fig. 7–12). On mucous membranes or moist body surfaces, the warts generally appear as firm, red-brown tumors with a smooth surface because much of the superficial hyperkeratosis found in common warts is absent (Fig. 7–13). When present on the foot, lesions tend to be endophytic with a smooth hyperkeratotic surface (Fig. 7–14). Skin markings are absent, which helps differentiate the plantar wart from a callus.

Diagnosis is made by clinical inspection and biopsy. Large plantar warts of many years' duration in adults should be biopsied to rule out verrucous carcinoma. Treatment is directed not only at destroying the wart but also at stimulating host response against the wart. Salicylic acid plasters (Occlusal, Tra-sal, Mediplast, Wart-Off), formalin soaks (3%–20% formalin), 5-fluorouracil (Effudex, Fluoroplex Solution 1%), cantharone (0.7% cantharidin), podophyllin (Pod-Ben 25), dichloroacetic acid, trichloroacetic acid, flexible collodion and lactic acid (Duofilm), retinoic acid (Retin-A 0.05% liquid), cryotherapy, and electrodesiccation all may be used with fairly good success. Subcutaneous interferon alpha injections may be used to treat genital warts. Women with genital warts should be evaluated for cervical or vulvar dysplasia because human papillomavirus infection has been associated with cancers in these areas. Surgery and radiotherapy should not be used because these therapies may be quite destructive and leave a painful wound which can compromise athletic performance.

FUNGAL AND YEAST INFECTIONS

Tinea Versicolor

Tinea versicolor is a very common yeast infection among athletes. Heat and moisture allow the yeast to proliferate. The upper chest and back are commonly involved with fine scaling macules. In light-skinned athletes, the lesions may appear reddish-brown (Fig. 7–15). In dark-skinned athletes, the lesions are typically hypopigmented because the organism produces a dicarboxylic acid, which inhibits normal tanning. The failure to pigment normally is usually what prompts the athlete to seek medical attention because lesions are usually asymptomatic. Diagnosis is made by clinical presentation and confirmed by potassium hydroxide (KOH) examination of lesional scrapings. Skin cultures for fungus are always negative.

Topical treatments usually suffice to eliminate infection. The most widely used treatment consists of applying selenium sulfide 2.5% lotion or shampoo. Two methods of application have been widely advocated. The medication may be applied to the affected areas at bedtime and left on overnight. In the morning, the medication is rinsed off in the shower. This method may lead to skin irritation in sensitive patients, but otherwise is easiest to use. Alternatively, the medication may be applied for 15 to 20 minutes each night before rinsing the medication off in the shower. This should be repeated each day for an entire week. The affected athlete should be told to expect only gradual repigmentation of the involved areas, however, because even when the causative organisms are eradicated, repigmentation has to occur by natural mechanisms. Other treatments have included 30% aqueous solution of sodium thiosulfate (Tinver Solution) applied twice daily for 10 days or topical azole preparations. Yet another method which has been shown to be effective is oral ketoconazole (Nizoral) 200 mg daily for 3 days prior to exercise. The increased sweating disperses concentrations of active fungitoxic drug on the skin. Unfortunately, ketoconazole may cause hepatic necrosis in rare cases.

Tinea Infections

A variety of dermatophytes may cause infection in athletes. These organisms live in the stratum corneum or in hair and elicit varying host responses. Infections of the hair and scalp with *Microsporum canis, Trichophyton mentagrophytes,* and *Trichophyton verrucosum* all create a strong inflammatory reaction (Fig. 7–16). Lesions appear as boggy erythematous alopecic plaques. Infections of the hair and scalp with *Microsporum audounini, Trichophyton tonsurans,* and *Trichophyton violaceum* produces much less of a reaction. *Microsporum audounini* produces alopecic plaques with short, stubby, broken hairs. This form of infection, although once common, is now exceedingly rare. *Trichophyton tonsurans* and *Trichophyton violaceum* infections produce areas devoid of hair in which hair shafts are broken near the skin surface giving the so-called black-dot or seborrheic dermatitis appearance.

Tinea corporis of the nonhairy skin is characterized by annular lesions. The advancing margin is erythematous and the central part of the lesion is often clear (Fig. 7–17). The most common causative organism is *Trichophyton rubrum.* Tinea cruris usually presents as a slightly scaly, erythematous patch with central clearing that spares the scrotum (Fig. 7–18). *Tricophyton rubrum* and *Trichophyton mentagrophytes* commonly cause this form of infection. Tinea infection of the feet can present as either a dry, scaling eruption in a "moccasin" distribution (Fig. 7–19) or as a moist, macerated infection of the interdigital web space. *Epidermophyton floccosum* and *Trichophyton rubrum* commonly cause interdigital infection. Onychomycosis commonly accompanies fungal infection of the hands and feet.

When fungal disease is suspected, potassium hydroxide examination allows for rapid confirmation. Culture may be useful, especially in cases of hair or nail infection. Localized dermatophyte infections may be treated by applications of a topical antifungal agent twice daily for a month (Table 7–2). Absorption is improved when the skin is well hydrated. The imidazoles are effective against dermatophytes, *Candida,* and tinea versicolor. The azole terconazole is especially effective at controlling *Candida* infection. Ciclopirox olamine may penetrate nails and help control onychomycosis. Naftifine controls dermatophytes effectively, but *Candida* species are controlled to a lesser extent. Eroded lesions in the intertriginous areas respond well to Castellani's paint.

Oral griseofulvin should be given for extensive dermatophyte infections or when treating onychomycosis. The usual adult dose is 5 mg/pound per day and infections of

TABLE 7–2. COMMON TOPICAL AGENTS EFFECTIVE AGAINST DERMATOPHYTES

Chemical Group	Generic Name	Brand Name
Allylamines	Naftifine	Naftin
Azoles	Clotrimazole	Lotrimin, Mycelex
	Econzole	Spectazole
	Ketoconazole	Nizoral
	Miconazole	Micatin, Monistat
	Oxiconazole	Oxistat
	Sulconazole	Exelderm
Pyridone	Ciclopirox olamine	Loprox
Tolnaftate		Dr. Scholl's Tinactin
		Aftate foot spray
Trichlorophenol	Haloprogin	Halotex
Undecylenic Acid		Cruex
		Desenex

the skin should be treated for approximately 1 month. Resistant infections may respond to ketoconazole. Nail infections need to be treated much longer than infections of the skin or hair because of the slow growth of the nailplate and, despite a complete course of therapy, the likelihood of long-term cure is low even with oral antifungal drugs.

Candidal Infection

Candidal infections are common in athletes and may mimic infection with dermatophytes. In general, candidal infections are found in intertriginous areas and appear "beefy red" because of the strong host inflammatory response they incite. Satellite pustules aid in establishing the diagnosis. Unlike tinea cruris, candidal infection of the groin commonly involves the scrotum (Fig. 7–20).

The finding of hyphae and pseudohyphae on potassium hydroxide examination is diagnostic. Kits are also now available to test for vaginal candidal antigens. Cool compresses and topical antifungal agents (clotrimazole, nystatin, haloprogin) are the treatments of choice. Scrotal or vulvar candidiasis also responds to gentian violet. Unlike ketoconazole, griseofulvin does not have activity against *Candida.*

INFESTATIONS

The most common infestations observed in athletes are those with the crab louse *(Pediculus humanus)* and the scabietic mite (*Sarcoptes scabiei*). Both are transmissible by intimate contact. Clothing and bedding should be washed and not used for 7 to 10 days.

Scabies

Scabies infection produces severe pruritus, which is usually the primary complaint. Often the pruritus is most severe at night. Scabies leave tortuous erythematous burrows in the epidermis, and a well-executed skin scraping can demonstrate the organism (Fig. 7–21) or its feces (which are known as scybala) under the microscope. Burrows and other lesions, such as inflammatory papules or nodules, may be observed on the lower abdomen, waist, hands, flexural areas, axillae, nipples, and umbilicus (Fig. 7–22). Late changes include eczematous allergic dermatitis. Folliculitis and furunculosis are rare but may be observed. At the time of diagnosis, infected individuals' personal contacts, teammates, and family members all need to be treated.

Lindane is the treatment of choice for eradicating adult scabietic infection. One percent lotion (Kwell, Scabene) is applied from the neck down to all body surfaces including under the nails. The lotion is left on overnight for approximately 8 hours and then washed off. After 1 week, the procedure is repeated. Because of concerns about neurotoxicity, crotamiton (Eurax) is often used for children and precipitated sulfur is used for treatment of pregnant women or babies. Recently, 5% permethrin (Elimite) cream has been shown to be effective in treating scabies. This medication is generally considered safe and may become the treatment of choice.

Pediculosis

The crab louse is transmitted mainly by intimate contact. The louse limits its excursions to the hairy areas of the body, such as the pubis, perineum, abdomen, axillae, and eyelashes. Pubic lice are rarely found in the scalp, but the head louse often inhabits this area.

The infected individual will experience severe pruritus or itching. Close inspection of the pruritic areas reveals nits (eggs), lice, or louse excretions (Fig. 7–23).

Permethrin (Nix 1% creme rinse) is the treatment of choice for eradicating lice, although pyrethrins (Rid, R & C), lindane (Kwell, Scabene) malathion, and DDT are also extremely effective. Permethrin should be applied to the affected areas for 10 minutes and then washed off. The treatment should be repeated once more in 7 days. Formic acid 8% creme rinse combined with a special nit comb (Step 2/Genderm) is especially helpful after permethrin treatment to ensure that all nits are removed. Although the nits may no longer be viable due to treatment with pediculocide, school-age children are often kept from school until all nits are gone, making the nit removal step particularly important.

INSECT BITES

The bites of most insects produce an immediate erythema at the site of the bite with subsequent itching or pain, depending upon the host's response to toxic saliva or body parts of the insect. These toxic lesions are painful and can produce fever and malaise. The lesions typically have a central area of infarction or blanching and peripheral edema. Extremely pruritic urticarial lesions may be seen if delayed-type hypersensitivity is present to saliva or body parts.

Treatment is dependent on the type of wound. It is not clear whether toxic wounds should be left alone or excised and injected with corticosteroids. Meat tenderizers may neutralize certain venoms and may be helpful immediately after the insect bite. Urticarial lesions are treated with antihistamine lotions or low-potency cortisone creams. Oral antibiotics are only helpful if secondary infection occurs.

Prevention of bites can be accomplished by avoiding use of perfumes and bright clothing. Heavily infested areas should be avoided and the use of pesticides in homes, gardens, and athletic training sites can also lower the numbers of stinging insects. Oral thiamine has been noted to lower the incidence of mosquito bites in some individuals. If severe reactions have occurred, the athlete should carry an anaphylaxis kit (Epi-Pen) and desensitization therapy should be considered.

CONTACT DERMATITIS

Contact dermatitis presents as either an acute or chronic inflammatory disorder of the skin that is secondary to irritation or allergy. Irritant contact dermatitis is a nonallergic reaction of skin resulting from exposure to an irritating substance or physical agent that produces skin damage, ulceration, and pain (Fig. 7–24). Allergic contact dermatitis is a skin disorder secondary to acquired hypersensitivity to a specific allergen such as poison ivy (Fig. 7–25).

Allergic reactions are predominantly due to contact with five major allergens: *Rhus* (poison ivy, oak, and sumac), paraphenylenediamine (blue and black dyes), nickel compounds (jewelry, metal protective gear), rubber compounds, and chromates (tanned leather and metal parts). Specific reactions to diethylthiourea in a wet suit, facial dermatitis in a scuba diver, and black rubber components on a windsurfer have all been reported as well. In addition, topical medications that have been used to treat athletic injuries have induced allergic contact dermatitis. These agents include benzocaine, nitrofurazone (Furacin), topical antihistamine preparations, ammoniated mercury, neomycin, sulfonamide, tincture of benzoin, and para-amino acids.

The therapy of contact dermatitis should be aimed at reducing exposure to the contactant responsible for the skin reaction. Patch testing is often needed to determine the identity of a contact allergen. Vesicular reactions should be treated with cool compresses or soaks and topical corticosteroids in vehicles that promote drying such as aerosol sprays, gels, lotions, solutions, and creams. Systemic antihistamines and aspirin will relieve pruritus. Limited short courses of systemic corticosteroids decrease the severity of the dermatitis. Disqualification of an athlete is totally dependent upon the degree of skin involvement and the severity of symptoms.

Chronic recurrent contact dermatitis can be treated by avoiding contact or by establishing a barrier between the athlete's skin and the offending agent. For example, contact dermatitis secondary to rubber material in foot gear can be treated by applying topical corticosteroid cream to the foot followed by talcum powder and heavy, absorbent, white socks. The socks should be changed whenever they become damp. Topical corticosteroids in emollient bases are most helpful in treating chronic contact dermatitis as the skin is often dry and scaly.

DISORDERS OF THE PILOSEBACEOUS UNIT

Acne

Physicians have long realized that mechanical irritation by helmets or other gear may exacerbate acne in athletes. Unfortunately, the widespread use of anabolic steroids among athletes is now responsible for producing resistant acne in patients who previously had only mild disease. Comedones, sebaceous cysts, and seborrhea also seem to be more common in these patients.

The affected athlete should be discouraged from continued use of anabolic steroids. The acne can otherwise be treated in much the same fashion as conventional acne. Acne vulgaris is initially a noninflammatory, noninfectious skin disease with open and closed comedones as the primary lesions. These lesions are caused by a defect in intrafollicular keratinization. Secondary lesions develop when the pilosebaceous unit becomes inflamed; this presents clinically as papules, pustules, and cysts. These lesions are observed in sites where the sebaceous glands are of greatest density, such as the face, scalp, and trunk (Fig. 7–26). Excessive heat, exogenous hormones, humidity, mechanical irritation, manual manipulation, stress, occlusive cosmetics, and medications can all exacerbate acne.

Mild acne can be treated by comedone extraction and reduction in the number of comedones by using agents such as tretinoin (Retin-A) or benzoyl peroxide (Table 7–3). Application twice daily gives the best results. Topical peeling agents such as keratolytics and cryotherapy may be helpful in select cases. Topical antibiotics such as clindamycin (Cleocin T), erythromycin (ATS, Staticin, Erymax, Erygel, Erycette, T-Stat), and tetracycline (Topicycline) can also be used. Oral antibiotics are indicated if many pustular or cystic lesions are present. Tetracycline, 250 to 500 mg twice daily, is often effective, but if no response is seen within 2 to 3 months, minocycline (Minocin), 50 to 100 mg twice daily, should be tried. If no response is seen with these therapies, isotretinoin (Accutane),

TABLE 7–3. ACNE TREATMENT

Type of Acne	Treatments
Comedonal	Topical preparations: astringent lotion, Retin-A, keratolytics
Papular	Topical preparations: benzoyl peroxide, topical antibiotics
Pustular	Oral agent (tetracycline, erythromycin, minocycline) and/or topical agent: sulfurated lime or any of the above-mentioned topicals.
Cystic	Oral agent and topical agent: oral antibiotics (if no response after adequate trial, consider isotretinoin after appropriate counseling)

1 mg/kg per day for 4 to 5 months, may be used. Isotretinoin is likely to cause severe birth defects when used in pregnant patients, so effective contraception and patient education is essential for women with childbearing potential. Liver abnormalities and elevations in triglycerides and cholesterol may be encountered, necessitating periodic blood tests. Oral or parenteral corticosteroids may be needed in rare cases of rapidly advancing, disfiguring acne, but this therapy should be used only by experienced physicians.

Some patients appear to have hormonal abnormalities that predispose to severe acne. Athletes with hirsutism, acne, and menstrual irregularities should undergo testing for DHEA-S and testosterone abnormalities. Agents such as spironolactone (Aldactone) or oral contraceptives may be helpful if abnormalities are found. Doses of 100 mg of ethinyl estradiol are often effective in reducing sebum production. Thromboembolic phenomena and water retention are unfortunate side effects of this form of therapy.

Alopecia

Exogenous anabolic steroids may lead to androgenic alopecia. The exogenous steroids lead to a male-pattern alopecia (balding) which is often permanent despite attempts at treatment. Early recognition and discontinuation of the causative agent is most important. Athletes may develop traction alopecia from wearing "walk-man"-type radios while jogging. This type of alopecia is often reversible.

STRIAE DISTENSAE

Striae represent tears in the dermis and present clinically as linear areas of thin skin with fine wrinkling. Striae are commonly seen when tissues expand rapidly, such as during adolescence, or due to the effects of exogenous anabolic steroids on underlying tissues. Although agents such as tretinoin (Retin-A) may be tried, results of treatment are usually disappointing.

SUMMARY

The skin disorders of athletes are varied. Correct diagnosis and prompt treatment is essential for maintaining peak performance. The skin disorders of athletes are often challenging to treat, but the innovative clinician has the opportunity to become an important part of a successful team.

REFERENCES

MECHANICAL INJURY

Basler RSW. Skin injuries in sports medicine. J Am Acad Dermatol 21:1257–1262, 1989.
Bergfeld WF, Taylor JS: Trauma, sports, and the skin. Am J Ind Med 8:403–413, 1985.
Gibbs RC: Tennis toe. Arch Dermatol 107:918, 1973.
Hien NT, Prawer SE, Katz HI: Facilitated wound healing using transparent film dressing following Mohs micrographic surgery. Arch Dermatol 124:903–906, 1988.
Houston SD, Knox JM: Cutis 19:487–491, 1977.
Itin P, Rufli T: Skin problems in joggers. Schweiz Med Wochenschr 116(35):1189–1194, 1986.
Levine N: Dermatologic aspects of sports medicine. J Am Acad Dermatol 3:415–424, 1980.
Levit F: Joggers' nipples. N Engl J Med 297:1127, 1977.
Ronchese F: Occupational Marks and Other Physical Signs. New York, Grune & Stratton, 1948.

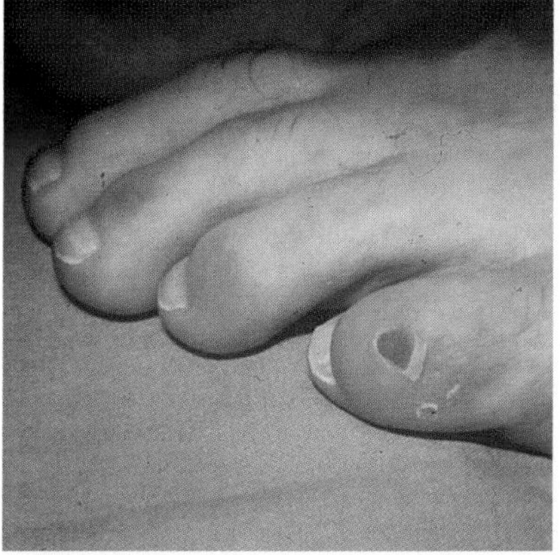

Figure 7–1.

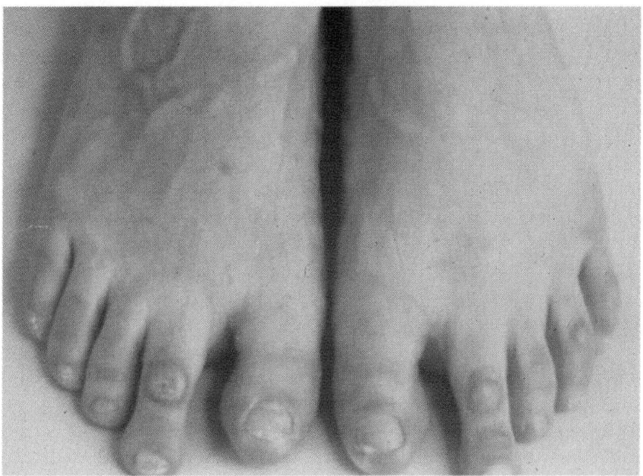

Figure 7–2.

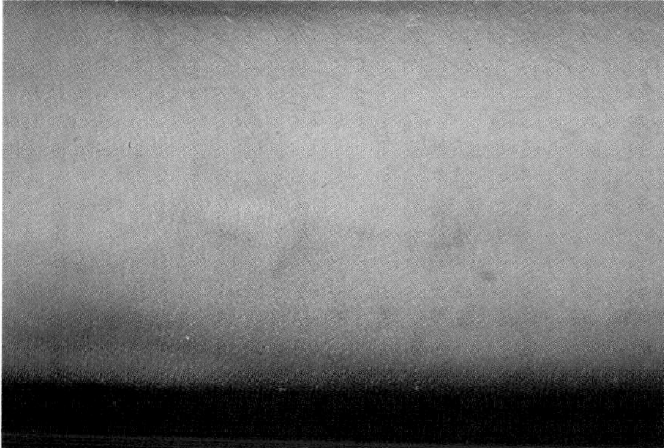

Figure 7–3.

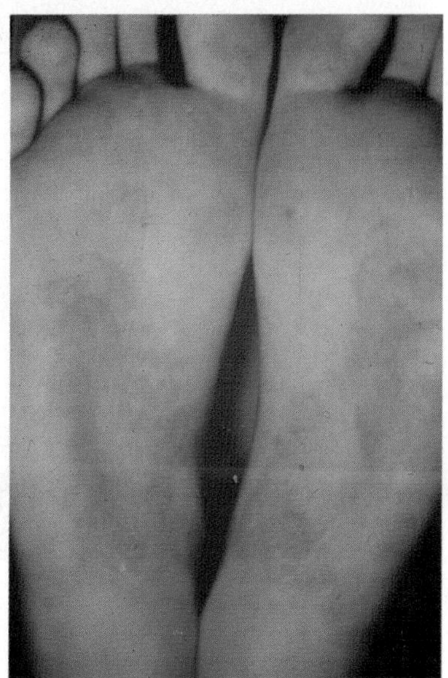

Figure 7–4.

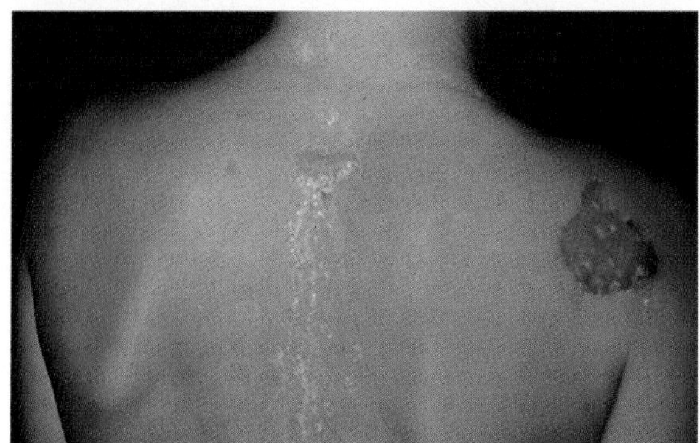

Figure 7–5.

Figure 7–1. Friction blister over the distal interphalangeal joint of the fifth toe.

Figure 7–2. Dystrophic nails and calluses from repeated trauma.

Figure 7–3. Typical urticarial lesions induced by the cold.

Figure 7–4. Erythema and edema of immersion foot resulting from prolonged exposure to low temperatures.

Figure 7–5. Third-degree sunburn with denuded blister and ulceration.

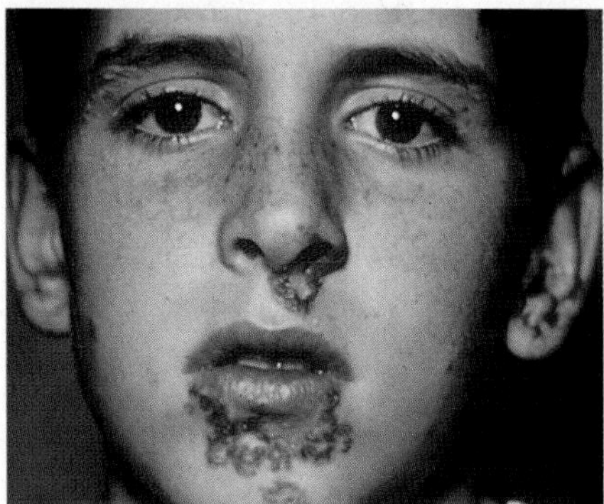
Figure 7–6.

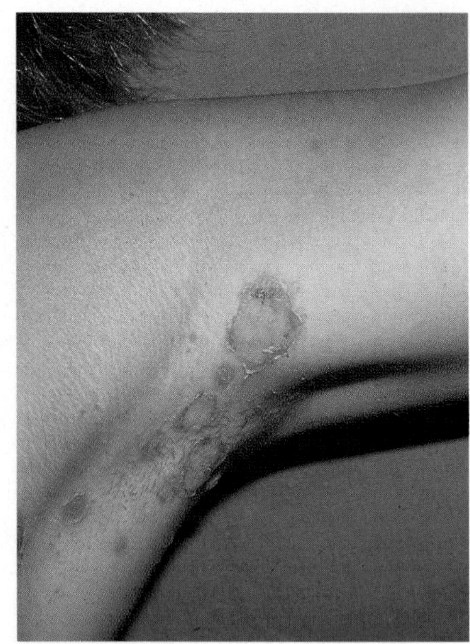
Figure 7–7.

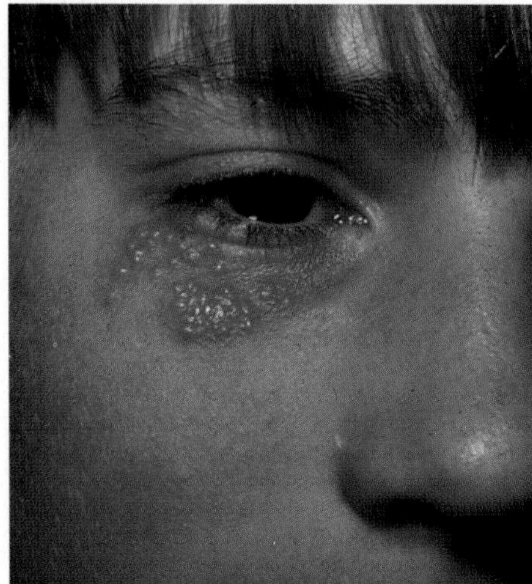
Figure 7–8.

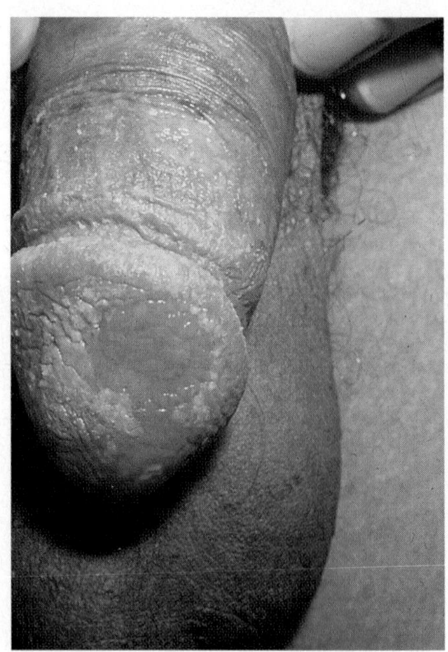
Figure 7–9.

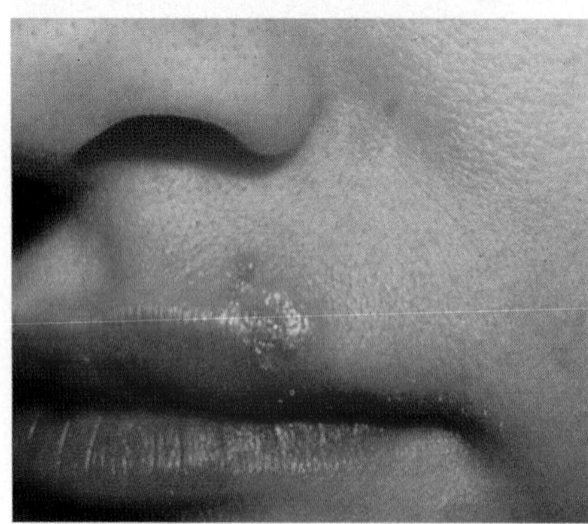
Figure 7–10.

Figure 7–6. Honey-colored crusts are characteristic of streptococcal impetigo.

Figure 7–7. Resolving bullae of staphylococcal impetigo leave annular lesions.

Figure 7–8. Lower eyelid involvement with herpes simplex virus 1.

Figure 7–9. Penile involvement with herpes simplex virus 2.

Figure 7–10. Characteristic labial herpes, which may be triggered by sunburn.

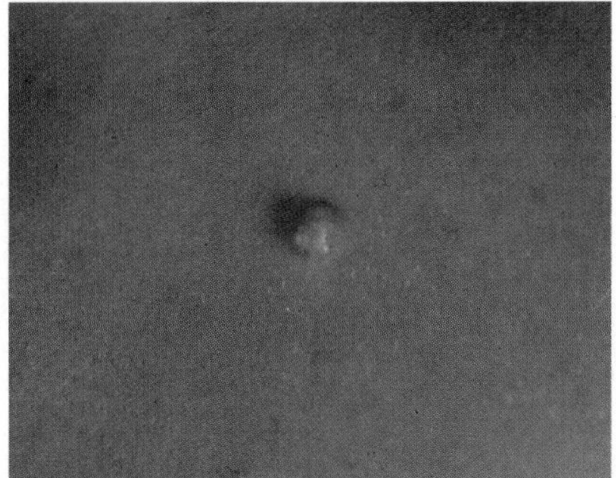
Figure 7–11.

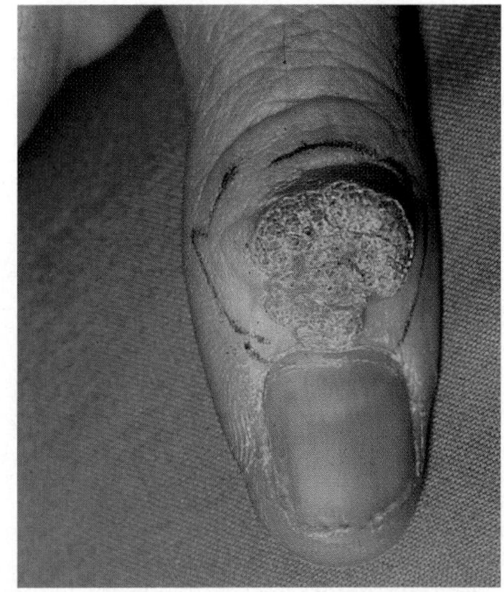
Figure 7–12.

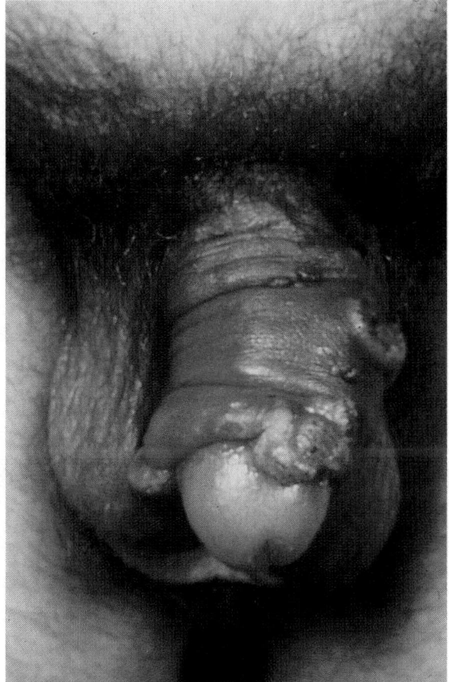
Figure 7–13.

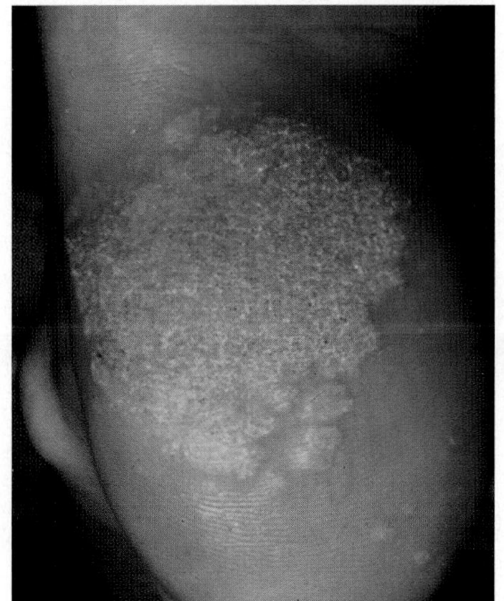
Figure 7–14.

Figure 7–11. Flesh-colored noninflammatory papule of molluscum contagiosum.

Figure 7–12. Verruca vulgaris on the right thumb.

Figure 7–13. Condyloma acuminata on the penis.

Figure 7–14. Endophytic appearance of plantar wart.

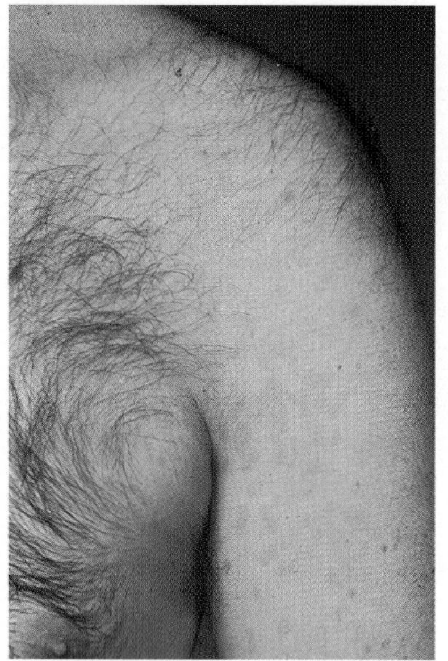

Figure 7–15.

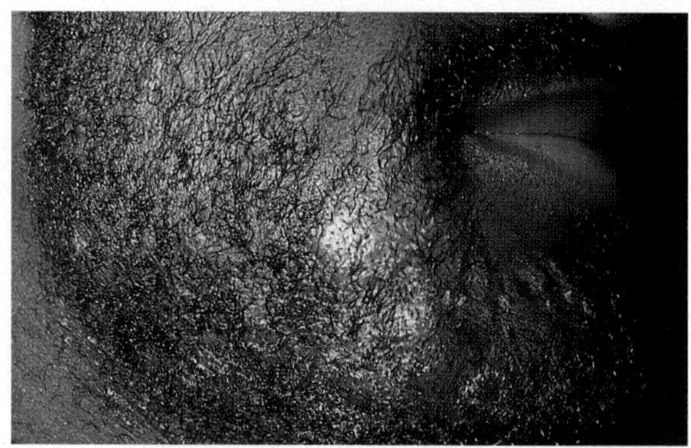

Figure 7–16.

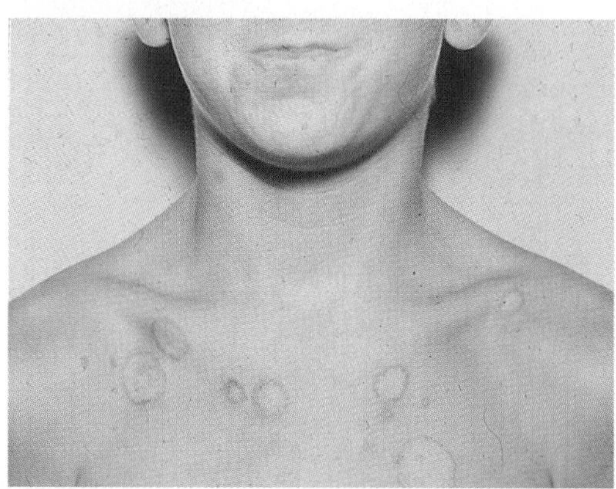

Figure 7–17.

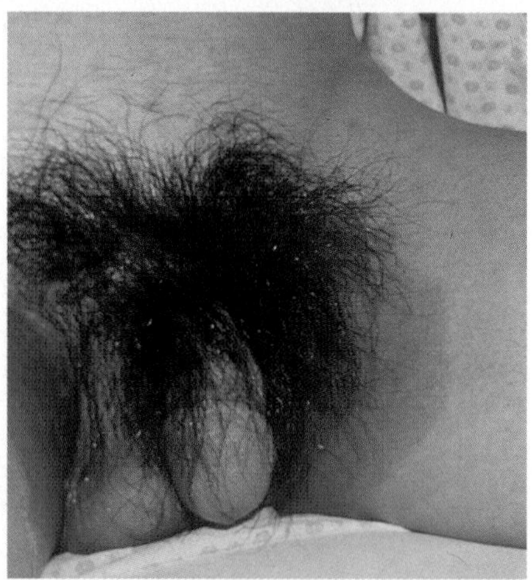

Figure 7–18.

Figure 7–15. Tinea versicolor with brown-red macules on a fair-skinned athlete.

Figure 7–16. Inflammatory sycosis barbae.

Figure 7–17. Annular lesion characteristic of tinea corporis.

Figure 7–18. Symmetric erythematous groin lesions of tinea cruris.

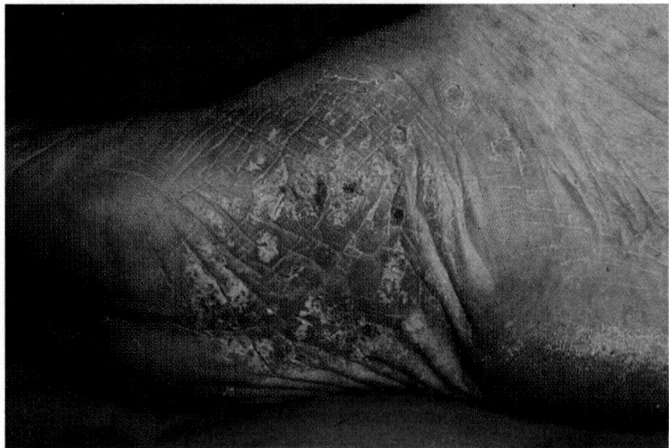
Figure 7–19.

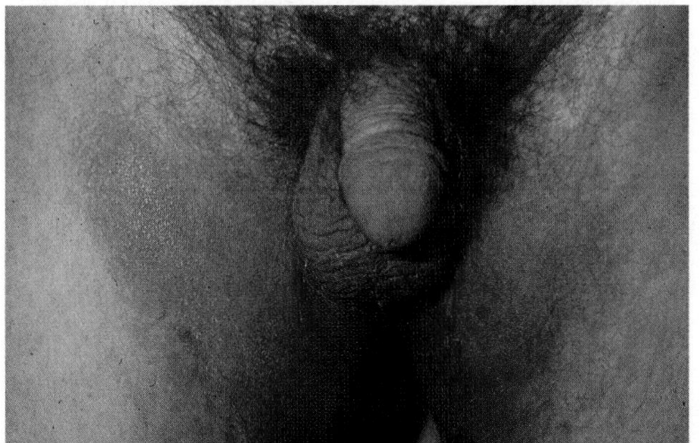
Figure 7–20.

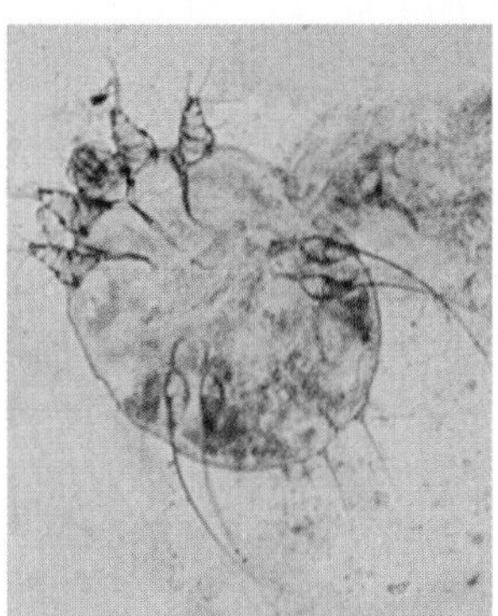
Figure 7–21.

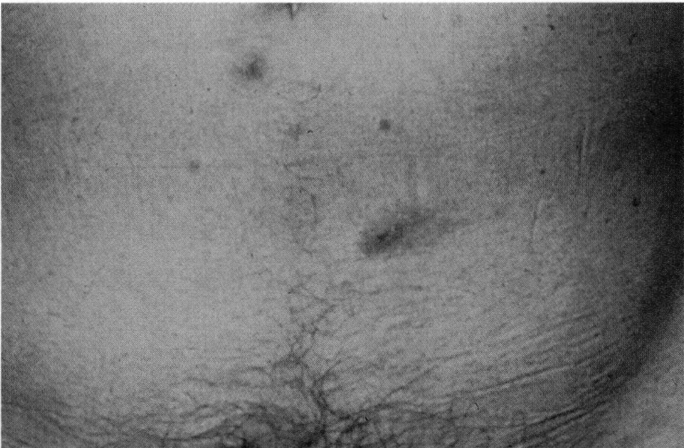
Figure 7–22.

Figure 7–19. Dry scaling appearance of "moccasin-type" tinea pedis.

Figure 7–20. Bright erythema of groin candidiasis.

Figure 7–21. Appearance of *Sarcoptes scabiei* under the microscope on a well-executed skin scraping.

Figure 7–22. Papular and eczematous lesions of scabies on the lower abdomen.

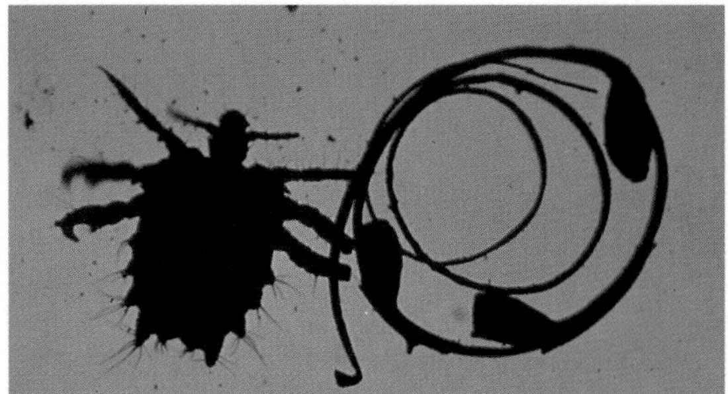

Figure 7–23.

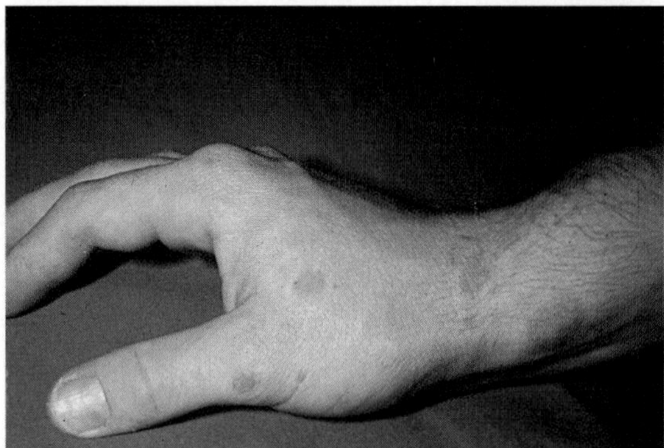

Figure 7–24.

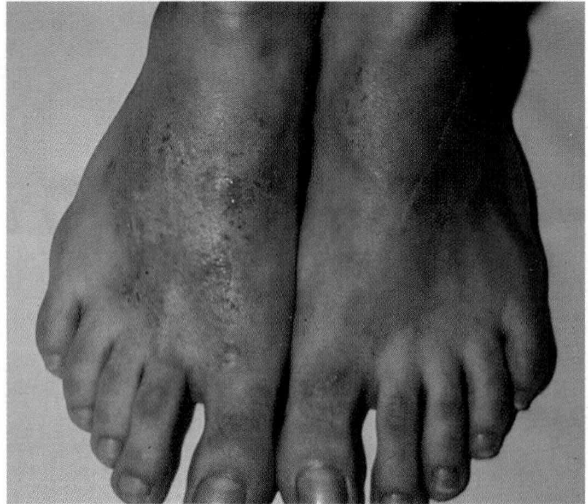

Figure 7–25.

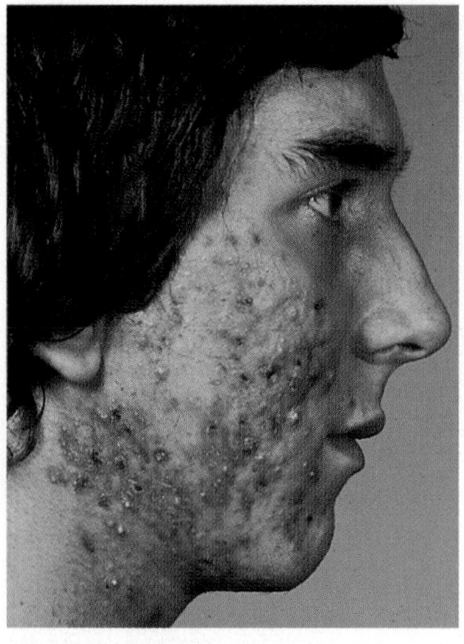

Figure 7–26.

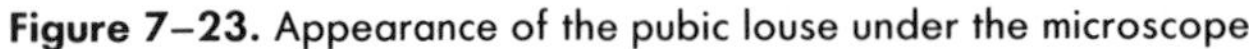

Figure 7–23. Appearance of the pubic louse under the microscope.

Figure 7–24. Nummular lesions of irritant eczema in a hockey player.

Figure 7–25. Contact dermatitis from athletic shoes.

Figure 7–26. Cystic acne with scarring.

Scott MJ, Scott MJ: Ping pong patches. Cutis 43(4):363–364, 1989.
Tomecki KJ, Mikesell JF: Rower's rump. J Am Acad Dermatol 1987; 16:890–891.
Wolf A, Gruber F, Jakac D: Painful piezogenic pedal papules and physical activity. Derm Beruf Umwelt 34(4):106–107, 1986.
Zitelli JA: Wound healing and wound dressings. *In* Roenigk RK, Roenigk HH (eds): Dermatologic Surgery: Principles and Practice. New York, Marcel Dekker, 1989, pp 97–135.

PHYSICAL FACTORS

Daniels F: Physiologic factors in the skin's reactions to heat and cold. *In* Fitzpatrick TB (ed): Dermatology in General Medicine. New York, McGraw-Hill, 1987, pp 1412–1424.
Herschkowitz M: Penile frostbite, an unforeseen hazard of jogging. N Engl J Med 296:178, 1977.
Kaplan AP, Garofalo J: Identification of a new physically induced urticaria: Cold-induced cholinergic urticaria. J Allergy Clin Immunol 68(6):438–441, 1981.
Nordlind K, Bondesson L, Johansson SG, et al: Purpura provoked by cold exposure in a skier. Dermatologica 167(2):101–103, 1983.

Sunburn

Arndt KA: Manual of Dermatologic Therapeutics. Boston, Little, Brown & Co, 1987.
Epstein JH: Polymorphous light eruption. Ann Allergy 24:397, 1986.
Lorencz AL: Physiological and pathological changes in skin from sunburn and sun tan. JAMA 173:1227, 1960.
Shupack JL, Gold JA, Stiller MJ, et al: Dermatologic Formulary. New York, McGraw-Hill, 1989, pp 211–216.
Singh KG, Singh RG, Girgla HS, et al: Incidence of sunburn during mountaineering expedition. J Sports Med Phys Fitness 26(4):369–372, 1986.

Impetigo/Furunculosis

Bartlett PC, Martin RJ, Cahill BR: Furunculosis in a high school football team. Am J Sports Med 10(6):371–374, 1982.
Dillon HC: Topical and systemic therapy for pyoderma. Int J Dermatol 19:443, 1980.
Ferrieri P, Dajoni A, Wannamaker LW, Chapman SS. Natural history of impetigo. J Clin Invest 51:2851–2862, 1972.
Kantor GR, Bergfeld WF: Common and uncommon dermatologic diseases related to sports activities. Exerc Sport Sci Rev 16:215–253, 1988.
Leyden J: Experimental infection with group A streptococci in humans. J Invest Dermatol 75:196, 1980.
Ludlam H, Cookson B: Scrum kidney: Epidemic pyoderma caused by a nephritogenic *Streptococcus pyogenes* in a rugby team. Lancet 2(8502):331–333, 1986.
Mertz PM, Marshall DA, Eaglstein WH, et al: Topical mupirocin treatment of impetigo is equal to oral erythromycin therapy. Arch Dermatol 125:1069–1073, 1989.
Steele R: Recurrent staphylococcal infection in families. Arch Dermatol 116:189, 1980.

Pitted Keratolysis

Zaias N: Pitted and ringed keratolysis. J Am Acad Dermatol 7:787–791, 1982.

Erythrasma

Schlapper OLA, Rosenblum GA, Rowden G, Phillips TM, et al: Concomitant erythrasma and dermatophytosis of the groin. Br J Dermatol 100:147–151, 1979.
Sokany I, Taplin D, Blank H: The etiology and treatment of erythrasma. J Invest Dermatol 37:283, 1961.

VIRAL INFECTIONS

Herpes Simplex

Jones BR, Fisan PN, Cobo LM, et al: Efficacy of acycloguanosine against herpes simplex corneal ulcer. Lancet 1:243, 1979.
Mattison HR, Reichmar R, Benedetti J, et al. Double-blind, placebo-controlled trial comparing long-term suppressive with short-term oral acyclovir therapy for management of recurrent genital herpes. Am J Med 85:20–25, 1988.

Oral acyclovir for genital herpes simplex infection. Medical Lett Drugs Ther 27(687):41–43, 1985.
Shelley WB: Herpetic arthritis associated with disseminated herpes simplex in a wrestler. Br J Dermatol 103:209–212, 1980.
Spruance SL, Hamill ML, Hoge WS, et al: Acyclovir prevents reactivation of herpes simplex labialis in skiers. JAMA 260(11):1597–1599, 1988.
Spruance SL, Overall JC, Kern ER, et al: The natural history of recurrent herpes simplex labialis: Implications for antiviral therapy. N Engl J Med 197:69, 1977.
Strauss RH, Leizman DJ, Lanesse RR, et al: Abrasive shirts may contribute to herpes gladiatorum among wrestlers. N Engl J Med 320:598–599, 1989.
White WB, Grant-Kels JM: Transmission of herpes simplex virus type I infection in rugby players. JAMA 252(4):533–535, 1984.

Warts/Molluscum Contagiosum

Bender ME, Pass F: Anogenital warts. *In* Maddin S (ed): Current Dermatologic Therapy. Philadelphia, WB Saunders, 1982, pp 483–486.
Beutner KR: Human papillomavirus infection. J Am Acad Dermatol 20:114–123, 1989.
Commens CA: Cutaneous transmission of molluscum contagiosum during orienteering competition. Med J Aust 146(2):117, 1987.
Eron LJ, Judson F, Tucker S, et al: Interferon therapy for condyloma acuminata. N Engl J Med 315:1059–1064, 1986.
Henaco M, Freeman RC: Inflammatory molluscum contagiosum. Arch Dermatol 90:479, 1964.
Massing AM, Epstein WL: Natural history of warts: A two-year study. Arch Dermatol 87:306, 1963.
Mobacken H, Nordin P: Molluscum contagiosum among cross-country runners. J Am Acad Dermatol 17(3):519–520, 1987.
Niizeki K, Kano O, Kondo Y: An epidemic study of molluscum contagiosum: Relationship to swimming. Dermatologica 169(4):197–198, 1984.

FUNGAL AND YEAST INFECTIONS

Tinea

Borgers M: Mechanism of actions of antifungal drugs with special reference to the imidazole derivative. Rev Infect Dis 2:520, 1980.
Catterall MD: Tinea versicolor. *In* Maddin S (ed): Current Dermatologic Therapy. Philadelphia, WB Saunders, 1982, pp 463–464.
Eaglestein WH, Pariser DM: Office Techniques for Diagnosing Skin Diseases. Chicago, Year Book Medical Publishers, 1978, pp 9–15 and 89–112.
Lesher JL, Smith JG: Antifungal agents in dermatology. J Am Acad Dermatol 17:383–396, 1987.
Robertson MH, Rich P, Parker F, et al: Ketoconazole in griseofulvin-resistant dermatophytosis. J Am Acad Dermatol 6:224–229, 1982.
Smith EB: New topical agents for dermatophytosis. Cutis 17:54, 1976.

INFESTATIONS

Pediculosis

Rasmussen JE: The problem of lindane. J Am Acad Dermatol 5:507, 1981.
Shacter B: Treatment of scabies and pediculosis with lindane preparations: An evaluation. J Am Acad Dermatol 5:517–527, 1981.
Van der Rhee HJ, Farquhar JA, Vermeulen NPE: Efficacy and transdermal absorption of permethrin in scabies patients. Acta Derm Venereol 69:170–182, 1989.

CONTACT DERMATITIS

Adams RM: Contact allergic dermatitis due to diethylthiourea in a wet suit. Contact Dermatitis 8(4):277–278, 1982.
Fisher AA: Contact Dermatitis, ed 3. Philadelphia, Lea & Febiger, 1986, pp 77–99.
Peystowski SB, et al: Allergic contact hypersensitivity of nickel, neomycin, ethylenediamine and benzocaine: Relationships between age, sex, history of exposure and reactivity to standard patch tests and use tests in general populations. Arch Dermatol 115:950, 1979.

Tennstedt D, Lachapelle JM: Windsurfer dermatitis from black rubber components. Contact Dermatitis 7(3):160–161, 1981.

Tuyp E, Mitchell JC: Scuba diver facial dermatitis. Contact Dermatitis 10(6):334–335, 1983.

DISORDERS OF THE PILOSEBACEOUS UNIT

Acne

Frank SB, Acne Vulgaris, American Lecture Series Publication Number 796. Springfield, IL. Charles C Thomas, 1971. pp 13–412.

Mills OH, Kligman A: Acne mechanica. Arch Dermatol 11:481, 1975.

Scott MJ, Scott MJ: Dermatologists and anabolic-androgenic drug abuse. Cutis 44(1):30–35, 1989.

Thomsen RR, Stanieri A, Knutson D, et al: Topical clindamycin treatment for acne. Arch Dermatol 116:1031, 1980.

8

THE RESPIRATORY SYSTEM

Carlos Vaz Fragoso, MD
David M. Systrom, MD

This chapter focuses on the special contributions of the respiratory system to exercise performance and on the relationships among exercise, pulmonary symptoms, and disease.

RESPIRATORY PHYSIOLOGY DURING EXERCISE

During exercise, the respiratory system must be able to accommodate a 30 to 40 fold increase in skeletal muscle metabolic rate by sufficiently "arterializing" mixed venous blood to prevent mitochondrial hypoxia and to mitigate tissue acidosis.[1] At exceedingly high rates of work, normal cardiopulmonary adjustments are remarkably adept at increasing O_2 uptake and CO_2 output to maintain arterial blood gas and acid-base homeostasis; the arterial partial pressure of oxygen (Po_2) is preserved near resting values and the pH falls only slightly.

Arterial pH is directly related to arterial concentration of bicarbonate buffer and indirectly to the arterial partial pressure of carbon dioxide ($Paco_2$), the variable directly controlled by pulmonary gas exchange. During submaximal exercise, alveolar (effective) ventilation perfectly matches increased CO_2 production produced by substrate metabolism in muscle. At more intense work loads, the lungs must also excrete "nonmetabolic" CO_2 generated from bicarbonate-buffering of lactic acid and depress arterial Pco_2 to compensate for the loss of buffer. This is achieved by increasing tidal volume to about 60% of the vital capacity and by increasing respiratory frequency. Improved perfusion of the apices of the upright lung occurs as pulmonary vascular pressures and cardiac output rise during exercise. When combined with larger tidal volumes, ventilation becomes more efficient (ie, the dead space/tidal volume ratio, (V_D/V_T, falls). Matching of ventilatory drive to metabolism is likely achieved through a combination of humoral (eg, CO_2, acid, catecholamines, potassium) and both central and peripheral neuronal pathways.

Except for the world-class athlete exercising at maximum metabolic rates, arterial O_2 content does not normally fall during exercise. This is quite remarkable given a mixed venous PO_2 which may be returned to the lung from working muscle in the 10- to 20-mm Hg range, and the fact that at high cardiac outputs, red cell contact with alveolar gas is diminished. Compensatory mechanisms during exercise include alveolar hyperventilation, an increase in the respiratory exchange ratio, increased diffusing surface area due to dilation and recruitment of pulmonary capillary beds, increased affinity of hemoglobin for O_2 following CO_2 unloading, hemoconcentration due to extravascular fluid shifts, improved matching of ventilation and perfusion at the lung bases, and a reduction in the right-to-left shunt fraction.

Athletes performing endurance events such as the marathon are generally limited by substrate; the cardiopulmonary unit operates at only approximately 80% of its capacity in such cases. Conversely, the maximum oxygen uptake ($\dot{V}O_{2max}$) during incremental exercise is thought to be largely limited by convective (blood flow) and diffusional transport of O_2 to active muscle. In untrained normal individuals, the respiratory system is endowed with sufficient functional redundancy to obviate a rate-limiting status. High levels of aerobic training, however, have been associated with depressed ventilatory chemosensitivity and an inordinate increase in cardiac output during exercise, which on rare occasions beget rate-limiting respiratory acidosis and hypoxemia.[2]

RESPIRATORY SYMPTOMS

Dyspnea

The etiology of breathlessness is not yet perfectly understood, but seems to be closely related to both the reflex stimulation of respiration and increased levels of outgoing motor command to the ventilatory pump.[3] Thus, dyspnea commonly results from conditions that increase ventilatory demand, work of breathing, or respiratory muscle weakness. When these three factors are subclinical at rest early in the course of disease, dyspnea may be elicited by the increased demands of exercise.

Ventilatory demand is increased when CO_2 production is increased, when the $PaCO_2$ "set-point" is decreased and when there is excessive "wasted" (dead space) ventilation. Excess CO_2 production occurs in hyperthyroidism, when work is inefficient (eg, in obesity), after a high-carbohydrate diet, and as newly produced lactic acid is being buffered by bicarbonate. The onset of lactic acidosis (lactate threshold) occurs at a lower metabolic rate in the untrained individual or a patient with cardiovascular disease when compared with normal and may cause exertional dyspnea. Arterial or arterialized venous lactate may be directly measured during an incremental exercise protocol, or an indirect "ventilatory threshold" may be assessed by gas exchange.[4] A lactate or ventilatory threshold below $\dot{V}O_2 = 1.0$ L/min or 40% of the predicted $\dot{V}O_{2max}$ is considered abnormal.

Hyperventilation during exercise occurs in response to hypoxemia, anemia, and lactic acidosis, and due to stimulation of lung stretch receptors (eg, interstitial disease). Exercise O_2 desaturation is often seen before resting hypoxemia and may therefore be an early marker of disease. During an incremental exercise protocol, gradual O_2 desaturation is characteristic of pulmonary disease (eg, interstitial and pulmonary vascular disease, emphysema). A rare patient with a patent foramen ovale and increasing right atrial pressures during exercise will abruptly increase venous admixture, causing sudden O_2 desaturation. O_2 desaturation with exercise is exceedingly rare in congestive heart failure, and should point the clinician toward alveolar hypoventilation or precapillary pulmonary vascular disease. Occasionally, a patient with psychogenic hyperventilation will defend a chronically depressed $PaCO_2$ set-point during exercise at the cost of markedly exaggerated and often erratic minute ventilation ($\dot{V}E$).

Increased dead space ventilation is seen in the restrictive lung (sarcoidosis, idiopathic pulmonary fibrosis) and chest wall disorders (kyphoscoliosis) and with pulmonary vascular disease due to excessive absolute dead space, inadequate tidal volumes, or both. Both O_2 desaturation and elevated dead space may be measured directly or inferred from increased ventilatory "equivalents" ($\dot{V}E/\dot{V}CO_2$ and $\dot{V}E/\dot{V}O_2$) during submaximal exercise.

Excessive work of breathing is due to increased elastic or resistive forces on the lung or chest wall. It is well known that chronic obstructive pulmonary disease imparts increased resistive work of breathing, but less commonly appreciated that the elastic work of breathing is significant for such patients. At high respiratory rates achieved during exercise, there may be insufficient time for expiration; breath-stacking and "auto–positive end-expiratory pressure (PEEP)" may ensue, decreasing lung compliance. The latter is also seen in the interstitial and chest wall disorders, pulmonary vascular disease (the stiff pulmonary vasculature provides an endoskeleton), and congestive heart failure. When the elastic work of breathing is high, the patient often develops a characteristic high-frequency, low tidal volume (<60% vital capacity) respiratory pattern.

Over the past decade, it has become increasingly evident that disorders of respiratory muscle strength and mechanics produce breathlessness, even when ventilatory demand and impedance are low. Respiratory muscle weakness is seen with neuropathies, myopathies, metabolic disorders, and malnutrition. The hyperinflation of chronic obstructive pulmonary disease decreases the preload of the diaphragm, rendering it an ineffective inspiratory muscle. When faced with increased demand (exercise, worsening obstruction), the diaphragm may decrease its activity, leading to the clinical finding of inspiratory abdominal retraction (abdominal paradox). Weakness or fatigue may also be confirmed in the laboratory by depressed maximal inspiratory, expiratory, and transdiaphragmatic forces, a fall ≥20% of the vital capacity when the patient assumes the supine versus the upright position, or a characteristic electromyogram (EMG) of the diaphragm.

Most often, the etiology of exertional dyspnea is readily apparent from the history, physical examination, resting pulmonary function tests, and radiographic data. When questions remain after an initial noninvasive investigation, cardiopulmonary exercise testing should be considered. Measurements can include ventilation and gas exchange, systemic and pulmonary artery blood gases and pressures, respiratory muscle strength, and cardiac output.

Ideally, treatment of dyspnea will reduce ventilatory demand (supplemental O_2, exercise training), decrease respiratory impedance (bronchodilators, intermittent positive-pressure breathing for extrapulmonary restriction), and improve respiratory muscle strength through a combination of endurance training and rest therapy (eg, nocturnal ventilation). Nonspecific pharmacologic efforts (eg, codeine, benzodiazepines) at decreasing dyspnea have met with little success.

Second Wind

A sudden easing of dyspnea during heavy exercise has been coined the "second wind."[5] Coincidental objective findings include a sudden increase in respiratory rate with a decrease in neural stimulation of the diaphragm by EMG. No changes are seen in pressures developed by the diaphragm, lung volumes, chest configuration, or recruitment of accessory muscles of respiration. It has been postulated that the second wind is related to improved contractility of the diaphragm due to increased circulating catecholamines or changes in diaphragmatic blood flow.

Chest Pain

Noxious mechanical or inflammatory stimulation of unmyelinated "C" neuronal fibers arising from thoracic and abdominal musculoskeletal strctures and viscera gives rise to "chest" pain.[6] When chest pain is associated with exertion, the differential diagnosis may be significantly narrowed. The most common cause of chest pain in the athlete is musculoskeletal, but it can occasionally be an important marker of significant pathology of the respiratory, cardiovascular, or gastrointestinal systems.

Pulmonary disorders are associated with chest pain through involvement of the parietal pleura, as both visceral pleura and pulmonary parenchyma are devoid of sensory nerve endings.[6] Pleuritic chest pain is typically abrupt in onset, unilateral, made worse by cough or deep breathing, and often, therefore, made worse by exercise. The pain will usually be referred to the overlying chest wall, but in cases of involvement of the dome of the diaphragm, it may be referred to the ipsilateral shoulder.

The most common variety of chest pain in the healthy athlete is probably the "stitch." It is described as a sharp respirophasic pain over the inferolateral chest wall and is usually related to exertion. Its genesis may be related to spasm and/or ischemia of the diaphragm.

Chest pain may also be a marker of more serious underlying disease.[6] Infection, connective tissue disorders, neoplasia, pulmonary embolism, and pneumothorax can all be associated with pleuritic pain. In the young athlete, the most common infectious etiology is viral, often coxsackievirus or echovirus, but bacterial and tuberculous causes are also possible. Systemic lupus erythematosus (SLE) occurs in young women, and lymphoma and germ cell tumors should be thought of in young people with mediastinal masses and pleuritic chest pain. Athletes on the birth control pill or at bed rest following surgery or immobilization of fractures are at risk for pulmonary embolism. Chest pain in this setting is due to pulmonary infarction, a rare event in the absence of preexisting congestive heart failure. It has been taught that the sudden onset of pleuritic chest pain during vigorous exertion suggests pneumothorax, but in reality, most pneumothoraces occur with walking or sedentary activity. A minimal investigation of pleuritic chest pain should include careful auscultation for a pleural friction rub and chest radiographs with bilateral decubitus views to rule out associated pleural effusion. If pleural effusion is present, and the diagnosis is in doubt, a thoracentesis should be performed.

Chest pain related to the cardiovascular system, especially that due to left ventricular ischemia, is dealt with in detail elsewhere in this book. Myocarditis is occasionally responsible for sudden death during exercise during or following a viral syndrome. Forty percent of patients with myocarditis complain of pleuritic chest pain, while another 20% report exertional pain consistent with angina. Chest pain due to pulmonary hypertension may mimic angina and, in fact, is likely due to an ischemic, pressure-overloaded right ventricle (see below). The pain of aortic dissection may begin suddenly in a hypertensive individual during exercise because of increased aortic sheer pressures. The pain may be anterior with radiation into the back, is generally most severe at its onset, and may have a tearing quality. It may be associated with new neurologic deficits, absent or diminished pulses, aortic insufficiency, or myocardial infarction. When the inflammation of pericarditis involves contiguous parietal pleura, sharp, anterior, pleuritic chest pain may result, which is classically relieved by assuming the upright position.

Chest pain related to the gastrointestinal system is commonly referred to the thoracic spinal segments and may be confused with that due to primary disorders of the cardiopulmonary system. In the young athlete, reflux esophagitis, with or without associated spasm, may worsen during exercise because of increases in abdominal pressure generated as expiratory muscles are recruited at high levels of $\dot{V}_E$. A relationshp to diet, body position, odynophagia or dysphagia, and relief after antacids suggests pain of esophageal origin. In contact sports, tremendously positive transesophageal pressures may result in an esophageal tear (Boerhaave's syndrome) often characterized by pain that is excruciating and steady. The athlete taking nonsteroidal anti-inflammatory medications may suffer gastritis or peptic ulcer disease with pain referred to the epigastrium or lower chest.

Musculoskeletal chest pain is exceedingly common in the athlete population. Viral or idiopathic costochondritis usually involves the second, third, or fourth costochondral junctions. Its pain varies with respiration, may worsen with exercise, and is reproduced by palpation. Degenerative arthritis of the cervical or thoracic spine may compress spinal roots, resulting in chest pain that sometimes worsens with truncal movement.

In general, healthy, exercising individuals will have a "benign" cause of their chest pain. If it persists, occurs in the setting of coronary artery disease risk factors, or is associated with deterioration in performance, a prompt and thorough evaluation is indicated.

Cough

The cough reflex likely evolved to protect the lungs from a variety of environmental insults.[7] Receptors linked to the medullary cough reflex center by means of the trigeminal, vagal, glossopharyngeal, and phrenic nerves are omnipresent. Their stimulation may occur from irritants in the ear canal, nose, sinuses, pharynx, trachea, bronchi, pleura, pericardium, diaphragm, and stomach.[7]

In the otherwise healthy population, causes of cough include rhinitis, sinusitis, and bronchial hyperreactivity.[7] The nose must be ruled out as the etiology of cough before an elaborate pulmonary workup is embarked upon. Clues to a nasal etiology include a history of nasal discharge, postnasal drip, facial pain, headache, sinus tenderness, and "cobblestoning" of the posterior pharyngeal mucosa. A positive response of the cough to nasal decongestants may secure the diagnosis. For up to 6 weeks following a viral upper respiratory tract infection, previously normal individuals may have hyperresponsiveness to respiratory epithelial heat and water loss during exercise or after aerosolized methacholine. Subjects may react to either challenge in this setting with cough, wheezing, dyspnea, and a significant (≥20%) fall in flow rates (usually measured as the forced expiratory volume in 1 second or FEV_1). These findings overlap with those in the asthmatic population (see below) and are separated from those of true asthma by their transience and less severe airway obstruction.

Cough may also be a cardinal symptom of serious underlying cardiopulmonary disorders that are not specifically related to the athlete or to exertion; a comprehensive discussion of these is beyond the scope of this chapter, but would include drug-induced pulmonary disease, chronic aspiration, chronic bronchitis, interstitial lung disease, bronchogenic carcinoma, foreign body, and congestive heart failure. Such diagnoses can be differentiated by history, pulmonary function testing, radiographic studies, nocturnal esophageal pH manometry, fiberoptic bronchoscopy, and cardiac echocardiogram or radionuclide studies. It should be emphasized that the frequency of daily cough varies in direct proportion to the number of cigarettes smoked per day and that passive smoking may be associated with chronic cough, especially in a susceptible individual. Psychogenic cough is found in the young individual. It is usually absent at night, may increase under emotional stress, and is a diagnosis of exclusion.

Hemoptysis

Hemoptysis is defined as expectorated blood arising from the respiratory tract below the larynx.[8] Confirmation of these criteria is critical, but sometimes difficult, as pulmonary aspiration of blood from an upper airway source is common, and hematemesis may mimic hemoptysis. A thorough ear, nose, and throat (ENT) examination on presentation may rule out the former, while a gastrointestinal source is suggested if the expectorated material has an acid pH. Bona fide hemoptysis is usually related to anatomic abnormalities of the pulmonary or bronchial blood vessel walls, pulmonary arterial or venous hypertension, or disorders of blood clotting. Although the differential diagnosis is a wide one in the general population, hemoptysis in the exercising population is rare and is usually due to one of a few relatively benign diagnoses.

Transient blood-streaked sputum in a nonsmoking individual less than 40 years of age is generally due to acute bronchitis.[8] If the chest radiograph is normal, no further workup is necessary. If purulent sputum, fever, leukocytosis, and an alveolar infiltrate are present, bacterial pneumonia is likely. If, after gathering appropriate culture data and administering adequate antibiotic treatment, the infiltrate resolves (normally within 6 weeks), no further testing need be done. Mycobacterium tuberculosis and fungal diseases are relatively rare causes of hemoptysis in the exercising population.

Gross hemoptysis is an uncommon event in the athlete. Occasionally, congenital arteriovenous malformation, bronchogenic cyst, pulmonary sequestration, or coagulopathy may be first manifested during an athletic event when intravascular pressures rise. Acquired coagulopathies, thrombocytopenia, or platelet dysfunction, most often due to drugs, may also present as hemoptysis during exertion. "Benign" bronchial adenomas are often vascular and tend to cause recurrent hemoptysis. When hemoptysis varies with the menstrual cycle, ectopic endometriosis is suggested. Pulmonary hypertension of any cause, with or without the capillaritis associated with connective tissue disorders (eg, SLE) and related disorders (eg, Goodpasture's syndrome, Wegener's syndrome, pulmonary hemosiderosis), can cause bloody sputum in a young person. For pulmonary embolism to be associated with hemoptysis, infarction—a rare event in the previously healthy individual—is required. Blunt or penetrating trauma acquired in the course of athletic competition may cause hemoptysis and is sometimes associated with hemothorax, which requires immediate chest tube evacuation. Aspiration of a foreign body may occur without any history of the same.

A comprehensive review of hemoptysis in the elderly population and in smokers is beyond the scope of this chapter. Chronic bronchitis, bronchiectasis, broncholithiasis, primary and (rarely) metastatic carcinoma of the lung, congestive heart failure, and mitral stenosis should be included in such a differential diagnosis.

Important historic information includes a familial or personal history of bleeding diathesis or hypercoagulable states, the quantity and duration of blood-streaked sputum, presence of purulent sputum, and any associated symptoms. The physical examination should rule out extrapulmonary sources of blood, and a careful search should be made for cutaneous or mucosal arteriovenous malformations, purpura and petechiae, abdominal organomegaly, and clubbing. Laboratory work should include indices of renal and hepatic function, a complete blood and platelet count, coagulation and bleeding times, urinalysis with examination of the spun sediment for the presence of red-cell casts, chest radiograph, microscopic and cytologic sputum analysis, and a tuberculin skin test with control. In selected cases, a serologic screen for connective tissue disorders, anticytoplasmic (Wegener's syndrome) or antiglomerular basement membrane antibodies (Goodpasture's syndrome), color flow Doppler of the lower extremities, ventilation/perfusion lung scan, pulmonary angiogram, and CT or MRI scan of the chest may narrow the differential diagnosis. Routine pulmonary function tests will differentiate obstructive from restrictive disorders and may provide clues to upper airway pathology. Arterial blood gases most often reflect hypoxemia due to the development of low ventilation-perfusion (V/Q) areas and right-to-left shunting. The diffusing capacity for carbon monoxide may be transiently elevated soon after a significant pulmonary parenchymal bleed. Although early direct visualization of the airways by bronchoscopy localizes the site of bleeding to a segment in most (93%) cases, it may not change diagnostic or therapeutic decision-making.

Treatment of hemoptysis is directed at the underlying cause. In mild cases, antitussives and bed rest may suffice. The most common cause of death with massive hemoptysis ($\geq$600 mL per 16 to 24 hours) is asphyxia, not exsanguination. Nonspecific therapeutic measures in this setting include placing the bleeding lung in the dependent position, supplemental O_2, and antitussives. Occasionally, rigid bronchoscopy with Fogarty catheter balloon tamponade of a segment, bronchial arteriography with embolization, or resectional surgery is needed.

Wheezing

Turbulent airflow through narrowed airways causes a continuous high-pitched musical sound known as wheezing.[9] Since high flow rates beget both turbulent flow and airway constriction, wheezing is often reported during or immediately following exercise.[9] Episodic, polyphonic, expiratory wheezing is likely due to asthma and is discussed below. Before labeling a patient as asthmatic, however, a rigorous search should be made for other disease entities that may mimic asthma.[9] In the young, exercising population, this list includes cystic fibrosis, alpha-1-protease inhibitor deficiency, upper airway obstruction (eg, goiter, epiglottitis, angioedema), fixed lower airway obstruction (eg, foreign body, adenoma), pulmonary embolism, and the carcinoid syndrome. The latter is suggested when hypotension, abdominal cramping, and diarrhea wax and wane with wheezing. Factitious asthma usually occurs in the young individual with a psychiatric history, is related to inappropriate apposition of the vocal cords, and may be responsive to speech therapy. Clues to its presence include a depressed peak flow out of proportion to the FEV_1, plateauing or "sawtoothing" of the inspiratory flow-volume loop, and a normal alveolar-arterial difference for Po_2 during exacerbations.

RESPIRATORY DISEASES

Exercise-Induced Asthma

Reversible airway obstruction that occurs during or following exertion has been termed exercise-induced asthma (EIA). Because of its increased resistance at high (turbulent) flow rates, the nose, a major mechanism for the conditioning of inspirate, is bypassed during exercise. In addition, a rise in mean pulmonary artery and left atrial pressures during exercise recruits and dilates pulmonary capillaries, which act as efficient heat exchangers. This combination leads to respiratory epithelial cooling and water loss. When combined with rapid endobronchial rewarming, reflex and mediator-related bronchospasm and airway inflammation result. EIA is exceedingly common; 15% of the 1984 U.S. Olympic team were reported to have exercise-induced bronchospasm.[10]

Individuals with EIA characteristically complain of dyspnea, cough, and/or wheezing 10 to 15 minutes following exercise of at least moderate intensity ($\geq$60% of $\dot{V}o_{2max}$) and duration (6 to 8 min). Symptoms are generally worse during exercise in cold, dry air and are mitigated by exercise in warm, humid environments (eg, swimming). Although controversial, there may occasionally be a "late-phase" reaction producing bronchoconstriction several hours after exercise. Much more often ($\geq$50% of patients), a refractory period of up to 4 hours follows the initial episode of bronchoconstriction, resulting in attenuated decrements in airflow with repeated exercise bouts. This may account for some patients' claim that "warm-up" exercise helps decrease or avoid subsequent EIA symptoms. In the laboratory, a prolonged (30-min) submaximal ($\dot{V}o_2 \simeq 30\ mL \cdot kg^{-1} \cdot min^{-1}$ exercise bout induces refractoriness to EIA without marked antecedent airflow obstruction.[11] The refractory period seems to be due to a product of the cyclooxygenase pathway and may be blocked by the ubiquitous nonsteroidal antiinflammatory medications. Uncomplicated EIA seems to be at the mild end of the asthma spectrum; such patients complain of symptoms only after exercise. Conversely, 90% to 95% of chronic asthmatics will have evidence of increased bronchospasm if they perform sufficiently long and intense exercise. They may be particularly susceptible, as airways inflammation probably increases heat and water loss from the respiratory epithelium.

The diagnosis of EIA is based on a compatible history, objective measurements of airflow obstruction after provocation, and a positive bronchodilator response. Classically, the FEV_1 or peak expiratory flow rate is measured before and at 5-minute intervals for a period of 30 to 60 minutes following exercise. A significant decrease ($\geq$20%) in either index of airflow obstruction suggests EIA. The test may be made more sensitive by asking the patient to breathe cold, dry air during and warm air after the exercise bout. If the diagnosis remains in question after exercise testing, bronchoprovocation with increasing concentrations of aerosolized methacholine may be performed. If negative, alternative diagnoses should be sought.

Preventive measures for patients with EIA include limiting exercise intensity and duration during periods of increased air pollution (see below), during and up to 6 weeks after episodes of respiratory infections, and, if possible, avoiding cool dry air.

First-line medical prophylaxis for EIA in the 1990s consists of a β_2-adrenergic agonist or cromolyn by way of a metered dose inhaler (MDI). The β-agonists work by increasing airway smooth muscle cAMP, whereas cromolyn probably prevents mast cell degranulation and exerts anticholinergic effects. The β-agonists may be preferable because they may also be used as treatment if EIA "breaks through" prophylactic attempts. Newly available β-agonists eg, Bitolterol (Tornalate, Winthrop Pharmaceuticals, New York, NY) and Pirbuterol (Maxair, 3M Riker, Northridge, CA) have increased β_2 specificity (lower incidence of cardiovascular and neurologic toxicity) and a prolonged duration of action. Their onset of action is slightly delayed compared with that of older preparations, however, and they should therefore be administered at least 30 minutes prior to exercise. The most common cause of failure of the MDIs in patients with EIA is their improper use. Patients should be instructed to exhale to functional residual capacity, to place the MDI 3 to 5 cm away from an open mouth, and to activate the MDI just as they begin a 5-second inhalation to total lung capacity. If the patient has difficulty timing the inspiration with MDI activation, a spacing mechanism such as the Inspirease device should be prescribed. These recommendations have been shown to facilitate drug delivery to the distal airway. Only rarely will chronic asthma medications such as theophylline and steroids be indicated for the patient with uncomplicated EIA.

Hyperventilation Syndrome

In a young individual, the association of dyspnea with lightheadedness, paresthesias, syncope, aerophagia, and anxiety is very suggestive of the hyperventilation syndrome.[12] The physical examination, radiographic studies, and pulmonary function tests are normal. A resting electrocardiogram can show nonspecific ST-segment and T-wave abnormalities, while the arterial blood gas reflects a compensated respiratory alkalosis. Lactate, if measured, may be high owing to activation of glycolysis by alkalosis. Cardiopulmonary exercise testing often reveals erratic hyperventilation at rest and submaximal exercise, but normal, regular breathing patterns at heavier work loads, when the respiratory system reflexly compensates for a lactic acidosis. Such testing will also rule out significant cardiopulmonary disease.

The patient should be reassured by the demonstration of normal heart and lung function at rest and with exercise. Therapy may include psychological counseling, anxiolytics, and episodic CO_2 rebreathing.

Primary Pulmonary Hypertension

Primary pulmonary hypertension (PPH)[13] and pulmonary embolism (discussed below) are two forms of pulmonary vascular disease that may occur in the relatively young age group. Symptoms from either disease entity may be first noticed during exercise. The common pathophysiology is related to a fixed increase in pulmonary vascular resistance (PVR) and mismatching of ventilation and perfusion. Failure of the increased cardiac output to dilate and recruit pulmonary vasculature results in worsening pulmonary hypertension during exercise. Diversion of blood flow from high to normal resistance pulmonary vessels causes overperfusion of relatively normal alveoli and arterial hypoxemia. Underperfusion of lung units affected by disease creates wasted ventilation. Pulmonary hypertension per se increases ventilation through a vagal reflex. An underfilled left ventricle may not be able to support the normal forward cardiac output, which causes both fatigue and yet another demand on ventilation through an early lactate threshold. It is not surprising that exertional fatigue and dyspnea are hallmarks of these disorders.

PPH is most common in 20- to 39-year old women and is defined by the presence of idiopathic pulmonary hypertension [mean pulmonary artery pressure (PAP) $\geq$20 mm Hg] at rest. Pathologic features include intimal fibrosis, medial smooth muscle hypertrophy and hyperplasia, and "plexiform" lesions as well as in situ thrombosis of small pulmonary arteries. A definitive diagnosis may be difficult and requires both documentation of the pulmonary hypertension and ruling out of secondary causes. Thus, the routine workup should include a thorough familial and personal history of hypercoagulable states, drug use, rheumatic heart disease or murmur, Raynaud's phenomenon, snoring, and daytime somnolence. On physical examination, pulmonary hypertension may be reflected by an increased P_2, right ventricular heave or S_3, and the murmur and jugular venous pulsations of tricuspid regurgitation. The skin examination may reveal cyanosis, arteriovenous malformations, or clues to the presence of cirrhosis. Polycythemia may reflect longstanding hypoxemia and a prolonged partial thromboplastin time (PTT) ("lupus anticoagulant"), a hypercoagulable state. The antinuclear antibody (ANA) is positive in 30% of PPH patients. A chest radiograph may show enlarged pulmonary arteries, a paucity of peripheral blood vessels, and right ventricular enlargement. Pulmonary function tests usually show mild restriction in PPH. A reduction of the diffusing capacity for CO out of proportion to lung volume is expected with precapillary pulmonary hypertension. The resting arterial blood gas uniformly shows hypoxemia and a compensated respiratory alkalosis. The V/Q scan is most often read as "low probability" in PPH, and a pulmonary angiogram may be necessary to rule out chronic pulmonary emboli. The ECG will usually show right axis deviation (79%) and right ventricular hypertrophy (87%) in symptomatic patients. Two-dimensional color flow echocardiography with pulsed Doppler estimation of pulmonary artery pressures will confirm pulmonary hypertension and eliminate secondary causes such as atrial septal defect and mitral stenosis. A pulmonary artery catheter study will document elevated PAP, PVR, and normal or low pulmonary capillary wedge pressure. The right atrial pressure may be normal or increased and the cardiac index high, normal, or depressed, depending on whether right heart failure or tricuspid regurgitation have developed.

Cardiopulmonary exercise testing elicits a distinct pattern of physiologic responses in the patient with PPH. The maximum O_2 uptake is depressed and sometimes associated with a terminal plateau when plotted against increasing work. A high heart rate as a percentage of predicted maximum is generally achieved and there is evidence for an early anaerobic threshold. As opposed to the patient with postcapillary pulmonary hypertension, abnormalities of gas exchange, including O_2 desaturation and a blunted fall in the V_D/V_T ratio, are common. Although ventilation is excessive throughout exercise, there is usually significant ventilatory reserve (maximum predicted-achieved $\dot{V}_E$) at peak exercise. If radionuclide studies of the heart are performed, a depressed resting or exercise right ventricular ejection fraction may be found.

Treatment includes O_2 supplementation sufficient to preserve arterial O_2 saturations $\geq$88% at rest and with exercise. If right heart failure has supervened, careful treatment with diuretics and digoxin should be considered. Although controversial, most patients with PPH should probably undergo a vasodilator drug trial with pulmonary artery hemodynamic monitoring in an intensive care unit. Most centers begin with O_2 and then proceed to an intravenous agent with a short half-life (eg, prostacyclin, prostaglandin E_1) to demonstrate vasoreactivity and to avoid side effects. If there is a fall in PAP > 20% or in PVR > 30%, which is greater than any fall in systemic vascular resistance, a real effect on pulmonary vascular tone is likely and one may be unjustified in pursuing a chronic oral regimen. Lesser changes are seen as a part of the natural history of PPH and may not be significant. Often, industrial doses of an oral agent (eg, verapamil) are necessary for beneficial symptomatic and hemodynamic effects. Heart-lung transplantation is the only definitive treatment at present.

Pulmonary Embolism

It has been recognized for more than 100 years that venous thromboembolism occurs in the setting of trauma to or decreased flow in the deep veins of the extremities and in hypercoagulable states. The young athlete may meet these criteria following injury or prolonged travel, or if oral contraceptives are used. The source of the embolus is usually the deep venous system of the legs above the popliteal fossa. Little can be done about the 10% of patients who die within 1 hour of pulmonary embolism (PE). Of the remainder, a correct diagnosis is made in only 30%, who when treated have a 92% survival. Conversely, 30% of patients whose PE is not diagnosed or treated subsequently die of recurrent PE.[14]

Diagnosis of deep vein thrombophlebitis (DVT) and PE requires a high index of suspicion because of the insensitivity of the physical examination and routine laboratory studies.[14] Symptoms of DVT include lower extremity pain, swelling, and redness. Although tenderness, warmth, edema, and a palpable "cord" may be present, the physical examination is normal in over half of patients with documented DVT. Patients with PE may complain of the sudden onset of dyspnea and sometimes cough. As noted above, hemoptysis and pleuritic chest pain imply infarction. The physical examination may reveal a respiratory rate > 16, fever, inspiratory crackles, and rarely, wheezing and a pleural friction rub (with infarction). A massive clot lodged downstream of an untrained right ventricle may result in lightheadedness, syncope, signs of right ventricular failure, and an "S_I,Q_{III},T_{III}" pattern on the ECG. The chest radiograph is most helpful in ruling out other diagnoses. A normal room air alveolar-arterial gradient for O_2 is more helpful in excluding PE than a normal Pao_2.[15]

A definitive diagnosis of proximal DVT can be made noninvasively by color flow Doppler.[16] Sensitivity, specificity, and positive and negative predicted values for the technic are all > 95% and compare favorably to contrast venography, with less risk. A normal ventilation/perfusion lung scan is generally thought to rule out PE, and a high probability scan (multiple subsegmental or segmental unmatched defects) is usually sufficient to begin treatment. Intermediate and low probability scans with a good history for PE require pulmonary angiography for the diagnosis to be made.

The major goal of therapy for DVT and PE is to prevent propagation and life-threatening embolization of residual blood clot in the leg, whereas endogenous thrombolysis and venous reendothelialization are ongoing. Since the latter occurs over approximately 1 week, patients should be asked to remain at bed rest for this amount of time. If there are no contraindications (eg, central nervous system pathology, bleeding diathesis), heparin is given intravenously in a bolus of 5000 to 10,000 units followed by continuous infusion sufficient to raise the activated partial thromboplastin time (a-PTT) to at least 1.5 times the control for 7 to 10 days, while carefully watching for heparin-induced thrombocytopenia. Recent studies have suggested that oral Coumadin (DuPont Pharmaceuticals, Wilmington, DE) can be begun safely and cost-effectively on the first or second day of heparin therapy in an effort to prolong the PT (off heparin) to 1.5 times control. The latter may be discontinued as soon as 3 months following institution of anticoagulation if the risk factors for DVT are no longer present, but must be continued indefinitely if they are. Athletes should be advised to avoid contact sports while they are anticoagulated. Thrombolytic therapy (streptokinase, urokinase, or recombinant tissue plasminogen activator) has been advocated by some to reduce the incidence of the postphlebitic syndrome, to promote more rapid clot lysis and hemodynamic improvement in the setting of massive PE, and to improve the diffusing capacity for CO measured 1 year after the event. Unfortunately, thrombolytic therapy has not been clearly shown to improve survival, it is associated with a higher incidence of bleeding, and the clinical relevance of a modest depression of diffusing capacity for CO, even in the athlete, is not currently known. If DVT or PE is proved and anticoagulation contraindicated, percutaneous placement of an inferior vena cava filter should be considered. Vena caval interruption is no longer necessary in such settings and has been associated with compromised (lower extremity) exercise performance, probably due to decreased venous return to the heart.

An athlete who has suffered long-bone fractures is at risk for pulmonary fat embolism. The diagnosis is suggested by dyspnea, fever, petechiae, hypoxemia, diffuse infiltrates on chest radiograph, hypocalcemia, and lipuria. It may be confirmed by searching for fat globules in pulmonary capillary blood obtained from the distal port of a pulmonary artery catheter in the wedged position. One study has suggested that prophylactic steroids reduce the incidence of fat embolism syndrome when given to patients at risk.[23]

Spontaneous Pneumothorax

Primary spontaneous pneumothorax (SP) often occurs in previously healthy young adults in the third or fourth decades of life.[17] There is a 4:1 male predominance with a tendency to involve tall, thin individuals and cigarette smokers.[17] The disease process is characterized by spontaneous air leaks from alveoli into the pleural space due to rupture of small blebs on the visceral pleural surface. These blebs represent a form of emphysema called distal acinar emphysema, which spares the remainder of the lung.[17] Secondary SP occurs in patients with interstitial or obstructive lung disease and in certain connective tissue disorders. SP most commonly occurs while individuals are sedentary, but may sometimes be associated with strenuous activity or with a forceful cough or sneeze.

Symptoms include pleuritic chest pain, dyspnea, and cough, with severity dependent on the presence of underlying cardiopulmonary disease, size of the SP, and presence of positive intrathoracic pressure. Physical examination reveals tachypnea, tachycardia, and decreased breath sounds with tympany on the affected side. If air has dissected to the mediastinum, a precordial crunching sound (Hamman's sign) and subcutaneous crepitus may be detected. The ECG may show axis shifts and the chest radiograph may show absence of peripheral lung markings with a pleural line. Tension pneumothorax is manifested by hypotension, cyanosis, jugular venous distension, and contralateral tracheal and mediastinal shift.

Residual air in the pleural cavity will be absorbed spontaneously at a rate of 1.25% per day. This process can be accelerated more than three times if elevated fractions of inspired O_2 are administered.[18] If the patient is stable and the SP occupies more than one third of the chest cavity, evacuation with a small-bore (no. 9 French) catheter is indicated. In general, this is placed in the second or third intercostal space in the midclavicular line. Successful treatment is usually accomplished by venting the proximal catheter opening through a Heimlich flutter valve and asking the patient to repeatedly cough. An occasional patient (usually with pulmonary parenchymal or airways disease) will require manual or wall suction. The catheter is removed only when full evacuation of pleural air has been accomplished and when there is no evidence of a continuing air leak. A 14-gauge intravenous catheter can be placed in the same anatomic position, with the hub connected to a 12-mL syringe if tension pneumothorax is suspected.

Fifty percent of affected individuals will experience a recurrence of SP, with an even higher percentage of recurrence after a second event. Surgical intervention is recommended for recurrent or bilateral SP even if the latter occur metachronously. Surgical options include chemical pleurodesis and parietal pleurectomy.

Recurrent pneumothoraces coinciding with the onset of menses suggests catamenial pneumothorax. This entity may be associated with endometrial implants on the pleura or solely within the abdomen. Nonsteroidal anti-inflammatory medications or hormonal suppression of ovulation may be of help.

Drowning and Near-Drowning

Each year, there are approximately 8000 drowning deaths and over 90,000 episodes of near-drowning (ND) in the United States.[19] Drowning is the most common cause of accidental death in the 1 to 24 year age group and it is the most frequent cause of accidental death in divers.

Autopsy studies of drowning victims reveal surprisingly small volumes of aspirated fluid. In fact, 10% to 20% of victims die of asphyxia due to laryngospasm with no evidence of aspirated liquid. Small amounts of aspirated fresh water are rapidly absorbed into the circulation and cause alveolar surfactant disruption, atelectasis, low V/Q areas, increased right-to-left shunting, and hypoxemia. Hypertonic sea water, on the other hand, leads to hypoxemia through pulmonary edema formation. Unusually large volumes (>22mL/kg) of aspirated fresh water can cause a depression of serum electrolytes, hemolysis, and disseminated intravascular coagulation, whereas similar volumes of sea water cause hemoconcentration and hypovolemia. Death may occur as a result of anoxic ventricular fibrillation or brain damage and from complications of the adult respiratory distress syndrome.

Key predictors of meaningful survival in near-drowning are the duration of anoxia and the temperature of the water. Full neurologic recovery has been reported after 40 min of submersion in cold water, owing to the protective effects of hypothermia on brain and cardiac function. Following warm-water submersion, 15 min of anoxia, a plasma pH ≤7.10, coma, and fixed, dilated pupils upon arrival suggest a poor prognosis. Admission chest radiographs are sometimes normal, with evidence of atelectasis and/or pulmonary edema developing hours later.

Therapy for near-drowning victims is largely supportive and includes restoration of an adequate airway, ventilation, oxygenation, circulation, electrolytes, and body temperature. Nasogastric tube evacuation of the stomach facilitates gas exchange and helps prevent further aspiration. Prophylactic steroids and antibiotics have not yet been shown to be of benefit. Ambulatory patients should be observed in the hospital for at least 24 hours because of the possibility of delayed pulmonary edema.

Exercise-Induced Allergic Syndromes

Urticaria and full-blown anaphylaxis have both been linked to exercise.[20] Cholinergic urticaria is reported most often by adolescents and young adults. Although exercise is the most common precipitating factor, emotional stress and spicy foods have also been linked to the syndrome.[20] Pruritic wheels and flares arise following exercise sufficiently intense to raise the core temperature 1°C and cause perspiration.[20] An individual attack lasts from 20 to 90 min. The disease is characterized by spontaneous remissions. High-dose, prophylactic antihistamines show the most promise for symptomatic individuals. Astemizole (Hismanal; Janssen Pharmaceutica Inc., Piscataway, NJ), a once-daily preparation, and Terfenadine (Seldane; Merrell Dow, Cincinnati, OH), a twice-daily preparation, are both relatively nonsedating and may therefore be particularly useful in the athletic population.

Anaphylaxis may follow even mild exercise in the rare susceptible individual. The syndrome usually includes urticaria, hypotension, and life-threatening laryngeal edema. Interestingly, wheezing is uncommon. Victims are generally young and a peculiar relationship to exercise during the postprandial state has been identified in many. Attacks are often sudden and totally unpredictable. Patients should be advised to avoid exercise for at least 2 hours following their last meal and to exercise with a partner. They should always carry Epi-Pen (Center Laboratories, Port Washington, NY) (epinephrine 0.3 mL subcutaneously) or epinephrine MDI (eg, Primatene; Whitehall Laboratories, New York, NY) 10–20 puffs), which can abort an attack.

Air Pollution

Incomplete combustion of fossil fuels produces a variety of airborne, respirable pollutants, several of which may affect exercise tolerance in normal individuals and patients with cardiopulmonary disorders.[21] Mouth breathing and the high levels of ventilation achieved during exercise increase the dose of gaseous and particulate matter delivered to distal airways. Predictably, respiratory symptoms and decrements in pulmonary function are worse when individuals are exposed to common pollutants such as ozone and sulfur dioxide during exercise as compared with rest.

Ozone (O_3) is a ubiquitous, highly reactive gas, which, because of its insolubility in water, is delivered to the alveolocapillary membrane, where it may cause edema and impair gas exchange.[21] Exposures of 0.1 ppm for only 1 hour cause eye and respiratory tract irritation. At levels as low as 0.2 ppm, increased frequency of asthma attacks is found in resting patients, and decrements in flow rates are found in *normal* endurance athletes following competition. O_3 at 0.1 to 0.4 ppm is associated with decreased performance in student cross-country track teams. Levels of up to 0.5 ppm are sometimes reached in Los Angeles air! "Adaptation" (attenuated decrements in lung function with successive O_3 exposures) has been described, but it is short-lived (7 days).

Sulfur dioxide (SO_2), as opposed to O_3, seems to predominantly affect patients with preexisting asthma or chronic obstructive pulmonary disease. Decreases in flow rates are 3 to 22 times as great when asthmatics are exposed to SO_2, 1.0 ppm, during exercise as opposed to rest.

Carbon monoxide (CO) binds to hemoglobin with 250 times the avidity of O_2. Increases in carboxyhemoglobin of even 2%, often achieved during a morning commute and easily obtainable by cigarette smoking, may sufficiently depress the O_2-carrying capacity of blood to compromise exercise tolerance in patients with coronary artery and peripheral vascular disease. Recent work with normal volunteers suggests that the lactate threshold during incremental exercise occurs at a lower metabolic rate after breathing CO. These changes would be expected to affect maximal athletic performance.

Pulmonary Rehabilitation

In patients with chronic obstructive pulmonary disease, the $\dot{V}O_{2max}$ is limited by excessive demands on ventilation (hypoxemia, wasted ventilation) and decreased maximal breathing capacity (increased work of breathing, malnutrition, and respiratory muscle fatigue).[22] Thus, such patients usually terminate an incremental exercise protocol when the dyspnea index ($\dot{V}E_{max}$/maximum breathing capacity) approaches 1.0. The reasons for compromised *submaximal* exercise tolerance in patients with chronic obstructive pulmonary disease are less clear, but as opposed to resting pulmonary function and $\dot{V}O_{2max}$, submaximal exercise tolerance seems to respond to endurance exercise training.

Pulmonary rehabilitation programs include endurance training, patient education, nutritional modifications, occupational and chest physical therapy, bronchodilator medication, O_2 supplementation, and sometimes, respiratory muscle training. They have been shown to increase patients' sense of well-being, to improve the 6- and 12-min walk distance, and to reduce hospital admissions in a cost-efficient manner. Recent work has suggested that patients with chronic obstructive pulmonary disease who generate lactic acid during incremental exercise are more apt to improve exercise tolerance than those who do not.

REFERENCES

1. Wasserman K, Hansen JE, Sue DY, et al: Principles of exercise testing and interpretation. Philadelphia, Lea & Febiger, 1987, pp 3–46.
2. Dempsey JA: Is the lung built for exercise? Med Sci Sports Exerc 18:143–155, 1986.
3. Jones NL: Dyspnea in exercise. Med Sci Sports Exerc 16:14–19, 1984.
4. Wasserman K: The anaerobic threshold measurement to evaluate exercise performance. Am Rev Respir Dis 129:S35–40, 1984.
5. Scharf SM, Bark H, Heimer D, et al: "Second wind" during inspiratory loading. Med Sci Sports Exec 16:87–91, 1984.
6. Donat WE: Chest pain: Cardiac and noncardiac causes. Clin Chest Med 8:241–252, 1987.
7. Irwin RS, Corrao WM, Pratter MR: Chronic persistent cough in the adult: The spectrum and frequency of causes and successful outcome of specific therapy. Am Rev Respir Dis 123:413–417, 1981.
8. Adelman M, Haponik EF, Bleecker ER, et al: Cryptogenic hemoptysis. Ann Intern Med 102:829–834, 1985.
9. Hollingsworth HM: Wheezing and stridor. Clin Chest Med 8:231–240, 1987.
10. Sheppard D: What does exercise have to do with "exercise-induced" asthma? Am Rev Respir Dis 136:547–549, 1987.
11. Reiff DB, Choudry NB, Pride NB, et al: The effect of prolonged submaximal warm-up exercise on exercise-induced asthma. Am Rev Respir Dis 139:479–484, 1989.
12. Magarian GJ: Hyperventilation syndromes: Infrequently recognized common expressions of anxiety and stress. Medicine 61:219–236, 1982.
13. Rich S, Dantzker DR, Ayres SM, et al: Primary pulmonary hypertension. Ann Intern Med 107:216–223, 1987.
14. Moser KM: Pulmonary embolism. *In* Murray JF, Nadel JA (eds): Textbook of Respiratory Medicine. Philadelphia, WB Saunders, 1988, pp 1299–1327.
15. Cvtanic O, Marino PL: Improved use of arterial blood gas analysis in suspected pulmonary embolism. Chest 95:48–51, 1989.
16. White RW, McGahan JP, Daschbach MM, et al: Diagnosis of deep-vein thrombosis using duplex ultrasound. Ann Intern Med 111:297–304, 1989.
17. Light RW: Pneumothorax. *In* Murray JF, Nadel JA (eds): Textbook of Respiratory Medicine. Philadelphia, WB Saunders, 1988, pp 1745–1759.
18. Chadha TS, Cohn MA: Noninvasive treatment of pneumothorax with oxygen inhalation. Respiration 44:147–152, 1983.
19. Modell JH, Graves SA, Ketover A: Clinical course of 91 consecutive near-drowning victims. Chest 70:231–238, 1976.
20. Casale TB, Keahey TM, Kaliner M: Exercise-induced anaphylactic syndromes: Insights into diagnosis and pathophysiologic features. JAMA 255:2049–2053, 1986.
21. Pierson WE, Covert DS, Koenig JQ, et al: Implications of air pollution effects on athletic performance. Med Sci Sports Exerc 1986; 18:322–327, 1986.
22. Make BJ: Pulmonary rehabilitation: Myth or reality? Clin Chest Med 7:519–540, 1986.
23. Schonfeld AS, et al: Fat embolism prophylaxis with corticosteroids. Ann Intern Med 99:438–443, 1983.

9

HEMATOLOGY

Marvin M. Adner, MD

This chapter describes the physiologic changes in the cellular elements of the blood and in blood coagulation produced by exercise, and the effects that certain diseases of the blood have on exercise performance. A comprehensive description of these disorders can be found in several excellent textbooks of hematology.[1,2]

THE RED BLOOD CELL

The function of the red blood cell is to transport oxygen from the pulmonary alveoli to metabolically active tissue. The oxygen is carried by the hemoglobin molecule within the red cell. The process of oxygen association and dissociation from the hemoglobin molecule is regulated by a variety of factors including oxygen, tension, blood pH, temperature, and quantitative and qualitative changes in the hemoglobin molecule. The normal red cell mass, plasma volume, and total blood volume measured by isotopic techniques are presented in Table 9–1. The greater red cell mass in men is attributed to the stimulatory effect of the male hormone testosterone. Because of the complexity of the technology, it is impractical to determine red cell mass and plasma volume routinely. Commonly, the red cell mass is described in terms of hemoglobin content or volume of red cells per 100 mL of blood, the latter being referred to as the hematocrit. Total blood volume is not considered in this calculation. Therefore, the hemoglobin and hematocrit levels do not reflect the total red cell mass.

Pseudoanemia Caused by Exercise

A number of investigators have noted that trained athletes have hemoglobin and/or hematocrit levels in the lower range of normal or occasionally, slightly below normal. This phenomenon has been referred to as "sports anemia."[3] In another study,[4] there was a progressive decrease in hemoglobin concentration in runners participating in a 20-day, 312-mile road race. Martin and colleagues[5] found significantly lower hematocrit levels in elite and good runners than in nonrunners, although hemoglobin levels were not significantly different. Other studies fail to demonstrate the differences in hemoglobin and hematocrit levels in athletes versus those in sedentary individuals.

Differentiation of true anemia (an absolute decrease in red cell mass) from a pseudoanemia (a relative but not absolute decrease in red cell mass) cannot be made from hemoglobin and hematocrit determinations alone; information on the total red cell mass is required. There is considerable evidence that athletes have a greater total blood volume than nonathletes. Brotherhood and associates[6] found a 25% increase in total blood volume in male distance runners compared with a control group. However, there was a pro-

TABLE 9–1. NORMAL HEMATOLOGIC VALUES FOR ADULTS

	Men	Women
Red cell mass*	32	25
Plasma volume*	40	38
Total blood volume*	72	63
Hemoglobin†	14–18	12–16
Hematocrit‡	40–54	37–47

*In mL/kg body weight.
†In g/dL.
‡In %.

portional increase in both red cell mass and plasma volume. In another study,[7] sedentary males placed in a 1-month running program developed a 6% increase in total blood volume caused by an increase in plasma volume without change in red cell volume. Therefore, decreased hemoglobin and hematocrit levels found in individuals participating in sports may, in some cases, represent a pseudoanemia caused by expansion of plasma volume alone.

The mechanism of plasma volume expansion as an adaptation to exercise training is not well understood. Crowell and Smith[8] found that, as the hematocrit increased to 40%, there was an increase in oxygen delivery that declined with higher hematocrit levels resulting from increase in blood viscosity. Similar conclusions were made based on experimental studies in dogs.[9] This "optimal hematocrit" corresponds to the values found in "sports anemia."

True Anemia Caused by Exercise

EXERTIONAL HEMOLYSIS

The forces exerted on the red cells of the capillaries of the feet may rupture the cells after prolonged marching, running, cross-country skiing, and aerobic dancing.[10,11] Effort-related intravascular hemolysis has also been observed in cyclists, rowers, and swimmers.[12] Free hemoglobin is liberated into the plasma. Haptoglobin is the principal plasma protein that binds the free hemoglobin during intravascular hemolysis. The haptoglobin-hemoglobin complex is rapidly cleared by the liver. When the hemoglobin-binding capacity of the haptoglobin is exceeded, free hemoglobin may be found in the urine. It is likely that the contribution of hemolysis to a decrease in hemoglobin concentration of the blood is quite small.

EXERTIONAL HEMATURIA

Exercise-related hematuria has been reported in association with many athletic events.[13] It is not uncommon to find red blood cells in the urine of distance runners. It has been postulated that the cause for this is traumatic lower urinary tract injury. It has also been proposed that the hematuria is renal in origin, due to a rupture in renal capillaries associated with increased renal-vascular resistance occurring during excessive physical stress. Exertional hematuria clears rapidly and should not be present 48 hours after the athletic event. Persistent hematuria is an indication for a search for other etiologies.

GASTROINTESTINAL BLOOD LOSS

Eichner's review of gastrointestinal bleeding in athletes indicates that in a large survey of marathoners, about 2% of the respondents noted bloody stool occasionally or frequently after running.[14] Occult blood loss may occur in up to 10% of runners before races and in up to 30% of runners after the event. There are several causes for the blood loss: (1) Ischemic gastritis and colitis (especially the cecum) due to shunting of blood from the gastrointestinal (GI) tract to the muscles in response to exercise. Gut ischemia may also be the cause for GI bleeding seen in endurance cyclists. (2) Gastritis caused by stress and the use of salicylates and nonsteroidal anti-inflammatory drugs so commonly used by athletes for analgesia. Although the amount of blood loss is trivial in most cases, there are individual accounts of massive life-threatening bleeding episodes during running.

IRON-DEFICIENCY ANEMIA

Although iron deficiency is a common cause for anemia in nonathletes, both men and women who exercise are at greater risk for being iron-deficient than their sedentary counterparts due to inadequate iron intake and increased iron loss.[15] It has been estimated that as high as 80% of young female athletes and 30% of elite male athletes are iron-deficient.[16] The sedentary male must eat a 2000-calorie balanced diet (containing 10 mg of iron) daily to absorb 1 mg of iron and remain in iron balance. The sedentary menstruating woman must eat a 3000-calorie balanced diet (containing 18 mg of iron) daily to absorb 1.5 mg of iron and remain in iron balance. The athlete's diet is often iron-deficient. It contains little red meat, a major source of dietary iron, and it is high in natural foods that are not iron-supplemented. Athletes often restrict calories in an attempt to reduce body fat and improve performance.

Increased iron loss also contributes to the negative iron balance. Although the amount of iron loss from the GI tract, urinary tract, and sweat is small, it is often enough to deplete the iron reserves. One third of a group of female cross-country runners became iron-deficient during a 75-day running season due to a combination of initially low iron stores and gastrointestinal bleeding.[17] When iron stores are decreased in the absence of anemia, the term latent phase of iron deficiency is used. When the reserves are totally depleted, continued iron loss will initially result in normocytic, normochromic anemia and then, hypochromic, microcytic anemia.

Iron stores can be assessed by several techniques: measurement of serum iron, total iron-binding capacity of the transport protein transferrin, percent of iron saturation (serum iron divided by total iron-binding capacity), erythrocyte protoporphyrin, and serum ferritin; and assessment of stainable iron in bone marrow aspirates and biopsies.[18] Each test has its limitations, but the serum ferritin is perhaps the best single noninvasive measure of iron stores; levels of less than 12 ng/mL are diagnostic of iron deficiency. However, the diagnosis is less certain when there is an associated inflammatory process which may increase ferritin. Muscle injury incurred during heavy training may have such an effect. In patients with ferritin levels ranging between 12 and 50 ng/mL, clinical history and use of multiple tests may be necessary to determine the status of body iron reserves.[19]

Even in the absence of anemia, a decrease in body iron may cause a diminished exercise performance unrelated to the oxygen-carrying capacity of the hemoglobin concentration.[20] Tissue iron compounds such as cytochrome c and myoglobin may be decreased in cases of iron deficiency that have not progressed to anemia. Cytochrome c is important in electron transport involved in oxidative metabolism, and myoglobin stores oxygen for use in muscle contraction. The ability to utilize oxygen is important in the capacity to perform endurance-type submaximal exercise, whereas the ability to deliver oxygen to the tissues by hemoglobin is the critical factor in maximal work load activities. The data, however, is controversial. Iron therapy improved treadmill running endurance in iron-deficient nonanemic rats.[21] A controlled study of administration of iron to nonanemic iron-deficient adolescent runners produced significant improvement in treadmill endurance time compared with controls.[22] In subjects who were made iron-deficient by phlebotomy and then transfused to a nonanemic state, there was no evidence of impaired treadmill exercise performance or change in iron-dependent muscle enzymes.[23] Even if latent iron deficiency does not result in decreased performance, its recognition is important as an early sign of negative iron balance. This may lead to early diagnosis and treatment before true anemia develops. True anemia will result in decreased performance in maximal aerobic activities.

If iron deficiency is found in an athlete, it is inappropriate to presume that the deficiency state is due to inadequate diet or exercise-related occult blood loss. The many causes for blood loss must be ruled out. The first sign of colon cancer, especially of the ascending colon, may be iron deficiency. Many athletes are of the age group in which this disease is common, a disease which is curable in its early stages.

The strategy for treatment of iron deficiency due to an inadequate intake of iron includes:

1. *Increase dietary iron.* Dietary iron comes in two forms: heme iron, which is readily absorbed; and nonheme iron, which is poorly absorbed. Heme iron is found in high amounts in protein such as lean red meat, pork chops, and the dark meat of poultry. Good sources of nonheme iron include dry fruits, beans, nuts, iron-fortified cereals and breads, and black strap molasses.
2. *Increase vitamin C.* Increased intake of vitamin C will facilitate iron absorption. Foods such as orange juice (fresh or frozen), potatoes, and fresh vegetables (broccoli, green peppers, tomatoes) are excellent sources.
3. *Avoid substances that inhibit iron absorption.* Some substances, such as tannic acid found in tea, inhibit iron absorption.[24]

If there is a large negative iron balance, increasing dietary iron is usually not sufficient to provide a correction of the deficiency. In a 70-kg woman whose normal hemoglobin of 14 g/dL decreases to below 12 d/gL, there is a 300-mg deficit in circulating hemoglobin iron. When the hemoglobin is 10 g/dL, the deficit is about 600 mg. In addition, there is a 1000- to 2000-mg deficit in iron stores. In such cases, use of iron-containing compounds, such as ferrous sulfate or ferrous gluconate, in doses of two or three tablets per day between meals is usually adequate. It is rare to have a patient who cannot tolerate iron. The side effects (nausea, constipation, and diarrhea) are dose-related and can be reduced by decreasing the number of tablets per day or by using the gluconate form (12% elemental iron) as compared with the sulfate form (20% elemental iron). Treatment with intramuscular or intravenous preparations does not result in more rapid repair of the iron depletion, but it is associated with the definite risk of anaphylaxis.

Assuming the source of iron loss is no longer present, iron repletion using oral compounds usually takes 4 to 6 months to bring the hemoglobin and storage iron to normal levels. Too often, iron is given only a month or so to replete hemoglobin iron, but this does not result in repletion of storage iron.

Anemia from Other Causes

Individuals participating in sports may develop anemia from a number of causes unrelated to the sporting activity. Selected disorders are described in the next five sections.

VITAMIN B_{12} DEFICIENCY

This is a very rare cause of anemia in athletes. Vitamin B_{12} is found in all animal tissues. The dietary requirement of vitamin B_{12} is 1 μg/day, and body stores are approximately 4000 μg. Vitamin B_{12} deficiency from a dietary lack will occur only in those individuals who are true vegetarians and will take a number of years to develop. The most common cause for vitamin B_{12} deficiency is the inability of the parietal cells of the stomach to produce intrinsic factor. Intrinsic factor binds with dietary vitamin B_{12} and facilitates its absorption in the ileum. The absence of intrinsic factor resulting from degeneration of the parietal cells is called pernicious anemia and it is quite rare in the young.

Other causes of vitamin B_{12} deficiency include surgical removal of part or all of the lower ileum. The use of vitamin B_{12} injections to improve athletic performance in individuals without such a deficiency has no physiologic basis, and any improvement in performance that occurs must be attributed to placebo effect alone.

FOLIC ACID DEFICIENCY

Whereas vitamin B_{12} deficiency from inadequate dietary intake is rare, folic acid deficiency secondary to decreased dietary intake is common in the general population. Folic acid is found in large amounts in green vegetables such as peas and beans, and in liver, yeast, figs, dates, and nuts. The body stores are relatively small, and folic acid deficiency will develop in 1 or 2 months on a folate-poor diet. Even on a folate-rich diet, malabsorption of ingested folate may occur in a variety of circumstances, such as with the use of anticonvulsant drugs, several antibiotics, or oral contraceptives.

In individuals found to be anemic, use of folic acid in the absence of demonstrative folic acid deficiency is not recommended. Large doses of folic acid may improve the anemia associated with a vitamin B_{12} deficiency, but it will not improve the neurologic abnormalities that may develop in individuals with decreased vitamin B_{12} levels. The symptoms related to the anemia will not be present, and by the time the patient presents with other manifestations of vitamin B_{12} deficiency, the neurologic damage may be irreversible, resulting in permanent dementia and serious sensory and motor loss.

SICKLE CELL DISEASE

Sickle cell disease is an example of a hemolytic disorder associated with a structural defect of the hemoglobin molecule. It is due to production of an abnormal hemoglobin, hemoglobin S, caused by a single amino acid substitution. The abnormal molecule aggregates under states of reduced oxygen tension and produces a deformity in the usual biconcave disc-shaped cell, transforming it into a rigid spindle-shaped cell. This cell will not traverse easily through blood vessels, especially at openings of a capillary or points of bending where the abnormal red cells will spontaneously obstruct the flow of blood.

In sickle cell disease, both parents transmit an abnormal sickle cell gene. Most of the hemoglobin is of the sickle cell type. Patients with sickle disease commonly have a chronic, severe, hemolytic anemia; cardiovascular decompensation; and painful organ infarctions. The ability of individuals with sickle cell disease to participate in sports is limited. However, under close supervision, exercise programs can be undertaken with avoidance of those factors that precipitate the sickle cell phenomenon and allowing activities that will help preserve good muscle and joint function.

Sickle cell trait is a common disorder with an incidence of approximately 6% to 9% in the black population. In this disorder, the individual receives one abnormal gene from a parent. Less than 50% of the hemoglobin is abnormal. Usually, there is no anemia, and no formation of sickle cells in vivo. However, physiologic changes caused by exercise such as acidosis, hydration, and fever, may promote the sickling phenomenon. Exercising in altitudes higher than 10,000 feet may increase the risk of splenic infarction. Whether sickle cell trait increases risk of exercise-induced death is controversial.[25] Four deaths occurred in black soldiers with sickle cell trait during basic training in an altitude of 4000 feet. This may be due to sickle cell crisis precipitated by hypoxia and acidosis or it may possibly represent exertional rhabdomyolysis. In his extensive review of the morbidity of sickle cell trait, Sears[26] concludes that it is not possible to define the role of the hemoglobinopathy in these rare reports of exertion-induced syndromes in patients with sickle cell trait.

THALASSEMIA

The term thalassemia refers to a heterogeneous group of hereditary disorders in which there is a decreased rate of synthesis of one or more of the hemoglobin polypeptide chains. The most common type is the heterozygote form of Mediterranean anemia in which there is decreased production of normal hemoglobin by one of the beta chains. The disease received its name because of the wide distribution of the disorder in that area of the world. However, it is also found in a relatively high frequency in the Middle East, India, Pakistan, and Southeast Asia, and it occurs throughout the world. The individual with beta thalassemia trait has a mild hypochromic anemia with hemoglobin in the range of 10 to 12 g/dL. The red cell count is normal. The cells appear similar to those seen in iron-deficiency anemia and the disease may be misdiagnosed and treated inappropriately with iron.

DECREASED PRODUCTION BY BONE MARROW

Anemia may develop as a result of a decrease in red cell production by the bone marrow. The decreased production may be due to cellular damage from drugs, unknown factors, or replacement of the normal cells by abnormal malignant cells as may occur in leukemia, lymphoma and metastatic tumor. Finally, anemia may result as a bodily response to a number of illnesses such as chronic infection, arthritis, renal failure, malignancy, and hypothyroidism. This has been termed the anemia of chronic disease.

Acquired Erythrocythemia

BLOOD DOPING

Increasing the red cell mass to elevated levels provides the potential to increase arterial oxygen content and systemic oxygen transport. If cardiac output is unaffected by the corresponding increase in blood viscosity, and muscle can extract and utilize increased oxygen, maximal aerobic power will be increased.[27] This state of normovolemic erythrocythemia can be achieved during high altitude acclimatization, with hypoxia enhancing erythropoietin production, principally by the kidney. The hormone stimulates the proliferation, differentiation, and maturation of red cell precursors in the bone marrow.[28]

In recent years, considerable attention has been given to the hypothesis that normovolemic expansion of the red cell mass may produce an enhancement of aerobic work capacity.[29,30] Because of the risk of transfusion-induced infection, most of the experimental studies have been performed using autologous transfusions. The subject is phlebotomized and the blood is stored in the frozen state. After the hemoglobin concentration returns to prephlebotomy levels, usually with the assistance of iron supplementation, the stored blood is then transfused back into the subject to achieve erythrocythemia.

Many of the initial studies failed to demonstrate enhanced performance by hypertransfusion, but study design may explain the results. Factors such as insufficient transfusion volumes, limited time from phlebotomy to transfusion, as well as training factors may have flawed the results. However, in recent years, a number of studies have demonstrated that transfusions do increase maximal exercise performance and probably submaximal performance as well, with the minimal critical volume being the equivalent transfusion of 900 mL of whole blood. Berglund and Hemmingson[31] reinfused 1350 mL of autologous blood into well-trained cross-country skiers and significantly increased performance both at 3 hours and at 14 days after the transfusion. Buick and associates[32] produced an increase in hemoglobin levels from 1.2 to 1.5 g/dL following infusion of 900 mL of blood. This resulted in a significant improvement in aerobic performance in highly conditioned runners, with a mean overall increase of 5% maximum oxygen uptake.

An unexpected finding was the persistence of this increase in maximum oxygen uptake in the 4 months following infusion when hemoglobin had returned to prephlebotomy levels.[32] In a well-designed study, infusion of freeze-preserved red blood cells from the product of two units of blood produced an average 1.3 g/dL increase in hemoglobin levels, with nearly all individuals experiencing an increase in maximal oxygen uptake. The magnitude of the hemoglobin increase did not relate to the magnitude of the oxygen uptake. Moderately fit individuals seem to benefit most from the transfusion, but a blunted response was seen in unfit and maximally fit subjects. The authors suggest that a factor which may modify the effect of transfusion may be the capacity to extract and utilize oxygen at a skeletal muscle level.[33] The increase in viscosity associated with expansion of red cell mass by transfusion with red cells derived from up to 1500 mL of whole blood does not appear to be a limiting factor in oxygen transport.

ERYTHROPOIETIN

Expansion of the red cell mass by administration of erythropoietin represents a new method of enhancing athletic performance. With successful cloning and expression of the erythropoietin gene, there is now available enough erythropoietin for human use. Although erythropoietin is used primarily for the treatment of anemia of chronic renal disease in which there is decreased hormone production, it appears to be effective in other anemic disorders, such as that associated with chronic infection and inflammation.[34]

Healthy individuals with normal hemoglobin levels will develop a significant increase in red cell mass when given erythropoietin.[35] Although there are no published clinical studies of potential enhancement of athletic performance with use of erythropoietin, the results should be comparable with those achieved by transfusion-induced erythrocythemia. With use of transfusion, there is a predictable expansion of red cell mass. However, with the use of erythropoietin, the response is less predictable; the subjects could develop hematocrits above 60% and hyperviscosity, imposing significant risk for thrombosis.[36] The risk is even greater during strenuous exercise when sweating will produce a concomitant plasma volume decrease and raise the hematocrit even higher.

The International Olympic Committee defines blood doping as the use of physiologic substances in abnormal amounts and with abnormal methods with the exclusive aim of obtaining an artificial, unfair increase in performance in competition. Transfusion and erythropoietin-induced erythrocythemia are examples of blood doping. Both the International Olympic Committee and the American College of Sports Medicine have banned blood doping.

HEMOSTASIS AND COAGULATION

Platelets are produced in megakaryocytes in the bone marrow and circulate in the blood. When a blood vessel is damaged, platelets are exposed to collagen, to which they adhere, and are activated, releasing aggregating agents such as adenosine diphosphate and thromboxane to form a platelet plug. The thromboxane also produces vasospasm, which assists in arresting the bleeding. The action is modulated by the release of prostacyclin from the intact endothelium, which antagonizes the platelet plugging by inhibiting platelet aggregation and causing vasodilatation.

Vascular injury also activates the coagulation system, which is a complex series of sequential activations of protease clotting factors enhanced by cofactors, converting prothrombin to thrombin, which in turn converts fibrinogen to fibrin monomers that polymerize to form a fibrin clot. This process is antagonized by the fibrinolytic system in which a proenzyme, plasminogen, is converted to the enzyme plasmin by activators, the most important of which is tissue plasminogen activator (TPA), derived from the endothelial cells. The resultant plasmin digests the fibrin clot.

Exercise produces alterations in the hemostatic coagulation and fibrinolytic mechanisms.[37–39] In individuals participating in strenuous exercise, there is a transient increase in the platelet count from 20% to 100% over baseline, probably due to platelet mobilization from the spleen, bone marrow, and lungs. There is considerable controversy as to whether these platelets are activated. This is likely to be dependent on two competing forces: a tendency for platelet activation due to an increase in exercise-induced plasma catecholamines; and increase in the antiaggregating effect of prostacyclin, which is also increased by exercise. Strenuous exercise also results in a transient increase in factor VIII and Von Willebrand factor, with shortening of the whole blood clotting time and partial thromboplastin time, suggesting the presence of a hypercoagulable state. There is increased fibrinogen activation, probably as a result of increased release of tissue thromboplastin activator from vascular endothelium without significant increase in inhibitors of TPA.[40] The magnitude of the fibrinolytic enhancement increases in proportion to the intensity and duration of the exercise and can be enhanced by physical conditioning.[41]

What is the clinical significance of these exercise-induced alterations in the blood coagulation system? Does strenuous exercise increase the risk of coronary artery thrombosis? Platelet activation has been implicated in resting and exercise-induced myocardial ischemia. Tofler and co-workers[42] have demonstrated a temporal relationship between enhanced platelet aggregation in the morning and increased frequency of myocardial infarction and sudden cardiac death. Platelet aggregation occurs during spontaneous ischemia in patients with unstable angina.[43] Green and colleagues[44] define a subset of patients with coronary artery disease who had exercise-induced platelet activation and secretion with myocardial ischemia.[44] Other investigators have failed to demonstrate such a correlation.[45] Stratton and coworkers[46] concluded that platelet factor 4 and beta-thromboglobulin increase minimally but significantly in normal subjects during maximal exercise. In patients with coronary artery disease and exertion-induced myocardial ischemia, platelet factor 4 increased significantly but to a lesser extent than in normal subjects, and beta-thromboglobulin, not at all.[46]

Other data suggest exercise is antithrombotic.[47] The enhancement of fibrinolysis due to increased release of tissue plasminogen activator could decrease the incidence of thrombotic disease. Exercise reduces whole blood viscosity by decreasing hematocrit and plasma viscosity, and increasing red cell deformability. In addition, the reduced hematocrit causes a decreased adherence of platelets to underlying arterial subendothelium.[48] However, there is still no definitive demonstration that these exercise-induced alterations actually enhance or inhibit the incidence of clinical thrombosis.

REFERENCES

1. Williams WJ, Beutler E, Erslev AJ, et al: Hematology, ed 4. New York, McGraw-Hill, 1990.
2. Wintrobe MM, Lee GR, Boggs DR, et al: Clinical Hematology, ed 8. Philadelphia, Lea & Febiger, 1981.
3. Williamson MR: Anemia in runners and other athletes. Physician Sports Med 9:73–79, 1981.
4. Dressendorfer RH, Wade CE, Amsterdam EA: Development of pseudoanemia in marathon runners during a 20-day road race. JAMA 246:1215–1219, 1981.
5. Martin RP, Haskell WL, Wood PD: Blood chemistry and lipid profiles of elite distance runners. Ann NY Acad Sci 301:346–360, 1977.
6. Brotherhood J, Brozovic B, Pugh LGC: Hematologic status of middle and long distance runners. Clin Sci 48:139–145, 1975.
7. Oscai LB, Williams BT, Hertig BA: Effect of exercise on blood volume. J Appl Physiol 24:622–624, 1968.
8. Crowell JW, Smith EE: Determination of the optimal hematocrit. J Appl Physiol 22:501–504, 1967.
9. Guyton AC, Jones CE, Coleman TG: Circulatory Physiology: Cardiac Output and Its Regulation, ed 2. Philadelphia, WB Saunders, 1973.
10. Davidson RJ: March or exertional hemoglobinuria. Semin Hematol 6:150–161, 1969.
11. Schwellnus MP, Penfold GK, Cilliers JF: Intravascular hemolysis in aerobic dancing: The role of the floor surface and type of routine. Physician Sports Med 17:55–67, 1989.
12. Selby GB, Eichner ER: Endurance swimming, intravascular hemolysis, anemia and iron depletion: New perspectives on athlete's anemia. Am J Med 81:791–794, 1986.
13. Hoover DL, Cromie WJ: Theory and management of exercise related hematuria. Physician Sports Med 9:90–95, 1981.
14. Eichner ER: Gastrointestinal bleeding in athletes. Physician Sports Med 17(5):128–140, 1989.
15. Clement DB, Sawchuk LL: Iron status and sports performance. Sports Med 1:65–74, 1984.
16. Clement DB, Asmundsun RC: Nutritional intake and hematological parameters in endurance runners. Physician Sports Med 10:37–43, 1982.
17. Nickerson JH, Holubets MC, Weiler BR, et al: Causes of iron deficiency in adolescent athletes. J Pediatr 114:657–663, 1989.
18. Cook JD, Skikne BS, Lynch SR, et al: Estimates of iron sufficiency in the U.S. population. Blood 68:726–731, 1986.
19. O'Toole ML, Iwane H, Douglas PS, et al: Iron status in ultra-endurance triathletes. Physician Sports Med 17:90–102, 1989.
20. Dallman PR, Beutler E, Finch CA: Effects of iron deficiency exclusive of anemia. Br J Haematol 40:179–184, 1978.
21. Dallman PR: Manifestations of iron deficiency. Semin Hematol 19:19–30, 1982.
22. Rowland TW, Deisroth MB, Green GM, et al: The effect of iron therapy on the exercise capacity of non-anemic iron deficient adolescent runners. Am J Dis Child 142:165–169, 1988.
23. Celsing F, Blomstrand E, Werner B, et al: Effects of iron deficiency on endurance and muscle enzyme activity in man. Med Sci Sports Exerc 18:156–161, 1986.
24. Clark N: Increasing dietary iron. Physician Sports Med 13:131–132, 1985.
25. Eichner ER: Sickle cell trait, exercise, and altitude. Physician Sports Med 11:144–157, 1986.
26. Sears DA: The morbidity of sickle cell trait: A review of the literature. Am J Med 64:1021–1036, 1978.
27. Gledhill N: Blood doping and related issues: A brief review. Med Sci Sports Exerc 14:183–189, 1982.
28. Smith MH, Sharkey BJ: Altitude training: Who benefits? Physician Sports Med 12:48–62, 1984.
29. Williams MH: Blood doping: An update. Physician Sports Med 9:59–62, 1981.
30. Eichner ER: Blood doping: Results and consequences from the laboratory and the field. Physician Sports Med 15:121–129, 1987.
31. Berglund B, Hemmingson P: Effect of reinfusion of autologous blood on exercise performance in cross country skiers. Int J Sports Med 8:231–233, 1987.
32. Buick FJ, Gledhill AB, Froese L, et al: Effect of induced erythrocythemia on aerobic work capacity. J Appl Physiol 48:636–642, 1980.
33. Sawka MN, Young AJ, Muza SR, et al: Erythrocyte reinfusion and maximal aerobic power: An examination of modifying factors. JAMA 257:1496–1499, 1987.
34. Zanjani ED, Ascensao JL: Erythropoietin. Transfusion 29:46–57, 1989.
35. Abels RI, Ortho Pharmaceutical Corporation, Raritan, NJ: Personal communication, 1989.
36. Cowart VS: Erythropoietin: A dangerous new form of blood doping? Physician Sports Med 17:115–118, 1989.
37. Colwell JA: Effects of exercise on platelet function, coagulation and fibrinolysis. Diabetes Metab Rev 1:501–512, 1986.
38. Bourey RE, Santoro SA: Interaction of exercise, coagulation, platelets and fibrinolysis—a brief review. Med Sci Sports Exerc 20:439–446, 1988.

39. Sinzinger H, Virgolini I: Effect of exercise on parameters of blood coagulation, platelet function and the prostaglandin system. Sports Med 6:238–245, 1988.
40. Stratton JR, Chandler WL, Cerqueira MD, et al: Exercise training increases tissue plasminogen activator activity [abstract]. Circulation 80(suppl II):610, 1989.
41. Ferguson EW, Bernier LL, Banta GR, et al: Effects of exercise and conditioning on clotting and fibrinolytic activity in men. J Appl Physiol 62:1416–1421, 1987.
42. Tofler GF, Brezinski D, Schafer AI, et al: Concurrent morning increase in platelet aggregability and the risk of myocardial infarction and sudden cardiac death. N Engl J Med 316:1514–1518, 1987.
43. Fitzgerald DJ, Roy L, Catella F, et al: Platelet activation in unstable coronary disease. N Engl J Med 315:983–989, 1986.
44. Green LH, Seroppian E, Handen RI: Platelet activation during exercise induced myocardial ischemia. N Engl J Med 302:193–197, 1980.
45. Mathis PC, Wohl H, Wallach SR, et al: Lack of release of platelet factor 4 during exercise-induced myocardial ischemia. N Engl J Med 304:1275–1278, 1981.
46. Stratton JR, Malpass TW, Ritchie JL, et al: Studies of platelet factor 4 and beta thromboglobulin release during exercise: Lack of relationship to myocardial ischemia. Circulation 66:33–43, 1982.
47. Eichner ER: Antithrombotic effects of exercise. Physician Sports Med 36:207–211, 1987.
48. Aarts PA, Bolhuis PA, Sakariassen KS, et al: Red blood cell size is important for adherence of blood platelets to artery subendothelium. Blood 62:214–217, 1983.

10

RENAL ABNORMALITIES DURING EXERCISE

Robert C. Goldszer, MD
Arthur J. Siegel, MD

Abnormalities in the urine associated with prolonged strenuous exercise have created justifiable concern about the consequences of such physical activity on the kidney. Many studies[1–4] describe hematuria and proteinuria occurring after physical exertion in a high proportion of apparently healthy subjects without underlying renal or genitourinary abnormalities. Such urinary findings are identical to presenting signs in a wide variety of renal disorders from glomerulonephritis and infection to stones and malignancy.[5–7] Exercise-related abnormalities have not been shown to predispose or progress to fixed renal disease, although specific prospective studies have not yet been reported.

The athlete with abnormal urinary findings presents a complex dilemma to the office physician, who must exclude significant underlying renal disease but must avoid expensive and potentially harmful invasive testing if it is unnecessary. A direct temporal relationship between exercise and onset of such findings and prompt clearing of all abnormalities after rest are the hallmarks of benign exercise-related urinary changes. The specific clinical setting in each patient, such as symptoms and age-related risks of tumor, must be taken into account in staging the extent of any workup. Exercise-related abnormalities, ultimately, are diagnoses of exclusion. This chapter discusses hematuria and proteinuria as the two most common urinary findings requiring exclusion of underlying disease. Acute renal failure in the setting of prolonged strenuous exercise, a rare but life-threatening and preventable complication, is also discussed.

HEMATURIA

There have been varied reports of the frequency of hematuria after exercise. Both gross and microscopic hematuria are described in association with a variety of sports and in trained as well as novice athletes. In general, a relationship exists between the duration and intensity of exercise and the proportion of athletes showing such abnormalities.[8–11] Bailey and colleagues[12] reported that 42 of 369 athletes in the 1974 Commonwealth Games had positive urine dipstick tests for occult blood. Blacklock[13] coined the phrase "10,000-meter hematuria" for male runners with these findings after running at such intermediate distances. A survey of marathon runners completing the 1979 Boston Marathon showed either gross or microscopic hematuria in 18% of 50 trained runners after a 26.2-mile race.[14] Of 31 runners, 63% showed microscopic hematuria after the 54-mile Comrade's Marathon.[9] Most of these findings have been reported in men, but similar findings are being reported in a significant number of women as well.[15]

TABLE 10–1. POSSIBLE CAUSES OF EXERCISE-RELATED HEMATURIA

Kidney	**Bladder**
Ischemia	Contusion
Acute renal failure	Stone
Increased vascular fragility	Infection
Trauma	**Urethra**
Nephroptosis	Contusion
Stone	Stone
Ureter	Infection
Stone	Trauma
	Cold

The direct relationship between degree of exertion and frequency or incidence of hematuria was best described by Kachadorian and Johnson[16] in data collected on men exercising at various rates on a treadmill. As the intensity of work was increased from 5.6 to 8.0 and 10.5 km/hr, there were more episodes of microscopic hematuria as well as the presence of urinary casts.

A number of etiologies for exercise-related hematuria have been proposed. It is possible that red blood cells may enter the urinary tract anywhere between the glomerulus and the urethra (Table 10–1). Transient pathologic changes from exercise may occur at any level of the genitourinary tract.

The early reports of postexercise hematuria implicated the kidney as the site of probable pathology. Gardner,[7] the first to use the term athletic pseudonephritis, described hematuria, proteinuria, and cylinduria in 45% of 424 urine samples from 47 football players. Direct trauma to the kidney may certainly cause hematuria in contact sports such as boxing or football, and indirect trauma may occur from impact during running. Hematuria is also described in sports such as long-distance swimming and rowing,[10] situations in which there is no high-impact component to cause renal trauma. Most athletes who demonstrate hematuria after exercise show rapid disappearance of this abnormality, making injury on a glomerular level an unlikely cause.

Other structures in the kidney may be the site of leakage of red blood cells into the urine. Hoover and Cromie[3] described blood flow changes in the renal pelvis as a possible source. They implicate ischemia in the small, corkscrew-like vessels surrounding the renal papillae and damage to these vessels. Goldberg[17] described jogging as a cause of nephroptosis in a patient with weak ligamentous attachments of the kidney, suggesting exercise-related displacement of the kidney.

The lower urinary tract is regarded as the most common source of hematuria after prolonged, severe exertion. Either gross or microscopic hematuria may occur as a result of contusions from running, although stones and infection must be excluded. In Blacklock's study of 10,000-meter hematuria, 18 runners were seen with this condition after running this distance.[13] Episodes were either asymptomatic or accompanied by dull pressure or suprapubic pain. All 18 runners had normal upper urinary tracts as demonstrated by intravenous pyelography. In eight of these athletes, contusions of the bladder mucosa were shown by cystoscopy, most often involving the intraureteric bar and the posterior rim of the internal meatus. There were also contracoup lesions in the lower posterior bladder and at the trigone. Hematuria on the basis of mucosal injury might be facilitated by an empty bladder at the time of exercise, although no relationship was reported to the amount or time of last voiding prior to exercise. Blacklock implicated such repeated trauma of the anterior bladder mucosa against the fixed posterior wall as the probable cause of the hematuria. Hematuria from some other source must occur in patients without bladder trauma.

Other sites in the lower urinary tract, such as prostatic or urethral inflammation, may also be a source of red blood cells in the urine. Exercise-induced irritation of the urethral meatus from contusion or cold exposure may be a rare cause of hematuria.[18] Such problems would be exacerbated by irritation from the urinary stream. Divided samples collected during a single urination may show clearing of blood in late-void aliquots.

The presence of casts in a postexercise urinalysis has also been described. Casts containing red or white blood cells, or hyaline, granular, and pigmented features have been occasionally observed.[1,5,7,19–21] The incidence and significance of casts in postexertional urine are yet to be elucidated, but they were not seen after careful search[14] in a study of marathon runners with hematuria. The presence of casts generally signifies underlying renal disease, and such patients should have a meticulous evaluation of additional urine samples to exclude persistence of such formed elements.

Hematuria associated with exercise alone is benign in nature. In most cases the urine becomes totally free of red blood cells within 24 to 48 hours. Several investigators[4,9,14] stress the importance of prompt resolution of hematuria, whether gross or microscopic. Even recurrences in the same individual may be isolated events after prolonged exertion, although such patients should receive more careful evaluations.

Proof of reversion to a normal urine after exercise-related hematuria is important to exclude such diseases as nephritis, nephrolithiasis, or tumors occurring elsewhere in the urinary tract. Papillary necrosis, infection, and vascular disease (vasculitis, renal artery or vein obstruction) must also be considered if abnormalities persist. Microscopic analysis of the urinary sediment is the first step in evaluating pigmentary change. In younger athletes (less than 40 years old) who have asymptomatic hematuria after exercise, we suggest a repeat urinalysis at 24 and 48 hours. A clean-voided urine may be cultured if cystitis or infection is suspected. If the repeat urinalyses are negative, no further tests are indicated. However, if the hematuria persists, is recurrent, or is associated with continued symptoms such as pain, dysuria, or fever, further investigations should be considered. Such indications are listed in Table 10–2. Consideration of the possible sources of persistent hematuria in the athlete (Table 10–1) highlight the need for extended workup while individualizing decisions in each case.

Figure 10-1 illustrates an approach to the diagnostic evaluation of hematuria in the nonexercising adult, and these same considerations should apply to the athlete with persistent hematuria as well. The follow-up urinalysis is the critical branch point indicating the need for medical evaluation if gross or microscopic hematuria persists. Measurement of serum creatinine to assess renal function and, if that is normal, intravenous pyelogram are appropriate at this juncture. If it is normal, excretory urography might be followed by cystoscopy to exclude bladder lesions, especially in individuals beyond age 40. A negative workup at this level is sufficient and need not be repeated after subsequent episodes of exercise-related hematuria as may occur in some individuals, provided that symptoms and signs clear with rest. Abnormalities on excretory urography or cystoscopy would be pursued in the conventional fashion, as shown in the diagram. Patients with negative tests but with persistent hematuria should have additional investigation for causes of intrinsic renal disease such as creatinine clearance. Renal biopsy should be considered when the workup shows persistent abnormalities without an established cause. Therapy will be

TABLE 10–2. RENAL ABNORMALITIES IN ATHLETES REQUIRING FURTHER EVALUATION

1. Progressive symptoms: colic or flank pain.
2. Persistence of hematuria or proteinuria beyond 48 hours after exercise.
3. Urinary casts: red or white blood cell; pigmented.
4. Positive urine culture for bacterial infection.
5. Oliguria after prolonged, strenuous exercise.

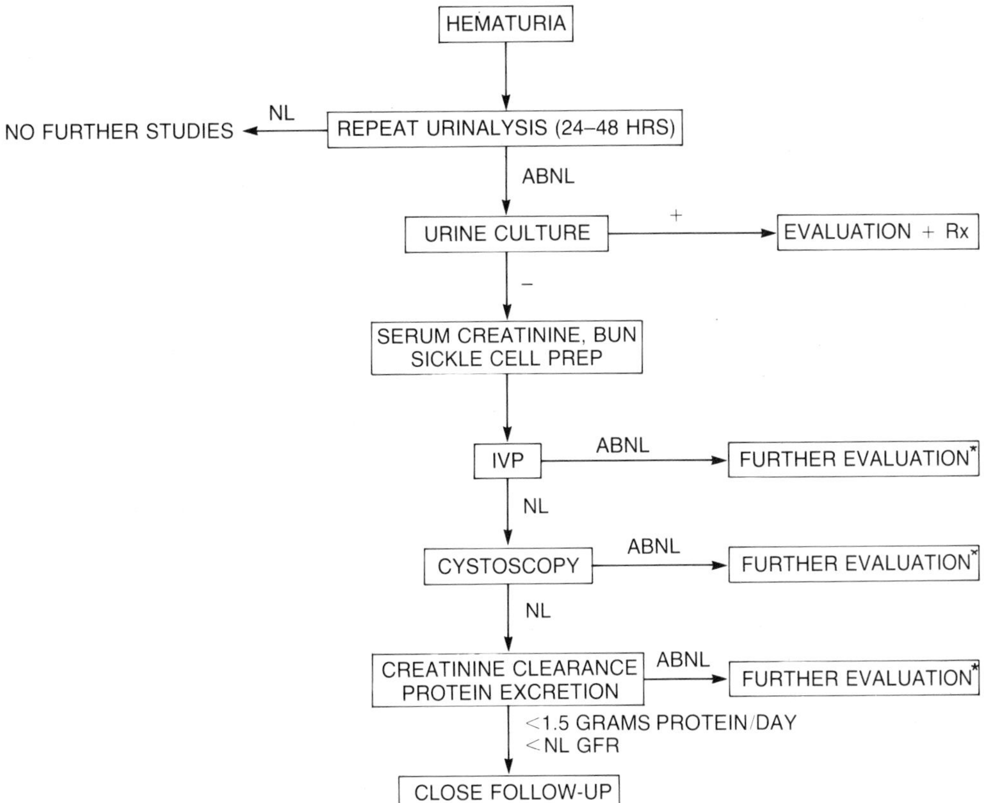

Figure 10–1. Evaluation of the patient with hematuria. (NL = normal, ABNL = abnormal, BUN = blood urea nitrogen, IVP = intravenous pyelogram, GFR = glomerular filtration rate.)

based on the specific diagnosis. Patients with benign hematuria related to exercise may continue to be active but should drink copious fluids before exercise and avoid dehydration.

In summary, microscopic or gross hematuria is a common occurrence in people who exercise strenuously and may occur in up to 20% of marathon runners after competition. The source of the red blood cells may be anywhere from the kidney to the urethra but most commonly arises from the lower urinary tract. Hematuria that has completely cleared within 24 to 48 hours, even if recurrent, has a benign prognosis. In-depth evaluation is reserved for those with persistent hematuria or symptoms.

PROTEINURIA

Proteinuria, like hematuria, has been shown to occur following many forms of strenuous exercise such as rowing, football, track and long-distance running, swimming, and calisthenics.[22–24] The incidence of exercise-induced proteinuria has also been reported to occur at different rates. Like hematuria, its occurrence is more frequent with more severe strenuous and prolonged exertions. Collier[25] reported the occurrence of albuminuria in oarsmen after strenuous exercise. Reports of renal abnormalities in military recruits after severe exercise in tropical weather conditions frequently demonstrate proteinuria.[26] In his studies of various degrees of exertion, Kachadorian and coworkers reported proteinuria only after the most strenuous treadmill exercise.[16,27] The degree of exertional proteinuria is usually 2+ to 3+ by dipstick determination and is always transient if it is due to exercise alone.[10,28] Quantitative measurements over 24 hours are in the range of 100 to 300 mg or less.

The pathogenesis of exercise proteinuria is more precisely described than it is for hematuria. The work of Poortmans and colleagues[29–31] has established that the proteins found in urine after exercise are of plasma origin. There may be a slight decrease in reabsorption of proteins, but the major component is albumin of plasma origin.

Renal hemodynamic alterations associated with exercise are the accepted source of this proteinuria. The work of several investigators has shown that prolonged, severe exercise is associated with a decrease in intravascular volume from acute dehydration.[32–34] This decrease in circulating plasma volume causes a rise in plasma renin,[35] angiotensin II,[36] aldosterone, and antidiuretic hormone (ADH).[37] Wade and Claybaugh in earlier work[32] involving treadmill exercise and in a later study[37] of ten men taking part in a 20-day road race showed acute elevations in plasma renin activity and plasma antidiuretic hormone. Their studies of subjects during prolonged, daily exercise showed increases in urinary aldosterone as well.[37]

In several reports of renal function in athletes, the most commonly observed pattern is an acute decrease in renal blood flow (RBF) with maintenance of glomerular filtration rate (GFR) because of autoregulation of blood flow within the kidney.[38–40] This results in a rise in filtration fraction (FF), the ratio of glomerular filtration rate to renal blood flow (FF = GFR/RBF).[41] Neviackas and Bauer[42] studied renal function in marathon runners and showed that alterations in these relationships depend upon the magnitude and duration of decreased renal blood flow. In cold weather, runners showed minimal alterations in renal function. In warm weather, with severe dehydration, there was a sustained decrease in RBF during prolonged exercise and a decrease in GFR as measured by clearance of para-amino-hippurate and inulin, respectively. Urinalyses were abnormal in all runners, showing red blood cells and 2+ proteinuria as the most common findings. Runners were retested at 1 week postmarathon, at which time measurements of renal function had returned to normal.

The hormonal response to sustained vigorous exercise includes elevations of renin, angiotensin II, and ADH, which cause alterations in renal hemodynamics. The efforts of Bohrer and associates[43] and Brenner and co-workers[44] have elucidated the mechanism of proteinuria associated with elevations of angiotensin II. Using micropuncture techniques in Munich-Wistar strain rats with surface glomeruli that are available to direct puncture and thus direct pressure measurement, the investigators showed that during angiotensin II infusion, pressure in the glomerulus is increased; the single nephron GFR is normal owing to a decrease in glomerular blood flow, and the FF is elevated. As a result of this increased FF, there is an increased concentration of plasma proteins along the glomerular membrane that permits increased passage of proteins by convection and diffusion into Bowman's space. Hemodynamically mediated hormonal changes in urinary flow may result in transient proteinuria on a similar basis.

The usual time course or duration of exercise-induced proteinuria is similar to that of hematuria, since clearing may be expected within 24 to 48 hours.[42,45–47] When proteinuria is due to exercise alone, it carries a benign prognosis with no long-term sequelae.

Proteinuria detected initially after exertion may be independent of exercise or secondary to underlying renal disease. If the urine of an athlete is not clear within 24 to 48 hours after exercise, further investigation is indicated (Fig. 10–2). A personal or family history of renal disease or other signs of illness such as hypertension, edema, or anemia would also suggest a need for further testing. If proteinuria persists in a resting urine specimen, we begin the evaluation by collecting overnight or supine and upright urine samples to exclude benign orthostatic proteinuria. If proteinuria persists while in the supine position, serum tests for renal function and a 24-hour urine collection for creatinine and total protein are useful. Determination of serum creatinine or urea nitrogen level, a fasting blood glucose level, and complete blood counts are relevant.

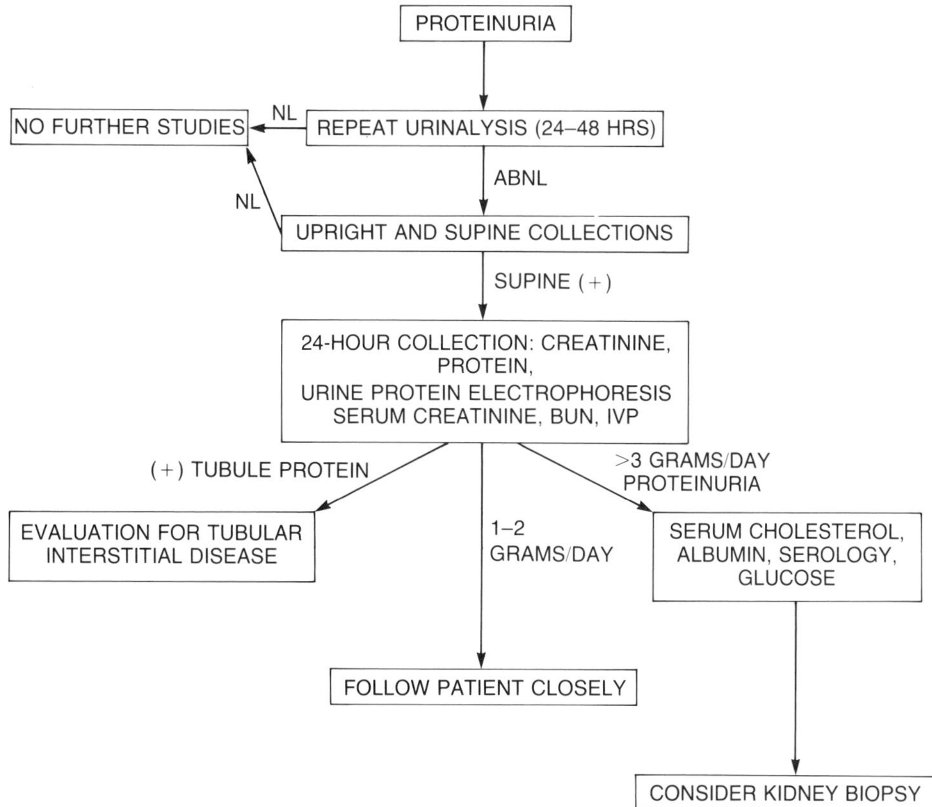

Figure 10–2. Evaluation of the patient with proteinuria. (NL = normal, ABNL = abnormal, BUN = blood urea nitrogen, IVP = intravenous pyelogram.)

Urinary protein electrophoresis may be helpful, including a measure of beta$_2$-microglobulin, a protein of low molecular weight that is normally reabsorbed in the renal tubule. Glomerular injury results in proteinuria with low levels of this protein, whereas tubular pathology may produce elevations of beta$_2$-microglobulin as a component of proteinuria.[48] Assessment of renal size, number, and function is important and may be accomplished by intravenous pyelography if renal function is normal as measured by the creatinine clearance. Patients showing greater than 1g of albumin in a 24-hour collection might be referred to a nephrologist for consultation and consideration of a diagnostic renal biopsy.

Whereas exercise-induced proteinuria is likely to be recurrent in a given subject after a specific level of exertion, there is no evidence of increased risk for chronic renal disease and no reason to limit physical activity. Such individuals should have a medical checkup and a urinalysis for protein on a yearly basis, but no other evaluation is necessary unless further abnormalities occur as described.

ACUTE RENAL FAILURE

Acute renal failure is the least common but most serious renal complication associated with exercise. Prolonged strenuous exercise, especially in the heat, produces profound physiologic decrements in RBF and urine production.[42,49–51] Mechanisms for the occurrence of self-limited hematuria and proteinuria during these low-flow states have been reviewed. Reports by Schrier and colleagues,[52] Vertel and Knochel,[53] and Knochel and associates[54] in military recruits confirm the risk of acute renal failure among previously healthy subjects after prolonged, strenuous exercise in the heat. These authors observed that acute renal failure occurred most commonly in the summer months, during the initial 2 weeks of basic training, and primarily among recruits from more temperate climates who were not acclimated to heat stress. Acute renal failure in this setting was precipitated by uncorrected dehydration, hyperpyrexia, rhabdomyolysis, and myoglobinuria. Acute renal failure during exercise results from a combination of a profound renal ischemia and nephrotoxins generated during heat injury.[55,56]

The magnitude and duration of dehydration during prolonged strenuous exercise convert the physiologic decrease in RBF to severe tissue injury. Autoregulation of blood flow on the glomerular level serves to protect the filtration rate during the stress of dehydration. Profound and sustained decreases in RBF drop perfusion pressure below a critical threshold and result in decreased GFR. Ischemic injury to the kidney may follow and result in acute tubular necrosis and renal failure.[57,58]

Hyperpyrexia and substrate depletion in muscle during such physiologic stress decrease blood flow to exercising muscle despite maximal vasodilation. Hypoxemia at a cellular level results in membrane damage and release of muscle enzymes into the circulation.[59–61] Myoglobin is released with muscle enzymes; this is an added insult to the hypoxic renal tubular cell.[62–64] These phenomena are shown diagrammatically in Figure 10–3.

Studies in asymptomatic marathon runners after competition show elevations of creatine kinase greater than 30 times the upper limits of normal without evidence of renal injury.[61] It remains unclear as to why renal injury remains rare if rhabdomyolysis is so commonplace in this setting. Grossman and coworkers[64] and Knochel[65] have summarized the clinical findings in patients with rhabdomyolysis, myoglobinuria, and acute renal failure. In most cases, there is an initial period of decreased RBF leading to intrarenal ischemia. Myoglobin precipitates in the renal tubules, causing obstruction to flow, and may be the central toxin to the renal tubules.

Hemolysis accompanying heat injury releases hemoglobin to the circulation, which adds to this toxic stress. Intravascular hemolysis as part of the syndrome of disseminated intravascular coagulation may occur in profound heat stroke. Hemoglobinuria and other as yet undefined toxins may contribute to tubular necrosis and acute renal failure.[66–69]

Nephrotoxic drug effects should also be considered in the pathogenesis of acute renal failure, since commonly used drugs may play a role in development of renal insufficiency.[70] Analgesics in the class of nonsteroidal anti-inflammatory drugs such as aspirin,

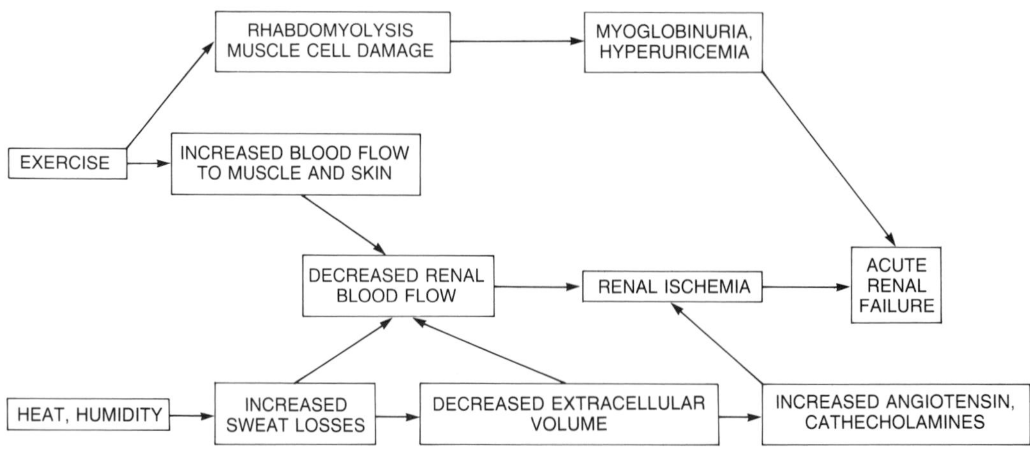

Figure 10–3. Possible pathogenetic mechanisms in acute renal failure.

ibuprofen, and indomethacin have been reported to decrease GFR and RBF under certain conditions.[71] This effect is mediated by inhibition of synthesis of prostaglandins, which are vasodilators. The penicillins and cephalosporins are rarely associated with interstitial nephritis on an allergic or immune basis.[72]

Each of these pathogenic stresses—myoglobinuria, hemoglobinuria, and nephrotoxic drugs—may compound renal ischemia from dehydration in association with exercise-induced heat injury. Prompt and adequate fluid replacement sufficient to restore urine flow is the specific antidote to such a crisis. Runners should consume sufficient fluids after competition to induce urination promptly (within 1 to 2 hours), or they should be evaluated by a physician. Intravenous fluids should be available for runners with hyperpyrexia when onset of vomiting may prevent adequate fluid repletion by mouth. Oliguric runners should be observed very closely; they may require short-term hospitalization for fluid repletion and treatment. If oliguria persists despite adequate fluid replacement, evaluation is indicated for threatened acute renal failure.[73]

Renal Responses to Dehydration During Prolonged Strenuous Exercise

DEFENSE AGAINST ACUTE RENAL FAILURE

One of the roles of the kidney is to defend plasma volume and maintain circulatory integrity against the dehydrating stress of prolonged strenuous exercise. Recent studies on urinary excretion of electrolytes during prolonged physical activity reflect the increase in plasma renin activity and levels of angiotensin II and aldosterone induced by volume contraction from the sweating response.[74] Specifically, potassium is released from muscle cells during the fatigue phase of exercise, which makes the use of specific potassium supplements during exercise inappropriate. The intrinsic sodium and potassium regulatory mechanisms of the normal kidney balance these electrolyte factors.

Added to the stress of dehydration is the additional evidence for intravascular hemolysis during distance running, which contributes to the risk for acute injury to the renal tubule. Recent studies document an acute decrease in haptoglobin levels during continuous running even at 1 hour with accentuation in fall of haptoglobin levels during downhill versus level or uphill running.[75] This may be due in part to the increase in mechanical trauma to red blood cells occurring at foot strike during these varied running configurations, but it may also reflect relative stresses on skeletal muscle. Free hemoglobin and myoglobin in the circulation during prolonged strenuous exercise are potential toxins that may cause renal tabular injury or dysfunction compounded by the relative degree of dehydration.[76]

Recent research indicates that the elevation of plasma atrial natriuretic factor induced by acute exercise may play a protective role in increasing sodium excretion during exercise to counteract the hormonal changes leading to a decrease in renal perfusion.[77] The body thus uses the kidney to protect and defend circulating plasma volume while the circulation, in turn, provides a peptide hormone to defend the kidney from tubular injury during stress of dehydration.

Hydration supplemented by these balanced endocrine mechanisms protects against acute renal failure from myoglobinuria and hemoglobinuria during a spectrum of exercise from military or police academy recruit training in the summer to extreme degrees of exercise, such as marathon running and triatholon participation up to the iron-man level. As an additional precaution, athletes should be counseled against optional or unnecessary analgesic use prior to competition, which can block prostaglandin synthesis and further compromise medullary blood flow.[78,79] Prophylaxis and prevention of acute renal failure depend on hydration and awareness of these risk factors.[80] Chronic analgesic use may contribute to fixed renal impairment in some cases.[81,82]

In summary, acute renal failure associated with exercise is an infrequent but preventable complication. Poorly acclimated persons who exercise to exhaustion in the heat are prime targets. The etiology is renal ischemia from uncorrected profound decreases in renal blood flow. Myoglobinuria from rhabdomyolysis, hemoglobinuria from intravascular hemolysis, and occasionally nephrotoxic drugs may be factors in precipitating tubular necrosis. Prompt rehydration is preventive and essential to avert this injury.

REFERENCES

1. Larcom RC, Carter GH: Erythrocytes in urinary sediment. J Clin Lab Invest 1:875, 1949.
2. Barach J: Physiological and pathological effects of severe exertion (marathon race) on circulatory and renal systems. Arch Intern Med 5:382, 1910.
3. Hoover DL, Cromie WJ: Theory and management of exercise-related hematuria. Physician Sports Med 9:91, 1981.
4. Fred HL, Natelson EA: Grossly bloody urine of runners. South Med J 70:1394, 1977.
5. Boileau M, Fuchs E, Barry JM, et al: Stress hematuria: Athletic pseudonephritis in marathoners. Urology 15:471, 1980.
6. Kudish HG: Determining the cause of hematuria. Postgrad Med 58:119, 1975.
7. Gardner KD: Athletic pseudonephritis—alterations of urine sediment by athletic competition. JAMA 161:1613, 1956.
8. Immergut MA: Urinary bleeding: When is it a danger signal? Modern Medicine, December 15, 1981, pp 68–77.
9. Dancaster CP, Whereat SJ: Renal function in marathon runners. S Afr Med J 45:547, 1971.
10. Alyea EP, Parish HH: Renal response to exercise—urinary findings. JAMA 167:807, 1958.
11. The hematuria of the long distance runner [editorial]. Br Med J July 21, 1929, p 159.
12. Bailey RR, Dann E, Gillies AHB, et al: What the urine contains following athletic competition. NZ Med J 83:309, 1976.
13. Blacklock NJ: Bladder trauma in the long distance runner: 10,000 metres haematuria. Br J Urol 49:129, 1977.
14. Siegel AJ, Hennekens CH, Solomon HS, et al: Exercise-related hematuria findings in a group of marathon runners. JAMA 241:391, 1979.
15. Fred HH: More on the grossly bloody urine of runners [letter]. Arch Intern Med 138:1610, 1978.
16. Kachadorian W, Johnson RE: Athletic pseudonephritis in relation to rate of exercise. Lancet 1:472, 1970.
17. Goldberg J: Jogger's kidney: A case of acquired nephroptosis. N Engl J Med 305:590, 1981.
18. Hershkowitz M: Penile frostbite, an unforeseen hazard of jogging. N Engl J Med 296:178, 1977.
19. Berman, LB: When the urine is red. JAMA 237:2753, 1977.
20. West CD: Asymptomatic hematuria and proteinuria in children: Causes and appropriate diagnostic studies. J Pediatr 89:173, 1976.
21. Barach JH: Evidences of nephritis and urinary acidosis. Am J Med Sci 159:398, 1920.
22. Leube W: Über Ausscheidung von Eiweiss im Hasn des gesunden Menschen. Virchows Arch 72:145, 1878.
23. West CD, Shapiro FL, Swartz CD: Proteinuria in the athlete. Physician Sports Med July 1981, pp 45–55.
24. Bozovic L, Castenfors J, Piscator M: Effect of prolonged heavy exercise on urinary protein excretion and plasma renin activity. Acta Physiol Scand 70:143, 1967.
25. Collier W: Functional albuminuria in athletes. Br Med J 1:4, 1907.
26. Schrier RW, Hano J, Keller HI, et al: Renal, metabolic and circulatory responses to heat and exercise. Ann Intern Med 73:213, 1970.
27. Kachadorian WA, Johnson RE: Renal responses to various rates of exercise. J Appl Physiol 28:748, 1970.
28. Taylor A: Some characteristics of exercise proteinuria. Clin Sci 19:209, 1960.
29. Poortmans J, Jeancoz RW: Quantitative immunological determination of 12 plasma proteins excreted in human urine collected before and after exercise. J Clin Invest 47:386, 1968.
30. Poortmans J, van Kerchoue E: La proteinuria d'effort. Clin Chim Acta 7:229, 1962.
31. Poortmans J: La protéinurie physiologique au repos et à l'effort. Ann Soc R Sci Med Natur Brux 17:89, 1964.
32. Wade CE, Claybaugh JR: Plasma renin activity, vasopressin concentration, and urinary excretory responses to exercise in men. J Appl Physiol 49:930, 1980.
33. Maher J, Jones L, Hartley L, et al: Aldosterone dynamics during graded exercise at sea level and high altitude. J Appl Physiol 39:18, 1975.

34. Kozlowski S, Szczepanska E, Zielinski A: The hypothalamohypophyseal antidiuretic system in physical exercises. Arch Intern Physiol 75:218, 1967.
35. Costill DL, Branan F, Fink W, et al: Exercise-induced sodium conservation: Changes in plasma renin and aldosterone. Med Sci Sports 8:209, 1976.
36. Kosunen KJ, Pakarinen AJ: Plasma renin, angiotensin II and plasma and urinary aldosterone in running exercise. J Appl Physiol 41:26, 1976.
37. Wade CE, Dressendorfer RH, O'Brien JC, et al: Renal function, aldosterone, and vasopressin excretion following repeated long distance running. J Appl Physiol 50:709, 1981.
38. Castenfors JA, Mossfeldt F, Piscator M: Effect of prolonged heavy exercise on renal function and urinary protein excretion. Acta Physiol Scand 70:194, 1967.
39. White HL, Rolf D: Effects of exercise and some other influences on the renal circulation in man. Am J Physiol 152:505, 1948.
40. Castenfors J: Renal function during exercise. Acta Physiol Scand 70:7, 1967.
41. Grimby G: Renal clearances during prolonged supine exercise at different loads. J Appl Physiol 20:1294, 1965.
42. Neviackas JA, Bauer JM: Renal function abnormalities induced by marathon running. South Med J 74:1457, 1981.
43. Bohrer MP, Deen WM, Robertson CR, et al: Mechanism of angiotensin II induced proteinuria in the rat. Am J Physiol 2:F13, 1977.
44. Brenner BM, Hostetter TH, Humes HD: Molecular basis of proteinuria of glomerular origin. N Engl J Med 298:826, 1978.
45. Rowe DS, Soothiu LL: The proteins of postural and exercise proteinuria. Clin Sci 21:87, 1961.
46. Glassock RJ, Cohen AH, Bennett CM, et al: Primary glomerular diseases. *In* Brenner BM, Rector FC (eds): The Kidney, ed 2. Philadelphia, WB Saunders, 1981, pp 1351–1492.
47. Starr I Jr: The production of albuminuria by renal vasoconstriction in animals and in man. J Exp Med 43:31, 1926.
48. Peterson PA, Evrin PE, Berggard J: Differentiation of glomerular, tubular, and normal proteinuria: Determinations of urinary excretion of beta$_2$-microglobulin, albumin, and total protein. J Clin Invest 48:1189, 1969.
49. Rowell LB: Human cardiovascular adjustments to exercise and thermal stress. Physiol Rev 54:75, 1974.
50. Castenfors J: Renal function during prolonged exercise. Ann NY Acad Sci 301:151, 1978.
51. Refsum HE, Stromme SB: Relationship between urine flow, glomerular filtration and urine solute concentration during prolonged heavy exercise. Scand J Clin Lab Invest 35:775, 1975.
52. Schrier RW, Henderson HS, Tisher CC, et al: Nephropathy associated with heart stress and exercise. Ann Intern Med 67:356, 1967.
53. Vertel RM, Knochel JP: Acute renal failure due to heart injury: An analysis of ten cases associated with a high incidence of myoglobinuria. Am J Med 43:435, 1967.
54. Knochel JP, Beisel WR, Herndon EG, et al: The renal, cardiovascular, hematologic and serum electrolyte abnormalities of heat stroke. Am J Med 30:299, 1961.
55. Demos MA, Gitin EL, Kagen LJ: Exercise myoglobinemia and acute exertional rhabdomyolysis. Arch Intern Med 134:669, 1974.
56. Howenstine JA: Exertion-induced myoglobinuria and hemoglobinuria. JAMA 173:493, 1960.
57. Hostetter TH, Wilkes BM, Brenner BM: Mechanisms of impaired glomerular filtration in acute renal failure. *In* Brenner BM, Stein JH (eds): Contemporary Issues in Nephrology, vol 6. New York, Churchill Livingstone, 1980, pp 52–78.
58. Smolens P, Stein JH: Pathophysiology of acute renal failure. Am J Med 70:479, 1981.
59. Magazanik A, Shapiro Y, Meytes D, et al: Enzyme blood levels and water balance during a marathon race. J Appl Physiol 36:214, 1974.
60. Siegel AJ, Silverman LM, Holman BL: Elevated creatine kinase MB isoenzyme levels in marathon runners. JAMA 246:2049, 1981.
61. Siegel AJ, Silverman LM, Lopez RE: Creatine kinase elevations in marathon runners: Relationship to training and competition. Yale J Biol Med 53:275, 1980.
62. DeLangen CD: Myoglobin and myoglobinuria. Acta Med Scand 124:213, 1946.
63. Meyer-Bietz F: Beobachtungen an einem Eigenartigen mit Muskellahmungen Verbundenen fall von Hämoglobinurie. Dtsch Arch Klin Med 101:85, 1910.
64. Grossman RA, Hamilton RW, Morse BM, et al: Nontraumatic rhabdomyolysis and acute renal failure. N Engl J Med 291:807, 1974.
65. Knochel JP: Rhabdomyolysis and myoglobinuria. Semin Nephrol 1:75, 1981.
66. Ferris EB, Blankenhorn MA, Robinson HW, et al: Heat stroke: Clinical and chemical observations in 44 cases. J Clin Invest 17:249, 1938.
67. Shibolet S, Coll R, Gilat T, et al: Heat stroke: Its clinical picture and mechanism in 36 cases. Q J Med 36:525, 1967.

68. Stahl WC: March hemoglobinuria: Report of five cases in students at Ohio State University. JAMA 164:1458, 1957.
69. Lalich JJ: The influence of available fluid on the production of experimental hemoglobinuric nephrosis in rabbits. J Exp Med 87:157, 1948.
70. Mudge GH, Duggin GG (eds): Drug effect on the kidney. Kidney Int 18:539, 1980.
71. Levenson DJ, Simmons CE, Brenner BM: Arachidonic acid metabolism, prostaglandins and the kidney. Am J Med 72:354, 1982.
72. Cotran RS: Tubulointerstitial nephropathies. Hosp Pract 17:79, 1982.
73. Ng RC, Suki WN: Treatment of acute renal failure. *In* Brenner BM, Stein JH (eds): Contemporary Issues in Nephrology, vol 6. New York, Churchill Livingstone, 1980, pp 229–274.
74. Lijnen P, Hespel P, Vanden EE, et al: Urinary excretion of electrolytes during prolonged physical activity in normal man. Eur J Applied Physiol 53:317–321, 1985.
75. Miller BJ, Pate RR, Burgess W: Foot impact force and intravascular hemolysis during distance running. Int J Sports Med 9:56–60, 1988.
76. Materson BJ, Preston RA: Myoglobinuria versus hemoglobinuria. Hosp Pract October 30, 1988, pp 29–38.
77. Donckier JE, deCoster PM, Buysschaert M, et al: Effects of exercise on plasma atrial natriuretic factor and cardiac function in men and women. Eur J Clin Invest 18:415–419, 1988.
78. Clive DM, Stoff JS: Renal syndromes associated with nonsteroidal anti-inflammatory drugs. N Engl J Med 310:563–566, 1984.
79. Patrono C, Dunn MJ: The clinical significance of inhibition of renal prostaglandin synthesis. Kidney Int 32:1–9, 1987.
80. Better OS, Stein JH: Early management of shock and prophylaxis of acute renal failure in traumatic rhabdomyolysis. N Engl J Med 322:825–829, 1990.
81. Sandler DP, Smith JC, Weinberg CR, et al: Analgesic use and chronic renal disease. N Engl J Med 320:1238–1243, 1989.
82. Bennett WM, DeBroe ME: Analgesic nephropathy—a preventable renal disease. N Engl J Med 320:1269–1271, 1989.

11

THE GASTROINTESTINAL SYSTEM

Stephen N. Sullivan, MD, FRCPUK, FRCPC

Exercise helps to throw down wind from the bowels and attenuates the contents of the stomach. It also serves at once as an evacuant and a diversion by which artifices the humours are put into condition of flying off without the danger of bringing on spasms. John Puch, 1794, A Treatise of the Science of Muscular Action.

Belatedly, modern man is rediscovering the benefits of exercise. Unfortunately, unlike John Puch, he is finding that it is not always good for the guts. Belching, heartburn, abdominal pain, and diarrhea may be the result. These troublesome gastrointestinal symptoms afflict mainly runners, being uncommon problems for cyclists, swimmers, and rowers. We have little knowledge of the prevalence of gastrointestinal symptoms in other sports. The cause of these symptoms is largely unknown, and even our knowledge of the effect of exercise on normal gastrointestinal physiology is scant. During the discussion which follows, I will comment on the effect of exercise on gastrointestinal physiology where it seems appropriate.

One clinically relevant effect of exercise on gastrointestinal function is its effect on gastric emptying. Vigorous exercise delays emptying of solids, but has little effect on the emptying of liquids until the work intensity exceeds 70% of $\dot{V}O_{2max}$, or until exhaustion is approached. Since water and electrolyte loss and glycogen depletion are the major factors that limit performance during severe, prolonged exertion, athletes often consume strange concoctions (one derived from the composition of sweat) to improve or sustain performance. Usually, water is all that is required. Cold water seems more palatable and may leave the stomach quicker.

For exercise lasting longer than 2 hours, the addition of carbohydrate to the sports drink will prevent hypoglycemia, improve performance, and delay exhaustion, but it can also slow gastric emptying. If the concentration of carbohydrate is kept below 10%, this seems to be a relatively minor problem. Attempts have been made to increase carbohydrate intake without slowing gastric emptying by using glucose polymer solutions, which have a lower osmolality while providing the same calories. As yet, I do not find the evidence convincing. The necessity of adding electrolytes to replacement fluids has not been proven, except perhaps for ultramarathons and Iron Man Triathlons where hyponatremia frequently develops.

THE GASTROINTESTINAL SIDE EFFECTS OF EXERCISE

Nausea and Vomiting

Nausea, vomiting, and retching (the "dry heaves") are experienced by 5% to 10% of competitive runners and triathletes. Usually these symptoms occur during maximal exertion, and it is not uncommon for the athlete to cross the finish line "heaving." Presumably, this is the result of "stress" in the physical sense. Stress in the mental sense can also cause troubles. Anxious athletes may vomit prior to competition. Eating before exercise or drinking too much and attempting to catch up on fluid, electrolyte, and carbohydrate depletion late in an endurance event, when gastric emptying may be delayed, are sometimes factors. Gastroesophageal reflux and heartburn may also precipitate nausea and vomiting.

Gastroesophageal Reflux

Vigorous exercise can induce gastroesophageal reflux. The symptoms of belching and regurgitation are particularly common whereas heartburn and chest pain are less frequent. The problem is more likely to occur if the athlete eats before exercising or if he or she already has a problem with reflux even when not exercising. Running and swimming are prime offenders and, to a lesser extent, it occurs with weight lifting and rowing. It is a minor problem for cyclists, except when they are "down on the drops" after recently eating or drinking. Esophageal pH monitoring studies confirm that asymptomatic reflux during exercise is a common event but fortunately, there is no evidence that it leads to any long-term problems such as esophagitis or peptic stricture.

Why does reflux occur during exercise? The answer is not known. It is very difficult to evaluate the function of the esophagus during exercise, and we do not have enough information to say with certainty what happens to the motility of the lower esophageal sphincter or the body of the esophagus during exertion. I suspect that purely mechanical factors such as posture, aerophagia, bodily agitation, and food and fluid in the stomach are more important than any exercise-induced changes in esophageal motility.

I can find no studies on the treatment of esophageal reflux that occurs during exercise. The treatment is therefore by trial and error. It consists of explanation to the athlete, avoiding heavy meals before exercising, and the use of antacids. The choice of antacid is individual preference. Foaming alginate-based antacids such as Gaviscon (Marion Laboratories, Kansas City, MO) can be used and they rarely cause bloating. One should avoid magnesium-containing antacids in athletes who are prone to diarrhea. For athletes with diarrhea, calcium-containing antacids tend to be constipating. One might also consider calcium-based antacids in thin, anorectic, amenorrheic female distance runners who are predisposed to osteoporosis. If these conservative measures are not successful and the problem is particularly troublesome, try an H_2-receptor antagonist such as ranitidine or famotidine an hour or so before exercising.

Abdominal Pain

The abdominal "stitch" is well recognized by athlete and coach. Its cause is unknown with suggestions ranging from trapped intestinal gas to diaphragmatic spasms or ischemia. Its sharp character, subcostal location, aggravation by breathing, onset with strenuous exertion, and quick relief with rest make the diagnosis easy. Any exercise-induced abdominal pain that does not have these features deserves a "second look." Other causes of exertion-associated abdominal pain include trauma, cecal volvulus, inguinal hernias, erosive gastritis, and ureteropelvic junction obstruction. I have seen athletes with Crohn's disease, and even one with cecal carcinoma, whose symptom of pain first manifested while exercising.

The approach to abdominal pain in the athlete is the same as that in the nonathlete. History is most important! Where is the pain? What does it feel like? Where does it radiate? What brings it on, relieves it, or aggravates it? What is its time course and what are the associated symptoms?

Usually physical examination is normal. Occasionally one finds hernias, masses, organomegaly, or abdominal bruits. Two diagnoses that are frequently missed are abdominal wall pain and the "slipping rib syndrome." The diagnosis of abdominal wall pain is made by demonstrating superficial tenderness with no relief and even worsening of pain during palpation when the abdominal musculature is tensed. "Slipping rib" can be diagnosed by hooking the fingers under the costal margin and causing the rib to "pop" with reproduction of the pain.

Runner's Diarrhea

The most common problem causing a distance runner or triathlete to interrupt exercise is the urgent need to have a bowel movement. Surveys reveal that approximately one third of distance runners have experienced the urge or need to defecate while running and that 20% to 25% suffer from troublesome cramps or diarrhea during or after competitive running.

Distance runner's diarrhea can be divided into four clinical subtypes. The first is the prerace urge, or the "nervous pooeys." Classic examples of this can be seen in the woods of Hopkington prior to the Boston Marathon, or in the continuous long queues in front of the "portapots" at any major competition. This is probably the athletic equivalent of a "nervous bowel."

Many runners will also experience the more troublesome second form of runner's diarrhea with lower abdominal cramps, rectal spasm, diarrhea, and not infrequently, fecal incontinence during or immediately following severe maximal exertion.

The third major form of distance runner's diarrhea is the "early morning dumps." This usually occurs if the morning run is held before the usual morning ablutions, but after a glass of orange juice or a muffin. This type of diarrhea can also occur at other times during the day, particularly if the runner has not had her (this is a more common problem for ladies) normal bowel movement for the day. Several miles into the run, vague lower abdominal disquietude is felt. This is progressive, culminating in severe rectal spasm and a dash to the bushes or a wild search for the nearest toilet.

The fourth and least common form of bowel dysfunction is that of bloody diarrhea. It is likely due to colonic ischemia from reduced blood flow to the bowel during maximal exercise. Alternatively, it might be due to traumatic contusion of the cecum or sigmoid colon in the pelvis (see GI Bleeding).

While we may have reasonable explanations for the "nervous pooeys" and for bloody diarrhea, it is not at all certain what causes the other forms of runner's diarrhea. The traditional explanation is that it is due to changes in gastrointestinal transit; however, there is little scientific evidence that exercise predictably affects small bowel or colonic motility. If motility is a factor, there are several possible explanations as to how and why. There is no doubt that blood flow to the bowel decreases with exercise. One can imagine situations in which profound hypovolemia secondary to sweating compounds the already decreased blood supply and results in ischemic gut injury. The explanation may be hormonal. With exercise, there are increased levels of motilin, vasoactive intestinal polypeptide, prostaglandins, and endorphins. These substances are known to affect small bowel and colonic function.

The explanation may be wholly mechanical, with the effect of gravity and jiggling on the colonic contents ensuring that stool passes readily into the rectum where it stimulates reflex defecation. The explanation may also lie in the area of increased dietary fiber. Runners traditionally like to stay slim and they may eat high-fiber low-calorie snacks to satisfy their appetite. In addition, the distance runner may consume 5000 to 10,000 more calories per week than his sedentary brother. These extra calories will contain an obligatory amount of extra dietary fiber.

Finally, there are a number of miscellaneous explanations such as "nerves," food allergies, food-associated exercise-induced anaphylaxis, psoas muscle hypertrophy, and lactase deficiency. The latter may be more common than we realise. More than half of adults do not digest milk sugar (lactose). This is a major problem for blacks, Orientals, and North American and Asian Indians. Lactose intolerance also affects approximately 10% of whites. Some of these milk-drinking, lactase-deficient athletes will get the symptoms of lactose malabsorption only when exercising.

Although running itself may cause bowel dysfunction, one must remember that, just as athletes are not immune to coronary artery disease, they are also not immune to gastrointestinal diseases such as infections, inflammatory bowel disease, malabsorption, or cancers. Some athletes with gastrointestinal diseases will first experience their symptoms while exercising. It is therefore prudent for the physician not to blame running as the cause until more serious conditions have been considered.

The management of runner's diarrhea is largely empiric as there are no scientific studies addressing the problem. The athlete should be encouraged to try to have a bowel movement before exercising. If this is not possible, a light meal a few hours before competition may stimulate the gastrocolic reflex and a bowel movement. Elimination of milk products or avoiding sugar-free gums that contain sorbitol or mannitol is worth trying. Some individuals who eat a lot of fruit may have difficulties with the sorbitol and fructose found in some fruits. Fructose is also used as a sweetener in many nondiet pops. Sometimes caffeine is the problem. Other dietary manipulations are all "trial and error," but excessive dietary restriction is inadvisable.

If the above measures are ineffective, and the physician is certain that there is no non–exercise-related gastrointestinal explanation for the diarrhea, then the occasional use of a prophylactic antidiarrheal is justified. Diphenoxylate (Lomotil; Searle & Co, San Juan, Puerto Rico) or loperamide (Imodium; Janssen Pharmaceutica, Piscataway, NJ) approximately 1 hour before competition is worth trying.

Gastrointestinal Bleeding

Exercise-associated gastrointestinal bleeding seems to be unique to running. Overt or visible blood loss is unusual, but when it occurs it may be dramatic—witness Derek Clayton's description of "vomiting black mucus" and "having black diarrhea" after his world's best marathon performance in Rotterdam in 1969. There are a number of reports of unexplained bloody diarrhea in distance runners and, more recently, cases of hematemesis have been described. A single jogging death has been attributed to hemorrhagic gastritis. In a recent survey of marathoners, 2.4% of those who answered a questionnaire reported "occasionally or frequently" having bloody stools. More commonly, however, runners are not aware of gastrointestinal bleeding and the blood loss is occult which, if it causes problems at all, presents as iron-deficiency anemia.

The incidence of occult gastrointestinal bleeding depends on the method used for its detection. If one uses a relatively insensitive method, such as the Hemoccult II guaiac cards (SmithKline Diagnostics, Sunnyvale, CA), 8% to 23% of distance runners will have stools positive for occult blood after a marathon. This may rise to as high as 85% following a 100-mile ultramarathon. If one uses more sensitive quantitative assays of gastrointestinal blood loss, then it can be shown that nearly all runners will have increases in fecal blood loss after a long distance race and that one third will have blood losses above the accepted upper limit of normal.

Why do runners bleed from their guts? Many use nonsteroidal anti-inflammatory medications for their aches and pains, but these do not appear to be a major factor. It seems that the bleeding is in some way related to the runner's level of fitness, intensity of training, and degree of exertion. Runners who experience abdominal cramps and diarrhea during running are more likely to have occult gastrointestinal bleeding. There are two major theories for its occurrence. The first proposes that bleeding is due to gastrointestinal ischemia. During severe exertion, splanchnic blood flow may decrease by as much as 80%. Even relatively mild exercise, such as walking on a slope at 5 km/hr may decrease superior mesenteric blood flow by 40% or more. Normally, the gut is tolerant of this decreased perfusion, but runners, like "mad dogs and Englishmen," may go out in the midday sun, and one can imagine situations where excessive fluid loss and hypovolemia compound the effects of physiologic splanchnic hypoperfusion.

The other theory proposes that gastrointestinal bleeding results from trauma or contusion to the lower gastrointestinal tract as a result of repeated jarring. This seems most likely to occur in the cecum and has been called the "cecal slap syndrome." A similar mechanism has been proposed as a cause of bladder contusion and hematuria.

If a runner bleeds from the gut, how can the problem be sorted out? There are several useful courses of action. The runner who vomits blood should, like any other person with an upper gastrointestinal hemorrhage, be stabilized and then endoscopy should be performed. The "dry heaves" may have caused a Mallory-Weiss tear. Nonsteroidal anti-inflammatory medications may cause gastric erosions. Stress or ischemia may cause hemorrhagic gastritis. The runner may have a coincidental peptic ulcer. If the problem is lower gastrointestinal bleeding, hemorrhoids can be quickly excluded by proctoscopy. If one is looking for either ischemic or traumatic injury to the colon, then colonoscopy is the investigation of choice. All of these endoscopic procedures should be performed as soon as possible after the onset of bleeding because the lesions we are looking for may be evanescent. In studies using these techniques, there are reports of hemorrhagic gastritis and colitis presumably due to ischemia or "stress."

Although running may cause gastrointestinal bleeding, there are many other causes of gastrointestinal blood loss that are unrelated to running and which, unlike running, are not conducive to good health. Runners may believe that they are immune to conditions that cause premature death in their sedentary neighbors, but there is no evidence that running prevents ulcers, colonic neoplasms (although it might reduce the odds), or inflammatory bowel disease. The prudent physician should ensure that the bleeding runner does not have a source of gastrointestinal blood loss unrelated to running.

EXERCISE AND GASTROINTESTINAL AND HEPATIC DISEASES

Liver Disease

What about exercise in patients with liver diseases such as hepatitis or cirrhosis? There is no evidence that rest is helpful or that exercise is harmful in any form of acute or chronic liver disease. Of course, it is prudent to advise a patient with a tender liver, big spleen, low platelet count, or a prolonged clotting time, to avoid contact sports or sports where they may be subjected to trauma. Theoretically, strain or performing a Valsalva maneuver might rupture an esophageal varix in a patient with portal hypertension, but there is no documentation of this in the literature.

The approach to sorting out abnormal liver tests in the athlete is no different than the approach in the nonathlete. However, remember that the elevated serum aspartate aminotransferase (AST, previously SGOT) level may be coming from muscle, rather than liver. This can be confirmed by measuring the creatine phosphokinase (CPK). Always ask about anabolic-androgenic steroid use as these drugs have been associated with cholestasis, peliosis hepatis, and benign and malignant liver tumors. Shared needles and heterologous "blood doping" might transmit hepatitis B or non-A, non-B viral hepatitis. Athletes traveling frequently to areas of the world where hepatitis B is endemic should consider being vaccinated.

Peptic Ulcer Disease

Previously, bed rest was part of the treatment of peptic ulceration. We now have much better therapies and there is no evidence that exercise will aggravate peptic ulceration or delay its healing. Indeed, there is some evidence that peptic ulceration is less common in individuals who exercise regularly. Perhaps this is because gastric acid secretion is decreased by moderate-to-vigorous exercise.

Constipation

There is a great deal of myth and very little fact surrounding the role of exercise in preventing or treating constipation. It is well recognized that bed rest may cause constipation, and I have yet to meet a constipated marathon runner; but, when diet is kept constant, and physiologically valid transit markers are used, it has not been possible to show that exercise consistently affects whole gut, small intestinal, or colonic transit. There is one report that physical activity after eating promotes mass movement of feces in the colon. My conclusion is that there is no proof that exercise can be used to treat constipation.

Traveler's Diarrhea

Athletic competition may involve international travel. For obvious reasons, "traveler's diarrhea" could be a catastrophe for the competing athlete. The standard precautions, such as eating in better establishments, not drinking the water, and avoiding ice cubes, salads, and unpeeled fruit, are sometimes not enough. If diarrhea develops, the athlete must ensure that hydration is maintained. This can usually be done by the oral route. If there is no blood in the stool, and the patient is afebrile, antidiarrheal drugs such as diphenoxylate (Lomotil) or loperamide (Imodium) can be used to control the symptoms. Symptoms can also be relieved with bismuth subsalicylate (Pepto-Bismol; Procter & Gamble, Cincinnati, OH), 30 to 60 mL every 30 minutes for eight doses. Warn the patient that with this regimen the stools will turn black. If trimethoprim, 160 mg, and sulfamethoxazole, 800 mg (Septra DS; Burroughs Wellcome, Research Triangle Park, NC), every 12 hours for 5 days is started with the first loose bowel movement, the illness can be shortened. Although they work, I do not recommend prophylactic antibiotics or prophylactic Pepto-Bismol. If the diarrhea persists after the athlete returns home, look for *Giardia* as most bacterial diarrheas are self-limited.

Anorexia and Bulimia

Endurance athletes are often very thin and some have anorexia nervosa or bulimia. Indeed, it has even been suggested that distance running may be an anorectic equivalent. Some young women use running and aerobics in their pathologic pursuit of thinness. Be especially attuned to this possibility when you see a very thin, not well muscled, nonelite athlete with amenorrhea and perhaps with findings that could be accounted for by vomiting or purging (hypokalemia, diarrhea or constipation, staining of the teeth, or esophagitis).

Colon Cancer

Finally, we will end on a note of optimism. The idea that physical activity may have a protective effect against colon cancer is supported by recent epidemiologic studies. Exercise may even decrease experimentally induced colon cancer in rats. A recent review of the literature suggests that physical exercise, particularly moderate aerobic exercise performed regularly and sustained throughout a lifetime, could confer protection against colon cancer, but by mechanisms as yet uncertain.

ACKNOWLEDGMENTS

My thanks to all the athletic "guinea pigs" who have participated in my research projects, and to Joyce Perry, who has faithfully typed my manuscripts and corrected my spelling.

BIBLIOGRAPHY

Bartram HP, Wynder EL: Physical activity and colon cancer risk? Physiological considerations. Am J Gastroenterol 84:109–112, 1989.

Hilsted J, Galbo H, Sonne B, et al: Gastroenteropancreatic hormonal changes during exercise. Am J Physiol 239:G136–G140, 1980.

Holdstock DJ, Misiewicz JJ, Smith T, Rowlands EN: Propulsion (mass movements) in the human colon and its relationship to meals and somatic activity. Gut 11:91–99, 1970.

Keeffe EB, Lowe DK, Goss JR, et al: Gastrointestinal symptoms of marathon runners. West J Med 141:481–484, 1984.

Larson DC, Fisher R: Management of exercise-induced gastrointestinal problems. Physician Sports Med 15:112–126, 1987.

Riddoch C, Trinick T: Gastrointestinal disturbances in marathon runners. Br J Sports Med 22:71–74, 1988.

Sullivan SN: The effect of running on the gastrointestinal tract. J Clin Gastroenterol 6:461–465, 1984.

Sullivan SN: Exercise-associated symptoms in triathletes. Physician Sports Med 15:105–110, 1987.

Sullivan SN, Champion MC, Christofides ND, et al: Gastrointestinal regulatory peptide responses in long distance-runners. Physician Sports Med 12:77–82, 1984.

Worobetz LJ, Gerrard DF: Gastrointestinal symptoms during exercise in Enduro athletes: Prevalance and speculations on the aetiology. NZ Med J 98:644–646, 1985.

12

THE NERVOUS SYSTEM

Robert C. Cantu, MD, MA

The central nervous system (brain and spinal cord) is unique in that nerve cells are not capable of regeneration. Injury to these structures takes on a singular importance because cells that die are forever lost. Whereas virtually every major joint (ankle, knee, hip, elbow, shoulder) and most of the body's organs can be replaced, the central nervous system housed in the skull and spine is not capable of regrowth, transplantation, or replacement with artificial hardware. With these sobering facts in mind, clinical evaluation of the head- or spine-injured athlete must be expeditious and precise, and the physician must be forever mindful of the Hippocratic prohibition: "First, do no harm."

Whenever an injury involves a loss of consciousness, several important simultaneous observations and assumptions must be made. It must be assumed that the patient has a fractured neck and the examination must be carried out with this in mind. First, it must be established that the patient has an adequate airway; then a rapid baseline medical and neurologic examination should be conducted. This should include blood pressure, pulse, respiratory rate, state of consciousness (alert, stupor, semicomatose, or comatose), pupillary size and reactivity, extremity movement spontaneously and in response to painful stimulation, and deep-tendon and Babinski reflexes.

This initial examination is crucial to subsequent evaluation and treatment. If the patient shows improvement within a few minutes, subsequent transportation and diagnostic evaluation can proceed in a routine manner. If, however, deterioration is seen, especially in the state of consciousness, transportation and subsequent treatment must be precipitous. Every unconscious athlete should be transported on a fracture board. The head should be secured in a neutral position with sandbags, four-poster collar, or traction device, if available.

If the unconscious athlete is wearing a helmet and has a good airway, the helmet should not be removed; this may precipitate quadriplegia if an unstable cervical fracture is present. The helmet should be removed only if the airway is questionable, and then never forcibly and always with the neck in a neutral (neither flexed nor extended) position. The helmet can be used for cervical traction, with the chin strap serving as the halter, and the earholes or immediately adjacent edge of the helmet as a site for attaching neutral traction. While the unconscious athlete is being moved onto the spine board, the earholes of the helmet may also serve as a convenient site to insert one's index finger to effect gentle neutral cervical traction. Only after appropriate cervical-spine radiographs have excluded a cervical–spine fracture, malalignment, or instability, can the helmet be safely removed from the unconscious athlete.

SPORTS MOST HAZARDOUS TO THE HEAD AND CERVICAL SPINE

Table 12–1 lists those athletic pursuits most likely to cause serious head and spine injuries. One study of automobile racing showed that during their first 2 years, 30% of new par-

TABLE 12–1. SPORTS MOST LIKELY TO CAUSE SERIOUS HEAD OR SPINE INJURY

Maximal Risk	High Risk
Automobile racing	Gymnastics
Diving	Horseback riding
Football (the only team sport)	Mountain climbing
Hang gliding	Parachuting
Motorcycle racing	Ski jumping
	Skydiving
	Sky gliding
	Snowmobiling
	Trampolining

ticipants were either killed or so seriously injured they could not compete again.[1,2] Motorcycles are even more dangerous. Eighty percent of the serious injuries occur to those with riding experience of 6 months or less. Hang gliding ranks at the top of the list in terms of fatalities or serious injuries per participant. Amazingly, the use of adequate helmets is not even uniformly seen in this "sport."

The most common mechanism of severe cervical-spine injury is illustrated in Figures 12–1 and 12–2. In neutral posture, the neck has a gentle S-shaped curve (Fig. 12–1). When the neck is flexed, the spine becomes straight (Fig. 12–2). With the vertebral bodies

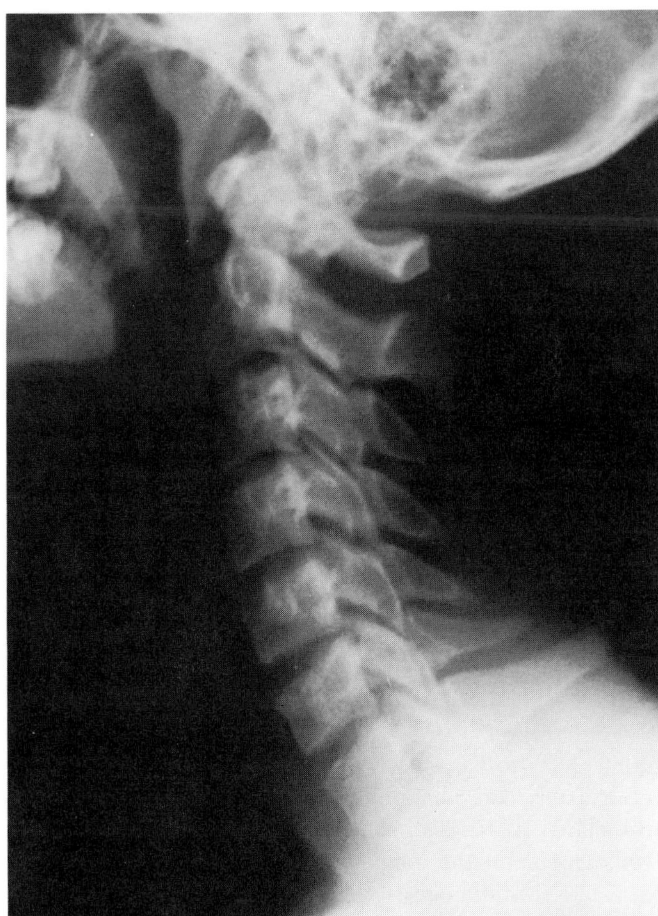

Figure 12–1. In neutral posture, the neck has a gentle S-shaped curve.

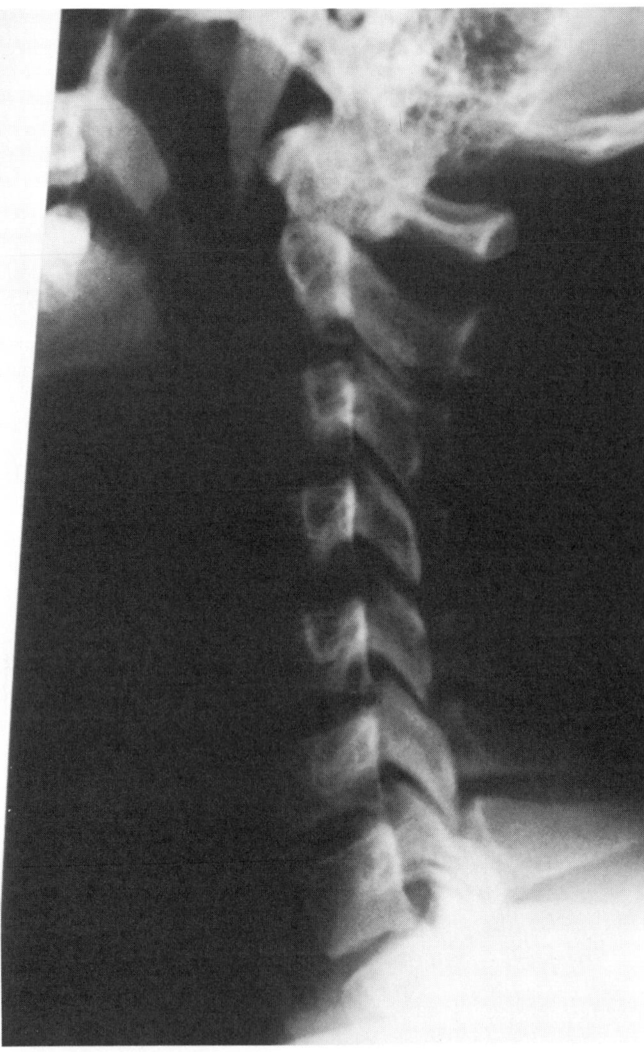

Figure 12–2. When the neck is flexed, the spine becomes straight.

lined up straight, vertical-impact force is directly transmitted from one vertebra to the next, allowing minimal dissipation of the impact force to be absorbed by the muscles. If the impact force exceeds the strength of the bone, it compacts the bone at one or more levels, causing a compression fracture. If the fractured vertebra malaligns and is driven back into the spinal cord, quadriplegia may result.

It is when tackling with the head, especially in the open field where momentum is greatest, that most serious neck injuries occur.[3] The small defensive back is the most susceptible player. The fast but light safety is injured trying to bring down a larger, heavier back with a head tackle. The high-school athlete, who has the greatest degree of variation in physical maturation and athletic ability, is at greatest risk.

Other direct causes of head and neck injuries include the knee-to-head or, more commonly, knee-to-face guard hyperextension injury. In rare instances, this can result in vertebral artery compression at C1 and the occiput with fatal cord infarction.[4,5] The practice of "piling on" has also been shown to contribute to head and neck injury.

At present, the incidence of catastrophic football head and neck injuries is at the lowest level in the last 18 years, with fatalities being 0.5 per 100,000 athletes.[2] This rep-

TABLE 12–2. FATALITY RATES IN SELECTED SPORTS

Sport	Annual Fatality Ratio (Deaths/ 100,000 Participants)
Powerboating	16.7
Auto racing	120.0
Horse racing	133.3
Motorcycling	178.6

Adapted from Clarke K, Braslow A: Football fatalities in actuarial perspective. Med Sci Sports 10:94, 1979; with permission.

resents a greater than 600% reduction from the peak years in the late 1960s. Keeping in mind the present death rates, football is more than 100 times safer than auto, horse, or motorcycle racing (Table 12–2).[6] Why has there been a decrease in football fatalities and paralysis in the last 15 years?

The answers are found in two main areas: (1) rules requiring changes in coaching techniques; and (2) improvements in conditioning, especially of the neck muscles, equipment, and medical supervision. It was first necessary to understand that most football fatalities were due to head and neck injuries sustained while tackling or being tackled with the point of contact being the top or crown of the helmet.

Thus, perhaps the most important changes were in rules which, in 1976, eliminated the head as a primary or initial contact area for blocking and tackling. Specifically, spearing and butt-blocking were made illegal. In addition, coaches were instructed to discourage players from using their heads as battering rams when blocking or tackling and to teach their athletes the proper fundamentals of blocking and tackling, including keeping one's head up at all times.

The wisdom of Earl "Red" Blaik came to be accepted. In 1960, the former army coach said: "But no matter the rules, football is not for the player without strong neck muscles, especially if his neck conformation is unusually long. After S's death I never allowed the boy with a long neck to play no matter his desire, unless his neck muscularity was well above average. I emphasize more than ever the importance of neck strength in calisthenics and more than ever I hammer to the boy learning to block and tackle with his head up for, if the head is not bent, the neck cannot be broken."[7] Strengthening of the cervical muscles became part of the conditioning program.

Equipment improvement under the guidance of the National Operating Committee on Standards for Athletic Equipment (NOCSAE), whose research has led to improved and better fitting football helmets as well as recognition of the need to discard or renovate worn equipment, is another factor.

A final area resulting in the reduction of head and neck injury in football is improved medical supervision, especially in the areas of on-the-field recognition and treatment of head and cervical-spine injuries and guidance for return to competition after such injuries.

Although football fatalities and catastrophic injuries will never be totally eliminated, their occurrence is now rare. Most college football conferences go for decades without encountering these problems. However, yearly, almost each participating school has one or more fatalities or catastrophic injuries attributed to a car or motorcycle accident. For the high-school student, it is clearly more dangerous to drive a car or motorcycle than to play football.

INTRACRANIAL INJURIES

Concussion

What are the definitions and grades or severity of concussion? It must first be stated that universal agreement on the definition of concussion does not exist. This fact renders evaluation of epidemiologic data extremely difficult. A working definition of concussion that has gained acceptance is the one proposed by the Committee on Head Injury Nomenclature of the Congress of Neurological Surgeons.[8] As stated, a concussion is "a clinical syndrome characterized by immediate and transient posttraumatic impairment of neural function, such as alteration of consciousness, disturbance of vision, equilibrium, etc., due to brain stem involvement."[8] Maroon and associates,[9] in attempting to simplify the clinical problem, divided concussion into three grades based on the duration of unconsciousness: mild (no loss of consciousness), moderate (loss of consciousness with retrograde amnesia), and severe (unconsciousness for more than 5 minutes). Others have classified concussion according to duration of posttraumatic amnesia.[10] Finally, concussion severity has been graded by using the duration of both unconsciousness and posttraumatic amnesia: mild (transient or no loss of consciousness with posttraumatic amnesia for less than 1 hour), moderate (unconscious less than 5 minutes with posttraumatic amnesia for 1 to 24 hours), severe (unconscious more than 5 minutes with posttraumatic amnesia for more than 24 hours).[11] As a neurosurgeon and team physician, I have evaluated many football players who had suffered a concussion. Most were mild and retrograde amnesia was present in most cases. In fact, this helped me in making the diagnosis. Thus, combining some elements of the prior two definitions with my experience, I have developed a practical scheme for grading the severity of a concussion based on the duration of unconsciousness and/or amnesia (retrograde plus posttraumatic) (Table 12–3).

INCIDENCE

Concussion most often occurs while making a tackle (43%), being tackled (23%), blocking (20%), or being blocked (10%).[12] Football head injuries are twice as frequent as neck injuries. Nearly nine out of ten football head injuries are concussions,[3] and one out of five high-school varsity athletes can anticipate a concussion each season.[12] The incidence of reported concussion may be unquestionably low as many athletes do not associate a brief loss of awareness or a few minutes of amnesia with concussion. The comment from a player that "the coach took me out of the game to see if I had a concussion, but I did not" is not unique. Furthermore, in his desire to play, the athlete may deny or minimize symptoms. Since, following a "concussion," catastrophic brain injury is known to occur after a second apparently minor head impact in the same game, especially football, accurate documentation and treatment is of paramount importance.[4,5,12,13]

RECOGNITION AND MANAGEMENT OF CONCUSSION

There is certainly little difficulty in recognizing a grade 3 or severe concussion (unconsciousness for more than 5 minutes). Initial treatment should be the same as for a sus-

TABLE 12–3. SEVERITY OF CONCUSSION

Type of Concussion	Loss of Consciousness	Duration of Amnesia*
Grade 1 (Mild)	None	<30 min
Grade 2 (Moderate)	None or <5 min	>30 min but <24 hr
Grade 3 (Severe)	None or >5 min	>24 hr

*Retrograde or posttraumatic.

pected cervical-spine fracture. If the airway is adequate, the helmet should not be removed on the playing field for fear of worsening a cervical fracture dislocation. The face mask can be removed with bolt cutters or left intact if the athlete is stable. The athlete should be transported on a fracture board, with the head and neck immobilized, to a hospital with neurosurgical coverage. Radiographs of the cervical spine, including lateral flexion/extension views if the initial neutral view is normal, should be obtained. Skull radiographs should be taken to rule out fractures. A computed tomographic (CT) scan of the head should be done if the neurologic examination is abnormal; if a skull fracture is identified; if the athlete is still unresponsive; or if associated symptoms, such as headache, nausea, vomiting, visual impairment, or disequilibrium, persist for 12 hours.[11] Even if an initial CT scan is normal, if these associated symptoms are not markedly improved in 24 to 48 hours, a repeat CT scan should be considered. In this time interval, microscopic hemorrhages may coalesce to form a brain contusion or a subacute subdural hematoma may be in evolution. It is recommended that all patients with severe concussions be admitted to the hospital and placed under neurologic observation for intracranial bleeding.[11,14]

With a grade 2 or moderate concussion (unconscious less than 5 minutes), the athlete should initially be managed in the same manner as a patient with a grade 3 concussion. In this case, however, clinical judgment may dictate that if the period of unconsciousness is brief, and if the now conscious athlete has no neck complaints, removal on a fracture board may not be necessary. It is recommended that the athlete be removed from the contest and evaluated at a neurosurgery-staffed medical facility with a thorough neurologic examination as well as skull and cervical-spine radiographs. Results of these examinations and associated symptoms will dictate whether a head CT scan is necessary. A period of neurologic observation is recommended for most athletes and for all those with any central neurologic abnormality by examination, or persistent symptoms, such as headache or skull fracture.

It is the grade 1 or mild concussion that is the most difficult to recognize. This is when the most careful clinical judgment must be exercised. Here there is no lapse of consciousness, but an impairment of cortical function, especially for recent memory and assimilating and interpreting new information, is present. This grade of concussion is the most frequent (>50%) and, not infrequently, it escapes medical recognition.[15] It is not uncommon for a player to be "dinged" or have his "bell rung" and continue playing. Dave Meggyesy, a professional football player turned author, described this condition. "Your memory is affected although you can still walk around and sometimes continue playing. If you don't feel pain, the only way other players and the coaches know that you have been 'dinged' is when they realize you can't remember the plays."[16]

The initial treatment of the condition involves immediate removal from the game and observation on the bench. In those instances in which the athlete, after a period of time, has no headache, dizziness, or impaired concentration, including orientation to person, place, and time, and full recall for events just prior to injury, return to the contest may be considered.[9,17] Prior to return, the athlete should not only be asymptomatic at rest but also after demonstrating that he can move with his usual dexterity and speed. If an athlete has any of the above symptoms or signs, either at rest or during exertion, the player should not be allowed back into the game. Close neurologic observation is essential.

RETURN TO COMPETITION AFTER A CONCUSSION

Just as with the definition of concussion, presently there are no universally accepted criteria for when to allow the athlete to return to competition. Many physicians are today more conservative because the ability to process information has been shown to be reduced after a concussion,[18] and the severity and duration of functional impairment is greater with repeated concussions.[18–20] Though subject to confirmation, these studies suggest that the damaging effects of the shearing injury to nerve fibers and neurons are proportionate to the degree the head is accelerated and that these changes are cumulative.[20–22] There is also evidence to suggest that once players have suffered a first concussion, their chances of incurring a second concussion are more than four times greater than the risk of concussion for the nonconcussed player.[22] If this is not enough to make the physician wary, the "second impact syndrome," recently reported by Saunders and Harbaugh[23] but also described by Schneider,[4] most certainly should. In this condition, fatal brain swelling may occur following minor head contact in a player still symptomatic from a prior concussion. Although rare, because the consequences are so catastrophic, it suggests that athletes should not return to competition until they are asymptomatic following a concussion.

The following recommendations for return to competition after concussion are based on the grade of concussion and prior incidence of concussion. From the medical standpoint, the same standards should apply for high-school, college, and professional football players, but the implementation may not be as strict in the latter two groups.

For a first grade 1 concussion, if the athlete is asymptomatic at rest and during exertion as discussed above, return to the contest and subsequent games are permissible. If a second grade 1 concussion occurs in the same game, the player is removed from the game and not allowed to participate for at least 2 weeks provided the player is asymptomatic at rest and during exertion. If headache or other associated symptoms either worsen in the first 24 hours or persist for more than 24 hours, a CT scan is recommended. Magnetic resonance imaging (MRI) promises to be even more sensitive than a CT scan in detecting inferior frontal lobe and temporal lobe contusions. The electroencephalogram (EEG) has not been found to be a sensitive indicator of minor neuronal dysfunction. After a second concussion, a thorough review of the circumstances resulting in the concussion should be analyzed. If available, videotapes or game films should be reviewed by the player, coach, and trainer. It should be determined if the player was using the head unwisely, illegally, or both. This review will also show if the player was wearing the equipment correctly. Finally, neck strength and development as well as equipment fit and maintenance should be checked. A player with three grade 1 concussions in one season should not be allowed to play in the remaining games.[24,25] In fact, the player should be encouraged to give up the sport.

Following a first grade 2 concussion, return to competition may be as soon as 1 to 2 weeks after the player becomes asymptomatic at rest and during exertion. After a second grade 2 concussion in the same season, return to competition should be deferred for at least 1 month and termination of future participation should be considered. An athlete with a history of three grade 2 concussions in 1 year or over several seasons should not be allowed to play football. CT or MRI scan abnormalities caused by trauma also preclude future participation.

After a grade 3 concussion, the athlete is held from competition for at least 1 month, and may then return only if asymptomatic at rest and with exercise. A player with two grade 3 concussions should not be allowed to play football. An athlete who has had intracranial surgery for removal of a blood clot or who has developed posttraumatic hydrocephalus should not be allowed to return to competition.[26]

POSTCONCUSSION SYNDROME

This syndrome consists of headache, especially during exertion, dizziness, fatigue, irritability, and most importantly, impaired memory and concentration. Its true incidence is not known. In this author's experience, it is uncommon. The persistence of these symptoms reflects altered neurotransmitter function,[11] and usually correlates with the duration of posttraumatic amnesia.[27] When these symptoms persist, the athlete should be evaluated with a CT scan and neuropsychiatric tests. Return to competition should be deferred until all symptoms have abated and the diagnostic studies are normal.

Intracranial Hemorrhage

Intracranial hemorrhage is the leading direct cause of death in football and other contact sports. This was shown by Schneider[4] and remains true today.[5] The acute subdural hematoma accounts for almost all football-induced head injury deaths.[4,28] There are four types of hemorrhage the examining trainer or physician must look for in every instance of head injury. Since all four types may be fatal, rapid and accurate initial assessment as well as appropriate follow-up is mandatory after an athletic head injury.

An *epidural* or *extradural hematoma* is usually the most rapidly progressing intracranial hematoma. It is frequently associated with a fracture in the temporal bone and results from a tear in one of the arteries supplying the covering (dura) of the brain. The hematoma accumulates inside the skull, but outside the covering of the brain. It may progress quite rapidly and reach a fatal size in 30 to 60 minutes. Although not always present, there may be a lucid interval; that is, the athlete may initially regain consciousness after the head trauma, before starting to experience increasing headache and progressive deterioration in level of consciousness as the clot accumulates and the intracranial pressure increases. The lesion, if present, will almost always be apparent within 1 or 2 hours after the time of injury. The brain substance is usually free from direct injury; thus, if the clot is promptly removed surgically, a full recovery is to be expected. Because this lesion is rapidly and universally fatal if missed, all athletes receiving a head injury must be very closely observed for the next 24 hours, preferably where full neurosurgical services are immediately available.

A *subdural hematoma* occurs between the brain surface and the dura, that is, under the dura and directly on the brain. It often results from a torn vein running from the surface of the brain to the dura. It may also result from a torn venous sinus or even a small artery on the surface of the brain that is torn. With this injury, there is often associated injury to brain tissue. If a subdural hematoma requires surgery in the first 24 hours, mortality is high, not due to the clot itself, but because of the associated brain damage. With a subdural hematoma that progresses rapidly, the athlete usually does not regain consciousness, and the need for immediate neurosurgical evaluation is obvious. Occasionally, the brain itself will not be injured, and a subdural hematoma may slowly develop over a period of days to weeks. This chronic subdural hematoma, although often associated with headache, may initially present with a variety of very mild, almost imperceptible, mental, motor, or sensory signs and symptoms. Since its recognition and removal will lead to full recovery, it must always be suspected in an athlete who has previously sustained a head injury and who appears somewhat abnormal days or weeks later. A CT scan of the head will definitively show such a lesion.

An *intracerebral hematoma* is the third type of intracranial hemorrhage seen after head trauma. In this instance, the bleeding is into the brain substance itself, usually from a torn artery. It may also result from the rupture of a congenital vascular lesion, such as an aneurysm or arteriovenous malformation. Intracerebral hematomas are not usually associated with a lucid interval and may be rapidly progressive. Death occasionally occurs before the injured athlete can be moved to a hospital. Because of the intense reaction such a tragic event precipitates among fellow athletes, family, students, and even the community at large, and the inevitable rumors that follow, it is imperative to obtain a complete autopsy to fully clarify the causative factors. Often the autopsy will reveal a congenital lesion, indicating that the cause of death was other than presumed and ultimately unavoidable. Only by such full, factual elucidation of the cause of death will inappropriate feelings of guilt in fellow athletes, friends, and family be assuaged.

The fourth type of intracranial hemorrhage is *subarachnoid* or confined to the surface of the brain. Following head trauma, such bleeding results from disruption of the tiny surface brain vessels, and is analogous to a bruise. As in intracerebral hematoma, there is often brain swelling, and such a hemorrhage can also result from a ruptured cerebral aneurysm or arteriovenous malformation. Bleeding is superficial, and surgery is not usually required unless a congenital vascular anomaly is present.

All types of intracranial hemorrhages usually cause headache and, not infrequently, associated neurologic deficit, depending on the area of the brain involved. The irritative properties of the blood may also precipitate a seizure. If a seizure occurs in a head-injured athlete, it is important to logroll the patient onto his or her side. By this maneuver, any blood or saliva will roll out of the mouth or nose, and the tongue cannot fall back and obstruct the airway. A padded tongue depressor or oral airway can be inserted between the teeth. Under no circumstances should fingers be inserted into a seizing athlete's mouth, as a traumatic amputation can easily result from such an unwise maneuver. Traumatic seizure will usually last for only 1 or 2 minutes; the athlete will then relax and can be transported to the nearest medical facility.

"Malignant Brain Edema" Syndrome

"Malignant brain edema" syndrome is found in the pediatric athlete and consists of rapid neurologic deterioration from an alert conscious state to coma, and sometimes death, minutes to several hours after head trauma.[29,30] Whereas this sequence in adults is almost always due to an intracranial clot, in children, the pathologic studies show diffuse brain swelling with little or no brain injury.[29] Rather than true cerebral edema, Adams and Graham[31] and Langfitt and associates[32,33] have shown that the diffuse cerebral swelling is the result of a true hyperemia or vascular engorgement. Prompt recognition is extremely important because there is little initial brain injury and the serious or fatal neurologic outcome is secondary to raised intracranial pressure with herniation. Prompt treatment with intubation, hyperventilation, and osmotic agents has helped to reduce the mortality from this condition.[34,35]

NECK INJURIES

The traumatic lesions (concussion, contusion, and the various types of hemorrhage) just discussed for the brain may also occur in the spinal cord, primarily the cervical area. The major concern with a cervical-spine injury is the possibility of an unstable fracture that may produce quadriplegia. At the time of injury, the presence of an unstable fracture cannot be determined until appropriate radiographs are obtained. Also, if quadriplegia is present, the physician is unable to say whether it is reversible. If the patient is fully conscious, the presence of a cervical fracture or cord injury is usually accompanied by severe cervical muscle spasm and pain that immediately alerts the athlete and physician to the presence of such an injury. It is the unconscious athlete, unable to state that the neck hurts and whose neck musles are not in protective spasm, who is most susceptible to an "iatrogenic second injury" if the possibility of an unstable cervical spine fracture is not considered. It is imperative with an unconscious or obviously neck-injured athlete to prevent movement of the neck. Definitive treatment must await appropriate radiographs at a medical facility, and all the precautions discussed previously must be carried out. The most common neck injury is a sprain caused by damage to the musculotendinous units. Of importance is that many athletes who incur a neck injury with cord trauma have a prior history of neck "sprains." This data perhaps indicates a preexisting lesion such as spinal canal stenosis, the continued use of improper tackling or blocking techniques, or failure of the athlete to increase the strength of the neck muscles.

Spinal Cord Concussion

This injury was described by Obersteiner in 1978 as something "that happens after a single violent impact to the vertebral column when the function of the spinal cord is affected though no gross anatomical changes can be found."[36] Schneider[4] described this injury as transient motor or sensory symptoms and signs that entirely cleared within 24 hours. Radiographs of the cervical spine are usually normal. Because delayed spinal cord and peripheral nerve signs and symptoms have been shown to occur with this supposedly innocuous injury,[37–40] observation for several weeks is indicated. Return to competition should not only await this period, but also the subsidence of cervical pain, spasm, or limitation of movement. An athlete with a second spinal cord concussion should undergo a more complete radiographic evaluation including CT scans of the spine in flexion and extension and, perhaps, MRI studies to rule out congenital anomalies or an unrecognized subluxation. A player with a history of a second spinal cord concussion should avoid all collision sports even if the aforementioned studies are normal.

Spinal Cord Contusion

With spinal cord contusion, the signs and symptoms do not clear within 24 hours. This implies some cord damage. A careful review of cervical-spine radiographs, not only for fracture/dislocations or subluxation but also for spinal stenosis, is indicated. Myelography, contrast CT scanning, and, perhaps, MRI should also be considered to rule out ruptured discs, intraspinal hematomas, or hematomyelia. The occurrence of a spinal cord contusion should preclude competition for the remainder of the season and permanently if spinal stenosis is detected,[5] or if there is neurologic evidence of cord damage.

Central Cervical Cord Syndrome

Described by Schneider and associates[28] in 1954, this syndrome consists of a disproportionately greater motor loss in the upper extremities (distal greater than proximal) than in the lower extremities, and a variable sensory loss below the lesion. This occurs because the most mesial fibers of the corticospinal tract in the cervical cord subserve finger movement and, proceeding laterally, hand, arm, leg, and sacral functions, respectively. Thus, a central spinal cord injury will disproportionately affect the upper extremities.

This condition is usually caused by a hyperextension injury with fracture/dislocation, although this may not always be detected. Myelography or CT scanning may demonstrate cord swelling at the level of the lesion. Cord ischemia is considered to be the responsible mechanism. Recovery may be complete; however, a football player with this type of injury should not be allowed to compete again.

"Burning Hands" Syndrome

This condition is really a variation of Schneider's central cervical spinal cord syndrome[4,28] and can be explained anatomically. The spinothalamic tract is arranged as is the pyramidal tract with the fingers and hands positioned most medially and the legs and sacral segments most laterally. Of importance is the observation by Maroon[41] that dysesthesias or paresthesias in the hands ("burning hands") may be the only complaint of an athlete with a central cervical spinal cord injury. Maroon's cases did not have pain or tenderness.[41] In one instance, there was a fracture/dislocation at C5–6. Thus, the complaint of burning hands, even in the absence of neck pain, mandates on-the-field treatment as if a fracture/dislocation had occurred. The symptoms are transient and full recovery usually occurs. Disposition is similar to that for athletes with spinal cord concussion.

Spinal Cord Transection

This entity will not be difficult to recognize. Initial treatment of spinal cord transection mandates the assumption that an unstable cervical fracture/dislocation is present although, in some cases, subluxation alone appears to be the mechanism. Emergency management has already been discussed. Maintenance of an adequate airway is essential. Removal from the field should only be done by the paramedics or trauma team.

Vascular Syndromes

Football-induced injury to both the carotid and vertebral arteries has been reported.[4,5,42] By extremes of either lateral flexion or extension, or by a forceful direct blow, such as by a stiffened forearm or helmet, to the neck, the intima of the carotid artery may be torn. This can lead to dissection and clot formation at the injury site, resulting in either complete occlusion of the artery or a potential source of emboli. This may result in an internal carotid–middle cerebral transient ischemic attack (TIA) or stroke.

While a vertebral artery may be compressed by a fracture/dislocation at any cervical level, Schneider and associates[42] have shown that the vertebral arteries are most vulnerable to compression at the level of C1 and the occiput by hyperextension and compression injuries. They reported mild cases from secondary vasospasm with brief neurologic brain stem signs and symptoms, but they also described others with thrombosis resulting in cervicomedullary infarction and death.[13,42]

Athletes with transient ischemic symptoms related to head or neck trauma should not return to competition until the cause is definitely determined and judged not likely to recur. A possible exception to this rule is trauma-induced migraine headache. Although the athlete most likely would not wish to participate with a trauma-induced migraine headache, there is not any known increased medical risk for such participation.

Brachial Plexus Injuries

The lateral pinch syndrome or "burner" is caused by stretching the spine laterally often with a simultaneous depression of the opposite shoulder. For a blow to the side of the head to cause these symptoms alone, the neck usually must be stretched beyond its physiologic limits of 50 degrees.[43,44] Pain and prickly burning paresthesias radiating from the neck down the arm (often to the base of the thumb) are immediately experienced. Usually, symptoms last only a few seconds in the beginning, but with repeated episodes, proximal arm weakness, especially of the external rotators and abductors of the shoulder and flexors of the elbow, may occur. After 3 weeks, in more severe injuries, fibrillations and sharp waves may be seen on an electromyogram (EMG) in the deltoid, supinators, and biceps muscles, indicating an injury to the upper trunk of the brachial plexus.[45] Most cases will resolve with time once repeated trauma is avoided. In the occasional severe case, however, weakness persists with a fixed sensory loss and increased pain with use of the affected arm. The incidence of "burners" may be as high as 50% in football players as reported by a recent University of Wisconsin study.[46]

The player with a "burner" plexus injury usually can be reognized by the arm hanging by the side or by the vigorous shaking and rubbing of the affected wrist or hand. The player with an acutely ruptured disc, a far less common occurrence, tilts the head away from the affected side and experiences neck and radicular arm pain, which is intensified by extending the neck and tilting it toward the affected side. It is important to recognize the difference between an intraspinal root injury and a plexus injury, for allowing a player with a ruptured disc to continue playing subjects the athlete to serious spinal root or cord injury.

It is recommended that an athlete not return to competition after a neck injury until the player is free of any neck or arm pain at rest and has a full range of neck motion without discomfort or spasm. Rockett has described further criteria used at Harvard University.[47] Each athlete is measured as to the maximum weight he or she can pull with neck in flexion, extension, and to each side. This becomes the neck profile for that person. An athlete with a neck injury is not allowed to return to competition until he or she can perform to the level of the neck profile.

EPILEPSY AND ATHLETICS

Epilepsy is a common neurologic disorder with incidence and prevalence rates per 100,000 population estimated at 50 and 650, respectively.[48] Most individuals with epilepsy attend conventional schools. The prognosis for epilepsy with onset in childhood and adolescence is particularly favorable as is epilepsy with a provoked as opposed to unprovoked cause. Recognized provocative factors include an acute neurologic insult (ie, head injury or cerebrovascular accident); metabolic disturbance, such as hypoglycemia or electrolyte imbalance; alcohol or other drug withdrawal; sleep deprivation; fatigue; or emotional upset.

The sports medicine physician must address two salient questions: First, will exercise adversely affect seizure control? Second, is the athlete at risk for serious injury or death if a seizure occurs during the sporting event?

With regard to the first question, seizures rarely are experienced during exercise; rather, they most commonly occur during sleep, rest, or idleness.[49,50] In fact, there is some evidence that physical activity may actually prevent seizures.[51] If a seizure does occur during physical activity, an underlying structural abnormality, such as a brain tumor or arteriovenous malformation, is highly suspect.

With regard to the second question, although some controversy still exists, epileptic patients under good control are presently allowed to engage in all sports, including contact and collision sports, except boxing and certain aquatic sports (ie, scuba diving) in which a seizure during participation would place the athlete at serious risk. This is the current opinion of the American Medical Association Committee on Medical Aspects of Sports. It is based on the fact that seizures are rare during exercise; exercise may even inhibit seizures. There is no evidence that morbidity and mortality related to sports is increased in epileptics, nor are there clinically significant changes in the pharmacokinetics of anticonvulsants related to exercise. Therefore, it is seizure frequency that should determine if an individual with epilepsy may participate in sports.

HEADACHE AND VARIOUS SPORTS

Headache is a frequent reason for medical evaluation of athletes because it is one of the most common medical complaints of civilized people. The sports medicine physician should be familiar with headaches associated with specific sports, as well as cognizant of the fact that, uncommonly, headache in the athlete may be a sign of underlying organic cerebral pathology.

Matthews[52] described the headache associated with repetitive head trauma in soccer and boxing as "footballer's migraine." This generalized headache usually lasts for at least an hour. Athletes subject to migraine headaches have also had migraine attacks precipitated by head trauma.

Powell[53] and Ibbotson[54] have described an occipital headache associated with weight lifting, especially maximal lifts.

Jokl[55] and Massey,[56] among others, have described migraine headaches associated with running. Altitude, dehydration, and poor nutrition are thought to be provocative factors. These headaches are usually unilateral and have a typical migraine aura preceding the headache. Such headaches were common at the 1968 Summer Olympics at Mexico City.

Simons and Wolff[57] described several types of posttraumatic headaches. Clearly, these headaches require careful medical evaluation to rule out underlying organic pathology. As discussed previously, because of concern for the "second impact syndrome," no athlete with a head injury should be allowed to return to contact sports until even the most minor persisting symptoms of head injury have resolved.

CONCLUSION

Recent studies have shown a decrease in mortality from head and neck injuries. This has resulted from rule changes and their enforcement; equipment modifications; improved coaching and training techniques; and educational programs for coaches, trainers, and team physicians on the early recognition of head and neck injuries. However, morbidity data is not as complete, particularly as it applies to concussion, the most frequent type of head injury in football. Questions on this condition that still need to be answered before a sound medical disposition can be made are the possible cumulative damage from repeated concussions, and whether one concussion renders a player more susceptible to a second. Presently, decisions on when to allow an athlete to return to a game or to participate in future contests are arbitrary and based primarily on the experience of the team physician. Data on the incidence, mechanisms, and prognosis of transient spinal cord signs and symptoms, such as spinal cord concussion and the central cervical cord syndrome, are also incomplete. What is the long-term prognosis for players who suffer frequent "burners"? Certainly, further studies are necessary to definitively answer these questions. This chapter attempts to provide sound guidelines to make American football a safer sport. Clearly, the work of Richard Schneider needs to be continued.

REFERENCES

1. Bodnar LM: Sports medicine with reference to back and neck injuries. Curr Pract Orthop Surg 7:116–153, 1977.
2. Cantu RC: Catastrophic injuries in high school and college athletes. Surgical Rounds for Orthopedics 2:62–66, 1988.
3. Torg JS, Quedenfeld TC, Burstein A, et al: National football head and neck injury registry: Report on cervical quadriplegia. Am J Sports Med 7:127–132, 1979.
4. Schneider RC: Head and Neck Injuries in Football. Baltimore, Williams & Wilkins, 1973.
5. Schneider RC, Kennedy JC, Plant ML: Sports Injuries. Baltimore, Williams & Wilkins, 1985.
6. Clarke K, Braslow A: Football fatalities in actuarial perspective. Med Sci Sports 10:94, 1979.
7. Chrisman DO, Smook GA, Stanitis JM, et al: Lateral-flexion neck injuries in athletic competition. JAMA 192:117–122, 1965.

8. Committee on Head Injury Nomenclature of Congress of Neurological Surgeons: Glossary of head injury including some definitions of injury to the cervical spine. Clin Neurosurg 12:386–394, 1966.
9. Maroon JC, Steele PB, Berlin R: Football head and neck injuries: An update. Clin Neurosurg 27:414–429, 1980.
10. Jennet B: Late effects of head injuries. *In* Critchley M, O'Leary JL, Jennet B (eds): Scientific Foundations of Neurology. Philadelphia, FA Davis, 1971, pp 441–451.
11. Hugen Holtz H, Richard MT: Return to athletic competition following concussion. Can Med Assoc J 127:827–829, 1982.
12. Gerberich SG, Priest JD, Boen JR, et al: Concussion incidences and severity in secondary school varsity football players. Am J Public Health 73:1370–1375, 1983.
13. Schneider RC, Reifel E, Crislor HO, et al: Serious and fatal football injuries involving the head and spinal cord. JAMA 177:106–111, 1961.
14. Lindsay KW, McLatchie G, Jennett B: Serious head injuries in sports. Br Med J 281:789–791, 1980.
15. Gennarelli TA: Cerebral concussions and diffuse brain injuries. *In* Torg JS (ed): Athletic Injuries to the Head, Neck and Face. Philadelphia, Lea & Febiger, 1982.
16. Meggyesy D: Out of Their League. Berkeley, CA, Ramparts, 1970, p 125.
17. Yarnell PR, Lynch S: The "ding" amnestic states in football trauma. Neurology 23:196–197, 1973.
18. Gronwall D, Wrightson P: Delayed recovery of intellectual function after minor head injury. Lancet 2:605–609, 1974.
19. Gronwall D, Wrightson P: Memory and information processing capacity after closed head injury. J Neurol Neurosurg Psychiatry 44:889–895, 1981.
20. Symonds C: Concussion and its sequelae. Lancet 1:1–5, 1962.
21. Peerless SJ, Rewcastle NB: Shear injuries of the brain. Can Med Assoc J 96:577–582, 1967.
22. Strick SJ: Shearing of nerve fibers as a cause of brain damage due to head injury. Lancet 2:443–448, 1961.
23. Saunders RL, Harbaugh RE: The second impact in catastrophic contact-sports head trauma. JAMA 252:538–539, 1984.
24. Quigley TB, cited by Schneider RC: Head and neck injuries. *In* Football: Mechanisms, Treatment and Preventions. Baltimore, Williams & Wilkins, 1973.
25. Thorndike A: Serious recurrent injuries of athletes: Contraindications to further competitive participation. N Engl J Med 247:554–556, 1952.
26. Murphey F, Simmons JC: Initial management of athletic injuries to the head and neck. Am J Surg 98:379–383, 1959.
27. Guthkelch AN: Post-traumatic amnesia, post-concussional symptoms and accident neurosis. Eur Neurol 19:91–102, 1980.
28. Schneider RC, Charie G, Pantek H: The syndrome of acute central cervical spinal cord injury. J Neurosurg 11:546–577, 1954.
29. Pickles W: Acute general edema of the brain in children with head injuries. N Engl J Med 242:607–611, 1950.
30. Schnitker MT: A syndrome of cerebral concussion in children. J Pediatr 35:557–560, 1949.
31. Adams H, Graham DI: Pathology of blunt head injuries. *In* Critchley M, O'Leary JL, Jennett B (eds): Scientific Foundations of Neurology. Philadelphia; FA Davis, 1972, pp 478–491.
32. Langfitt TW, Kassell NF: Cerebral vasodilatations produced by brainstem stimulation: Neurogenic control vs. autoregulation. Am J Physiol 215:90–97, 1978.
33. Langfitt TW, Tannenbaum HM, Kassell NF: The etiology of acute brain swelling following experimental head injury. J Neurosurg 24:47–56, 1966.
34. Bowers SA, Marchall LF: Outcome in 200 consecutive cases of severe head injury treated in San Diego County: A prospective analysis. Neurosurgery 6:237–242, 1980.
35. Bruce DA, Schut L, Burno LA, et al: Outcome following severe head injuries in children. J Neurosurg 48:679–688, 1978.
36. Obersteiner H: Ueber Erschutterung des Ruckenmarks. Wien Med Jahrb 1879, quoted by Bickles: Obersteiner's. AR 3:102, 1895.
37. Baldwin RD: Spinal concussion: A histologic study of two cases. Archives of Neurology Psych 32:493–500, 1934.
38. Groat RA, Rambach WA, Jr., and Windle WF. Concussion of the spinal cord. An experimental study and a critique of the use of the term. Surg Gynecol Obstet 81:63–74, 1945.
39. Hassin GB. Concussion of the spinal cord: a case with the clinical picture. Arch Neurol Psychiatry 10:194–203, 1923.
40. Lhermitte J: Etude des lesions histologiques fines da la commotion de moelle epiniere. Ann Med 4:295, 1917.
41. Maroon JC: "Burning hands" in football spinal cord injuries. JAMA 238:2049–2051, 1977.
42. Schneider RC, Gosch HH, Norrell H: Vascular insufficiency and differential distortion of brain and cord caused by cervicomedullary football injuries. J Neurosurg 33:363–374, 1970.

43. Chrisman DO, Smook GA, Stanitis JM, et al: Lateral-flexion neck injuries in athletic competition. JAMA 192:117–122, 1965.
44. Pearl AM, Mayer RN: Neck motion in the high school football player. Am J Sports Med 7:231–233, 1979.
45. Sherk HH, Watters WC: Neck injuries in football players. J Med Soc NJ 78:570–581, 1981.
46. Feldick HG, Albright JP: Football survey reveals "missed" neck injuries. Phys Sports Med 4:77–81, 1976.
47. Rockett FX: Injuries involving the head and neck: Clinical and anatomic aspects. *In* Vinger PF, Hoerner EF (eds): Sports Injuries: The Unthwarted Epidemic. Littleton, MA, PSG Publishing, 1981, p 106
48. Kurtzke JF: Neuroepidemiology. Ann Neurol 16:265–277, 1984.
49. Korczyn AD: Participation of epileptic patients in sports. J Sports Med 19:195–198, 1979.
50. Gotze W, Kubicki ST, Munter M, et al: Effect of physical exercise on seizure threshold (investigated by electroencephalographic telemetry). Dis Nerv Syst 28:664–667, 1967.
51. Department of Health, Education and Welfare: Plan for Nationwide Action on Epilepsy [DHEW Publication NIH 78–276], 1978, pp 29–43.
52. Matthews WB: Footballer's migraine. Br Med J 2:326–327, 1972.
53. Powell B: Weightlifter's cephalgia. Ann Emerg Med 11:449–451, 1982.
54. Ibbotson SH: Letter. Br J Sports Med 21:3–8, 1987.
55. Jokl E: Olympic medicine and sports cardiology. Ann Sports Med 1:149, 1984.
56. Massey EW: Effort headache in runners. Headache 22:99–100, 1982.
57. Simons DJ, Wolff HG: Studies on headache: Mechanisms of chronic post-traumatic headache. Psychosom Med 8:227, 1946.

13

EAR, NOSE, THROAT, AND EYE

David E. Schuller, MD
Robert A. Bruce, MD

Nontraumatic health problems afflicting the athlete in the head and neck area primarily are the result of inflammatory and infectious etiologies. The fact that this area of the aerodigestive tract is always exposed to environmental alterations in temperature and humidity, irrespective of the sporting event, results in frequent stress. This chapter reviews the variety of otolaryngologic and ophthalmologic problems that commonly affect athletes of all ages. It is important to remember that most athletes, whether formally or informally involved in competition, have a strong desire to continue to train and to compete even when they are being treated for a health problem. Therefore, the physician must be aware of this consideration and try to plan a therapeutic program that indeed allows for this training as long as it does not compromise the successful resolution of the problem.

OTOLOGIC DISORDERS

Otitis Externa

One of the most common otologic disorders involving athletes is otitis externa. The incidence of this problem increases when the ear canal remains moist, as in competitive swimming, or when perspiration runs into the ear. Presenting symptoms usually include pain in the ear canal that is exacerbated by auricular movement but which rarely causes a concomitant hearing loss. Physical examination reveals an erythematous, edematous ear canal that usually contains debris composed of cerumen and squamous epithelium.

The epithelium of the ear canal extends onto and comprises the outer layer of the tympanic membrane. Therefore, it is not at all uncommon to find an erythematous tympanic membrane with otitis externa. However, this can be differentiated from otitis media because the tympanic membrane has normal mobility and there is no evidence of any middle ear effusion.

The cornerstone of proper initial treatment involves immaculate cleansing of the ear canal. This is usually least traumatically achieved with irrigations rather than attempts at mechanical removal, which often are painful and less efficient. The most common offending organisms are *Pseudomonas* and *Proteus*. If the infection is indeed confined to the ear canal, local medications are usually adequate after the ear canal has been cleaned. Acetic acid is bactericidal for the organisms commonly involved. Therefore, a typical regimen involves irrigations with acetic acid, 1% solution, followed by instillation of otic drops three or four times daily. Sometimes otitis externa is associated with periauricular cellulitis. In this situation, it is usually advisable to add systemic antibiotics to the regimen of local medications.

The patient is instructed to keep water out of the ear canal. This can be achieved with either a cotton ball in the ear canal covered with a generous amount of petrolatum ointment or an ear plug covered with ointment. Individually configured ear canal molds have not been found to provide any more water protection than the standard nonfitted variety. The athlete can usually continue to train as long as water-protective techniques are followed.

In extreme cases, the ear canal is so edematous that local medications cannot flow beyond the external auditory meatus. Expansile otic wicks are now available that can be gently insinuated into the inflamed ear canal; the wicks then expand with the instillation of the otic drops and provide an avenue of delivery for the medications.

Pain is the incapacitating symptom associated with otitis externa. Therefore, it is critical that the patient receive adequate analgesics, especially for the first 48 to 72 hours, which is the time prior to when antibiotics have any dramatic effect. In rare instances, hospitalization is necessary for a few days to deliver intramuscular analgesics and intravenous antibiotics.

For athletes with recurrent otitis externa, especially those involved with water sports, prophylactic irrigation of the canal after leaving the water is effective. Acetic acid, 0.25%, or 70% alcohol can be used.

Otitis Media

Otitis media does not involve athletes more frequently than normal populations. It is commonly seen in children below the age of 10 years. The presenting symptom is ear pain that often is accompanied by a sense of fullness or decreased hearing. Physical examination demonstrates that the external auditory canal is not inflamed. The examination will reveal an erythematous, dull, thickened, tympanic membrane that either has decreased mobility or is totally immobile with evidence of purulent secretions in the middle ear.

Systemic antibiotics represent the treatment of choice. In the athlete who is incapacitated as a result of the pain of otitis media, myringotomy may provide dramatic relief and can be performed under local anesthesia as an outpatient procedure.

Middle ear effusion usually clears spontaneously with resolution of the infection. However, a follow-up exam 14 to 21 days after treatment is necessary to assure that there is no residual middle ear fluid that could predispose to other bouts of otitis media. Use of an antihistaminic or decongestant for 3 to 4 weeks will usually clear any residual middle ear effusion. (The physician should not prescribe a decongestant or any other medication that may disqualify the athlete from competition at which drug testing is carried out. See chapter 17.) If the fluid does not clear with medication, it is advisable to proceed with simple myringotomy. In the nonathlete, it may be appropriate to insert a tympanostomy tube at this time. However, because of the possibility of infection with indwelling tympanostomy tubes, it is best to avoid aggressive use of such tubes in the athlete.

Eustachian Tube Dysfunction

Otitis media with effusion represents that condition characterized by the presence of a transudate within the middle ear cleft. Although there are many different thoughts about the basic pathophysiology of this clinical condition, there is no question that eustachian tube dysfunction plays an integral role in its development. Therefore, sporting events associated with barometric changes (scuba diving, skydiving) may result in the development of otitis media with effusion. It is important for athletes to understand that if they are engaged in such sports, any upper respiratory tract infection that causes eustachian tube edema and subsequent dysfunction may well predispose to the development of otitis media with effusion.

In the pediatric population, it was formerly believed that tonsil and adenoid pathology had a much closer relationship to middle ear effusion than is currently thought. Therefore, this otologic problem is not usually treated with surgical removal of lymphoid tissue unless there are specific indications (eg, recurrent tonsillitis) for the removal of that lymphoid tissue independent of the otologic problems.

Initial therapy is usually medical and involves the use of antibiotics and/or decongestants for an extended period of time. If the decongestants do not clear the middle ear fluid, and if there is no past history of such a problem, simple myringotomy might be the initial surgical approach instead of tympanostomy tube insertions for the reasons that were previously mentioned. If it becomes necessary to insert tympanostomy tubes, it is still permissible for the athlete to continue competing but only if there is a clear understanding of the importance of keeping water from entering the ear canal. Once again, this is achieved with the wearing of either cotton plugs or ear plugs thoroughly covered with petrolatum ointment while exposed to water or showering.

Bilateral involvement is so common that the identification of a *unilateral* otitis media with effusion in an adult athlete should be interpreted as a potential warning sign that there might be something other than the usual eustachian tubal dysfunction explaining the problem. The concern in a unilateral problem is that there may be a mass in the nasopharynx causing unilateral tubal obstruction. Therefore, a thorough nasopharyngeal examination is mandatory when a unilateral otitis media with effusion is present.

The Auricle

It is important to realize that the auricle is covered with relatively thin skin that is constantly being exposed to environmental factors. The athlete who trains outside regularly must be cognizant of the vulnerability of the auricle to extremes of temperature. Frostbite and sunburn are common occurrences in the athlete who unwittingly neglects to protect the auricles during prolonged exposure. Use of sun-blocking agents to avoid sunburn or proper coverage of the auricles provides effective protection. If vesicles develop on the auricle (Fig. 13–1) as a result of overexposure to either sun or cold, it is advisable to avoid rupturing the vesicles for fear of initiating infection with resultant deeper injury to the auricular skin. These vesicles usually resolve in a few days. Subsequently, the ear can be

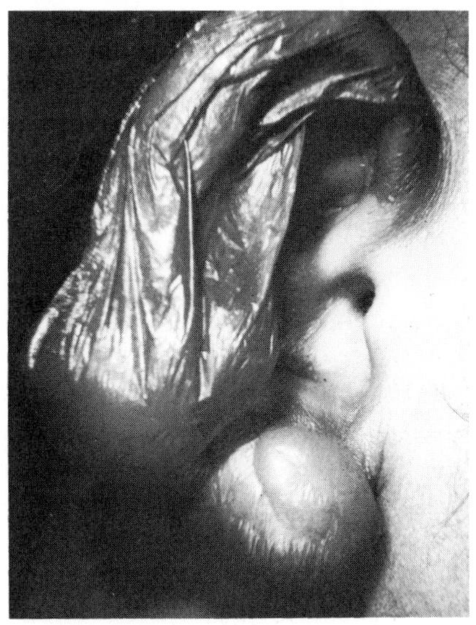

Figure 13–1. Auricular frostbite with development of massive vesicles that are beginning to resolve spontaneously.

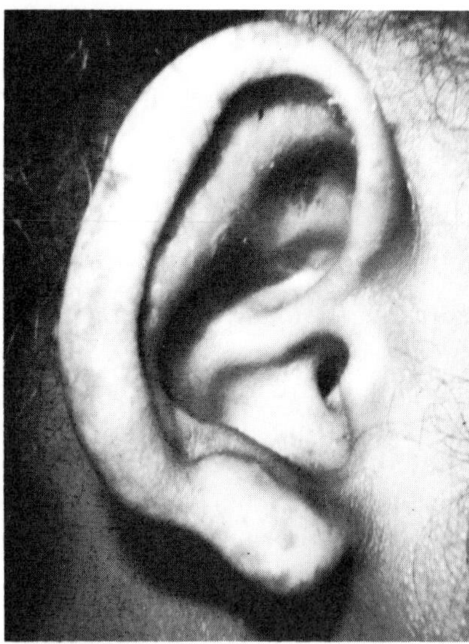

Figure 13–2. The appearance of auricle shown in Figure 13–1 after resolution of vesicles.

protected with fluffy dressings so that the athlete can continue training. If infection does not occur, recovery is usually excellent with little or no residual deformity (Fig. 13–2).

Dizziness

When the athlete develops dizziness, the physician must determine if it is true vertigo. If the individual feels that the room is spinning about him or if the athlete is spinning about the room along with nausea, vomiting, and sweating, these symptoms are most likely true vertigo originating from disorders of the semicircular canals. However, dysequilibrium is also called "dizziness." The athlete who is subjected to massive short-duration fluid changes as a result of training can precipitate metabolic disturbances that potentially could cause dysequilibrium. Dysequilibrium can best be described as a nonspecific feeling of unsteadiness.

Whenever there is a concomitant loss of consciousness associated with dizziness, it is infrequently, if ever, due to disorders involving only the semicircular canals. Atherosclerotic cardiovascular disease involving the carotid arterial system must be considered in the middle-aged or older athlete, who may be kinking or narrowing the lumen of an already partially occluded carotid artery as a result of exaggerated head, neck, or trunk movements during exercise, which subsequently produces transient ischemia and "dizziness."

If true vertigo is present, it is appropriate for an otolaryngologic evaluation to include an audiogram, electronystagmography, and possibly, radiographs and blood tests to ascertain the etiology. The majority of labyrinthine disorders are inflammatory and usually of viral origin. Therefore, therapy attempts to control symptomatology while vestibular compensation is occurring. Diazepam is a potent vestibular depressant and is routinely used to control vertiginous symptoms in the nonathlete. However, in the athlete, the use of such medication may impair performance.

Hearing Loss

When an athlete complains of a hearing problem, it is important to first determine whether it is a conductive or a sensorineural loss. This can be done with the basic tuning fork tests. The most common problem resulting in some loss of hearing in the athlete is impaction of cerumen in the canal. This is treated easily by irrigating the canal with tap water at body temperature. An agent to soften the cerumen can be used at the time of treatment but should be left in the canal for only a few minutes because it can cause severe irritation. An upper respiratory tract infection that has resulted in otitis media with effusion also can cause hearing loss.

Barotrauma can result in a transudate in the middle ear, blood (hemotympanum), or perforation of the tympanic membrane. When a perforation has occurred, it is important to prevent infection. The overwhelming majority of traumatic tympanic membrane perforations will heal spontaneously if they do not become infected. The primary preventive measure is to keep the area dry. Systemic or local antibiotics given prophylactically are not recommended for fear of altering the normal bacterial flora. Middle ear effusions are managed as previously described.

The athlete will sometimes complain of a "hollow feeling" within the ear. This is usually a transient complaint noted soon after vigorous exercise. Although not clearly established, the pathophysiology appears to involve a eustachian tube that remains abnormally patent as a result of fluid shifts in the mucosal lining. The athlete is aware of air passing in and out of the middle ear from the nasopharynx, in contrast to the normal condition in which the eustachian tube is closed most of the time.

If the tuning fork tests suggest a sensorineural hearing loss, the athlete should be questioned about any training activities involving Valsalva maneuvers, such as breath-hold diving or weight lifting. It has been demonstrated that a rupture of the membrane around either the oval or round window can occur as a result of the increased intracranial pressure associated with a Valsalva maneuver being transmitted to the perilymph, which communicates with the cerebrospinal fluid cavities. The loss of perilymph from the inner ear often results in a fluctuating hearing loss and may cause vertigo as well. It is critical to ascertain the possibility of this diagnosis because a perilymph leak necessitates urgent surgery. When this condition is diagnosed early enough and treated effectively, hearing is often preserved. The athlete usually cannot train during recovery.

SINONASAL DISORDERS

Nasal Obstruction

The athlete with compromised nasal passageways is forced to rely more on oral breathing than a healthy person. This may affect endurance.

Anatomic alterations are among the most common causes of obstruction. These can be the result of congenital or acquired deformities. Deflection of the nasal septum is a common problem in the general population. However, the increased demands of nasal airflow during exercise increase the significance of a nasal septal deflection that would normally not be a problem for the nonathlete. Such nasal septal deflections usually are effectively treated by surgical reconstruction.

Hypertrophic inferior turbinates and lymphoid tissue within the nasopharynx (adenoids) and tonsillar area can also cause nasal obstruction. The hypertrophic turbinates are often a result of engorged, edematous mucosa that may be allergic in etiology. Such patients often notice improvement in the nasal passages with the long-term usage of systemic antihistaminics and/or decongestants. Nasal steroid sprays have become popular for this condition and have minimal systemic side effects. Surgical reduction may be necessary and is accomplished by outfracture and cauterization of the inferior turbinates. Cryosurgery can be used to achieve the same results.

Inflammation of the nasal mucous membranes may also result in obstruction. Edematous mucous membranes of the nasal septum and turbinates restrict nasal airflow. Postnasal inflammatory problems are usually viral in origin and are treated symptomatically. The athlete with allergic rhinitis may develop nasal polyps. These represent outpouchings of edematous mucosa from the ethmoid sinuses. Many small polyps respond to nasal steroid sprays. If such medication is contraindicated, airway obstruction can be relieved surgically. However, the evaluation of the athlete with nasal polyps should include sinus radiographs to determine the extent of the sinusitis. The radiographs are usually computed tomograms, which provide the capability of assessing the osteomeatal complex when taken using coronal views. Endoscopic sinus surgery is a new approach to sinus disease which appears to improve the results and decrease the morbidity.

Some people will be bothered with nasal congestion and persistent rhinorrhea where there is no apparent inflammatory or allergic condition. If these symptoms persist, it may be advisable to obtain a sinus computed tomogram to rule out the possibility of occult sinus disease. If the radiographs are normal, these patients usually have vasomotor rhinitis and management of this problem relies heavily on the use of antihistaminics or decongestants. In addition, maintaining hydration and breathing humidified air from a vaporizer on a daily basis will provide symptomatic relief.

For the athlete participating in outside sports during temperature extremes, it is imperative to protect nasal skin from overexposure to heat or cold. Sun-blocking agents can be used during prolonged exposure to the sun, which includes sports such as skiing.

Epistaxis

The management of epistaxis in athletes usually requires a more aggressive approach than in the nonathlete. The most common cause of epistaxis is desiccation of the nasal mucous membranes. The anterior nasal septum on either side contains an area (Little's area) containing a confluence of vessels (Kisselbach's plexus) that is located just below the thin nasal mucosa. For the athlete performing in a low-humidity environment, rapid nasal airflow dries the mucous membranes and results in cracking with subsequent bleeding. Management of acute epistaxis involves direct pressure on the area by pinching the tip of the nose between the index finger and thumb while breathing through the mouth. If bleeding has not stopped following a few minutes of direct pressure, the affected side of the nose should be packed with cotton saturated with a vasoconstricting agent and direct pressure should be applied again. This cotton should not be removed but allowed to dry in position until it separates from the mucosa and can be removed without avulsing the clot.

The majority of recurrent bouts of epistaxis can be resolved by increasing humidification of the nose. This is best accomplished in the athlete by applying plain petrolatum to the nasal mucosa just prior to exertion. The use of a vaporizer while sleeping is recommended. If conservative treatment is not effective, nasal cautery under local anesthesia is usually effective.

The evaluation of recurrent epistaxis should rule out the possibility of more serious causes, such as hypertension, platelet disorder, hereditary hemorrhagic telangiectasia, or nasopharyngeal angiofibromas.

Sinusitis

Sinus infections can result in nasal obstruction coupled with copious amounts of mucopurulent secretions draining anteriorly from the nose and intermittent nasopharyngeal drainage, which can be especially troublesome to the person experiencing vigorous physical activity. Nasal drainage may be discolored and associated with nasal congestion and sensation of pressure over the sinuses. Radiography (computed tomography) will confirm

SECTION III

SELECTED TOPICS

14

CHRONIC FATIGUE AND STALENESS

E. Randy Eichner, MD

Fatigue is a common complaint among athletes of all ages, sizes, shapes, and abilities. Indeed, chronic fatigue is one of the most common complaints in medicine: One of every five patients who walks into a physician's office complains that fatigue is disrupting his or her life. Every year, it is estimated, fatigue accounts for 10 million office visits.

Fatigue, in fact, is a common complaint among apparently healthy people, athletes or not. For example, surveys find that if you stop 100 people on the street and ask them if they have had any symptoms that week, 90 will say yes. The five most common symptoms voiced, in decreasing order of frequency, are tiredness, headache, worries, muscular aches, and irritability.

It is no wonder, then, that sports medicine physicians often encounter athletes who complain of chronic fatigue. This fatigue can vary from pervasive, felt even at rest, to subtle, felt only during all-out competition. Such a complaint, of course, is vague, nonspecific, and wide-ranging in its implications. Because of these imponderables, one hesitates to expound a single, comprehensive diagnostic approach to chronic fatigue in the athlete. Indeed, such an approach would be cumbersome, costly, and inefficient.

Instead, this chapter covers the common etiologic categories of chronic fatigue. Within categories, the appropriate investigation and management, if not implicit, are addressed. To highlight the most common causes of fatigue at different stages of life, athletes here are arbitrarily divided into adolescents, adults, and seniors.

ADOLESCENT ATHLETES

Fatigue is a common complaint among adolescent athletes. Usually, it is benign and brief. Occasionally, it becomes chronic and generates increasing concern from athlete, parents, and coaches alike. Sooner or later, a physician is consulted.

Unfortunately, the roots of fatigue can be elusive because, in a sense, fatigue wears many masks. The complaint itself is devilishly subjective. Fatigue, after all, is easy to feel but hard to define and impossible to see. It defies easy measurement; we cannot really gauge its severity. And chronic fatigue has many metaphors: "no energy, pep, or stamina," "tired all the time," "can't concentrate," "can't peak," "lost interest," "never get enough sleep," "times falling off," "wake up tired," "I'm stale," and so forth. In the final analysis, fatigue can be as individual as the athletes themselves.

Even defining fatigue is not easy. For example, ponder these medical symptoms: tiredness, lethargy, listlessness, weariness, and lassitude, to name some in current use. Physiologists define fatigue as the failure to sustain the expected or required muscular force, but physicians define it both more vaguely and more broadly. Physicians might agree that fatigue is a subjective condition wherein patients feel tired before beginning activities, lack the energy to accomplish tasks requiring sustained effort and attention, and become unduly exhausted after normal activities.

Probably the most common causes of chronic fatigue or staleness in adolescent athletes are infection, psychological problems, and overtraining. In some young athletes, use of certain energy-sapping drugs contributes to fatigue. And, paradoxically, exercise-induced asthma can be an unrecognized cause of fatigue during sports play.

Infections

Infection, especially viral infection, is often considered as a possible cause of fatigue in adolescent athletes. When it comes to chronic fatigue, however, most of the common viral infections are not really valid candidates. Not only are they easy to diagnose, but they cause only transient fatigue, not chronic fatigue.

The common cold, for example, most often caused by a rhinovirus, is easily recognized by its upper respiratory symptoms and causes fatigue for only a few days. Similarly, influenza, with its high fever, myalgias, and hacking cough, along with its seasonality and epidemic occurrence, is easy to diagnose. To be sure, it causes profound fatigue at first, but it rarely causes fatigue for longer than 2 weeks.

Mycoplasmal pneumonia, too, is typically a subacute illness, not a chronic one. Although perhaps the most common community-acquired pneumonia in adolescents, it does not long remain undiagnosed and would not be a likely cause of chronic fatigue in an adolescent athlete.

INFECTIOUS MONONUCLEOSIS

In contrast, infectious mononucleosis is a common cause of chronic fatigue in young athletes.[1] One recent example in the literature described a 15-year-old runner whose primary illness was so mild that the presenting features were a loss of stamina, a decline in race performance, and an inability to manage his usual training regimen. After the diagnosis of infectious mononucleosis, he cut back on his training; 4 months later, he had regained his form.

Another example is an 18-year-old runner who complained only of loss of stamina. He recalled no recent illness but had mild hepatitis as reflected by abnormal serum chemistries. He also had infectious mononucleosis; 6 months later, he still complained of fatigue and he had not regained his prior level of performance.

Although such cases suggest that incipient or insidious mononucleosis can appear as performance-limiting chronic fatigue in a young athlete, it is far more common for chronic fatigue to follow a florid case of mononucleosis. The classic features, course, and management of infectious mononucleosis are covered in chapter 6.

If infectious mononucleosis can cause chronic fatigue, what are sensible guidelines for when the affected athlete can return to his or her sport? Activity should be individualized, but most patients feel much better within 1 week, so there is no basis for strict bed rest. In one college study, bed rest did not shorten symptoms, and moderate activity as desired seemed to hasten recovery, not impede it. Convalescence occurs gradually, with some waxing and waning of fatigue, but most patients are back to normal within 4 to 8 weeks. The highly trained athlete, however, may not regain top fitness for 3 months or more.

Some patients remain fatigued for many months after a bout of infectious mononucleosis. In fact, this slow, incomplete recovery from mononucleosis led to the birth of the "chronic fatigue syndrome," to be considered in the section on adult athletes. In general, however, athletes tend to recover faster from mononucleosis than do nonathletes. Research has shown, in fact, that the course of mononucleosis is influenced by personality: Fast recovery correlates with psychological health, whereas slow recovery correlates with depression.

Most experts seem to agree on a clinical timetable for returning to sports: The athlete who feels well can resume easy training (ie, jogging, swimming, cycling) after the third week of symptomatic illness. If splenomegaly is not evident on palpation, the athlete can probably return to contact sports after 1 month. Repeating the heterophil test is no help, because it stays positive too long. However, if the liver chemistries were abnormal initially, they should be back to normal or near-normal before the resumption of exhausting physical workouts. This timetable, of course, is only a guide—the physician must use clinical judgment for each athlete.[1]

OTHER VIRAL INFECTIONS

Other viral infections can cause chronic fatigue in young athletes. After infectious mononucleosis, the next most common, probably, is viral hepatitis, usually from the type A virus, occasionally from sporadic community cases of non-A, non-B hepatitis. It has even been suggested that athletes, as a group, are more susceptible to infectious hepatitis. That is, in one college outbreak, 90 of 97 members of the football team were affected, but no other students or staff.

But is it being an athlete that increases the likelihood of getting viral hepatitis, or is it being on a team? Studies of aseptic meningitis, for example, show that once an enterovirus is introduced into a team, the potential for transmission is enhanced.[2] It seems unlikely that athletes, per se, are at undue risk for hepatitis.

Once an athlete has infectious hepatitis, however, how should he or she be managed? In general, the guidelines are similar to those for infectious mononucleosis. On the one hand, volunteers with chronic active hepatitis have tolerated moderate, short-term physical activity such as cycling, and studies in the military have shown that even strenuous activity does not appear to worsen the acute course of infectious hepatitis.

On the other hand, it has also been shown that a mild, fever-producing viral infection decreases the subject's isometric muscular strength by up to 15% and also decreases ability and/or willingness to complete a submaximal exercise walk.[3] All considered, then, it seems prudent to allow an athlete with hepatitis to return to vigorous training only after his or her liver chemistries return to normal or near-normal levels.

Psychological Problems

"BURNOUT"

Burnout can cause chronic fatigue, among other symptoms, in adolescent athletes, especially those driven by intrusive parents and/or authoritarian coaches. Elite athletes are the most vulnerable; typical examples include female gymnasts, swimmers, and divers, who often retire from their sport during their midteens, long before they have reached their physical prime. What is burnout, and why do elite adolescent athletes burn out?

Burnout is a complex, negative psychological reaction to the increasing intensity of elite athletic training superimposed on the everyday agonies of being a teenager. Surely, burnout is composed of many parts: self-concept, increasing demands, unreachable goals, desire to please, increasing sacrifices, and separation from peers. Although it is difficult to define concisely, burnout seems to overlap with both depression and overtraining.

Burnout has three broad stages. In the first stage, athletes experience growing fatigue, loss of enthusiasm, irritability or anger, and diverse somatic symptoms. In the second stage, they are withdrawn and sullen and have severe fatigue, frequent colds, and changes in appetite and weight. In the third stage, by now convinced they are just not good enough, they become cynical and feel alienated. Obnoxious or escapist behavior emerges, and there are sudden, dramatic changes in values and beliefs.[4]

Most susceptible to burnout are those athletes who are perfectionists, have tremendous energy, are oriented toward others, and are not very assertive. Ironically, these quiet, intense, sensitive, malleable, achieving athletes are just the sort that coaches like best.

How can burnout be prevented? Parents and coaches can help athletes fight five common demotivators. To combat the law of diminishing returns from ever-increasing training, one can praise subtle improvements. To meet the need for self-determinism, one can foster independence. To respect the athlete's awareness of the increasing physical price required, one can scale workouts down. To keep the athlete from setting impossible goals, one can deemphasize winning and emphasize the diverse rewards from being an athlete. Finally, to adjust to the teenaged athletes' growing awareness of the social price required, one can help them find time for fun.[4]

DEPRESSION

Burnout merges into depression. Every adolescent feels "blue" at certain trying times of life; such a response is normal. But those who cannot "snap out of it" within 2 weeks may be suffering from the illness known as depression. Chronic fatigue is a cardinal feature of depression. In addition, the American Psychiatric Association characterizes a depressed person as feeling "pervasively sad, helpless, and hopeless." The telltale symptoms of depression are listed in Table 14–1. A diagnosis of depression should always be considered if a young athlete has had four or more of these symptoms for more than 2 weeks.

Depression is on the increase today, and it is increasing fastest among the young.[5] Why are the seeds of depression planted ever earlier in childhood? Experts speculate that contributors include the rising rate of divorce; the greater number of single parents; more time alone for the children, when they have to rely on themselves; and, even when both parents are in the home, less and less parent-child interaction. Some cases of depression, of course, have a genetic basis; others seem to be environmental. In general, the earlier and harder depression strikes, the more likely it is to be genetic, and the more likely it is that drug therapy will be needed.

Unfortunately, only one in five victims of depression seeks help. Most sufferers do not recognize the pattern; rather, they attribute the physical symptoms to a virus, the sleeping and eating problems to stress, and the emotional problems to lack of sleep or

TABLE 14–1. SYMPTOMS OF DEPRESSION

Change in appetite
Major weight loss or gain without dieting
Change in sleep pattern: too much or too little sleep
Waking in the morning at least 2 hours earlier than usual
Feeling sad
Moving slowly
Loss of interest in or pleasure from activities formerly enjoyed
Fatigue or loss of energy
Feeling worthless or inappropriately guilty
Inability to concentrate, decide, or think
Irritability
Thoughts of death or suicide

poor diet. Any young athlete with chronic fatigue may be depressed. With therapy (ie, counseling and/or medication), up to 90% can be cured.

Overtraining

Overtraining is a real but nebulous entity that is often considered in the evaluation of a young, competitive athlete who complains of fatigue or declining race performance. Everyone agrees that overtraining can cause chronic fatigue, but no one seems to know exactly what overtraining is. To be sure, it often contains elements of burnout or depression, but it can also include components of muscle damage and/or "underfueling."

Chronic fatigue, or "staleness" is widespread, for example, among college swimmers, for whom the yearly incidence approaches 10%, and among elite distance runners, for whom the lifetime incidence may approach 60%.[6] But is overtraining, per se, the key element here? Is it often difficult to be certain. Consider this recent case, in which overtraining was at first included in the differential diagnosis.

CASE 1

An 18-year-old state-ranked high school cross-country runner consults a sports medicine physician because of declining race performance. He has been used to winning all his races. Now, halfway through his senior year, he is beginning to place third or fourth in key, statewide meets. In the final few hundred meters of these 5-km races, he becomes pale, exhausted, and unduly dyspneic. He feels like dropping out; once, he did drop out near the finish.

He is now becoming nauseated before races; once he even vomited shortly before the start. He is eating reasonably well and is not losing weight. His coach is working with him to increase the percentage of carbohydrates in his diet. He is training harder than ever running 50 miles per week, many at a fast pace. In general, his training runs are uneventful. Indeed, his races are uneventful until near the end.

He has never had heart problems or arrhythmias. He has no cough or wheezing, and prerace inhalation of albuterol has made no difference. He takes no drugs. He feels a lot of pressure, because top colleges are looking at him for a track scholarship. Neither his father nor his coach seems to be the source of the pressure.

Physical examination is normal. Hemoglobin is 16 g/dL; mean cell volume, 90 fl; white blood cell count, 5000 μL; platelet count, normal; serum ferritin, 7 μg/L. Serum chemistries are normal; the muscle enzymes are at the upper limit of normal.

Is this young athlete overtraining? Are his muscles "underfueled"? Is he beginning to burn out? Or is it other factors? Arrhythmias? Race-induced asthma? Is the low ferritin level the culprit, even in the absence of anemia? Is he sensing pressure from his father or coach? Or is merely putting too much pressure on himself? Late in the race, when he sees he is not going to win, is he hyperventilating or giving up? Such were the considerations of his physician.

What, then, is overtraining? Mae West said that too much of a good thing is—wonderful! Obviously, she had never been overtrained. At its core, overtraining is an imbalance between training and recovery, between work and rest. But as implied by its synonyms (chronic fatigue, staleness, burnout), overtraining remains a subtle, mysterious phenomenon that ranges from muscles to motivation.

Regarding motivation, Morgan and colleagues[6] were able to link the chronic fatigue of overtraining with the athlete's mood. Over a span of 10 years, these investigators monitored 400 collegiate swimmers at intervals of 2 to 4 weeks during individual indoor seasons.[6] They used the Profile of Mood Scores, a self-assessment of tension, depression, anger, vigor, fatigue, and confusion. In general, they found that elite athletes score below the population average on tension, depression, anger, fatigue, and confusion, and above the population average on vigor (the "iceberg profile").

As their training progressively increases, however, the swimmers show "dose-related" mood disturbances; their "iceberg profile" tends to invert, with low scores for vigor. Conversely, when training is reduced ("tapered"), the mood profiles revert to baseline. In other words, the athlete's mood disturbance waxes and wanes with his or her training load.

Nonathlete, control students in the same environment do not show these mood swings. Morgan and associates[6] thus postulate that monitoring the mood states of elite athletes can provide one gauge of distress that coaches can use to titrate training loads so as to prevent overtraining.

Overtraining, in fact, quickly alters mood. For example, when 12 male college swimmers suddenly doubled their daily training distance for 10 days in a row, their mood scores changed to reflect the adverse physiologic signs of overtraining. In other words, short-term overtraining adversely affects both the body and the mind.[7]

This study of short-term overtraining also focused on the role of muscle dysfunction. Four of the 12 swimmers could not keep up with the heavier training demands. These four men, compared with the other eight, had significantly reduced muscle glycogen stores, which, in turn, were related to an abnormally low intake of carbohydrates.[8] In other words, some elite swimmers seem to experience chronic fatigue because they eat too little carbohydrate to meet the demands of heavy training. The same probably applies to some female distance runners.[9]

What are the most reliable clinical signs of overtraining? The lay literature touts ten "symptoms": heavy legs, sore muscles, rise in resting pulse rate, lack of motivation, sleep problems, diminished sex drive, frequent infections, weight loss, depression, and the perception that the usual workout is harder than normal. These ten symptoms, however, are more empiric than scientific. It seems unlikely that they offer a precise gauge of overtraining.

Perhaps the best documented among these "symptoms of overtraining" is the rise in resting pulse rate. For example, when 12 marathoners ran a 20-day road race, mean morning pulse rate fell during the first week of running, but rose steadily thereafter, becoming 10 beats per minute higher as the race ended.[10]

Another of these symptoms, diminished sex drive, is the subject of increasing research. We know that, in women, strenuous athletic training can impair the hypothalamic secretion of gonadotropin-releasing hormone. This, in turn, leads to low blood levels of estrogen and to amenorrhea, a "clinical sign" of hypogonadism. Now research is beginning to suggest that, in men, too, strenuous training can impair secretion of gonadotropin-releasing hormone. This may suppress testicular function and diminished libido may be a symptom.

For example, in a recent study, indicators of testicular function were followed in six endurance athletes before and after 2 weeks of strenuous training. Lasting fatigue developed in all six men. Mean plasma testosterone level fell 17%; sperm counts fell 29%; and all six men reported decreased libido and a decline in sexual activity.[11]

Another "neuroendocrine" system of interest as a possible gauge of overtraining is

TABLE 14–2. THE ACUTE PHASE RESPONSE: A REACTION TO THE INFLAMMATION OF EXHAUSTIVE EXERCISE

Fever and muscle wasting
Leukocytosis and thrombocytosis
Activation of leukocytes and lymphocytes
Fall in serum iron and zinc levels
Rise in serum copper levels
Rise in erythrocyte sedimentation rate and certain serum protein levels

thyroid function, that is, the "euthyroid sick syndrome." It is known that, like illness itself, starvation and/or strenuous exercise, perhaps in part by releasing cortisol, can inhibit the conversion of thyroxin (T_4) to T_3, the active thyroid hormone. This triggers a complex chain of events that seems to "reset the thermostat" that governs the thyroid gland.

Yet another aspect of overtraining is inflammation—in muscles—that triggers the acute phase response.[12] In other words, sore muscles often are inflamed muscles. The acute phase response is an age-old biologic defense mechanism that comprises fever, leukocytosis, muscle wasting, fall in serum iron and zinc levels, rise in serum copper levels and in the erythrocyte sedimentation rate, and activation of leukocytes and lymphocytes (Table 14–2).

Strenuous, prolonged exercise can trigger the acute phase response. As I have reviewed before, exercise can spur the release—from monocytes infiltrating damaged muscles—of interleukin-1, which can evoke all of the above features of the acute phase response as well as a feeling of sleepiness, or fatigue. This coordinated body response, in fact, seems designed to heal injury.[12]

One might, then, propose to gauge overtraining by monitoring indices of neuroendocrine function or of the acute phase response. At best, however, such monitoring would be cumbersome and costly. Over the past few years, working with a college track team, we have used more practical, clinical measures to try to distinguish overtraining from other causes of chronic fatigue in athletes.

Specifically, we monitor complete blood count, iron stores, and serum chemistries, focusing on the muscle enzymes. When the question of overtraining arises, we talk to the coach, review the training log, see the athlete, and recheck the blood studies. This practical approach can help distinguish overtraining from other common causes of fatigue in collegians, such as viral infection, anemia, sinusitis, asthma, jet lag, or social pressures.

A final word about muscle pain. If the myalgia the day after strenuous exercise is from muscle inflammation, the cramps during exercise, especially during hot-weather exercise, are "heat cramps." Heat cramps are brief, excruciating muscular cramps, as in the gastrocnemius. They tend to occur in heat-acclimatized athletes (eg, runners or tennis players), who play long and hard, drink copious amounts of water, but fail to replace losses of salt. The higher the sweat rate, the more sodium is lost; although the mechanism of heat cramps is unclear and debated, some experts think hyponatremia plays a role. If heat cramps are the only symptom of heat stress, sufficient treatment is rest, oral fluids, cooling, stretching, and massage.[13]

Lifestyle Problems

Lifestyle problems can also contribute to chronic fatigue in adolescent athletes. Pathogenic weight-control behavior is one example. Such behavior may be common among athletes who participate in the "low-weight sports," that is, running and gymnastics. In a survey of 182 female college athletes, one in three practiced self-induced vomiting or binging; or took laxatives, diet pills, and/or diuretics.[14] Studies of ballet dancers, swimmers, and wrestlers have yielded similar results.

Other behaviors (eg, getting too little sleep) can also contribute to chronic fatigue in some adolescent athletes. The total number of hours of sleep per week declines steadily between the ages of 12 and 18 years. Many teenagers may train and compete on too little sleep. "Situational deconditioning" may also be an occasional factor. For instance, a previously fit 16-year-old boy who now tires easily when playing basketball may have become "detrained" by a lifestyle more sedentary during his midteens than in his childhood.[15]

Drugs

In sports medicine today, we hear a lot about drugs believed to bestow energy or otherwise enhance performance. These drugs are termed "ergogenic." But what about drugs that sap energy? What about "ergolytic drugs"? Ergolytic drugs can impair athletic performance and, potentially, contribute to fatigue. Typical examples of ergolytic drugs for the adolescent athlete are alcohol, marijuana, and smokeless tobacco.[16]

Some athletes believe that small doses of alcohol, by reducing tension and enhancing confidence, will aid their performance. Alcohol, however, is ergolytic. Even at small doses, it temporarily weakens the contractility of the left ventricle. Furthermore, a recent study found that "social" amounts of alcohol slowed sprinting and middle-distance racing. Specifically, prerace alcohol significantly slowed the 200-m, 400-m, 800-m and 1500-m runs.

Marijuana, like alcohol, makes the heart work harder and curbs exercise performance. In one study, when ten healthy men cycled against increasing work loads, marijuana diminished peak performance. In another study, 161 young men and women given tetrahydrocannabinol (THC) showed decrements in steadiness, reaction time, and psychomotor skills. When 12 healthy young adults cycled to exhaustion 10 minutes after smoking a marijuana cigarette, exercise duration fell significantly, from 16 to 15 minutes.

Smokeless tobacco, commonly used by young football and baseball players, also curtails exercise performance. The nicotine therein narrows blood vessels and raises heart rate and blood pressure, making the heart work harder. In a recent study of young athletes, for example, the use of snuff during exercise caused a notable fall in cardiac stroke volume, along with a fall in cardiac output at a heart rate of 150 beats/min. The heavy use of smokeless tobacco, then, can contribute to fatigue, at least during all-out exertion.

Table 14–3 lists drugs that can be ergolytic. I will return to this topic in the section on adult athletes.

Asthma

Paradoxically, exercise-induced asthma can be an unrecognized cause of fatigue during athletic activity. Usually, asthma is identified by its characteristic wheezing, chest tightness,

TABLE 14–3. COMMON ERGOLYTIC DRUGS

Alcohol
Marijuana
Smokeless tobacco
Antihypertensives (beta-blockers)
Eyedrops (beta-blockers)
Diuretics

and breathlessness. But up to one third of athletes with it are unaware they have it, and sometimes its manifestations can be subtle. For example, a basketball player consulted a physician because of sneezing during the hay fever season.[17] An exercise test indicated that he had severe exercise-induced asthma. After treatment controlled his asthma, he realized for the first time that "the second quarter of the game does not have to be a wipeout."

ADULT ATHLETES

Adult athletes can suffer from many of the same causes of chronic fatigue that plague adolescent athletes. But certain causes of fatigue seem to be more common in adults than in adolescents. Among these are anemia, endocrine disorders, cardiac disorders, and especially, the "chronic fatigue syndrome."

Chronic Fatigue Syndrome

What is chronic fatigue syndrome (CFS)? Santayana said that those who cannot remember the past are condemned to repeat it. And CFS, it seems, is a repeat.[18]

Over the past 5 years, CFS has frustrated untold thousands of Americans (and their doctors). Previously termed "chronic mononucleosis" and "chronic EBV" (for chronic Epstein-Barr virus disease), our national pall of CFS began with an "epidemic" in a Lake Tahoe resort community. As word spread, a national wave of CFS ensued.

In the initial epidemic, CFS comprised a bewildering array of soft symptoms. Over several months, 200 sufferers reported to two internists that they had contracted "mono" or "flu." Some had been active athletes and had even run marathons just before becoming ill. Victims complained of sore throat, headaches, swollen lymph glands, myalgias, feverishness, and disabling fatigue that lasted for months. Many also had bizarre neurologic symptoms, although physical examinations were generally normal. Some fatigue victims quit work and became recluses.

Why did all the patients go to the same two internists? The other doctors in the area saw many of the same patients, found no evidence of a unique fatigue syndrome in these educated, ambitious, professional people, and thus, dubbed the illness "yuppie flu."

Meanwhile, the two internists found recent medical articles describing patients with long-lasting fatigue that, in many, seemed to follow infectious mononucleosis. As in the Lake Tahoe patients, physical and laboratory abnormalities were generally absent. Yet the articles tied this "syndrome" to the EBV because many patients had EBV antibody profiles suggesting reactivation of latent infection. In short, the articles said the EBV might cause a CFS.

Recognizing their patients' symptoms, the two doctors ordered EBV titer from commercial laboratories. Test after test came back "positive." Soon they thought they saw a pattern of contagion: a third of one high-school faculty; members of a casino staff; an entire girls' basketball team. They declared an epidemic and called in the federal government's Centers for Disease Control (CDC).

The CDC investigation brought insight and controversy. After studying 134 patients, they declared the "epidemic" iatrogenic, debunked any link between EBV and CFS, and implied CFS was a "wastebasket" diagnosis that included cases of anxiety and depression. Also, they cited several past "epidemics" of bizarre, fatiguing illnesses with elements of "social hysteria" and strong mind-body links.

And when it comes to CFS, the past is certainly prologue. Similar, false epidemics date back at least to 1934, and probably to the Civil War. The clinical features, if not identical to today's CFS, are hauntingly familiar. Research is closing in on psychosocial roots.

In fact, in many cases, it seems that anxiety and depression cause CFS. Studies from clinics in Boston, San Antonio, and Connecticut suggest (1) EBV testing to diagnose CFS is useless and should be abandoned; (2) CFS stems from a medical disease in only 5% of patients; and (3) psychiatric ailments (ie, mood disorders, somatization, anxiety disorders) account for at least two thirds of cases.

A key clinical trial also weakened the link between EBV and CFS. Acyclovir, which inhibits replication of the EBV, did not ameliorate CFS. In this trial, 24 patient with CFS and high titers to EBV were treated alternatively with either acyclovir or placebo. About 50% of patients improved—modestly and transiently—on acyclovir, but 50% also improved on placebo.

Neither acyclovir therapy nor clinical improvement correlated with changes in laboratory findings, including EBV titers. In contrast, subjective improvement correlated with less anger, anxiety, and depression. In other words, in CFS, the patient's mood shapes how well he or she feels.

This trial also shed light on the natural history of CFS. Relentless clinical deterioration, for example, was not seen. Indeed, as with insomnia, no one has ever died from CFS. Also, "feverishness" does not mean fever: patients, feeling sick or well, were generally afebrile. Finally, most patients (21 of 24) improved. Improvement was attributed to the cyclic nature of the syndrome and to a strong placebo effect.[19]

CFS remains vexing and controversial. Even its demographics are peculiar: two out of three patients are educated, adult white women. There is, in fact, considerable overlap with the "fibromyalgia" syndrome. Typical patients have been called "somatocentric." Many report prior excellent health, including sports competition, but display "unachievable ambition and poor coping skills." They "recite a litany of complaints" and can be "disabled by mild emotional or physical stress."

In evaluating new patients with CFS, some experts now first seek psychiatric explanations (eg, depression, anxiety, or panic disorder) and search for possible underlying medical causes only when no psychiatric cause is found. In treating patients, they stress counseling, good nutrition, adequate rest, judicious exercise, and, when necessary, psychotropic drugs. Low doses of antidepressants seem especially helpful.

Do elite athletes get CFS? Yes. That is, they are diagnosed as having it.[20] For example, from 1984 to 1987, six female cyclists on the U.S. Cycling Federation national team were diagnosed as having the syndrome. I have also seen elite female distance runners who were told they had CFS. In each athlete, however, overtraining, disappointment, frustration, and/or depression seemed to play major causative roles in the chronic fatigue. In time, most of these athletes recover fully and return to outstanding performances.

Chronic fatigue may be one reaction to the stress of midlife. CFS, it seems, has long been here, and may long stay. Each new generation of doctors rediscovers and renames it; each new generation of adults confronts and defeats it.

Anemia

Anemia is another common cause of fatigue in adult athletes, but it differs from the fatigue of CFS and from other common patterns of fatigue. In CFS, as in depression, patients feel tired on arising and are tired all day long, even without exercising. During recovery from infectious mononucleosis, patients feel strong in the morning but tire later and need a nap. But with anemia, as with insidious heart failure, fatigue occurs only during exertion. And the milder the anemia, the more exertion it takes to cause the telltale fatigue.

In other words, mildly anemic athletes note symptoms only when they race. Typical symptoms include labored breathing, "heavy" limbs, undue sweating, and (from high blood lactate levels) burning muscles, "tying up," nausea, and even retching.

What constitutes anemia in an athlete? As covered in the chapter on hematology, athletes, especially endurance athletes, are often falsely considered to have anemia due to a natural dilution of the hemoglobin that occurs in response to regular aerobic exercise. This dilution is caused by an expansion of the baseline plasma volume, a beneficial adaptation to the hemoconcentration that occurs during exercise. The resultant hemoglobin level, often at least 1 g/dL below "normal," causes no symptoms and needs no treatment.[21]

Athletes, however, can also develop true anemia, most commonly caused by iron deficiency. This true anemia causes the exercise-related fatigue described above.

Does athleticism, per se, cause iron-deficiency anemia? Probably not. Over the past decade, a spate of reports imply that (1) up to 80% of elite women athletes, for example, are deficient in iron; (2) athletes are uniquely susceptible to iron deficiency; and (3) a low serum ferritin level, even in the absence of anemia, impairs athletic performance. All three of these implications, it seems, are wrong.

Recent research, in fact, suggests that athletes, as a group, have serum ferritin values similar to those of carefully matched nonathletes, and that athletes do not necessarily lose more iron than nonathletes. The notion that a low serum ferritin level, alone, curbs performance is also ill-founded. Recent studies agree that, in the face of a low ferritin level, even all-out performance is normal unless anemia is also present.[21]

All considered, then, how can one recognize true anemia in an athlete? Clinically, the best definition of anemia is a hemoglobin concentration below normal for the athlete at hand. An athletic woman with a hemoglobin level of 13 g/dL, for example, is anemic if her usual hemoglobin is 15 g/dL. In other words, even though her hemoglobin level is within the broad range of "normal," she is anemic by her own standard.

If the "usual" or "normal" hemoglobin level for a given athlete is unknown, as it often is in clinical medicine, one has to use guidelines. In general, hemoglobin levels among healthy women athletes are often under 14 g/dL, commonly under 13 g/dL (especially in endurance athletes), rarely under 12 g/dL, and almost never under 11 g/dL. The corresponding values for male athletes are from 1 to 2 g/dL higher.

Although a low serum ferritin level alone does not impair athletic performance, anemia, even very mild anemia, does. When in doubt, then, the wise course is an empiric trial of iron therapy. For example, if the hemoglobin level is 12 g/dL and the serum ferritin value is borderline, so you are uncertain whether the correct diagnosis is early iron-deficiency anemia or dilutional pseudoanemia, give ferrous sulfate, 325 mg orally three times a day for 2 months. A rise in hemoglobin level (of 1 g/dL or more) proves that the anemia was due, at least in part, to iron deficiency.

Iron deficiency could be prevented in most athletes by paying more attention to diet. To boost iron supply, one can (1) eat more lean red meat or dark meat of chicken; (2) enhance iron absorption from bread and cereal by shunning coffee or tea with meals and consuming instead a source of vitamin C (eg, orange juice); (3) cook occasionally in cast iron skillets and pans; and (4) eat poultry or seafood with dried beans or peas—the animal protein here increases the absorption of the iron in the vegetables.

Endocrine Disorders

Thyroid disorders can cause fatigue in athletes. Margaret Groos, who won the 1988 U.S. Women's Olympic Trials Marathon, had experienced a slump in 1984 at the age of 24. Shortly after placing fifth in that year's trials, she developed tachycardia (250 beats/min) when she tried to run. She became so tired she could not run a mile in less than 8 minutes. A physician diagnosed hyperthyroidism (Graves' disease), and she was cured with radioactive iodine.

Hypothyroidism, too, can cause chronic fatigue. Thus, thyroid function tests are worth considering when evaluating fatigue in athletes. Another possible endocrine cause of fatigue is incipient diabetes mellitus. Usually, of course, one would expect the typical symptoms of hyperglycemia: thirst, polyuria, weight loss, blurred vision, irritability, and infections. Finally, Addison's disease is at least a plausible cause of fatigue in an athletic adult (eg, President John F. Kennedy). In young athletes, in fact, cryptic Addison's disease is a rare cause of collapse and death during sports play.

Cardiac Disorders

Certainly, in any middle-aged male athlete who complains of exertional fatigue, one must immediately suspect coronary heart disease. To be sure, fatigue, alone, is not a common prelude to heart attack or sudden cardiac death. But fatigue may connote silent myocardial infarction, undetected arrhythmia, or atypical angina. Indeed, fatigue can be the only harbinger of a catastrophic coronary event. For example, in a recent review of 36 cases of heart attack or sudden death in marathon runners, 20 athletes (71%) had noted premonitory symptoms; in one athlete that symptom was generalized fatigue.[22]

On the other hand, in athletes at least, fatigue seems not to be a sensitive or dependable index of cardiac reserve. To wit, the recent report of the 57-year-old lifelong, elite runner who set an age record in a distance race (ran 3 km in 10.5 min) and, 1 minute later, collapsed and died of coronary heart disease. The same applies to structural heart disease, as shown by the 28-year-old professional football player who denied exertional fatigue (and all other cardiac symptoms) despite moderately severe aortic regurgitation from a bicuspid aortic valve.[23]

In general, then, heart disease in athletes rarely presents solely as chronic fatigue. Paroxysmal tachyarrhythmias can, of course, cause brief bouts of exertional fatigue. Myocarditis, presumably viral in most cases, is a rare cause of exertional sudden death in athletes, but whether this event is routinely heralded by fatigue is unclear. Congestive cardiomyopathy, albeit rare, does cause chronic fatigue, as evidenced today by an esteemed ex–professional football player. Mitral valve prolapse can be associated with fatigue, as well as with dizziness, palpitations, and nonexertional chest pain. However, in some patients, these episodes may be panic attacks and, most often, mitral valve prolapse causes no symptoms.

Ergolytic Drugs

Ergolytic drugs (see Table 14–3) likely to be used by adult athletes include blood pressure pills, eyedrops, and diuretics. Several of the antihypertensives have been reported to curtail all-out performance, but the main culprits are the beta-adrenergic blockers, especially the nonselective beta-blockers, such as propranolol.[16]

Propranolol is ergolytic because it (1) attenuates the exercise-induced rise in heart rate and blood pressure; (2) reduces tidal volume during heavy exercise; (3) alters skin blood flow and sweat rate so as to raise exercising core temperature; and (4) possibly compromises fuel supply and/or muscle metabolism by inhibiting lipolysis and altering potassium metabolism.

When it comes to all-out exercise, the more fit the athlete, the more he or she will suffer from beta-blockade. Among elite athletes, beta-blockade can reduce maximal oxygen uptake by up to 15%. The same applies to race times in the field. In one study of 25 distance runners, 10-km race times averaged 36 minutes on placebo, 39 minutes on atenolol (a β_1-selective blocker), and 41 minutes on propranolol. In general, elite athletes perform better on β_1-selective blockers than on propranolol.

Even eyedrops can be ergolytic. In a double-blind, controlled study of healthy volunteers, ophthalmic timolol, a beta-blocker commonly used to treat glaucoma, significantly reduced maximal oxygen uptake and maximal exercise duration.[24]

Diuretics, of course, especially if first used shortly before competition, also can be ergolytic. For example, when eight healthy young men ran 5 km or 10 km, 5 hours after taking 40 mg of furosemide orally, their mean running times were significantly slowed by 1.3 and 2.6 minutes, respectively.[16]

Other drugs theoretically can be ergolytic. Examples include antihistamines, tranquilizers, sleeping pills, narcotic pain relievers, and, of course, hypoglycemics. Paradoxically, even caffeine, by creating peaks and troughs in alertness and by disrupting sleep, can be ergolytic. Recently, in a report from a sleep-disorder clinic, pathologic sleepiness induced by caffeine was reported in six adults, including a 43-year-old physician.[25]

Miscellaneous Conditions

Crohn's disease often begins with chronic fatigue, along with abdominal pain, bloody diarrhea, fever, and weight loss. Several prominent athletes have overcome the disease and enjoyed active sports careers. The same applies to Hodgkin's disease and certain other cancers that can appear initially as performance-sapping fatigue in athletes. Neuromuscular disease, such as myasthenia gravis or multiple sclerosis, could manifest as chronic fatigue. Finally, in a female athlete (eg, a marathon runner), fatigue can be caused by pregnancy.

SENIOR ATHLETES

Unfortunately, little is known about the common causes of chronic fatigue in senior athletes. It stands to reason that, compared with the adult athlete, the senior athlete is even more prone to diverse medical diseases, including cancer, that can present as chronic fatigue. But systematic studies in this area are lacking. I have seen individual cases of exertional fatigue in seniors from chronic renal disease, from chronic active hepatitis, and from apathetic hyperthyroidism.

Senior athletes, understandably, are slow to rebound from debilitating infections (eg, influenza). After such infections, it can take the dedicated senior jogger, for example, a year or more to return to his or her former level of athleticism.

Probably, in selected senior athletes, the acute phase response (Table 14–2), either from "too much, too soon" or from chronically pushing beyond limits (eg, running repeated marathons), contributes to chronic fatigue. Here, too, however, there is no systematic research. In general, the athlete most likely to push beyond his limits is not the senior, but the middle-aged man, who, when it comes to exhaustive exercise, hates to admit that, sometimes, more is less.[12]

Finally, it is worth noting that senior athletes seem to be "immune" to the chronic fatigue syndrome that is in vogue today among those who suddenly find themselves fighting the midstream of life.

REFERENCES

1. Eichner ER: Infectious mononucleosis: Recognition and treatment in athletes. Physican Sportsmed 15(12):61–72, 1987.
2. Moore M, Baron RC, Filstein MR, et al: Aseptic meningitis and high school football players. JAMA 249:2039–2042, 1983.
3. Daniels WL, Vogel JA, Sharp DS, et al: Effects of virus infection on physical performance in man. Milit Med 150:8–14, 1985.
4. Feigley DA: Psychological burnout in high-level athletes. Physician Sportsmed 12(10):108–119, 1984.
5. Klerman GL, Weissman MM: Increasing rates of depression. JAMA 261:2229–2235, 1989.
6. Morgan WP, Brown DR, Raglin JS, et al: Psychological monitoring of overtraining and staleness. Br J Sports Med 21:107–114, 1987.
7. Morgan WP, Costill DL, Flynn MG, et al: Mood disturbance following increased training in swimmers. Med Sci Sports Exerc 20:408–414, 1988.
8. Costill DL, Flynn MG, Kirwan JP, et al: Effects of repeated days of intensified training on muscle glycogen and swimming performance. Med Sci Sports Exerc 20:249–254, 1988.
9. Weight LM, Noakes TD: Is running an analog of anorexia? A survey of the incidence of eating disorders in female distance runners. Med Sci Sports Exerc 19:213–217, 1987.
10. Dressendorfer RH, Wade CE, Scaff JH: Increased morning heart rate in runners: A valid sign of overtraining? Physican Sportsmed 13(8):77–86, 1985.
11. Griffith RB, Dressendorfer RH: Effect of overwork on testosterone, sperm count, and libido [abstract 231] . Med Sci Sports Exerc 20:S39, 1988.
12. Eichner ER: The mararthon: Is more less? Physician Sportsmed 14(4):183–185, 1986.
13. Knochel JP: Heat stroke and related heat stress disorders. Disease-a-Month 35(5):306–377, 1989.
14. Rosen LW, McKeag DB, Hough DO, et al: Pathogenic weight-control behavior in female athletes. Physician Sportsmed 14(1):79–86, 1986.
15. Rowland TW: Exercise fatigue in adolescents: Diagnosis of athletic burnout. Physician Sportsmed 14(9):69–77, 1986.
16. Eichner ER: Ergolytic drugs. Sports Sci Exchange 2(15):1–4, 1989.
17. Miller RK, Katz RM, Kersee R, et al: Exercise and asthma. Physician Sportsmed 12(1):59–77, 1984.
18. Eichner ER: Chronic fatigue syndrome: Searching for the cause and treatment. Physician Sportsmed 17(6):142–152, 1989.
19. Straus SE, Dale JK, Tobi M, et al: Acyclovir treatment of the chronic fatigue syndrome. N Engl J Med 319:1692–1698, 1988.
20. Eichner ER: Chronic fatigue syndrome: How vulnerable are athletes? Physician Sportsmed 17(6)157–160, 1989.
21. Eichner ER: Anemia in female athletes. Your Patient & Fitness 3(2):3–11, 1989.
22. Noakes TD: Heart disease in marathon runners: A review. Med Sci Sports Exerc 19:187–194, 1987.
23. Pipe AL, Chan K, Rippe JM: Asymptomatic heart murmur in a professional football player. Physician Sportsmed 16(11):53–60, 1988.
24. Everitt DE, Avorn J: Systemic effects of medications used to treat glaucoma. Ann Intern Med 112:120–125, 1990.
25. Regstein QR: Pathologic sleepiness induced by caffeine. Am J Med 87:586–588, 1989.

15

DIABETES AND EXERCISE

John R. Sutton

This chapter describes the metabolic and hormonal responses to exercise in normal persons and in diabetic individuals. Because many insulin-dependent diabetics are active in athletic events and some have reached international standing in their respective sports, it is clear that diabetes is no longer a deterrent to maximal athletic performance. In fact, physical training appears to improve glucose tolerance and diminish insulin requirements of diabetics. However, there are certain precautions that must be taken when insulin-requiring diabetic individuals exercise. In contrast, more than 80% of diabetics are non–insulin-dependent, a condition notably associated with obesity.[1] Some practical details have been enunciated in a recent consensus conference on non–insulin-dependent diabetics[2] and also in insulin-dependent diabetics.[3]

EXERCISE AND DIABETES—HISTORICAL BACKGROUND

Physical exercise has been considered beneficial in the treatment of diabetes mellitus for many years and was one of the few therapies available in the preinsulin era. Aristotle was an advocate of the use of physical activity for the treatment of many disorders, including that of diabetes, while in the East, the Indian physician Sushruta suggested the use of exercise in the treatment of diabetic patients as early as 600 BC.[4] More recently, the great diabetologist Joslin emphasized exercise as one of the mainstays in the management of diabetic patients.[5] However, in spite of these recommendations, it was uncertain how exercise might be beneficial. Although we are well aware of the long-term cardiovascular effects of diabetes, this chapter discusses the more immediate factors regulating blood glucose and the supply of energy substrates during exercise in the diabetic. This topic has been the subject of several reviews.[1–4,6–9]

METABOLIC AND HORMONAL RESPONSES TO EXERCISE IN NORMAL SUBJECTS

Hypoglycemia

Hypoglycemia can be a problem during exercise even in nondiabetic people. Levine and coworkers[10] reported a number of such occurrences in well-conditioned athletes during the Boston Marathon. More recently, hypoglycemia has been described in joggers entering fun runs, and as these fun runs and marathons are now occurring on a scale quite unprecedented, it can be seen that hypoglycemia could well be a major medical hazard in such races (Figs. 15–1 and 15–2).[11]

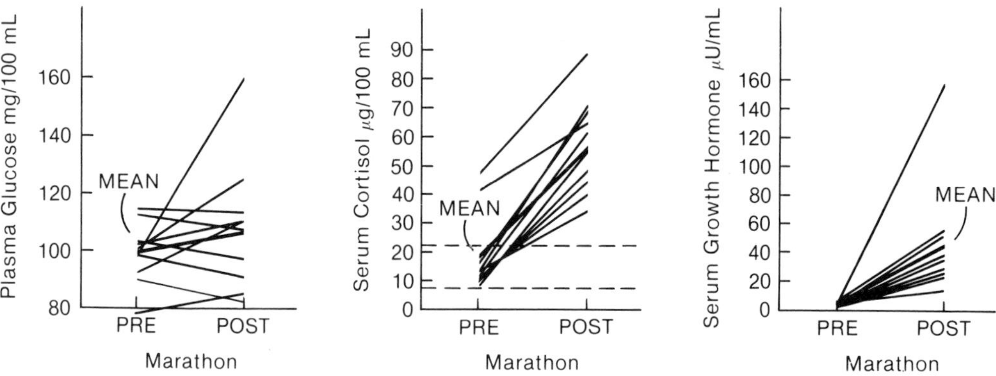

Figure 15–1. Blood glucose, plasma cortisol, and serum growth hormone levels before and after the marathon in trained athletes.

In a comprehensive study during prolonged laboratory exercise, Felig and colleagues[12] demonstrated that hypoglycemia (plasma glucose less than 45 mg/dL) occurs in a significant number of subjects. It is interesting to note in their work that on repeated occasions when plasma glucose was maintained at euglycemic levels by the administration of oral glucose, the time taken to develop exhaustion and the perceived exertion were unaltered. These observations are of interest because they are in apparent conflict with the early work of Christensen and Hansen,[13] who were able to increase performance in exhausted subjects by giving oral glucose.

Fuels for Exercise

The continuous production of adenosine triphosphate (ATP) is essential for prolonged exercise. The high-energy phosphates stored in muscle in the form of ATP or creatine phosphate will enable muscle contraction to continue only for a matter of seconds. For exercise lasting longer than a few seconds, continuous production of ATP by the metab-

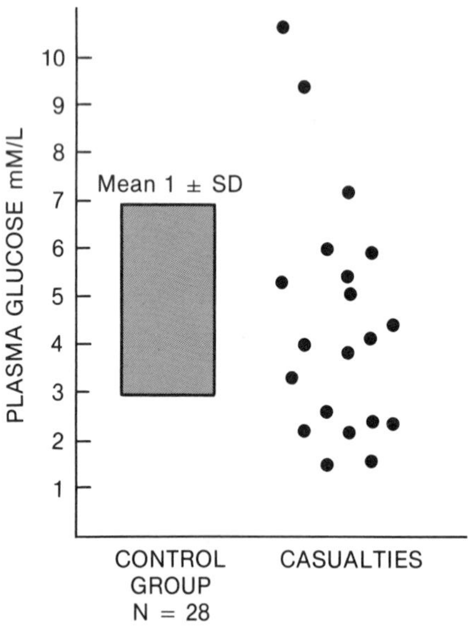

Figure 15–2. Blood glucose levels following a fun run in patients who "collapsed," compared with 28 control subjects. (*Data compiled from* Sutton JR, Coleman MJ, Millar AP: The medical problems of mass participation in athletic competition: The "City-to-Surf" race. Med J Aust 2:127, 1972 *and* Richards D, Richards RD, Richards PJ, Schofield PJ: Reducing the hazards in Sydney's The Sun City-to-Surf fun runs. Med J Aust 2:453–457, 1979; with permission.)

TABLE 15–1. SUBSTRATE STORES

	kg	kJ
Circulating Fuels		
Glucose (extracellular water)	0.020	300
Free fatty acids (plasma)	0.0004	15
Triglycerides (plasma)	0.004	150
Total		465
Tissue Stores		
Fat		
Adipose tissue triglycerides	15	560,000
Intramuscular triglycerides	0.3	11,000
Protein (mainly muscle)	10	160,000
Glycogen		
Liver	0.085	1,500
Muscle	0.350	6,000
Total		738,500

From Newsholme EA, Jones NL: Intermediary metabolism. *In* Sutton JR, Jones NL, Houston CS (eds): Hypoxia: Man at Altitude. New York, Thieme-Stratton, 1982, p 32; with permission.

olism of carbohydrate or fat is essential. The energy stores available for exercise are shown in Table 15–1. As can be readily seen, the stores of fat are predominantly in adipose tissue, while those of carbohydrate are in both muscle and, to a lesser extent, liver.

At the onset of exercise and certainly prior to the circulatory adaptations that increase oxygen transport, the anaerobic breakdown of glycogen to form lactate provides an immediate source of ATP. When exercise continues for more than a few minutes, blood-borne substrates from liver (in the form of glucose) or from adipose tissue (in the form of free fatty acids) become available. As exercise continues for more than 20 to 30 minutes, increasing dependence is placed on blood-borne sources of energy until, after 60 to 90 minutes, free fatty acids (FFAs) become the principal supplier of energy. The utilization of FFAs continues to increase as the duration of exercise increases (Fig. 15–3).

Under most circumstances, proteins (amino acids) are not an important source of energy. Under normal circumstances, they almost always contribute less than 10% of the total energy supply.

Occasionally, in normal people, significant hyperglycemia and clinically important hypoglycemia will occur. However, when exercising at moderate intensities (30% to 60% $\dot{V}O_{2max}$), plasma glucose remains within a relatively narrow range. This has been elegantly demonstrated by Chisholm and coworkers,[14] who looked at healthy subjects exercising at 60% $\dot{V}O_{2max}$ for 60 minutes. Using tritium-labeled glucose (^{3}H-glucose infusion), they were able to demonstrate that hepatic glucose output was precisely matched to glucose uptake independent of changes in insulin and glucagon concentrations.

Wahren and colleagues[15] have demonstrated that glucose uptake by muscle increases with exercise and is greater with greater exercise intensity. Also, as the intensity of exercise approaches the $\dot{V}O_{2max}$ of a subject, a relative hyperglycemia results. Laboratory studies have shown that the plasma glucose response to exercise will be dependent on the relative intensity of the exercise and the fitness of the subject (Fig. 15–4).[16] In women, it is also dependent on the phase of the menstrual cycle. At low levels of exercise, plasma glucose remains relatively unchanged and there is no phase difference. However, at 80% $\dot{V}O_{2max}$, there is an increase in plasma glucose concentrations with exercise; this is greatest in the follicular phase.[17] With high-intensity exercise, there is an increased production of lactate, which in itself may inhibit FFA release from adipose tissue.[18] However, with pro-

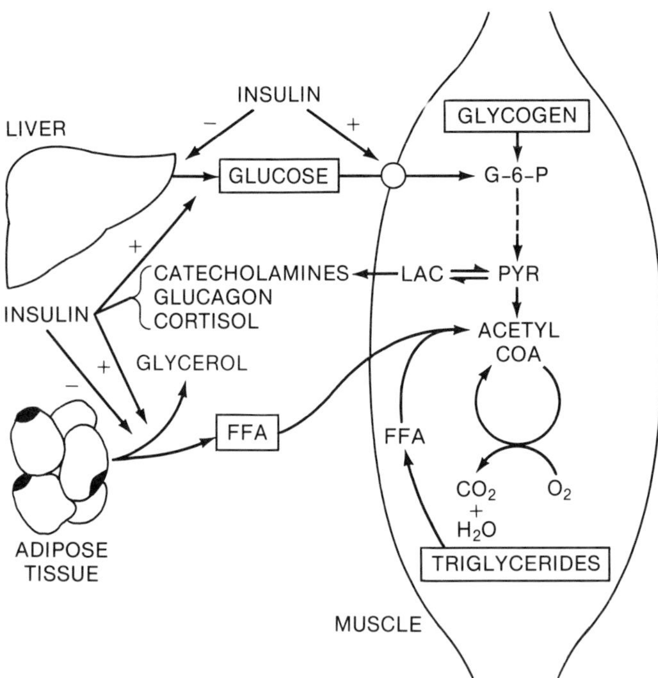

Figure 15–3. Intracellular and extracellular fuel sources during exercise. Fat and carbohydrate are present in muscle; glucose is transported from the liver following glycogenolysis. Lipolysis in adipose tissue will release free fatty acids, which are transported in combination with albumin to muscle. Also illustrated in this diagram are the effects of hormones, such as catecholamines, glucagon, and cortisol—which enhance hepatic glycogenolysis and adipose tissue lipolysis—and insulin—which enhances muscle glucose uptake but inhibits hepatic glycogenolysis and lipolysis in adipose tissue. (*Adapted from* Richter EA, Ruderman NB, Schneider SH: Diabetes and exercise. Am J Med 70:202, 1981; with permission.)

longed exercise and increased FFA concentration, the FFAs themselves may inhibit muscle glycogenolysis, as shown by Rennie and colleagues[19] in the rat and by Costill and coworkers[20] in humans.

Glucose Transport into Muscle; Insulin Receptors

The basis for the stimulation of glucose transport into muscle by exercise is unknown. In resting muscle, glucose transport occurs by facilitated diffusion and is modulated by insulin. For instance, transport is severely impaired in diabetic animals and is restored to normal by the administration of small quantities of insulin.[21] It is possible that insulin in some

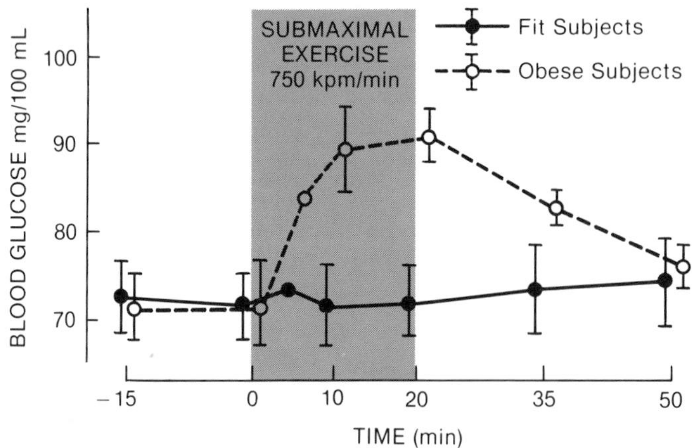

Figure 15–4. The effect of fitness on plasma glucose response to submaximal exercise in fit and obese subjects. (*From* Sutton JR: Hormonal and metabolic responses to exercise in subjects of high and low work capacities. Med Sci Sports 10:2, 1978; with permission.)

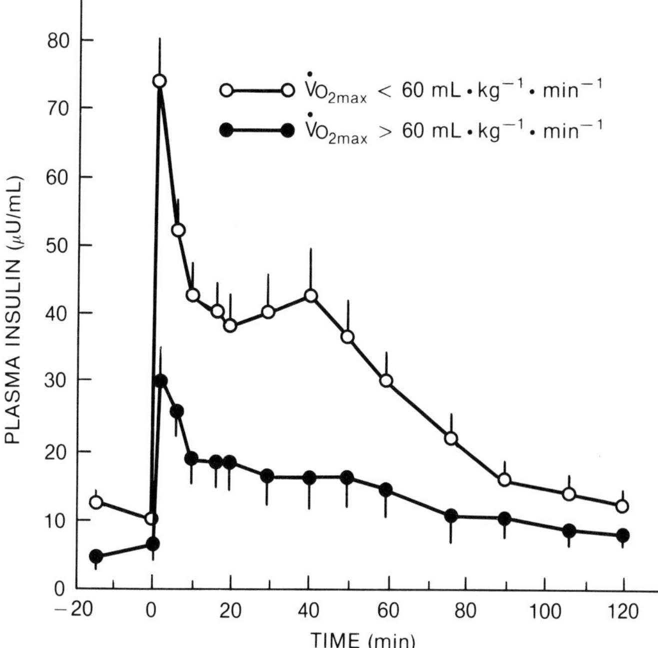

Figure 15–5. The effect of cardiorespiratory fitness on the insulin response to intravenous glucose (20 g/m² body surface) given over a 3-minute period. (*From* LeBlanc J, Nadeau A, Boulay M, et al: Effects of physical training and adiposity on glucose metabolism and ^{125}I-insulin binding. J Appl Physiol Respirat Environ Exerc Physiol 46:236, 1979; with permission.)

way maintains the muscle cell membrane so that it can increase glucose transport in response to contractions. Exercise may also enhance the insulin binding to receptor sites on the muscle cell because, in most studies of exercise, insulin concentration itself is either unchanged or diminished.[22] This hypothesis is supported by the observation that, in persons with euglycemic hyperinsulinism produced by an insulin-glucose clamp,[23] exercise results in an increase in glucose uptake at the same insulin concentration.

LeBlanc illustrated increased binding of insulin to monocytes in fit, as compared with unfit, subjects (Figs. 15–5 and 15–6).[24] Burstein[25] has shown that this difference may be due to the exercise sessions themselves rather than to an effect of training. Thus, a more complex regulatory process is emerging. This has been well expressed by Roth and Grunfeld:

> We are accustomed to the notion that hormone concentrations fluctuate widely in response to changes within the organism. With the advent of methods to measure directly the binding of hormone to its receptors, it has become evident that the concentration and affinity of receptors also change rapidly in response to signals from inside and outside the cell. Given that the receptors are at the crossroads between the interior and exterior of the cell, retrospectively it is not surprising that they are so responsive to the environment.[22]

Hormonal Control Mechanisms During Exercise

Exercise is associated with a number of significant changes in the plasma concentration of a variety of hormones. The hormones that are important in glucose homeostasis and their response to progressive exercise are reviewed in Table 15–2 and Figure 15–7. This topic has been considered in more detail in a recent review.[27]

With submaximal exercise, there is a steady decline in plasma glucose and also a decline in insulin[16,28] but a progressive increase in glucagon.[29] The increase in glucagon tends to increase hepatic glycogenolysis, which would increase plasma glucose, whereas the decrement in insulin would have three actions:

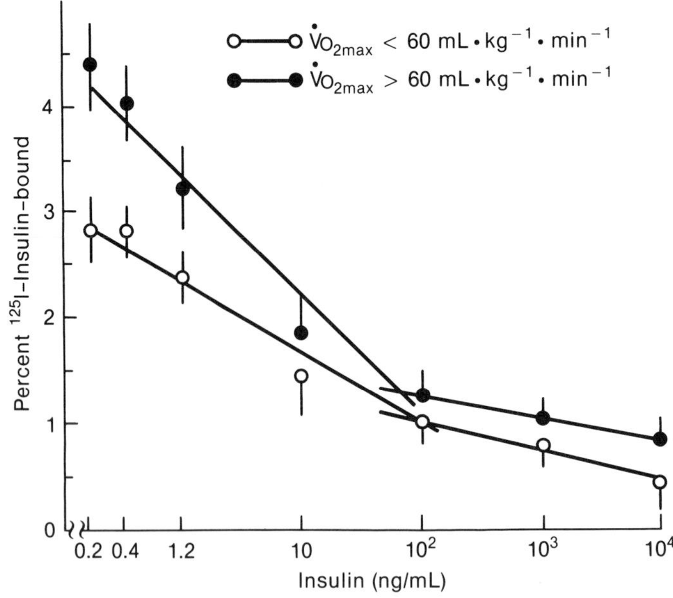

Figure 15–6. The effect of cardiorespiratory fitness on percent ^{125}I-insulin–bound/10^6 monocytes in the presence of various concentrations of unbound insulin. (*From* LeBlanc J, Nadeau A, Boulay M, et al: Effects of physical training and adiposity on glucose metabolism and ^{125}I-insulin binding. J Appl Physiol Respirat Environ Exerc Physiol 46:237, 1979; with permission.)

1. It would decrease glycogen synthesis in the liver and, therefore, facilitate hepatic glucose output.

2. It may also have an important effect on nonexercising tissues, diminishing glucose uptake.

3. Finally, the decrement in plasma insulin may be important in releasing the inhibition on FFA metabolism and enabling adipose tissue lipolysis to proceed.

An increase in catecholamines will occur early in the response to exercise, and the magnitude of the response will be dependent on the intensity of the exercise, being greatest with high-intensity exercise.[30] Norepinephrine is released from the sympathetic nerve endings and is also correlated to the increase in heart rate response to exercise. Christensen and colleagues[31] have shown a close relationship between plasma norepinephrine concentration and mixed venous-arterial oxygen saturation. We have shown (unpublished observations) that the response in plasma norepinephrine may occur within 30 seconds of the commencement of exercise and so be important in the early increase in hepatic glucose output. Plasma epinephrine is released from the adrenal medulla. Its levels increase in proportion to the intensity of the exercise. The greatest increases are seen when hypoglycemia occurs during exercise, and the increase will be minimized if glucose

TABLE 15–2. HORMONAL RESPONSES TO EXERCISE

↓ Insulin
↑ Glucagon
↑ Catecholamines
  ↑ Norepinephrine
  ↑ Epinephrine
  ↑ Sympathetic nervous system discharge
↑ Cortisol
↑ Growth hormone

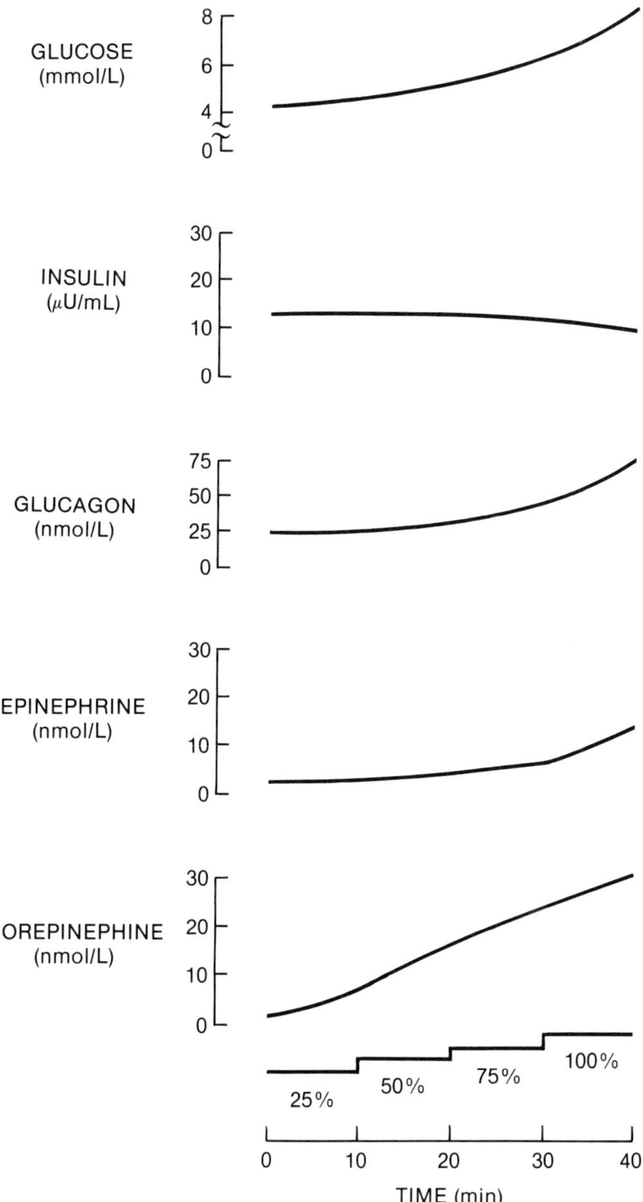

Figure 15–7. Hormonal response to progressive exercise in normal subjects. This is a composite graph. (*Data from* Sutton JR: Hormonal and metabolic responses to exercise in subjects of high and low work capacities. Med Sci Sports 10:1, 1978 *and* Rennie MJ, Jennett S, Johnson RH: The metabolic effect of strenuous exercise: A comparison between untrained subjects and racing cyclists. Q J Exp Physiol 59:201, 1974; with permission.)

concentration is maintained.[12] The important metabolic consequences of increased catecholamines in exercise are to provide the following energy substrates for contracting muscle: *fat,* by stimulating adipose tissue lipolysis and thereby increasing plasma FFAs; and *carbohydrate,* by (1) enhancing hepatic glycoglucolysis, (2) increasing muscle glycogen breakdown, and (3) inhibiting pancreatic beta cell secretion of insulin. All of these factors tend to result in the maintenance of euglycemia during exercise and the preservation of central nervous system function.

Other hormonal changes in exercise that have a bearing on fat and carbohydrate metabolism but that are not as significant as the foregoing are those of growth hormone and cortisol. With both, the increase with exercise[32] tends to be in proportion to the intensity of the exercise; with growth hormone, the response in plasma concentration may persist for several hours after exercise ceases.[33] Cortisol may potentiate the effect of epinephrine on hepatic glycogenolysis, and both cortisol and growth hormone may impair the cellular action of insulin—cortisol, by inhibiting the receptor affinity, and growth hormone, by decreasing insulin receptor concentration.

FACTORS THAT DETERMINE PLASMA GLUCOSE RESPONSE TO EXERCISE

The balance between peripheral glucose uptake and hepatic glucose output determines the plasma glucose response to exercise:

1. *Peripheral glucose uptake* (glucose disposal) will be determined by:
   a. Insulin concentration.
   b. Counterregulatory hormone concentrations: catecholamines, cortisol, and growth hormone.
   c. Changes at the insulin receptor site, both in receptor number and in insulin binding to the receptor.
   d. Postreceptor changes in muscle: cyclic adenosine monophosphate (AMP) and rate-limiting enzymes in the glycolytic pathway are altered, including changes in hexokinase, glycogen phosphorylase, phosphofructokinase, and pyruvate dehydrogenase.[34]
2. *Hepatic glucose output.* Regulatory factors are unknown but may be neuronal. Under steady-state conditions of moderate-intensity exercise, hepatic glucose output is perfectly matched to peripheral glucose output, independent of insulin or the counterregulatory hormones, at least in short-term exercise.[14, 35] However, under most physiologic situations of high intensity, short bursts of exercise result in hyperglycemia where hepatic glucose output exceeds glucose disposal rate.

METABOLIC AND HORMONAL RESPONSES TO EXERCISE IN DIABETIC INDIVIDUALS

In insulin-dependent (type I) diabetics, the chance of hypoglycemia during exercise is well known. Early in the postinsulin era, it was discovered that the insulin requirements of a juvenile diabetic decreased if the patient was physically active. In 1926, Lawrence[36] published a study indicating that the decrease in blood glucose following an insulin injection at rest was magnified when the insulin injection was followed by physical exercise. Figure 15–8 illustrates such a situation; blood glucose dropped from nearly 250 to 50 mg/dL. This patient experienced symptoms of hypoglycemia. Thus, although insulin requirements appeared to be lower in exercising diabetics, the interrelationship between insulin and exercise was thought to be a precarious one and certainly not unassociated with hazard. Two extremes were seen. Patients who were poorly controlled and ketotic seemed to be made worse by exercise; they became more hyperglycemic and more ketotic (Fig. 15–9). On the other hand, there were young physically active diabetics in whom the association of insulin and exercise produced significant hypoglycemia. These findings seemed to be quite paradoxical, and it was only many years later that we began to understand how such events could occur. This topic was recently reviewed.[37]

In moderately well-controlled diabetics, the responses in glucose, FFAs, ketone bodies, and glucoregulatory hormones are relatively similar to those in normal subjects.[38] As was well known in the preinsulin era, with regular exercise and training such individuals

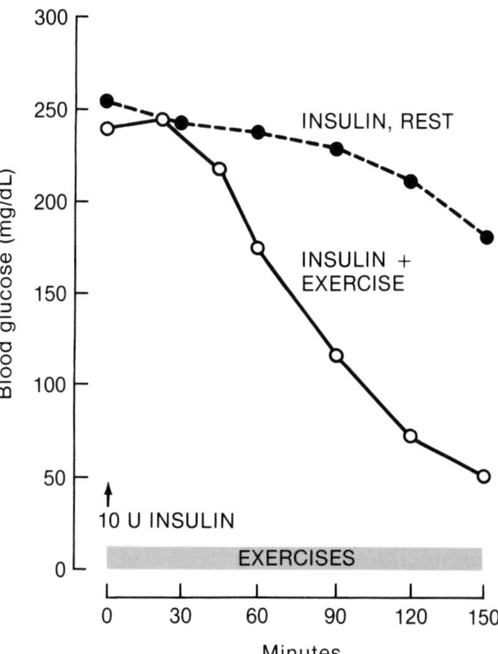

Figure 15–8. Blood glucose levels in a diabetic individual following subcutaneous injection of insulin (10 U). On one day, the subject rested; 2 days later, the same study was performed, but the subject exercised and developed symptoms of hypoglycemia between the 120th and 150th minutes. (*From* Lawrence RD: Br Med J 1:648–650, 1926.)

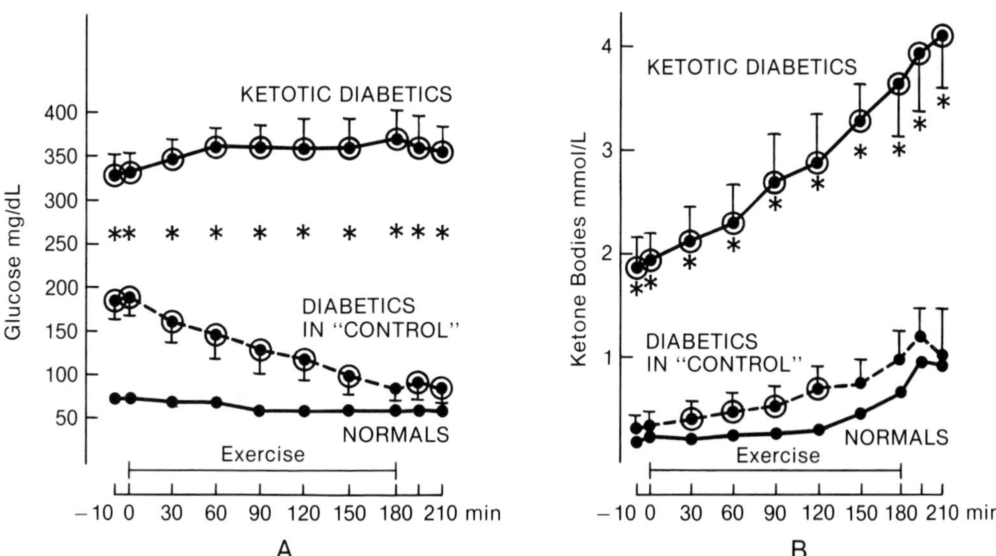

Figure 15–9. The effect of prolonged exercise on glucose and ketone bodies (acetoacetate and 3-hydroxybutyrate) in healthy control subjects, diabetic patients in moderate metabolic control, and diabetic patients who were ketotic. Asterisks indicate significant difference ($P < 0.05$). (*Adapted from* Berger M, Berchtold P, Cüppers HJ, et al: Metabolic and hormonal effects of muscular exercise in juvenile type diabetes. Diabetologia 13:355, 1977; with permission.)

decrease their daily insulin requirement. It is important that a permissive amount of insulin be present because it is required for glucose uptake in muscle. Studies in totally depancreatized dogs show that in the absence of any measurable insulin, exercise does not result in an increased muscle glucose uptake and, thus, the ketotic diabetic will become worse during exercise. Both Berger and coworkers[38] and Christensen[39] have demonstrated that the ketotic diabetic will have a greater response in glucagon, catecholamines, growth hormone, and glucocorticoids during exercise, all of which will tend to aggravate the hyperglycemic, hyperlipidemic, and ketotic states.

Hypoglycemia is one of the most common and important clinical problems for diabetics who exercise. In some brittle diabetics, the change from hyperglycemia to hypoglycemia can be very quick and dramatic. There is considerable individual variation in the predisposition to hypoglycemia during exercise in diabetics, and there has been some evidence from Zinman and colleagues[40] that exercise may increase the absorption of subcutaneously injected insulin. When insulin concentration is sufficiently high, the ability of hepatic glycogenolysis to respond to the increased glucose need is suppressed. Thus, exercise would enhance the muscle uptake of glucose but with insufficient hepatic glucose output, hypoglycemia would occur. The common occurrence of hypoglycemia in insulin-dependent diabetics thus appeared to have a rather simple explanation. When insulin was injected into the thigh rather than the arm or the abdomen, exercise resulted in a greater absorption of insulin and the delivery to liver and muscle provided the environment in which hypoglycemia occurred. This thought was supported by Dandona and colleagues[41] and by Koivisto and Felig.[42] However, such a simple explanation has been disputed by Kemmer and coworkers,[43] although there were some differences in the experimental protocols. Kemmer and colleagues[43] used approximately twice the amount of insulin, and the delay between the insulin injection and the beginning of exercise was 30 minutes rather than 5 minutes, as in the Koivisto and Felig experiment. Furthermore, studies by Chisholm and associates[14] have suggested that fourfold differences in plasma insulin concentration would have very little impact on the hepatic glucose output and peripheral uptake of insulin when subjects perform moderate exercise (about 60% $\dot{V}O_{2max}$). Perhaps the most detailed examination of the absorption kinetics and the biological effects of subcutaneously injected insulin was that performed by Berger and coworkers[44] in 1982. They again found very little influence of exercise on the rate of absorption of insulin from subcutaneously injected sites. However, other important aspects of their study include the fact that the rate of insulin absorption was greatest after injection into the abdomen rather than the arm or thigh; a hot bath and local massage dramatically increased insulin levels in the first 90 minutes after injection. These workers also performed studies on different types of insulin and, not surprisingly, found some slight differences in the rate of absorption of the various long-acting preparations and mixtures of short- and long-acting preparations. In general terms, it appears that the longer the duration of action of the insulin, the longer the time period following injection and the more its absorption may be altered by exercise; again, however, one must stress the great individual variation.

Interrelationships of Insulin Secretion with Other Drugs

Like many other endocrine organs, the membrane of the pancreatic beta cell contains adenyl cyclase. Activation of this system and the formation of cyclic AMP have a vital role in the control of insulin secretion. Beta-adrenergic stimulation enhances, whereas alpha-adrenergic stimulation inhibits, the secretion of insulin.[45] Thus, drugs such as isoproterenol will augment insulin secretion, but epinephrine would have an inhibitory effect and would be expected to aggravate the diabetic state. Both of these drugs are used in the treatment of asthma. Other drugs commonly used in the treatment of asthma are theophylline and its derivatives (eg, aminophylline). Theophylline inhibits the activity of phosphodiesterase, the enzyme responsible for the hydrolysis of cyclic AMP.[46] Consequently, the insulin response to a standard glucose challenge is augmented. Thus, it can be seen that in a diabetic asthmatic patient, these drugs can further complicate the picture.

More recently, it has been shown that other agents that are not obvious alpha or beta agonists or antagonists can impair the diabetic state. For instance, diphenylhydantoin (Dilantin [Parke-Davis, Morris Plains, NJ]), a drug used in the treatment of epilepsy, will suppress insulin secretion.[47,48] The picture becomes more complex when we find that serotonin-blocking agents, such as methysergide, interfere with insulin secretion,[49] as do potassium- and calcium-altering drugs (for example, diuretics).[47] Thus, in the management of diabetes, the interrelationship between drugs as well as exercise is important in assessing the overall glucose homeostasis.

Certain beta-blocking agents, such as propranolol, stimulate muscle glucose uptake.[50] However, in an elegant series of studies in depancreatized totally insulin-deprived dogs[51] and alloxan-diabetic dogs[50] with residual insulin secretion, Vranic's group concluded that there was a limited role of catecholamines in regulation of glucose uptake in exercise. Only when sufficient insulin was available to inhibit FFA mobilization did propranolol increase glucose metabolic clearance (Fig. 15–10).[52]

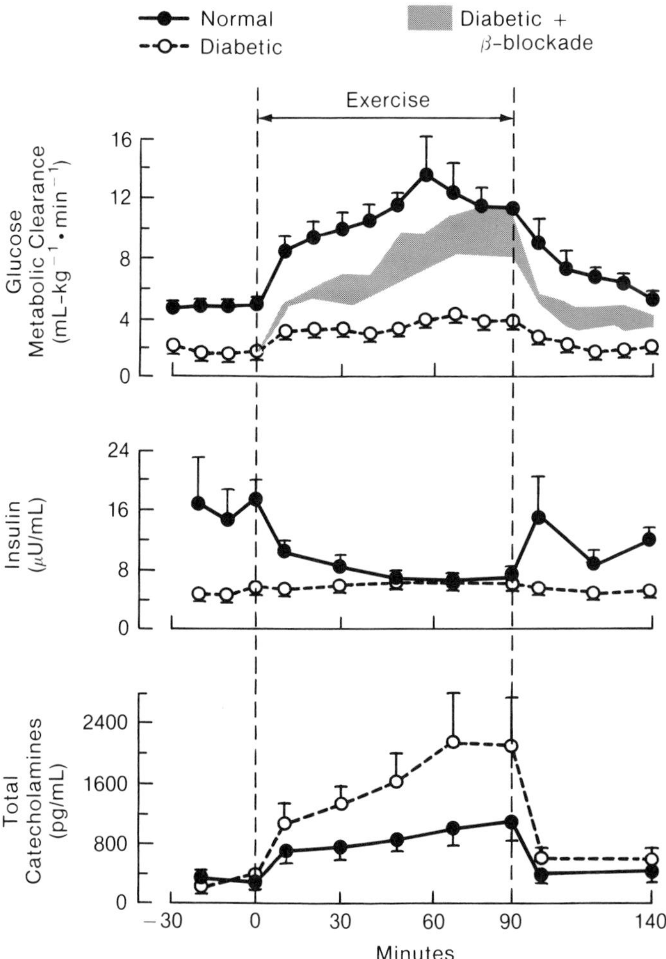

Figure 15–10. Effect of exercise on glucose metabolic clearance rate, immunoreactive insulin, and total catecholamines in normal dogs (n = 5; *solid line*) and alloxan-diabetic dogs (n = 6; *dashed line*). Stippled area in panel A represents the effect of exercise with beta-blockade in alloxan-diabetic dogs (n = 6). (*From* Wasserman DH, Vranic M: Interaction between insulin and counterregulatory hormones in control of substrate utilization in health and diabetes during exercise. Diabetes Metab Rev 1(4):159, 1986; with permission.)

In normal subjects, beta-blockade can be associated with significant metabolic effects. In normal subjects, there is no change in plasma glucose during exercise with the addition of propranolol but there is a further diminution in FFA levels, presumably related to the inhibition of lipolysis. However, in a comparison of the effects in diabetic subjects, propranolol affects both plasma glucose and FFAs. A number of diabetics who are hypertensive or who have angina, if treated with propranolol, will have not only hepatic glycogenolysis impairment and be unable to maintain glucose homeostasis but also will have an inhibition of FFA mobilization.[53] Thus, the usual sources of ATP generation will be impaired. In contrast, the more cardioselective beta-blockers do not appear to result in hypoglycemia.[54] Furthermore, cardioselectivity may affect the circulatory responses to hypoglycemia. With acute administration of propranolol, hypoglycemia is followed by sinus bradycardia and an increase in systolic and diastolic blood pressure, but this does not appear to be so with the more selective beta-blockers, such as metoprolol.[54] Thus, if a diabetic person prone to hypoglycemic episodes must be treated with a beta-blocker, a cardioselective agent is preferable because it may lessen the risk of hypoglycemia.

MANAGEMENT CONSIDERATIONS IN DIABETIC PATIENTS

The major treatment goals in diabetics are to optimize the regulation of blood glucose levels and to prevent and treat complications of diabetes. As diabetes is a lifelong disorder, optimum regulation of blood glucose levels will occur only if diabetic persons have a good understanding of the nature of their problem and work in association with a health care team. In young diabetics, education of the patients and their families is vital; this is becoming easier with the evolution of specific centers and diabetic day care clinics.

The objective of treatment of insulin-dependent diabetes mellitus patients is to maintain blood glucose levels within the physiologic range throughout the 24-hour period. This is almost impossible with the conventional once-daily insulin injection, and it is clear that home testing is the optimal way to monitor blood glucose levels. In so doing, it is also vital to understand the appropriate timing of the blood sample with reference to insulin injection, food intake, and exercise.

Urine testing of glucose provides only a rough guide because there is tremendous dependence on the renal threshold, rapidity of the change of blood glucose levels, and the time between voiding. Urine glucose testing is most useful in stable patients who usually have little glycosuria. However, urine testing for ketones cannot be overemphasized, particularly when diabetics develop an intercurrent illness, if they are unwell in any way, or if they develop persistent hyperglycemia.

Diet

Diet must provide sufficient energy for the activity of the individual, together with appropriate nutrients. It is important that the meals and snacks have a consistent amount of carbohydrate and are taken at regular times. One of the most common problems is an underestimation of the amount of carbohydrate needed for various sports and activities.

Insulin Requirements

There are several types of insulin commonly used. Each has a characteristic time of action that allows for a large number of different insulin strategies. The single morning dose of intermediate-acting insulin has been the custom, but the use of additional short-acting insulin at the same time tends to provide better control, particularly before lunch. However, it has now become clear that to maintain near-normal blood glucose levels, three or perhaps four injections of insulin daily are required, using combinations of shorter- and longer-acting insulin. As one strives to achieve normoglycemia, symptoms of mild hypoglycemia are bound to appear, especially asssociated with increased activity or decreased food intake. The diabetic patient should be aware of such possibilities and should always carry extra glucose.

Physical Activity

In the preinsulin era, physical exercise was one of the mainstays of treatment. The role of physical activity in the management of the diabetic patient is of no less importance today, as it will improve metabolic control in both the noninsulin-dependent and the insulin-dependent diabetic. This may result in a decreased insulin requirement.[55,56] It appears that this occurs by an enhanced insulin binding to receptor sites on monocytes and also, presumably, on muscle cells. However, the stability of blood glucose may not be improved by physical activity. Another potential benefit of physical activity in diabetics would be to minimize the impact of the cardiovascular complications.

Non–Insulin-Dependent Diabetes (Type II, or Maturity Onset Diabetes)

A defect in the peripheral response to insulin (insulin resistance) rather than an impaired insulin secretion is now considered to be the mechanism of glucose intolerance in non–insulin-dependent diabetic and obese patients. In fact, 80% of non–insulin-dependent diabetic patients are overweight. However, there are significant differences between the obese nondiabetic and the obese diabetic individual as demonstrated by Minuk and associates (Fig. 15–11).[57]

In non–insulin-dependent diabetes mellitus (NIDDM) patients with hyperglycemia of 11.0 mmol, plasma glucose fell by about 2.7 mmol in 45 minutes primarily because hepatic glucose production was impaired while glucose utilization remained normal. Thus, for a given increase in plasma insulin, glucose uptake is reduced compared with normal uptake. However, these subjects secrete insulin normally, or even in excess, in response to an oral glucose load. Thus, the glucose intolerance is due to a peripheral tissue resistance to insulin.

Because physical training enhances tissue sensitivity to insulin, it stands to reason that an activity program should be one of the mainstays of therapy in the management of any insulin-resistant state. However, improvements in glucose tolerance with moderate training have been either nonexistent or very modest.[58–60] Only if training is of high intensity and for a prolonged time will it improve glucose tolerance and then only briefly.[61] The acute effects of exercise on glucose tolerance in these subjects has been recently reviewed.[62]

NIDDM is a significant health problem and is closely associated with overeating. Epidemiologic studies show that the prevalence of NIDDM increases with body weight, especially in those with a family history. A recent consensus conference on NIDDM concluded that attempts to control body weight with diet and exercise were the cornerstones of treatment. The use of oral hypoglycemic agents and insulin was then additional. This group emphasized diet, concluding that specific dietary inclusion, such as high fiber, although helpful in certain individuals, was not as important as calorie restriction.

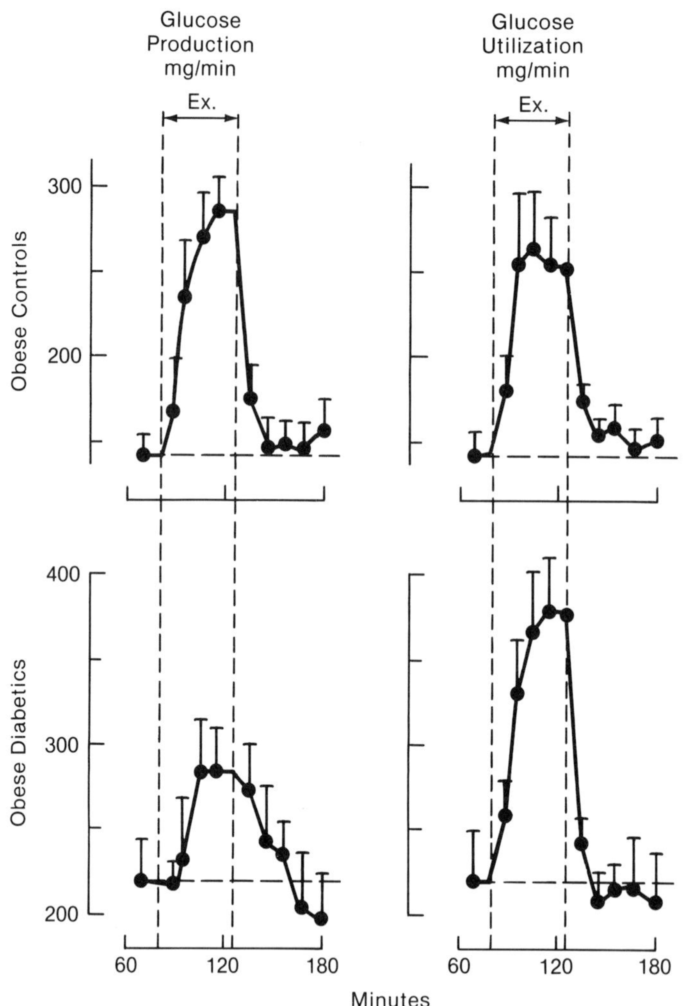

Figure 15–11. Glucose production and utilization in seven obese controls *(upper panel)* and ten obese non–insulin-dependent patients *(lower panel)* during rest, exercise (60% $\dot{V}O_{2max}$), and recovery. Means and standard errors are shown. (*From* Minuk HL, Vranic M, Marliss EB, et al: Glucoregulatory and metabolic response to exercise in obese non–insulin-dependent diabetes. Am J Physiol 240:E458, 1981; with permission.)

CONCLUSIONS

Exercise results in a 10 to 20 fold increase in metabolic rate. The energy for this is supplied principally by the metabolism of fats and carbohydrates. During moderate exercise, significant increases can occur in glucose uptake without a dramatic change in plasma glucose. Thus, there is a fine link between the peripheral uptake of glucose and hepatic glycogenolysis. In insulin-dependent diabetes mellitus (IDDM) patients, there is no contraindication to exercise, provided that they are well controlled and have an understanding of the relationship between insulin injections, dietary intake of food, illness, and exercise. However, the poorly controlled diabetic may become more hyperglycemic and ketotic with exercise, although hypoglycemia is a more frequent observation. General principles of diabetic control apply to the diabetic who wishes to become physically active and, in fact, a minimum of physical activity should be an essential ingredient in the optimum management of diabetics.

Additional difficulties arise in diabetic control if, for some other health reasons, the diabetic patient requires medication such as beta-sympathomimetic amines as for the control of asthma, or beta-blockers for the management of ischemic heart disease or hypertension. In general, beta-blockers, if used, should be the cardioselective type. As physical training increases tissue sensitivity to insulin, physical activity programs may provide effective therapy for insulin-resistant states, such as the NIDDM patient who, in 80% of cases, is also obese. Caloric restriction coupled with exercise is the cornerstone of treatment. Exercise might carry more difficulties for the insulin-requiring diabetic. However, there are significant short- and long-term benefits to be gained in both the maintenance of normoglycemia and the general psychological and physical well-being of diabetic persons who can see themselves participating along with their peers in various sports and activities. Especially in the NIDDM patient, exercise is valuable in preventing the cardiovascular complications.

REFERENCES

1. Ekoe JM: Overview of diabetes mellitus and exercise. Med Sci Sports Exerc 21:353, 1989.
2. Consensus development conference on diet and exercise in non–insulin dependent diabetes mellitus. Diabetes Care 10:639, 1987.
3. Horton ES: Role and management of exercise in diabetes mellitus. Diabetes Care 11:201, 1988.
4. Vranic M, Berger M: Exercise and diabetes mellitus. Diabetes 28:147, 1979.
5. Joslin EP: The treatment of diabetes mellitus. *In* Joslin EP, Root HF, White P, et al (eds): The Treatment of Diabetes Mellitus, ed 10. Philadelphia, Lea & Febiger, 1959, pp 243–300.
6. Richter EA, Ruderman, NB, Schneider SH: Diabetes and exercise. Am J Med 70:201, 1981.
7. Sutton JR: Drugs used in metabolic disorders. Med Sci Sports Exerc 13:266, 1981.
8. Terjung R: Endocrine response to exercise. *In* Hutton RS (ed): Exercise and Sports Sciences Review, vol 7. Philadelphia, Franklin Institute Press, 1979, pp 153–180.
9. Vranic M, Wasserman D: Exercise, fitness and diabetes. *In* Bouchard C, Shephard RJ, Stephens T, et al (eds): Exercise, Fitness and Health. Champaign, IL, Human Kinetics Publishers, 1990, pp 467–490.
10. Levine SA, Gordon B, Derick CL: Some changes in the chemical constituents of the blood following a marathon race. JAMA 82:1778, 1924.
11. Sutton J, Coleman MJ, Millar AP, et al: The medical problems of mass participation in athletic competition: The "City-to-Surf" race. Med J Aust 2:127, 1972.
12. Felig P, Cherif A, Minagawa A, et al: Hypoglycemia during prolonged exercise in normal men. N Engl J Med 306:895, 1982.
13. Christensen EH, Hansen O: Arbeitsfähigkeit und Ernährung. Skand Arch Physiol 81:160, 1939.
14. Chisholm DJ, Jenkins AB, James DE, et al: The effect of hyperinsulinemia on glucose homeostasis during moderate exercise in man. Diabetes 31:603, 1982.
15. Wahren J, Felig P, Ahlborg G, et al: Glucose metabolism during leg exercise in man. J Clin Invest 50:2715, 1971.
16. Sutton JR: Hormonal and metabolic responses to exercise in subjects of high and low work capacities. Med Sci Sports 10:1, 1978.
17. Sutton JR, Jurkowski JE, Keane PM: The effect of the menstrual cycle on the plasma catecholamine response to exercise in normal females. Clin Res 26:847A, 1978.
18. Issekutz B Jr, Paul P, Miller HI: Metabolism in normal and pancreatectomized dogs during steady state exercise. Am J Physiol 23:857, 1967.
19. Rennie MJ, Winder WW, Holloszy JO: A sparing effect of increased plasma fatty acids on muscle and liver glycogen content in the exercising rat. Biochem J 156:647, 1976.
20. Costill DL, Coyle E, Dalsky G, et al: Effects of elevated plasma FFA and insulin on muscle glycogen usage during exercise. J Appl Physiol Respirat Environ Exerc Physiol 43:695, 1977.
21. Vranic M, Kawamori R: Essential roles of insulin and glucagon in regulating glucose fluxes during exercise in dogs: Mechanism of hypoglycemia. Diabetes 28 (suppl 1):45, 1979.
22. Pedersen O, Beck-Nielsen H, Heding L: Increased insulin receptors after exercise in patients with insulin-dependent diabetes mellitus. N Engl J Med 302:886, 1980.
23. Soman VR, Koivisto VA, Grantham P, et al: Increased insulin binding to monocytes after acute exercise in normal man. J Clin Endocrinol Metab 47:216, 1978.

24. LeBlanc J, Nadeau A, Boulay M, et al: Effects of physical training and adiposity on glucose metabolism and ^{125}I-insulin binding. J Appl Physiol Respirat Environ Exerc Physiol 46:235, 1979.
25. Burstein R: Changes in insulin resistance in trained athletes upon cessation of training [thesis]. Hamilton, Ontario, Canada, McMaster University, 1982.
26. Roth J, Grunfeld C: Endocrine systems: Mechanisms of disease, target cells and receptors. *In* Williams RH (ed): Textbook of Endocrinology. Philadelphia, WB Saunders, 1981, pp 34–35.
27. Sutton JR, Farrell PA, Harber VJ: Hormonal adaptation to physical activity. *In* Bouchard C, Shephard RJ, Stephens T, et al (eds): Exercise, Fitness and Diabetes. Champaign, IL, Human Kinetics Publishers, 1990, pp 217–243.
28. Pruett, EDR: Plasma insulin concentrations during prolonged work at near maximal oxygen uptake. J Appl Physiol 29:155, 1970.
29. Böttger I, Schlein EM, Faloona, GL, et al: The effect of exercise on glucagon secretion. J Clin Endocrinol 35:117, 1972.
30. Galbo H, Holst JJ, Christensen NJ: Glucagon and plasma catecholamine responses to graded and prolonged exercise in man. J Appl Physiol 38:70, 1975.
31. Christensen NJ, Galbo H, Hansen JF, et al: Catecholamines and exercise. Diabetes 28 (suppl 1):58, 1979.
32. Sutton JR, Casey JH: The adrenocortical response to competitive athletics in veteran athletes. J Clin Endocrinol Metab 40:135, 1975.
33. Sutton JR, Young JD, Lazarus, L, et al: Hormonal response to physical exercise. Aust Ann Med 18:84, 1969.
34. Ward GR, Sutton JR, Jones NL, et al: Activation by exercise of human skeletal muscle pyruvate dehydrogenase in vivo. Clin Sci 63:87, 1982.
35. Vranic M, Wrenshall GA: Exercise, insulin and glucose turnover in dogs. Endocrinology 85:165, 1969.
36. Lawrence RD: The effect of exercise on insulin action in diabetes. Br Med J 1:648, 1926.
37. Wallberg-Henriksson H: Acute exercise: Fuel homeostasis and glucose transport in insulin-dependent diabetes mellitus. Med Sci Sports Exerc 21:356, 1989.
38. Berger M, Berchtold P, Cüppers HJ, et al: Metabolic and hormonal effects of muscular exercise in juvenile type diabetes. Diabetologia 13:355, 1977.
39. Christensen NJ: Plasma norepinephrine and epinephrine in untreated diabetics, during fasting and after insulin administration. Diabetes 23:1, 1974.
40. Zinman B, Murray FT, Vranic M, et al: Glucoregulation during moderate exercise in insulin treated diabetics. J Clin Endocrinol Metab 45:641, 1977.
41. Dandona P, Hooke D, Bell J: Exercise and insulin absorption from subcutaneous tissue. Br Med J 1:479, 1978.
42. Koivisto VA, Felig P: Effects of leg exercise on insulin absorption in diabetic patients. N Engl J Med 298:79, 1978.
43. Kemmer FW, Berchtold P, Berger M, et al: Exercise-induced fall of blood glucose in insulin-treated diabetics unrelated to alteration of insulin mobilization. Diabetes 28:1131, 1979.
44. Berger M, Cüppers HJ, Hegner H, et al: Absorption kinetics and biologic effects of subcutaneously injected insulin preparations. Diabetes Care 5:77, 1982.
45. Porte D Jr, Graber AL, Kuzuya T, et al: The effect of epinephrine on immunoreactive insulin levels in man. J Clin Invest 45:228, 1966.
46. Ensinck JW, Stroll RW, Gale CG, et al: Effect of aminophylline on the secretion of insulin, glucagon, luteinizing hormone and growth hormone in humans. J Clin Endocrinol Metab 31:153, 1970.
47. Arky RA: Diphenylhydantoin and the beta cell. N Engl J Med 286:371, 1972.
48. Malherve C, Burrill KC, Levin SR, et al: Effect of diphenylhydantoin on insulin secretion in man. N Engl J Med 286:339, 1972.
49. Quickel KE Jr, Feldman JM, Lebovitz HE: Enhancement of insulin secretion in adult onset diabetics by methysergide maleate: Evidence for an endogenous biogenic monoamine mechanism as a factor in the impaired insulin secretion in diabetes mellitus. J Clin Endocrinol Metab 33:877, 1971.
50. Wasserman DH, Lickley HLA, Vranic M: Role of beta-adrenergic mechanisms during exercise in poorly controlled insulin deficient diabetes. J Appl Physiol 59:1282, 1985.
51. Bjorkman O, Miles P, Wasserman DH, et al: Regulation of glucose turnover during exercise in pancreatectomized totally insulin-deficient dogs: Effects of beta adrenergic blockade. J Clin Invest 81:759–767, 1988.
52. Wasserman DH, Vranic M: Interaction betweeen insulin and counter regulatory hormones in control of substrate utilization in health and diabetics during exercise. Diabetes Metab Rev 1(1):159, 1986.
53. Hansen AP: The effect of adrenergic receptor blockade on the exercise-induced serum growth hormone rise in normals and juvenile diabetics. J Clin Endocrinol Metab 33:807, 1971.
54. Davidson NM, Corrall RJM, Shaw TRD, et al: Observations in man of hypoglycaemia during selective and non-selective beta-blockage. Scott Med J 22:69, 1976.

55. Ruderman NB, Ganda OP, Johansen K: The effect of physical training on glucose tolerance and plasma lipids in maturity-onset diabetes. Diabetes 28 (suppl 1):89, 1979.
56. Saltin B, Lindgärde F, Houston M, et al: Physical training and glucose tolerance in middle-aged men with chemical diabetes. Diabetes 28 (suppl 1):30, 1979.
57. Minuk HL, Vranic M, Marliss EB, et al: Glucoregulatory and metabolic response to exercise in obese non–insulin-dependent diabetes. Am J Physiol 240:E458, 1981.
58. Krotkiewski M, Lonnroth P, Mandroukas K, et al: The effect of physical training on insulin secretion and effectiveness and on glucose metabolism in obesity and type 2 (non-insulin–dependent) diabetes mellitus. Diabetologia 28:881–890, 1985.
59. Leblanc J, Nadeau A, Richard R, et al: Studies on the sparing effect of exercise on insulin requirements in human subjects. Metabolism 30:1119–1124, 1981.
60. Ruderman NB, Ganda OP, Johansen K: Effects of physical training on glucose tolerance and plasma lipids in maturity onset diabetes mellitus. Diabetes 28(suppl):89–92, 1979.
61. Holloszy JO, Schultz J, Kusnierkiewicz J, et al: Effects of exercise on glucose tolerance and insulin resistance. Acta Med Scand(Suppl) 711:55–65, 1986.
62. Rogers MA: Acute effects of exercise on glucose tolerance in non-insulin–dependent diabetes. Med Sci Sports Exerc 21:362–368, 1989.

16

NUTRITION

Nancy Clark, MS, RD

This chapter offers practical sports nutrition information that addresses the nutrition questions athletes commonly ask. The information will help you guide your clients toward selecting a high quality sports diet that (1) fuels the muscles for top performance, (2) nourishes the body, and (3) contributes to current health and future longevity.

CARBOHYDRATES—THE FOUNDATION OF THE SPORTS DIET

Athletes should eat a 60% to 70% carbohydrate diet on a daily basis to get adequate carbohydrates for both training and competing. These carbohydrates get stored (1) as muscle glycogen, needed to perform exercise; and (2) as liver glycogen, needed to maintain normal blood glucose level. Unfortunately, misconceptions about carbohydrates—what they are and what they aren't—keep many athletes from making the best carbohydrate selections.

Carbohydrates include both sugars and starches; both get stored as glycogen but have differing abilities to nourish the athlete with vitamins and minerals. The carbohydrates in sugary soda pop or sports drinks get stored as glycogen but provide little or no vitamins or minerals. The carboyhdrates in wholesome fruits, vegetables, and grains also get stored as glycogen *plus* provide vitamins and minerals—the spark plugs that help the athlete's "engine" to perform at its best.

The average 150-lb active man has about 1800 calories of carbohydrates stored in his liver, muscles, and blood in approximately the following distribution:

Muscle glycogen	1400 calories
Liver glycogen	320 calories
Blood glucose	80 calories

These carbohydrate stores determine how long an athlete can exercise. Depleted muscle glycogen results in "hitting the wall" and the inability to exercise energetically. Depleted liver glycogen results in a low blood glucose level and causes the athlete to "bonk" or "crash," feeling lightheaded, uncoordinated, unable to concentrate, and overwhelmingly fatigued. Proper preexercise nutrition, which includes adequate carbohydrates, can reduce the likelihood of becoming glycogen-depleted. (This will be discussed in the section on preexercise nutrition.)

Carbohydrates are important for all athletes regardless of sport; both runners and body builders alike need this fuel for performing their desired type of exercise. Weight-conscious athletes, such as runners and figure skaters, often try to "stay away" from carbohydrates, believing them to be fattening. Carbohydrates are *not* fattening. They supply only 4 calories per gram, as compared to fats, which offer 9 calories per gram. Carbohydrates can become fattening if eaten with fatty foods, such as *butter* on bread, *gravy* on potato, and *mayonnaise* on a sandwich. Because carbohydrates are likely to be burned off rather than stored as fat, even weight-conscious athletes can and should include them as the foundation of their sports diet.

To consume a daily sports diet that provides 60% to 70% of its calories from carbohydrates, the athlete should opt for more grains and starches, and fewer fatty, greasy foods. By working with a sports nutritionist, the athlete can learn the appropriate food choices, such as having bagels instead of croissants, pancakes instead of eggs, pasta instead of steak (Table 16–1).

Food labels, which list the grams of carbohydrates per serving can assist with appropriate food selection. Some dedicated athletes "count carbohydrates" to reach their daily quota. For example, an athlete who eats 3500 calories/day should eat at least 60% of those calories in the form of carbohydrates:

60% × 3500 calories = 2100 calories of carbohydrates
= 525 grams of carbohydrates (approximately 4 calories per gram carbohydrate)

A second way of estimating carbohydrate needs is to multiply body weight by 3 to 4 grams carbohydrate per pound.[1] Hence, a 150-lb runner who burns about 2800 to 3700 calories when running 7 to 15 miles per day would get 65% of those calories from carbohydrates by eating 3 to 4 g carbohydrate/lb (450 to 600 g carbohydrate). When sitting down to breakfast and reading the food labels, the athlete can calculate his or her carbohydrate intake: ½ cup Grapenuts, 46 g; 1 cup milk, 8 g; 1 cup orange juice, 25 g. This educational exercise will enhance both food knowledge and appropriate food selections.

FAT

For both cardiovascular health and optimal sports performance, athletes should reduce their intake of fatty, greasy foods such as donuts, pastries, butter, mayonnaise, french fries, and ice cream. These foods tend to fill the stomach but leave the muscles unfueled; they also may contribute to elevated blood cholesterol levels. Since the typical American diet is about 40% fat but only 45% carbohydrate, the athletes need to trade in fat calories for more carbohydrates to bring their sports diet to 25% fat, 60% carbohydrate—that is, eat two plain bagels (400 calories of primarily carbohydrates) as opposed to one bagel with cream cheese (approximately 400 calories, 50% from fat).

Although eating *too much* fat is the standard problem among athletes, overly compulsive personalities commonly try to cut *all* fats out of their diet. They often become overly restrictive with their food choices, eating only fat-free foods such as rice cakes, broccoli, and nonfat yogurt. This restrictiveness, at times, may border on an eating disorder. Since 20% to 25% of the calories in a sports diet can appropriately come from fat, this entitles the athlete to a small amount of fat, as can be easily consumed in the hidden fats in wholesome muffins, lean meats, and other popular foods.

Athletes with high caloric demands who severely restrict their fat intake may have trouble consuming adequate calories and maintaining their weight if they don't replace the deleted fat calories with adequate carbohydrates. For example, instead of having one baked potato drenched with butter and sour cream (400 calories), the athlete would need to eat two plain potatoes (400 calories). Sometimes the sheer volume of food poses a problem because the athlete may tire of chewing before being adequately fed. By working with a sports nutritionist, athletes can be taught how to include appropriate amounts of heart-healthy fats, such as peanut butter and olive oil, into their 60% to 70% carbohydrate sports diet.

TABLE 16–1. SAMPLE HIGH-CARBOHYDRATE, FAST-FOOD MEALS*

	Total Cal	CHO Cal	
Breakfast			
McDonald's Fast Food			
Orange juice, 6 oz	85	80	
Pancakes, syrup	420	360	
English muffin, jelly	155	120	
TOTAL	660		85% carbohydrate
Muffin House, Bakery			
Bran muffin, large	320	205	
Hot cocoa, large	180	100	
TOTAL	500		61% carbohydrate
Family Restaurant			
Apple juice, large	145	145	
Raisin Bran, 2 sm boxes	220	200	
Low-fat milk, 8 oz	110	80	
Sliced banana, medium	125	120	
TOTAL	600		91% carbohydrate
Lunch			
Sub Shop			
Turkey sub, no mayo	655	340	
Fruit yogurt, Dannon	260	200	
Orange juice, half-pint	110	105	
TOTAL	1025		63% carbohydrate
Wendy's Fast Food			
Plain baked potato	240	200	
Chili, 1 cup	230	100	
Chocolate shake	390	220	
TOTAL	860		60% carbohydrate
Salad Bar			
Lettuce, 1 cup	15	10	
Green pepper, ½	10	8	
Broccoli, ½ cup	20	15	
Carrots, ½ cup	20	17	
Tomato, large	50	45	
Chick peas, ½ cup	170	120	
Feta cheese, 1 oz	75	0	
Italian dressing, 2 T	100	0	
Bread, 1″ slice	200	180	
TOTAL	660		60% carbohydrate
Dinner			
Pizzeria			
Cheese pizza, 4 sl, 13″	920	520	
Large cola, 12 oz	150	150	
TOTAL	1070		63% carbohydrate
Italian Restaurant			
Minestrone soup, 1 cup	85	60	
Spaghetti, 2 cups	400	320	
Tomato sauce, ⅔ cup	120	60	
Parmesan cheese, 1 T	30	0	
Rolls, 2 large	280	240	
TOTAL	915		74% carbohydrate
Family Restaurant			
Turkey, 5 oz white meat	250	0	
Stuffing, 1 cup	200	160	
Mashed potato, ½ cup	95	60	

TABLE 16–1. SAMPLE HIGH-CARBOHYDRATE, FAST-FOOD MEALS* *Continued*

	Total Cal	CHO Cal	
Dinner			
Family Restaurant			
Peas, ⅔ cup	70	60	
Cranberry sauce, ¼ cup	100	100	
Orange juice, 8 oz	110	105	
Sherbet, 1 scoop	120	110	
TOTAL	945		63% carbohydrate

*These menus are sample sports meals that offer at least 60% carbohydrates. Some of the food items (eg, soft drinks, milk shakes) are not generally recommended as part of an optimal daily diet, but they can be incorporated into a fast-food meal on the road from time to time. The purpose of these sample meals is simply to offer the concept of what a 60+% carbohydrate diet "looks like," so that athletes can use it to guide their food choices. The menus are appropriate for active women and men who need 2000–2600+ calories per day. Food portions may be adjusted to suit individual needs.

Abbreviations: CHO = carbohydrates, cal = calories, oz = ounces, sm = small, mayo = mayonnaise, T = tablespoon, sl = slice.

PROTEIN

Traditionally, athletes have eaten high-protein sports diets, believing that if they eat extra meat, they'll build extra muscle. Excess protein does *not* build muscle; exercise does. To bulk up, the athlete needs to perform resistance exercise, such as weight lifting and push-ups, in addition to eating a wholesome diet. To have adequate energy to perform the muscle-building exercise, the diet should be approximately 60% carbohydrate, 15% protein.

Strange as it may sound, both body builders and marathon runners should eat the same sports diet. Because body builders have comparatively more muscle mass than runners, they generally eat more calories and hence larger protein servings:

- 15% of the 2600 calories a 140-lb marathoner might need are 390 protein-calories, or 97 grams protein, the amount in about 13 ounces of meat
- 15% of the 3600 calories a 170-lb body builder might need are 540 protein-calories, or 135 grams protein, the amount in about 18 ounces of meat

It is hard to specify the exact protein requirement for athletes because their needs vary according to type of sport (endurance athletes need more protein/kg than body builders), total calorie intake (dieters need more protein/kg than athletes eating their full complement of food), and level of growth and training (athletes rapidly building muscles have higher protein needs). To help calculate a client's protein needs, use the following generous yet safe protein recommendations:

Active adult	1.0–1.5 g/kg body weight/day
Growing athlete	1.5–2.0 g/kg body weight/day

This amount is generally consumed through the typical American diet.

When it comes to protein intake, athletes seem to fall into two categories: *protein-pushers,* the body builders, weight lifters, and football players who think they can't get enough protein; and *protein-avoiders,* the runners, triathletes, and dancers who never eat meat in their efforts to bolster their carbohydrate calories as well as eat a low-fat, heart-healthy diet. Both groups can perform poorly due to dietary imbalances. Protein-pushers, such as high-school athletes who frequently eat fast-food burgers and french fries, generally consume a high-fat, high-cholesterol diet that not only leaves their muscles unfueled but also contributes toward heart disease. Protein-avoiders, such as runners who think that meat is bad for their health, tend to be deficient in not only protein, but also iron and zinc, two minerals important for top performance. The trick is to teach athletes how to get *adequate* but not excess portions of *lean* protein. If you suspect a problem imbalance, you might want to refer the client to a sports nutritionist who will evaluate the current protein intake and teach the athlete how to make appropriate adjustments.

Vegetarian athletes who eat no meat tend to differ from the protein-avoiders in that they make the effort to incorporate adequate vegetarian sources of protein into their diet. Rather than simply avoiding meat, they conscientiously include beans, lentils, tofu, nuts, and other vegetarian proteins to fulfill their protein needs. Yet, their diets are still likely to be deficient in iron and zinc, two minerals found primarily in animal proteins, and particularly in red meats. Iron is important for preventing anemia; zinc is important for healing.

IRON

Athletes who become anemic due to an iron-deficient diet are likely to experience needless fatigue upon exertion. Those at highest risk of suffering from iron-deficiency anemia include female athletes, who lose iron through menstruation; athletes who eat no red meats; marathon runners, who may damage red blood cells through "footstrike hemolysis"; endurance athletes, who may lose a significant amount of iron through heavy sweat losses; and teenage athletes, who are growing quickly and may consume inadequate iron to meet their expanded requirements.

TABLE 16–2. IRON IN FOODS*

Food Sources	Iron (mg)	Food Sources	Iron (mg)
Animal			
Liver, 4 oz cooked	10†	Baked beans, ½ c	2
Beef, 4 oz roasted	6†	Kidney beans, ½ c	2
Pork, 4 oz roasted	5†	Bean curd, ¼ cake	2
Turkey, 4 oz roasted dark meat	3†	***Grains***	
Tuna, 6.5 oz light	2†	Cereal, 100% fortified, ¾ c	18
Chicken breast, 4 oz	1†	Kellogg's Raisin Bran, ½ c	18
Fish, 4 oz broiled haddock	1†	Cream of Wheat	9
Egg, 1 lg	1	Wheat Chex, ⅔ c	4.5
Fruits		Spaghetti, ½ c cooked, enriched	1
Prune juice, 8 oz	3	Bread, 1 sl enriched	1
Apricots, 12 halves dried	2	***Other***	
Dates, 10 dried	1	Molasses, 1 T blackstrap	2
Raisins, ⅓ c	1	Brewer's yeast, 1 T	2
Vegetables/Legumes		Wheat germ, ¼ cup	2
Spinach, ½ c cooked	2		
Green peas, ½ c cooked	1		
Broccoli, ½ c cooked	1		

*The recommended daily allowance (RDA) for iron is 10 mg for men and 15 mg for women. This target intake is set high because iron is poorly absorbed. The best iron sources are from animal products.

†This iron is best absorbed.

Abbreviations: mg = milligrams, oz = ounces, lg = large, c = cup, sl = slice, T = tablespoon.

From Clark N: Nancy Clark's Sports Nutrition Guidebook. Champaign, IL, Leisure Press, 1990; with permission.

To boost and/or maintain a high iron intake, an athlete can eat the following foods:

1. Lean cuts of beef, pork, and lamb (4-ounce portions) and the dark meat of chicken and turkey three to four times per week. (The heme iron in these animal proteins is more bioavailable than the iron found in vegetable foods, such as spinach and raisins.)

2. Enriched and fortified breads and cereals (by reading the food label, the athlete can determine if the product has added iron) as well as whole grains, beans, and legumes. (The nonheme iron found in these plant foods has poor bioavailability.)

3. A food rich in vitamin C with each meal, such as a glass of orange juice or a vegetable. (Vitamin C enhances iron absorption from both heme and nonheme iron sources.)

4. Foods cooked in cast iron skillets, particularly acidic foods such as spaghetti sauce. The acid attracts the iron and significantly increases iron content of a food.)

Athletes who do not eat meat or iron-rich foods (Table 16–2) may wish to take an iron supplement as a "health insurance" to possibly reduce their risk of becoming anemic. They should be educated that the iron from a supplement may be poorly absorbed compared with that found in animal proteins, and that they are likely to still have a diet that is deficient in zinc because the two minerals tend to be found in similar foods (Table 16–3). Hence, a supplement that contains both iron and zinc is the better choice but, nevertheless, an imperfect solution.

TABLE 16–3. ZINC IN FOODS*

Animal Sources	Zinc (mg)	Vegetarian Sources	Zinc (mg)
Beef, steak, 4 oz	7	Almonds, 1 oz	0.7
Beef, liver, 4 oz	6	Cashews, 6–8	0.6
Chicken leg, 4 oz	3.5	Peanut butter, 1 T	0.5
Chicken breast, 4 oz	1		
Chicken liver, 4 oz	4	Garbanzo beans, 1 c	2
Pork, 4 oz	4.5	Lentils, 1 c	2
Turkey leg, 4 oz	5	Bread, white, 1 sl	0.2
Turkey breast, 4 oz	2	Bread, whole wheat, 1 sl	0.5
Cheese, cheddar, 1 oz	1	Rice, white, 1 c	0.6
Cheese, cottage, 1 c	1	Rice, brown, 1 c	1.2
Milk, 1 c	1	Oatmeal, 1 c	1.2
Yogurt, 1 c	1	40% Bran flakes, 1 oz	1
		Wheat germ, ¼ c	3.2
Egg, 1 lg	0.5	Shredded wheat, 1 oz	0.8
Clams, 4–5	1	Apple, 1 med	0.1
Crab, 1 c	6.5	Banana, 1 med	0.3
Fish, white, 4 oz	1	Raisins, ¼ c	0.1
Oysters, 2–4	75		
Tuna, 1 can (6.5 oz)	2	Potato, 1 med boiled	0.3
		Spinach, 1 c raw	0.5

*The RDA for zinc is 15 mg. This recommended intake is set high and may be hard to consume, but it should be a target intake, particularly for athletes who sweat heavily and may incur subsequent zinc losses.

Abbreviations: mg = milligrams, oz = ounces, c = cup, T = tablespoon, sl = slice, med = medium, lg = large.

Note: Nutrient data adapted from Pennington J, Church H: Bowes and Church's Food Values of Portions Commonly Used, ed 14. Philadelphia, JB Lippincott, 1985; with permission.

From Clark N: Nancy Clark's Sports Nutrition Guidebook. Champaign, IL, Leisure Press, 1990; with permission.

VITAMIN SUPPLEMENTS

The vitamin business is big business among athletes and Americans in general. For example, 90% of the nation's top female runners take supplements, as do 40% to 60% of the general population. The reasons for taking supplements vary. Some take supplements to compensate for poor eating; others as "health insurance." Many athletes swallow the advertising claims that promise enhanced athletic prowess. Unfortunately, they don't understand that if a claim sounds too good to be true, it probably is!

Supplement-takers often fail to understand that they still need to eat a well-balanced diet, regardless of the amount of vitamins they take, because a pill may contain only 8 to 12 of the more than 50 nutrients they need for top performance. Many athletes spend significant amounts of money on assorted pills and potions, when they could better put that money toward wholesome foods. If they are taking supplements because they question the adequacy of their diet, they should have a nutrition checkup with a registered dietitian, who can teach them to get the nutrients they need through the foods they eat.

Although it seems logical that an active person would need more vitamins than a sedentary person, the research to date shows no evidence of dramatically increased vitamin needs that cannot be met through a wholesome diet. An athlete who takes extra vitamins is unlikely to notice increased performance, strength, or stamina, unless he or she was nutritionally deficient to start with, or else experiences a placebo effect.

Most athletes easily consume more than enough vitamins through 1500 to 2000 calories of a variety of wholesome foods each day. Hence, the hard-training athlete who consumes 4000+ calories can easily get more vitamins than needed. For example, the cyclist who drinks a small 6-oz glass of orange juice gets 100% of the recommended daily allowance (RDA) for vitamin C. If thirsty, such as after a workout, the athlete is more likely to drink 24 oz of juice and get 400% of the RDA for vitamin C from this one snack alone, to say nothing of what is consumed in other fruits and vegetables throughout the day.

AMINO ACID AND PROTEIN SUPPLEMENTS

Athletes who strive to develop muscles and increase strength often look to amino acid pills and protein supplements for beneficial effects. To date, there is no evidence that these result in greater muscular bulk. Exercise, not extra protein, is the key to building bigger muscles. Athletes who want to bulk up should spend time lifting weights and performing other forms of resistance exercise, rather than spending their money on expensive amino acid supplements.

The amount of protein or amino acids in the special powders or pills is far less than that which you might easily get from foods. For example, an athlete would have to eat five tablespoons of one popular brand of protein powder at an approximate cost of $1.10 to get the same amount of protein in a small (3.5 oz) can of tuna at half the price (Table 16–4).

FLUIDS

Drinking adequate fluids is essential for top sports performance. Fluids transport nutrients to and from the working muscles, dissipate heat, and eliminate waste products. Unfortunately, many athletes neglect this aspect of their sports diet and consequently hurt their performance. To maintain optimal hydration, athletes should follow these guidelines:

TABLE 16–4. AMINO ACIDS: FOOD VERSUS PILLS*

Food or Protein Supplement	Amount	Arginine (mg)	Tryptophan (mg)	Amount Needed for 25 g Protein	Approximate Cost ($)
Chicken breast	4 oz (raw)	2100	400	3 oz (cooked)	0.30
Eggs	2	780	200	4	0.35
Skim milk	1 c	300	120	3 c	0.55
Amino Fuel	1 svg	120	75	7 wafers	1.45
Coach's Formula	1 svg	410	170	5 T	1.10
Dynamic Muscle	1 svg	680	240	4 T	0.70

*This table compares the milligrams (mg) of two amino acids, arginine and tryptophan, as available in food and in several popular protein supplements. The second part lists the approximate cost for 25 g of protein.

Abbreviations: oz = ounces, c = cup, svg = serving, T = tablespoon.

Note: Nutrient data adapted from Pennington J, Church H: Bowes and Church's Food Values of Portions Commonly Used, ed 14. Philadelphia, JB Lippincott, 1985; with permission. Protein supplement data is taken from product labels.

From Clark N: Nancy Clark's Sports Nutrition Guidebook. Champaign, IL, Leisure Press, 1990; with permission.

1. *Prevent dehydration during training* by drinking adequate fluids on a daily basis—lots of water, juices. Athletes can determine whether or not they're drinking enough fluid by monitoring their patterns of urination: the urine should be clear-colored and copious, and they should be urinating frequently. Dark-colored, scanty urine is a sign of dehydration and a signal for the athlete to consume more fluids.

To increase awareness of sweat losses during exercise, athletes should weigh themselves before and after a hard workout. Each pound of weight lost represents 2 cups (16 ounces) of sweat. They should replace this accordingly, and strive to lose no more than 2% of their weight during a workout (ie, 3 lb or 6 cups sweat for a 150-lb athlete). If they become 2% dehydrated, they have reduced their work capacity by 10% to 15%.

2. *Before an event,* athletes should drink extra water, juice, and other fluids to be sure the body is well hydrated. They should drink 2 to 3 large glasses of fluid up to 2 hours before the start. Since the kidneys require about 90 minutes to process fluids, this allows time to empty the bladder prior to the event. Five or ten minutes before start time, athletes should drink another 1 or 2 cups of water or sports drink.

3. *During hard exercise,* athletes should drink as much as they comfortably can, ideally 8 to 10 ounces every 20 minutes. Because they may be sweating off three times this amount, they may still have a water deficit. They should start drinking early in the event, *before* they are thirsty, to prevent dehydration.

4. *After exercise,* athletes should drink enough fluids to quench their thirst, plus more. The thirst mechanism inadequately indicates whether the body is optimally hydrated; monitoring urination is safer. If several hours pass before an athlete has urinated, he or she is still dehydrated.

For the recreational athlete, water is always an appropriate fluid replacer before, during, and after exercise. For endurance athletes and those exercising for more than 90 minutes, a sports drink or diluted juice that contains 60 to 100 calories per 8 ounces is best during exercise because it will help to maintain normal blood glucose levels. The best recovery fluids include juices, because the juice replaces not only fluids but also carbohydrates and electrolytes. Commercial fluid replacers are generally weak sources of carbohydrates and electrolytes and hence are better suited for consumption during the event (Table 16–5).

TABLE 16–5. FLUID REPLACERS

Drink	Calories per 8 oz	Potassium (mg) per 8 oz	Sodium (mg) per 8 oz
Gatorade	50	25	110
Recharge	50	25	15
Vitalade	85	90	—
Exceed	70	45	50
Coke	95	—	8
Pepsi	100	8	6
Orange juice	110	475	2
Apple juice	115	300	5
Cranberry juice	150	60	10
Grape juice	155	335	5
Cranapple	175	70	5
Orange, 1 lg	120	440	0
Fruit yogurt	225	400	120
Possible losses in a 2-hour workout:	1000 calories	180 mg potassium	1000 mg sodium

Abbreviations: oz = ounces, lg = large, mg = milligrams.

Note: Nutrient data adapted from Pennington J, Church H: Bowes and Church's Food Values of Portions Commonly Used, ed 14. Philadelphia, JB Lippincott, 1985; with permission.

From Clark N: Nancy Clark's Sports Nutrition Guidebook. Champaign, IL, Leisure Press, 1990; with permission.

Coffee

Coffee is often used as a preexercise "perk me up." For some athletes, coffee makes the effort seem easier. For others, it makes them needlessly nervous and jittery, and plagues them with a "coffee stomach" and excessive trips to the bathroom. Although the original research studies suggested that caffeine might have an ergogenic effect that enhances endurance performance, the more recent studies challenge this finding.[2] If an athlete is well fed, rested, and nutritionally prepared for competition, coffee is unlikely to have any beneficial effects.

If athletes ask about caffeine, they should be reminded that every person has a unique reaction to caffeine. Some "perk up" with a cup or two; others don't want to touch the stuff. Hence, each athlete has to experiment with preexercise caffeine to determine if he or she experiences any ergogenic benefits. Athletes should also be reminded that caffeine has a dehydrating effect and is a drug limited by the Olympic Committee.

Beer

Beer may be a popular beverage for thirsty athletes, but it is certainly an inappropriate choice in terms of physiologic needs. Despite popular belief, beer is a poor source of carbohydrates, electrolytes, and fluids. Of the 150 calories in a can of beer, only 50 are from carbohydrates; light beer has even fewer carbohydrates. The alcohol content has a diuretic effect that contributes to increased fluid losses rather than fluid replacement.

Athletes who are destined to drink beer after an event should first drink 2 or 3 large glasses of water, have something to eat (so they aren't drinking on an empty stomach), and then, if they desire, relax with a beer or two for social value rather than for a thirst quencher and fluid replacement. They should also make plans to have a designated driver because alcohol consumed on an empty stomach when the athlete is dehydrated can quickly have a depressant effect. Encourage all athletes to enjoy the "natural high" that follows hard exercise rather than seek out alcohol.

PRECOMPETITION NUTRITION

The precompetition meal has several goals:

1. To help prevent hypoglycemia with the symptoms of light-headedness, blurred vision, needless fatigue, and indecisiveness—all of which can interfere with top performance.
2. To abate hunger feelings, help settle the stomach, and absorb some of the gastric juices.
3. To provide energy for the muscles.
4. To provide adequate fluids to fully hydrate the body.

In preparation for competition, an athlete should eat a 60% to 70% carbohydrate-rich diet (ideally, this is the same as the daily training diet) and drink additional fluids both the day(s) *prior* to the event and the *day of* the event, in combination with tapering off from exercise in order to allow the muscles the opportunity to store the carbohydrates as glycogen.

- Athletes participating in endurance sports that last for longer than 90 minues, such as marathoning or long-distance bike racing, should reduce exercise and emphasize carbohydrates for 3 days prior to the event.
- Athletes participating in events less than 90 minutes in duration can store adequate glycogen with 1 or 2 rest days and a carbohydrate-rich diet.

Because a single precompetition meal inadequately compensates for a poor training diet, athletes should eat a carbohydrate-rich sports diet *every day* to enhance daily muscle glycogen storage. The precompetition meal should simply be an extension of the tried-and-true daily training diet. The primary focus of the precompetition preparation should be to reduce exercise so that the athlete's muscles can store the carbohydrates and optimally replenish depleted glycogen stores.

Although an athlete may want to know exactly when, what, and how much to eat, specific recommendations are hard to make due to metabolic differences from person to person. For example, some runners can eat within an hour of racing; others avoid food to reduce the risk of gastrointestinal distress. Some gymnasts want a small snack to absorb gastric juices; others are so nervous they feel sick and unable to eat. Precompetition food preferences also vary from sport to sport. For example, cyclists are likely to eat more than runners who fear gastrointestinal problems related to the jostling that occurs with running. Since each athlete has unique food preferences and aversions, it is impossible to recommend a single food or meal that will insure top performance. The better plan is to encourage the athlete to experiment with different foods *during training* to determine what settles best and enhances performance.

Although many athletes have traditionally competed on an empty stomach, current research supports the benefits of precompetition food eaten within 4 hours of the event. Contrary to popular belief, food eaten within 4 hours of exercise *is* used for fuel. In one study,[3] five male athletes who consumed 400 calories of sugar 3 hours before running for 4 hours (45% $\dot{V}O_{2max}$) oxidized 68% of the glucose. In another study,[4] cyclists who consumed 400 calories of sugar 1 hour before cycling for 2 hours (35% $\dot{V}O_{2max}$) oxidized 41% of the glucose.

Precompetition food is especially important before morning events. Athletes who enter competition after an overnight fast have depleted their liver glycogen stores; they are likely to have less stamina and endurance as compared with exercising after having eaten a light snack/meal, which replenishes the liver glycogen stores and helps maintain normal blood glucose levels. Some popular food choices include bagel, toast, cereal, fruit and/or juice, about 100 to 400 calories as tolerated.

Meal Timing

When planning the time of the precompetition meal, the athlete should allow adequate time for the food to empty from the stomach, so that he or she can exercise comfortably without feeling weighed down. Because high-calorie meals take longer to leave the stomach than lighter snacks, the general rule-of-thumb is for an athlete to allow:

- 3 to 4 hours for a large meal to digest
- 2 to 3 hours for a smaller meal
- 1 to 2 hours for a blended or liquid meal
- less than an hour for a light snack, as tolerated

Because fatty foods delay gastric emptying, the meal should focus on carbohydrates, with small portions of lean protein also being appropriate as an accompaniment, such as spaghetti with a little bit of extra lean hamburger in the tomato sauce, or a turkey sandwich with thickly sliced bread and a thin layer of turkey.

The night before *morning events,* athletes should eat a hearty, high-carbohydrate dinner and bedtime snack. That morning, they should eat a light snack/breakfast to abate hunger feelings, replenish liver glycogen stores, and absorb some of the gastric juices. For example, a runner who is going to participate in a 10 AM road race will want only a light breakfast (eg, small bowl of cereal with low-fat milk, about 300 calories) because the primary fueling was done the night before by the hearty carbohydrate-rich dinner. Before *afternoon events,* athletes should plan a hearty carbohydrate-rich dinner and breakfast, to be followed by a light lunch. A runner racing at noon can enjoy a heartier breakfast (eg, four or five pancakes, about 600 calories) as compared with when he races earlier in the day. Before *evening events,* athletes should plan a hearty carbohydrate-rich breakfast and lunch, followed by a light snack 1 to 2 hours prior to the event. In addition to focusing the meals on carbohydrates, the athletes should also consume an additional glass of fluid with each meal, as well as between meals, to insure complete hydration. Water, low-fat milk, and juices are the recommended choices, although the less nourishing soft drinks and sports drinks are also popular, acceptable choices.

Some athletes who are overly nervous or stressed or have sensitive stomachs may prefer to abstain from food the day of competition. They should make a special effort to eat extra food the day before to be well fueled for competition. They may want to experiment the day of the event with simple liquids, such as apple juice, canned liquid diets, or sports drinks.

Liquid Meals

Liquid foods leave the stomach faster than solid foods; thus, the athlete may want to experiment with blenderized meals to determine if they offer any advantage. Reports of one research study[5] indicate that a 450-calorie meal of steak, peas, and buttered bread remained for 6 hours in the stomach. A blenderized version of the same meal emptied from the stomach in 4 hours. Before converting to blenderized meals, the athlete should keep in mind anecdotal reports that too much liquid may "slosh" in the stomach and contribute to a nauseous feeling. Hence, any new meal should be experimented with *during training* to determine if it settles well.

Preexercise Sugar

Historically, athletes have been advised to stay away from sugary foods before exercise, with the belief that the "sugar high" will trigger a rebound hypoglycemic effect that will hinder performance. More recent studies suggest that precompetition sugar may actually enhance stamina and endurance. Sherman and associates[6] reported that cyclists who ate about 1200 calories of carbohydrates 3 hours prior to 95 minutes of intermittent exercise improved their performance. Gleeson and co-workers[7] similarly reported that subjects who ate about 280 calories of carbohydrate 45 minutes prior to hard exercise (73% $\dot{V}O_{2max}$) improved their time to exhaustion by 12%.

For some athletes, preexercise sugar does result in a negative hypoglycemic feeling with light-headedness, confusion, and fatigue. Hence, athletes who perceive themselves as being sugar-sensitive should abstain from concentrated sweets and rely more upon hearty meals than sugary snacks for energy.

The best advice regarding preexercise sugar is to *avoid the need* for a quick-energy fix by having appropriately timed meals before the event. The high-school athlete who craves a sugary quick-energy fix before an afternoon event could remedy the need for quick energy by having a wholesome breakfast and lunch, rather than skimping on those meals and then looking for a last-minute energizer. Not only would this pattern invest in better performance but also in better nutrition, and eliminate the risk of possibly hurting performance with rebound hypoglycemia.

Psychological Value of Food

Precompetition food may have beneficial effects both physiologically and psychologically. If an athlete firmly believes that a specific food/meal such as the traditional steak and eggs enhances performance, then it probably does. The mind has a powerful effect upon the body's ability to perform at its best. Athletes who believe in a "magic food" that ensures competitive excellence should take special care to be sure this food/meal is available preevent. This is particularly important for athletes who travel. They should bring along tried-and-true precompetition foods, such as a favorite cereal, muffin, or sandwich. By doing this, athletes will be worry-free about what they are going to eat and will be better able to focus on performance.

Practice Precompetition Eating

Experience has shown that each athlete has to learn through trial and error during training and competitions what foods work best for his or her body, when they should be eaten, and in what amounts. Food preferences vary depending on the type of exercise, level of intensity, and time of day. Hence the above-mentioned guidelines regarding precompetition eating should be viewed as simply considerations to be pondered and experimented with *during training*. The bottom line is that each athlete has to experiment to learn which combinations of food work best for his or her body.

EATING DURING EXERCISE

Athletes who exercise for more than 90 minutes at a time will have greater stamina and enhanced performance if they consume carbohydrates *during* the event. These carbohydrates help to maintain a normal blood glucose level as well as provide a source of energy for the exercising muscles. Trained cyclists (150 lb) can metabolize about 1 gram of carbohydrate per minute; this equals 240 calories of carbohydrates per hour of endurance exercise. This breaks down into 60 calories per 15 minutes (about 8 ounces of sports drink)—much more than most athletes are likely to consume.

The harder an athlete exercises, the less likely he or she is to want to consume food. During intense exercise (>70% $\dot{V}O_{2max}$), the stomach may get only 20% of its normal blood flow.[5] This slows the digestive process; any food in the stomach may feel uncomfortable or be distastefully regurgitated. Sports drinks or sugar solutions (5% to 7%) tend to be most readily accepted. Other popular choices include diluted juices, tea with honey, and defizzed cola taken along with water.

During moderate-intensity exercise, the blood flow is 60% to 70% of normal; the athlete can still digest food.[5] Hence, the solid food snacks, such as bananas, fig bars, and bagels, that recreational skiers, cyclists, and ultrarunners eat during exercise do get digested and contribute to lasting energy during long-term, moderate-intensity events.

Because some athletes more than others can tolerate food/fluids during exercise, it is important to experiment during training with different snacks to determine what works best, and how much is tolerated.

POSTCOMPETITION EATING: RECOVERY FOODS

Many of the same athletes who carefully select a high-carbohydrate diet before competition neglect their recovery diet. Because muscles are most receptive to replacing muscle glycogen within the first 2 hours after a hard workout, a low-carbohydrate postevent diet can hinder optimal recovery. This, in turn, limits the athlete's readiness to compete again, particularly important in the case of repeated events in the same day, such as with swimming or track meets. A poor recovery diet can also delay the athlete's ability to return to intense training.

A carbohydrate-deficient recovery diet is commonly selected by athletes who eat:

- too much protein, such as may happen at a postevent dinner that focuses on steak as a change from the precompetition pasta meal
- too many greasy foods, such as cheeseburgers and french fries that are popularly eaten by athletes who frequent fast-food restaurants
- too many "sweets," when the "sweets" are actually fat-laden cookies, ice cream, and brownies that get at least half their calories from butter or margarine
- too few calories, such as may happen with diet-conscious athletes who skimp on carbohydrates (thinking that carbohydrates are fattening) and instead sustain themselves on protein-rich cottage cheese, tuna, and chicken

To optimize the recovery process after a hard workout, an athlete should eat 200 to 400 calories of carbohydrates within 2 hours of the exercise bout, then repeat this another 2 hours later.[8] This "dose" comes to about 0.5 gram carbohydrate per pound of body weight. For a 150-lb person this would be the equivalent of 300 calories of carbohydrates (75 g) in a postexercise snack (eg, juice) followed by a carbohydrate-rich meal after having stretched, showered, and recovered from the workout. Examples of 300-calorie snack/meal include:

- 2 cups (16 oz) of orange juice and a banana
- an average-sized bowl of cereal with fruit
- a dinner with generous servings of starch and vegetables

For those who report that exercise "kills their appetite," juices can provide adequate carbohydrates, as well as quench the thirst and supply fluids. The popularly advertised carbohydrate supplements are generally unnecessary after exercise, because a hungry athlete can easily consume the recommended amount of carbohydrates, and benefit from the nutritional value of wholesome foods as compared to the empty calories of the supplements.

In addition to replacing carbohydrates, the athlete should be careful to replace fluids lost through sweat. Carbohydrate-containing fluids, such as juices, replace both muscle glycogen and water losses; they are the best choice from a vantage of both overall health and performance. Although many athletes may be tempted to drink sports drinks after an event, commercial fluid replacers are a poor choice because they tend to be very dilute and thereby are poor sources of carbohydrates. For example, an athlete may have to drink 48 ounces of a commercial fluid replacer when he could more easily (and less expensively) get the same amount of carbohydrates in 16 ounces of cranapple juice.

To determine how much fluid an athlete needs to replace, he or she can be weighed before and after the event. Since each pound lost represents 2 cups of sweat losses, the athlete should drink enough to cover those losses, plus more. Thirst inadequately signals dehydration; an athlete may not feel thirsty but can actually still be dehydrated. As mentioned before, the better way to monitor hydration is to pay attention to patterns of urination. An athlete is adequately hydrated if the urine is clear-colored and voluminous. Dark-colored urine is still concentrated with metabolic wastes.

Although many athletes are concerned about replacing the sodium and potassium that are lost in sweat, few athletes are at risk of depleting their body stores. They can easily replace these minerals with the foods and fluids they eat after the event without needing special supplements. Based on the assumption that athletes who exercise a lot also eat a lot, healthy athletes who are concerned about electrolyte replacement can be assured that they will consume more than enough sodium, potassium, and other minerals in their subsequent meals. Electrolyte replacement becomes more of a concern for ultraendurance athletes who exercise for more than 5 hours. They should consume sodium during the event, as well as afterwards, to replace significant losses.

WEIGHT GAIN

When seemingly thin young athletes seek advice regarding weight gain, remind them that light athletes can be swift, skilled, and effective, and caution them that with age, they will undoubtedly bulk up. Efforts to gain weight by eating overindulgent portions of steak, french fries, and ice cream may have negative future effect in terms of not only heart disease but also food preferences. Many once-thin high-school athletes grow into obese businessmen with heart disease who love to eat fatty foods. Recommending healthful, high-energy diets in addition to appropriate exercise and a weight lifting program is by far preferable to encouraging fatty, and fattening, diets.

Many athletes who desire to gain weight simply need to *consistently* eat three meals per day plus additional snacks. Thin athletes commonly are "too busy" to eat adequately to support their caloric needs for growth and training. With regular meals and snacks that include generous portions of wholesome foods, they can consume adequate calories to resolve their problem.

Some athletes do indeed have trouble gaining weight, despite their abundant food intake. In theory, athletes who eat an additional 500 calories per day will enjoy 1 lb of weight gain per week. In reality, some people are "hard gainers" and need to eat far more calories than that.[9] For them, food becomes a medicine, and they must eat even if they don't feel hungry.

The trick to gaining weight is to add 500+ calories/day to the baseline diet. This can be done by incorporating:

- an extra snack, such as a bedtime peanut butter sandwich with a glass of milk
- larger-than-normal portions at meal time, such as two potatoes instead of one
- higher-calorie foods, such as cranberry-raspberry juice instead of orange juice

A sports nutritionist can suggest quick and easy snacks and meals that will help the busy athlete easily accommodate the higher calorie intake.

WEIGHT LOSS

Many athletes—not just those in weight-related sports, such as running, dancing, and gymnastics—strive to lose weight. They believe that a lighter body will enhance performance, if not self-image.[10] However, they commonly hurt their performance due to crash diets and inappropriate weight reduction techniques.

"Diets" typically do not work. The best approach for successful weight loss that allows the athlete to both lose fat and maintain energy for training is to incorporate appropriate portions of healthful, high-carbohydrate, low-fat foods. Strict diets based on sheer willpower result in feelings of denial, to say nothing of poorly fueled muscles. Gradual weight loss (½–1 lb/week for women; 1–2 lb/week for men) offers greater long-term success.

A first step to successful weight reduction is for athletes to keep food records and become aware of what, when, and how much they eat. Typically, weight-conscious athletes "diet" during the day, then "blow it" at night. They are likely to have greater success if they eat the majority of their calories during the day so that they have energy to train, and then "diet" at night. The higher daytime caloric intake prevents feelings of fatigue, to say nothing of the ravenous hunger that often results in overeating in the evening. Generally speaking, once dieters become too hungry, they don't care about what they eat—nor how much—and can too easily overeat.

A second step is to know how many calories per day are appropriate to eat. To roughly estimate caloric needs for weight maintenance, multiply the desired weight by 12 to 15 calories/lb for moderate activity; 15 to 20 calories/lb for higher levels of activity. This number offers a very rough estimate of daily caloric needs; the actual requirements will vary greatly, depending upon individual metabolic differences.

From this estimate of calories needed to maintain weight, the third step is to determine the number of calories appropriate for weight reduction by subtracting 300 to 1000 calories/day (subtract fewer calories for smaller athletes). Divide this number into three, and you'll have a calorie target for each meal. For example, a 110-lb female runner who is moderately active with daily activities plus runs 5 miles/day may need 110 lb × 17 cal/lb = 1870 cal per day to maintain weight. To create a calorie deficit for weight loss, subtract about 350 to 400 calories, bringing the total to 1500 calories per day or 500 calories per meal.

By reading food labels for calorie content and by working together with a registered dietitian, athletes can learn more about calories, nutrient-dense food choices, and successful weight reduction techniques, as well as develop meal plans that suit their likes and lifestyles while contributing to steady weight loss. The dietitian's goal is to educate the athletes about lifelong weight control and healthful low-fat, carbohydrate-rich choices, because the weight problem is likely to be a chronic cause of concern.

Body-fat measurements can be helpful to determine an appropriate weight for athletes. The measurements are best used to reflect changes in body composition, rather than precisely give a measurement of percentage of fat.

SPECIAL NUTRITIONAL NEEDS OF WOMEN

Female athletes should be particularly aware of their intake of iron (to replace menstrual losses) as well as calcium (to optimize bone mineralization). Unfortunately, many women are overly weight-conscious, think of food as the "fattening enemy" rather than a nourishing fuel, eat a very restrictive diet, and cheat themselves of important vitamins, minerals, and protein. Women who severely restrict their diets to the point of becoming amenorrheic place themselves at a much higher risk of suffering stress fractures and premature osteoporosis.[11]

Although there is no proof that the thinnest athlete will be the best athlete, most American women—athletes included—think of themselves as being too fat. This social problem has particularly detrimental effects upon female athletes, as evidenced by the surveys which suggest that about one third of female athletes struggle with some type of pathogenic eating problem.[10] To help reduce the incidence of eating disorders, sports nutrition counseling (which includes discussion of body image and differences in body types) should be an integral part of women's athletics, to help women determine their healthy weight (as opposed to a self-imposed ideal weight) and fuel themselves optimally.

CONCLUSION

Each athlete is metabolically unique and has personal food preferences and special "magic foods"; thus, it is hard to make specific rules and regulations regarding sports nutrition. During training, the athlete should experiment to determine the foods and fluids that settle best and contribute to top performance.

To insure optimal sports nutrition among your athletes, I recommend that you, the physician, work together with a registered dietitian/sports nutritionist, who has the time and expertise to educate the athletes about their nutritional needs and to answer their nutrition question with practical "how to" food suggestions. This sports nutritionist should be available for individual counseling with weight-conscious and eating-disordered athletes, and for group discussions with teams. The job of the sports nutritionist is to teach the athletes how to eat to win. Your job, as a physician, is to reinforce that information and remind the athletes that *everyone* wins with good nutrition.

To find a local sports nutritionist, contact the American Dietetic Association (1-800-877-1600) and ask to be referred to a member of SCAN (their practice group of Sports and Cardiovascular Nutritionists). You may also ask for a referral from your state's dietetic association or your local hospital's nutrition department.

REFERENCES

1. Williams C: Diet and endurance fitness. Am J Clin Nutr 49:1077, 1989.
2. Weir J, Noakes T, Myburgh K: A high carbohydrate diet negates the metabolic effects of caffeine during exercise. Med Sci Sports Exerc 19:100–105, 1987.
3. Jandrain B, Krzentowski G, Pirnay F, et al: Metabolic availability of glucose ingested three hours before prolonged exercise in humans. J Appl Physiol 56:1313–1319, 1984.
4. Rvussin L, Pahus P, Dorner A, et al: Substrate utilization during prolonged exercise preceded by ingestion of 13C-glucose in glycogen-depleted and control subjects. Pflugers Arch 382:197–202, 1979.
5. Brouns F, Saris W, Rehrer N: Abdominal complaints and gastro-intestinal function during long-lasting exercise. Intl J Sports Med 8:175–189, 1987.
6. Sherman W, Simonsen J, Wright D, et al: Effect of carbohydrate in four hour pre-exercise meals. Med Sci Sports Exerc 20:S157, 1988.
7. Gleeson M, Maughan R, Greenhaff P: Comparison of the effects of pre-exercise feedings of glucose, glycerol and placebo on endurance and fuel homeostasis in man. Eur J Applied Physiol 55:645–653, 1986.
8. Ivy J: Muscle glycogen synthesis after exercise and effect of time of carbohydrate ingestion. J Appl Physiol 64:1480–1485, 1988.
9. Sims E: Experimental obesity, dietary induced thermogenesis and their clinical implications. Endocrinol Metab Clin North Am 5:377–395, 1976.

10. Rosen L, McKeag D, Hough D, et al: Pathogenic weight control behavior in female athletes. Physician Sportsmed 14:79–86, 1986.
11. Clark N, Nelson M, Evans W: Nutrition education for elite women runners. Physician Sportsmed 16:124–135, 1988.

ADDITIONAL READINGS

American Dietetic Association: Sports Nutrition: A Manual for Professionals Working with Active People, American Dietetic Association, PO Box 10960, Chicago, IL 60610–0960.

Belko A: Vitamins and exercise—an update. Med Sci Sports Exerc 19:S191–S196, 1987.

Clark N: Nancy Clark's Sports Nutrition Guidebook. Champaign, IL, Leisure Press, 1990.

Clark N: The Athlete's Kitchen, 1981. (Available by mail order only through New England Sports Publications, PO Box 252, Boston MA 02113.)

Coleman E: Eating for Endurance. Palto Alto, Bull, 1987.

Evans W, Hughes V: Dietary carbohydrates and endurance exercise. Am J Clin Nutr 41:1146–1154, 1985.

Lemon P: Protein and exercise: Update 1987. Med Sci Sports Exerc 19:S179–S190, 1987.

Williams M: Vitamin and mineral supplements to athletes: Do they help? Clin Sports Med 3:623–637, 1984.

Williams M: Nutritional Aspects of Human Physiology and Performance. Springfield, IL, Charles C Thomas, 1985.

18

TRAVEL

Robert S. Hillman, MD
Robert P. Smith, MD

Domestic and foreign travel is often required of athletes engaged in competitive sports. Trips limited to the United States generally present no major difficulties for the individual athlete or athletic team. No unusual health hazards are involved, and the best health care facilities of the area are easily identified. Travel to more distant locales, however, can present problems. Minor annoyances such as jet lag from changing time zones and gastrointestinal upsets caused by differences in local diet are well known. Unfamiliarity with local health hazards and a lack of knowledge of available emergency health care facilities can be a much bigger problem. For athletic teams traveling to a domestic or foreign city, the team physician can help organize the trip medically and may accompany the team for the purpose of coordinating health care. The athlete traveling alone must take personal responsibility both for being aware of potential health hazards and for being sufficiently knowledgeable about a foreign health care system to find immediate, professional medical attention. While domestic and international travel usually pose no greater health risks than those at home, even a simple illness or sports injury can be devastating for the athlete who needs to be in top form for a competition.

Awareness of the differences in health care systems in other cities and countries, together with a certain amount of preparation, is the best safeguard for any traveler. No one plans a trip without researching travel arrangements, hotel accommodations, and sightseeing activities. At the same time, Americans tend to be extremely complacent about the availability of health care facilities within their own country and abroad. For example, many do not know whether their medical insurance policy covers health care in foreign countries, whether they need extra travel insurance in case of an accidental injury, whether their prescription drugs will be easy to find in the distant city or country, whether a good sports medicine facility will be available, or where the best full-service hospital is located. The answers to such questions are as important as any of the other travel arrangements required in a trip. For foreign travel, such preparation can be a lifesaver.

PREPARING FOR A MAJOR TRIP

There are a number of general considerations that apply to anyone planning a major trip, including amateur and professional athletes. These include arrangements that can easily be made before a trip to solve potential problems that are almost impossible to achieve from a distance.

Paying for Medical Emergency

Even though emergency medical care for a traveler may on occasion be free in a foreign city, most physicians and hospitals require immediate payment for all medical bills just as in the United States. Moreover, health care insurance plans such as Blue Cross and Blue Shield require travelers to pay physician and hospital bills in cash, with reimbursement granted after returning home contingent upon presentation of properly itemized bills. For the athlete traveling abroad, this can involve a major financial outlay. Furthermore, some insurance plans may not cover health care abroad at all. Medicare and Medicaid do not cover care abroad as so stated on the back of the U.S. government passport. Thus, an important consideration before any trip is to check on whether medical insurance plans provide coverage while traveling abroad.

It is also important to consider whether the insurance plan is adequate. This is of special significance for the athlete who is at risk for a major sports injury. Will an injury be covered by the health insurance policy? If not, can temporary additional coverage be arranged with that company or should a separate policy with another company be obtained? Institutions that sponsor team sports and competitions may be aware of this problem and can arrange for a group policy for sports injuries. Obviously, it should be the responsibility of the team physician to be sure of the adequacy of the coverage for a group of traveling athletes. For the individual athlete who does not have access to a group policy, travel agencies can provide information about such policies. But it is always important that the buyer beware; the extent of coverage must be carefully examined.

In the case of trips abroad in which flying is the only means of travel, it may also be advisable to take out insurance that covers emergency evacuation. For travelers not covered by special insurance, emergency evacuation from a foreign country is extremely expensive. Commercial airlines may or may not be able to accommodate an injured person according to the availability of airplanes and the nature of the equipment. If stretcher accommodation is required, it can be very costly. Usually four first-class seats need to be purchased and it may be necessary to purchase a round trip fare for an accompanying nurse or doctor before the airline will accept the injured traveler. Evacuation by U.S. military aircraft is not an alternative. Not only is it extremely difficult to arrange, it also bears a stiff price tag in excess of $10,000 for most international trips.

Insurance plans that cover emergency evacuation can be purchased from companies such as International SOS Assistance, 1420 Walnut Street, Philadelphia, Pennsylvania 19102. Generally, these plans involve transport by air ambulance if a commercial carrier will not accept the injured traveler; they may also identify physicians in various foreign countries who can help arrange for the evacuation. For such service, insurance is important, if not essential. Transport by a private air ambulance without coverage is extremely expensive, and most companies will not put a plane in the air until payment has been guaranteed.

Finally, a note of warning may be given regarding the handling of physician and hospital payments outside the United States. If services of a physician or hospital are required, the traveler must obtain an itemized bill before leaving the country. American health plans, particularly Blue Cross and Blue Shield, require itemization of service for reimbursement. This can be a problem for both hospital and patient. Daily hospital fees abroad are often based on a flat daily rate that includes physician fees, radiographic examination, laboratory procedures, and a number of other services. This is quite different from the system used in the United States, where each item is separately billed. It is not always easy to solve this problem. The hospital may be able to translate and itemize its bill and sometimes the nearest U.S. consul will have had experience in dealing with the problem. Even if it is a difficult thing to do, it is far better to put in the effort while in the foreign country. After returning home, it will be an impossible feat.

Carrying Personal Medical Supplies

The easiest and best way of handling a minor medical problem when traveling is to be able to take care of it personally. To do this, the traveling athlete should have a well-stocked kit of medical supplies. Just what should be in such a kit depends on personal health care needs. It may include the simplest of medications, such as aspirin or another non-narcotic analgesic, prescription drugs for well-recognized past medical problems, and a range of medical supplies, such as elastic bandages, gauze, and tape, for the management of recurrent sports injuries.

For team travel, a well-prepared kit of medical supplies for the management of sports injuries is essential. It should be organized and maintained by the team physician. If a team is traveling without a physician, the trainer, coach, or a team member experienced in the management of sports injuries should take responsibility.

The importance of a good medical kit can not be overstressed. It may seem to be an easy thing to replace a medication or medical supply while in a familiar United States city. In the United States, the selection of drugs is standardized and names are easily recognized. This is not true, however, for foreign countries and foreign cities. Even the simplest of over-the-counter drugs can be difficult to recognize, and the traveler may have great difficulty in locating and using a foreign pharmacy. Differences in pharmacies in various foreign countries are striking. In some, most drugs, except narcotics, can be purchased without prescription. In others, extremely rigid laws control all drug purchases. In some countries, a prescription is required to obtain a refill. Even a U.S. prescription may be inadequate, forcing a trip to a local physician or hospital. Finding the same or equivalent drug may also be difficult. Even when the personnel in a pharmacy speak excellent English, and this is not the rule, they may be unable to match an American trade name drug to a local drug simply because there are no publications that identify comparable drug preparations.

The best course of action is always to have more than an adequate supply of prescription medications in hand. In hand means in one's hand luggage, not stowed in a suitcase that can easily be lost during international travel.

Avoiding Health Hazards

The best way to avoid health hazards while traveling is to know about them ahead of time. This may take some research. Although travel agencies are eager to tell a traveler about sightseeing opportunities and the enjoyable aspects of a trip, they are understandably loath to describe potential health hazards. Such information must be obtained from word-of-mouth contacts with other travelers and athletes. A few major U.S. teaching hospitals now offer clinics for travelers at which health care professionals provide advice about immunizations, health hazards, and preventive measures to avoid certain problems.

A physician accompanying a team abroad should take responsibility to research the hazards in a foreign trip both in terms of prophylactic measures, such as immunizations, and potential health problems that should be avoided in the foreign country. For example, differences in diet and the quality of water are always to be considered. It may seem like a great adventure to live "like the natives" and taste all the local foods, but no one wants to spend the better part of a week getting over an attack of diarrhea or return home only to have a bout of infectious hepatitis a month or more after the trip. For the athlete, such problems can be a disaster. Therefore, the more that is known about the health hazards of a particular country, the better one is equipped to avoid a problem.

Checking Shots and Immunizations

There are no required immunizations for travel to most of the major cities of the world. Smallpox vaccination is no longer needed for travel anywhere. Immunizations for diseases such as cholera, typhoid, and yellow fever are only necessary for trips to remote tropical areas. Detailed information regarding the need for such immunizations is provided by the U.S. Public Health Service and most county or city public health departments. These organizations may also sponsor clinics that provide a full range of immunizations and the necessary documentation for travel.

While there are no required immunizations for travel to major cities, it is important to have routine immunizations up to date. The following may be recommended:

1. All children should be current for their diphtheria-pertussis-tetanus (DPT) vaccination.
2. Adults should have had a tetanus-diphtheria booster within the last 10 years.
3. Travelers born in or after 1957 should be revaccinated for measles with either monovalent measles vaccine or measles-mumps-rubella vaccine (MMR) unless they have already received a measles booster vaccination.
4. Travelers of all ages should not leave the United States without being fully immunized against polio. A polio vaccine booster is recommended if the primary series was completed 5 years prior to the trip. For adults who have never received oral polio vaccine (OPV), booster doses of enhanced inactivated polio vaccine (eIPV) are preferred.
5. For travel to coastal resorts or to areas with poor sanitation, passive immunization with immune globulin (human gamma globulin) for prevention of infectious hepatitis is also recommended. Immune globulin can be given concomitantly with most other vaccinations, but should be given no sooner than 3 to 4 weeks following a dose of MMR, OPV, or eIPV.

When a trip is planned to any country where malaria may be present, prophylactic chemotherapy is recommended. The traveler should first check with a physician, the American Consulate, or the U.S. Public Health Service as to the type of malaria in the area to be visited, especially whether the chloroquine-resistant *Plasmodium falciparum* type is present. When resistant malaria is not the problem, adults and children weighing more than 120 lb should take a single 500-mg tablet of chloroquine phosphate once a week, beginning a week before the trip and continuing 6 weeks after. Recommendations for areas with endemic chloroquine-resistant *P. falciparum* malaria vary depending upon the local risk of malaria, length of stay, and the presence of multiple resistant strains. Up-to-date information on appropriate measures for malaria prevention can be obtained by calling the CDC's Malaria Prevention and Prophylaxis phone line (404-639-1610). Travelers to malarious areas must remember that no chemoprophylaxis regimen is 100% effective. The importance of measures to prevent mosquito bites (ie, use of DEET-containing insect repellants, screened sleeping areas, and appropriate clothing) cannot be overstated.

Traveling with a Known Health Problem

Any athlete who has a known chronic illness or recurrent health problem should make special preparations to manage that problem while traveling. If it may be necessary to consult a foreign physician or use a health care facility while abroad, the traveling athlete should always carry a letter from an American physician or a detailed medical history that describes the condition and makes recommendations for medical management. If medications are required, the generic name and recommended dosages should be clearly stated. Finally, if a special portion of the medical record, such as an electrocardiogram or a radiographic examination, may be of crucial significance in the management of a medical problem, a copy of these records should be carried.

When a recurrent health problem may involve a sudden loss of consciousness or mental confusion, for example, with diabetes or allergic condition, it can be extremely important to have a bracelet or neck tag prepared that describes that condition. Med-ident bracelets and neck tags are sold in drug stores for less than $10.00. A full selection of bracelets is available, including ones that say Diabetic, Drug Allergy, See Wallet, Epilepsy, Heart Condition, Allergic to Penicillin, and so on. Blank tags can also be purchased and mailed to Med-ident, P.O. Box 1686, Buffalo, NY 14216 to be marked for other conditions.

Medic Alert bracelets and necklaces can also be purchased from the Medic Alert Foundation, P.O. Box 1009, Turlock, CA 95380. Generally, it takes 3 weeks to obtain one. However, as a part of the fee for purchasing a Medic Alert bracelet, the organization maintains a record of the purchase and a certain amount of medical information on file. Engraved on the bracelet is a phone number that can be called from anywhere in the world in an emergency to gain information about the bracelet's owner.

TRAVELING HEALTH TIPS

Respiratory Infections

Getting there can be half the fun if a few simple rules are followed. There really is little risk associated with air travel. However, for the traveler with an upper respiratory tract infection and a blocked eustachian tube, changes in cabin air pressure can cause considerable discomfort. In such a situation, the use of a nasal decongestant one half hour before flight is recommended. This will open the eustachian tube and permit free equilibration of the air in the middle ear with the cabin air pressure.

Jet Lag

Air travel across several time zones is also associated with jet lag. How bothered a traveler is with jet lag varies from person to person and may be less severe for younger individuals. However, it is doubtful that anyone is invulnerable; thus, mental and physical performance may well be substandard for several days after arriving in a foreign country. As a rule, the more time zones crossed, the longer it takes for an individual to reorient the sleep cycle to the new time zone. Avoidance of alcohol and a light diet on the day of travel may help reduce the symptoms of jet lag.

Intestinal Disturbances

Minor disturbances in appetite and bowel function may also occur. This may be another manifestation of changing time zones or a response to the change in diet. A few loose bowel movements or mild diarrhea does not rank as classic "turista" or traveler's diarrhea. Generally, a diarrhea caused by a virus or a toxigenic *Escherichia coli* (the bacterium often responsible for traveler's diarrhea) is accompanied by nausea, frequent watery bowel movement, and 1 or 2 days of low-grade fever. A short, mild episode of traveler's diarrhea requires no medical attention or specific therapy other than eating lightly and drinking plenty of fluids. More severe diarrhea with nausea, vomiting, and dehydration should be treated. With the appearance of high fever with chills or blood in the stools, a physician should be consulted immediately.

For mild-to-moderate traveler's diarrhea, self-treatment is a reasonable approach. A number of therapies have been recommended, including short courses of a broad-spectrum antibiotic, such as trimethoprim/sulfamethoxazole (Bactrim), ciprofloxacin or norfloxacin, or even a single 2.5-g (five 500-mg capsules) dose of tetracycline. Another popular treatment is to take frequent doses of Pepto-Bismol (up to a bottle a day). When athletes travel to an area where traveler's diarrhea is a frequent problem, some physicians recommend prophylaxis with either bismuth subsalicylate (Pepto-Bismol, 2 tablets four times a day) or a single daily dose of an antibiotic such as doxycycline, Bactrim, or norfloxacin. Although these regimens are 60% or more effective in reducing the incidence of traveler's diarrhea, the possibility of side effects from each of these medications must be weighed in the balance. Severe diarrhea should not be self-treated. The attention of an expert physician is necessary, and the traveler may need a full-service hospital.

If possible, the medications required for treating mild diarrhea should be carried by the traveler. If a medication, especially an antibiotic, is recommended by a foreign physician or the personnel in a foreign pharmacy, great care must be exercised. Certain antibiotics commonly used in foreign countries to treat diarrhea are unsafe. For example, chloramphenicol, iodochlorhydroxyquin (Entero-vioform), and neomycin not only are contraindicated in the treatment of diarrhea but also can be extremely dangerous. Finally, gut-paralyzing drugs such as diphenoxylate (Lomotil), loperamide (Imodium), and paregoric should be used with caution. Although these drugs are useful in controlling the intestinal cramps associated with diarrhea, they can prolong the episode by trapping the toxic products in the intestine. They should not be used in the treatment of diarrhea associated with high fever or blood in the stool. Further, paregoric, an opium derivative, is illegal in some countries.

Of course, the best way to handle the whole problem of traveler's diarrhea is not to experience it in the first place. The key to this lies in what is eaten and drunk. Experienced travelers drink bottled mineral water exclusively wherever they go, with few exceptions. It is not difficult to know when to drink bottled water; one only has to watch what everyone else is doing. If bottled water is nowhere to be seen in public places, the tap water is usually of high quality and safe to drink. On the other hand, if everyone in restaurants is ordering bottled water or if it is offered by the waiter, the message should be clear. In a number of European countries, including France, Italy, Spain, and Greece, travelers should drink bottled water exclusively and brush their teeth with it as well. Experienced travelers buy a bottle at the bar before going to bed.

Accidental injury is the most common serious health problem experienced by college-aged travelers to foreign countries. Young travelers should be reminded that vehicular accidents (motorcycles in particular) remain the gravest health hazard while abroad. Particular care should be used when driving in an unfamiliar country where road conditions may differ markedly from those in the United States.

FINDING HEALTH CARE ABROAD

Success in finding health care in a foreign city or country depends on a number of factors, including the level of development of health care in that country, the size of the city or town, the knowledge and experience of the traveler, and, perhaps most importantly, the effort put in by the traveler or companions to find the right health care facility. One law of probability that applies anywhere in the world is that the bigger the city, the better the health care. The more remote the area, the harder it will be to find professional help. It is also true that good health care can be provided only by a well-trained professional with adequate equipment. This is especially true for the athlete who is trying to care for a sports injury. Paramedical personnel or physicians who come to a hotel room with a black bag are not capable of providing high quality care. Therefore, it is up to the traveling athlete to get up and go to the appropriate medical facility for the problem.

Self-treatment or Care by a Team Physician

For a minor problem or recurrent difficulty with a known chronic illness or sports injury, self-treatment is the best course of action. When a physician travels with a team, the majority of minor problems can be handled outside the local health care system as long as sophisticated diagnostic or therapeutic equipment is not required. When traveling alone, self-treatment for many problems is a possibility. However, this will depend on the athlete's knowledge of the management of common health problems. Usually, a great deal can be accomplished if there was good preparation before leaving the country. If the traveling athlete is aware of common local health hazards, these can either be avoided or dealt with by carrying appropriate medication. For example, traveler's diarrhea is such a common problem in some countries that an athlete should go prepared for self-treatment if not on a prophylactic regimen.

Finding a Physician

The traditional entry point for any traveler into a foreign health care system is through a doctor provided by the hotel or host institution. Hotel doctors are usually selected because they speak English well and are willing to come to the hotel at any time day or night. For a minor complaint, this is quite satisfactory. When an athlete travels to a major competition in a foreign country, there will usually be no difficulty in identifying skilled medical personnel. Medical professionals experienced in the management of sports injuries will be on call if not in attendance at major sports events.

Other dependable sources of English-speaking physicians are lists provided by the Health and Welfare section of the American Consulates abroad. These may be obtained either by visiting the consular services section or by calling the duty officer. The list is free, updated yearly, and usually carefully checked. Although the government assumes no responsibility for the results of one's choosing a physician from the list, consular services personnel work hard to keep the list current and dependable. Usually, there are many physicians to choose from according to the common medical and surgical specialties. This is a major advantage over the use of the hotel physician.

Although there are regional medical officers attached to certain of the U.S. embassies abroad, these physicians do not generally treat travelers. However, they can be a source of information and advice in the case of an extended or critical health care problem. There are U.S. embassy physicians, for example, in Bonn, Belgrade, Vienna, Panama City, Athens, and Moscow. The one in Moscow is perhaps the greatest potential resource. Any traveler who becomes seriously ill should contact the American embassy physician before following the advice of a Soviet physician and entering a Soviet hospital. The embassy can help arrange for alternative care in Helsinki, Finland.

Finally, full-service university teaching hospitals are a prime source of English-speaking physicians. During business hours, they can be consulted in various outpatient departments. In an emergency, they can be found in the emergency room. Most foreign cities set up a rotational system for emergency room coverage on a 24-hour basis.

Choosing a Hospital

The best place to be hospitalized is always in the traveler's own hometown. If hospitalization is required while in a foreign country, the athlete must take the responsibility to check on the nature of the hospital recommended. In most foreign countries, there are a wide range of hospitals and clinics that vary greatly in size and capability. Furthermore, European hospitals can be a physical puzzle for American travelers. Often they are large complexes of buildings of varying size, shape, and age, each offering a differing medical or surgical service. In fact, in some hospitals there may be two or more emergency rooms, one for medical and one for surgical emergencies, and the traveler must make the decision as to which emergency room to use. Often at the front entrance there will be a porter who knows where everything is but who rarely speaks English. Therefore, it can be extremely important for the American traveler to have the assistance of a foreign national to serve as a translator in an emergency.

In most foreign countries, there are a number of different kinds of medical institutions, including public, private, military, and university-affiliated teaching hospitals. In Europe and elsewhere, private hospitals or clinics are usually small and rarely provide a full range of services or 24-hour house staffs and emergency rooms. Rather, they are hospitals of choice for specialized elective procedures and noncritical conditions. At the same time, they are frequently listed by U.S. and other consular services as available facilities. The reason for this is that these hospitals request that the consul include them on the list.

Although there are still a few U.S. military hospitals abroad, they are restricted to members of the U.S. armed forces, government employees, and dependents of both. Only in the case of serious emergency is a military hospital permitted to provide limited assistance to an American traveler. The critically ill traveler who seeks help at such a hospital is usually stabilized and then transferred to a foreign hospital as soon as possible.

Public hospitals in foreign countries can vary greatly in size and quality of services. In poorer countries, public hospitals can be extremely crowded and in poor condition. However, in other countries, the public hospital may be the best of available facilities with modern buildings and a full range of services. Often, the public hospital is also a university or teaching hospital. This can be most desirable because any hospital that trains physicians, nurses, and other health professionals maintains high standards. Furthermore, it is the full-service teaching hospital that is most accustomed to dealing with a full range of complaints from exotic to routine. This situation is further strengthened by the fact that hospital staffs of teaching hospitals maintain a worldwide contact with other physicians. They often speak English and can be expected to be current on recent scientific developments. Furthermore, full-service teaching hospitals generally have well-equipped intensive care and coronary care units and rehabilitation medicine services.

Success in using a foreign hospital always depends on the traveler's ability to communicate within a different cultural system. Foreign hospitals look like American hospitals, but the relationship of physician and medical personnel to the patient may be quite different. Physicians abroad may have the equivalent of training available in the United States, but they will probably not have the same bedside manner. In most foreign countries, physicians are not accustomed to having to explain much to their patients. Therefore, if a physician seems cool, distant, uncommunicative, or even arrogant, he (more rarely she) is really just functioning in the expected and acceptable way. Again, the help of a foreign national can be very valuable in gaining information and managing the problems that arise during a hospitalization. Sometimes U.S. consular personnel—even the consuls themselves—visit American patients hospitalized abroad.

SUMMARY

In conclusion, travel abroad should present no major risk to the athlete if a few simple rules are followed. The most important of these is to go prepared. This includes learning as much as possible about potential health hazards in the countries to be visited, being knowledgeable about minor health problems, including recurrent sports injuries, and carrying a kit of personal medical supplies. If professional health care is required while abroad, the team physician, the athlete, or a companion should take the time to research the local health care facilities before selecting a physician or hospital. American consular services or a host institution may help in this regard. In the case of an emergency, the best rule is always to go to the emergency room of the largest, full-service hospital in the city.

BIBLIOGRAPHY

Dawood R: How to Stay Healthy Abroad. New York, Penguin Books, 1988.
Hill DR, Pearson RD: Health advice for international travel. Ann Intern Med 108:839–852, 1988.
Hilman SH, Hillman RS: Traveling Healthy. New York, Penguin Books, 1980.

19

PHYSIOLOGY OF EXERCISE AND TRAINING

James S. Skinner, PhD

There are two types of adaptation to exercise. *Functional* adaptations are characterized by changes in efficiency or functioning of various tissues or systems (eg, a reduction in heart rate at a given power output), whereas *structural* adaptations are characterized by changes in the number or size of the functional units within a body system (eg, muscle hypertrophy in weight lifters or an increased number and size of mitochondria in distance runners). Generally speaking, functional adaptations occur earlier but are also lost sooner. Structural adaptations take longer but also last longer when training is decreased or is stopped; the time required to reverse a structural change also depends on how long it had been present.

The responses and adaptations to exercise are logical (ie, they do not occur without a good reason) and specific (eg, weight lifting primarily involves responses by the nervous and muscular systems, whereas prolonged, continuous running requires responses by the nervous, muscular, cardiovascular, respiratory, hormonal, and thermoregulatory systems). The study of the functional effects of physical activity is therefore related to the description and explanation of the logical acute responses and chronic adaptations by the body to single or repeated bouts of exercise. It is the specificity factor that makes the study of these functional effects so complex, challenging, and interesting.

A number of books and reviews have been written on various aspects of the physiology of exercise and training. The reader should refer to these for more details.[1–6]

BASIC CONCEPTS OF ENERGY AND ITS SOURCES

The energy needed for the functioning of each cell in the body (eg, muscle contraction, transmission of nervous impulses, hormone synthesis) is produced by chemical reactions. These chemical reactions are either aerobic (occurring in the presence of oxygen) or anaerobic (without oxygen).

Some energy is stored in the muscle in a form (adenosine triphosphate, ATP) that can be used immediately, especially when energy is needed rapidly (eg, at the onset of exercise or activities that are more intense). Phosphocreatine (PC) is another form of stored energy that can be broken down to supply very limited amounts of ATP. Both of these high-energy phosphate bonds are metabolized by anaerobic reactions and can be used for very brief, very high-intensity exercise requiring as much as 80 to 90 times the energy required at rest. However, these phosphagen reserves are extremely limited and must be continually resynthesized if exercise is to continue.

Even though the aerobic system resynthesizes ATP more efficiently than the anaerobic system, the cardiorespiratory system adjusts too slowly to provide adequate amounts of oxygen to muscle. As a result, ATP must be resynthesized by the faster, less efficient system of anaerobic glycolysis (ie, anaerobic degradation of carbohydrates). This mechanism can provide the majority of the energy necessary to exercise at a power output (PO) ranging from 70 times that required at rest for 20 sec to 30 times resting energy requirements for 120 sec.

With increases in pulmonary ventilation, oxygen diffusion into the blood, and blood flow, a greater amount of oxygen is transported to muscle. After several minutes, the aerobic system becomes the major producer of ATP for muscular contractions. This energy is produced by the breakdown of carbohydrates (CHO) and fats. Fats can be degraded only by aerobic processes, whereas CHO can be metabolized by aerobic and anaerobic reactions. Proteins are generally not a direct source of energy. They are the structural components of cells and a major element of hormones and enzymes. They can be converted to fat or CHO and either stored or used for energy in that form.

With adequate amounts of oxygen available to oxidize the abundant energy stored in the body in the form of CHO and fats, these aerobic reactions will continue as long as the requirements for ATP are not too high. However, if there is sudden increase in energy expenditure that cannot be met by the slower aerobic reactions or if the exercise intensity exceeds 60% to 80% of the maximal aerobic power ($\dot{V}O_{2max}$) of the average person, then anaerobic glycolysis also provides some energy.

It is a basic rule in exercise physiology that a given PO requires a given amount of energy, regardless of the source of that energy. The relative contribution of aerobic and anaerobic energy production depends on the type, intensity, and duration of exercise. Thus, brief, high-intensity, static and intermittent activities that emphasize speed and strength tend to be anaerobic (using only CHO), whereas prolonged, low-intensity, dynamic and continuous activities that emphasize endurance tend to be aerobic (using both CHO and fat). Exercise is not so simple, however, and many factors can influence which energy sources are used.

Based on findings from many studies, Skinner and associates[7] proposed a classification system that included two aerobic, one mixed (aerobic and anaerobic), and two anaerobic types of activity:

1. *Aerobic* activities requiring <65% to 80% $\dot{V}O_{2max}$ that can be continued for 2 hr or more.
2. *Aerobic* activities requiring <90% to 95% $\dot{V}O_{2max}$ that can be done for 10 to 60 min.
3. *Aerobic and anaerobic* activities requiring >90% to 95% $\dot{V}O_{2max}$ that can be sustained for up to 8 min but <200% $\dot{V}O_{2max}$ that can last up to 1 min.
4. *Anaerobic* activities requiring 200% to 300% $\dot{V}O_{2max}$ that can be done for 20 to 45 sec.
5. *Anaerobic* activities requiring 250% to 450% $\dot{V}O_{2max}$ that can be done for 1 to 10 sec.

Figure 19–1 is a schematic diagram of this classification system, expressed as a percentage of the $\dot{V}O_{2max}$ for an average individual. The diagonal line in the upper figure shows that a given PO requires a given amount of energy. The areas below the diagonal represent an estimate of the relative contribution of stored energy (ATP and PC), anaerobic glycolysis, and aerobic metabolism at each PO. At low intensities requiring 75% to 90% $\dot{V}O_{2max}$, most energy is derived from aerobic metabolism. As the intensity increases, the anaerobic system provides more and more energy until about 200% to 250% $\dot{V}O_{2max}$. Finally, for activities requiring very high levels of energy (300% to 400% $\dot{V}O_{2max}$), the phosphagens are the main source.

The solid curve in the lower part of Figure 19–1 depicts the maximal duration of exercise that can be done at each intensity. At low intensities, the energy source is pri-

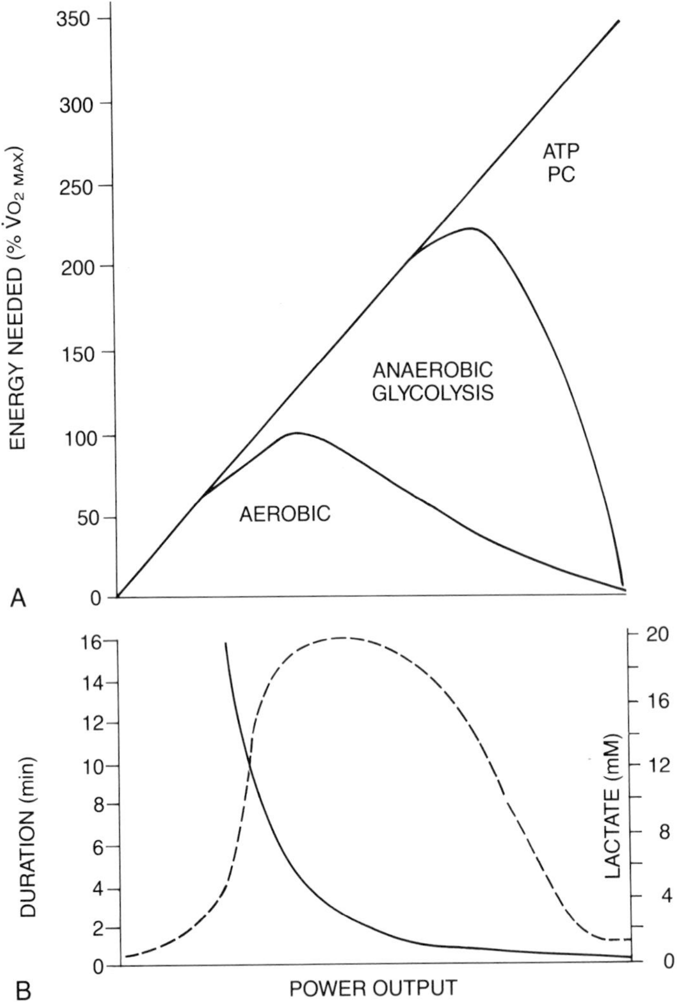

Figure 19–1. Schematic representation of energy needed, duration of exercise, and levels of blood lactate relative to power output. **A:** Energy needed, expressed as a percentage of the maximal aerobic power ($\dot{V}O_{2max}$), and the relative contribution of aerobic metabolism, anaerobic glycolysis, and phosphagens (ATP and PC). **B:** Duration of exercise possible and the associated blood lactate level at the various power outputs. (ATP = adenosine triphosphate, PC = phosphocreatine.)

marily aerobic and one can exercise for a long time. For example, it has been shown that one can work continuously at about 50% $\dot{V}O_{2max}$ for 8 hr per day with no problems or fatigue. At the other extreme, if intensity is very high, then duration is very short because limited amounts of ATP and PC are available. For intensities that can be maintained for a maximum of 1 to 8 min, energy is provided by both aerobic and anaerobic sources. As can be seen, there is a gradual transition from one source to another and no abrupt threshold.

The dashed curve in Figure 19–1 shows the association between blood lactate (LA) levels and the various types of exercise. At low intensities and long durations, as well as at high intensities and short durations, low levels of blood LA are seen, suggesting that the energy sources are aerobic in the first case and phosphagens at the other extreme. The highest levels of LA are obtained during high-intensity activities lasting 1 to 8 min that involve both the aerobic and anaerobic systems. Because both systems are providing energy, one can exercise long enough to accumulate high levels of LA.

From Figure 19–1, it can be seen that few activities are purely anaerobic or aerobic and these few occur only at the extremes of the intensity-duration continuum (eg, sprinting and slow walking, respectively). Thus, intermittent activity can be aerobic (eg, golf is low intensity) and prolonged activity can have anaerobic periods (eg, sprinting in soccer).

The fuels used during continuous aerobic exercise vary with exercise duration (Fig.

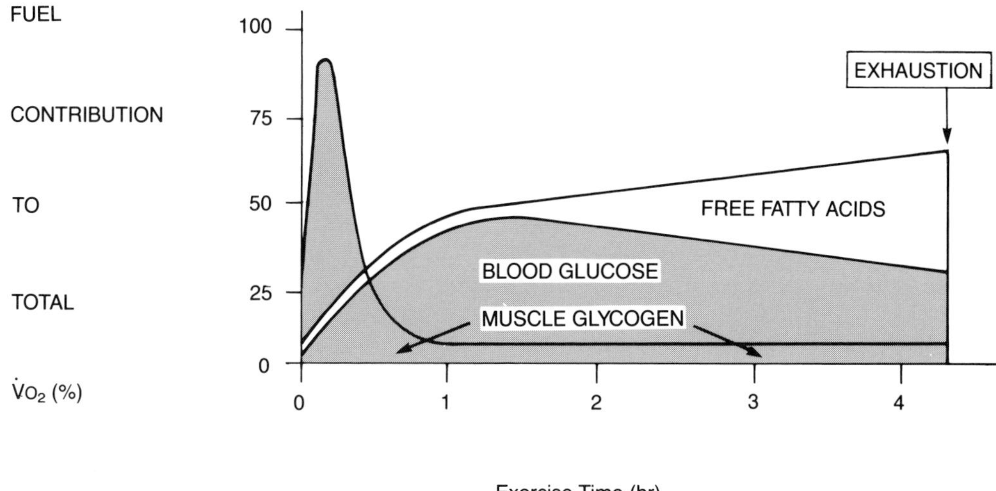

Figure 19–2. Relative contribution of various fuel sources to the total oxygen intake ($\dot{V}O_2$) during 4 hours of exercise to exhaustion.

19–2). During the first 20 min, the main fuel source is the glycogen present and available in muscle. The contribution of fat and blood glucose is relatively small but increases continuously, so that they each provide about 40% of the total fuel at 60 min. The release of fat from the fat cells in the form of free fatty acids (FFA) and its use by muscle continues to rise, while the contribution of blood glucose drops.

Intensity is also an important factor in the types of fuels used by the body during exercise (Fig. 19–3). As FFA can be metabolized only in the presence of oxygen, whereas CHO can be metabolized aerobically and anaerobically, it is not surprising that the main energy source during low-intensity exercise is fat oxidation. With increasing intensity, more and more CHO are used (aerobic glycolysis). At about 60% to 80% $\dot{V}O_{2max}$, anaerobic glycolysis occurs and small amounts of LA are present in the blood. Thus, different fuels are used and different energy systems will be stimulated at different exercise intensities.

The relative contribution of aerobic and anaerobic energy is also influenced by muscle blood flow. In order to sustain a high exercise intensity, muscle tension must be raised by increasing the number of activated motor units and muscle fibers. When the tension within a muscle or muscle group reaches 15% to 20% of its maximal voluntary contractile force (MVC), the intramuscular tension begins to exceed the pressure within the arteries that run parallel to the fibers. The resulting mechanical compression of the arteries produces a drop in blood flow and reduces the delivery of oxygen to the working muscle fibers. As the % MVC increases, anaerobic glycolysis is used more and more to provide energy within the muscle. When intramuscular tension exceeds 60% to 70% MVC, local circulation is completely blocked and anaerobic glycolysis is the only available source of energy. Thus, different systems and fuel sources are associated with the intensity of contraction (% MVC) within a given muscle group.

Similarly, different muscle fiber types are recruited at different intensities of exercise (Fig. 19–4). When a small amount of force is needed at slow speeds or light resistances, the slow-twitch (ST), oxidative muscle fibers are used. With moderate amounts of force, some fast-twitch muscle fibers (FT_a) are also used; these tend to be intermediate fibers, in that they have oxidative and glycolytic properties. Finally, the FT glycolytic muscle fibers (FT_b) are added at high levels of force, such that all muscle fibers are used at maximal tensions.

The recruitment of muscle fibers depends on the kind of activity being performed. At the onset of exercise of moderate intensity, FT fibers are selectively recruited to over-

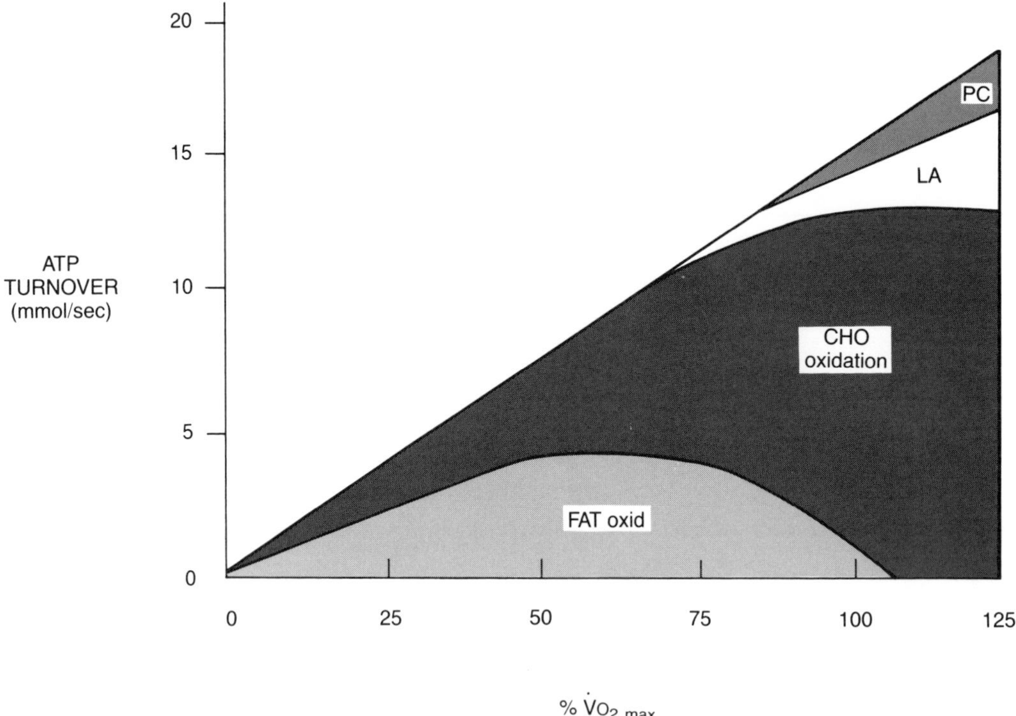

Figure 19–3. Contribution of aerobic metabolism (oxidation of fat and carbohydrates) and anaerobic metabolism (lactate formed by glycolysis and phosphocreatine stored in muscle) to total ATP turnover at various intensities of exercise (% $\dot{V}O_{2max}$). (PC = phosphocreatine, LA = lactate, CHO = carbohydrate, oxid = oxidation.)

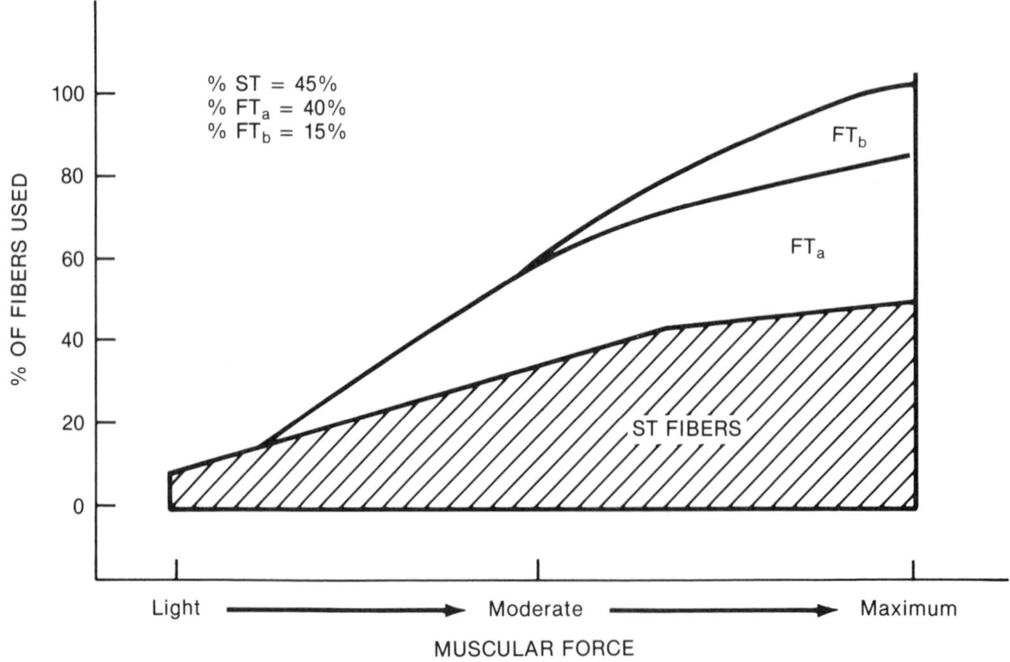

Figure 19–4. The ramp-like recruitment of muscle fibers at varied levels of muscular effort. Whereas light force requires only slow-twitch fibers, heavy loads on the muscle causes the recruitment of all three types of muscle fibers. (ST = slow-twitch, FT_a = fast-twitch, FT_b = fast-twitch glycolytic.) (*From* Wilmore JH, Costill DL: Training for Sport and Activity, ed 3. Copyright © 1988 William C Brown Publishers, Dubuque, Iowa. All rights reserved. Reprinted by permission.)

come the initially high resistance. After a few seconds, the body is in motion, less force is required, and the ST fibers take over. If the exercise continues for a long time, however, the glycogen stores in the ST fibers are reduced, such that more and more FT fibers have to be recruited. Once the glycogen reserves of the FT fibers also reach low levels, one must either reduce the intensity of the exercise (thereby allowing the slower aerobic system to metabolize more fat) or stop because of exhaustion.

Of course, the recruitment pattern of the different muscle fiber types will also be affected by their relative distribution in each person. There is a wide distribution of FT and ST fibers, with sprint athletes tending to have more FT fibers and endurance athletes more ST fibers (Fig. 19–5), with most people being somewhere in between. Even within

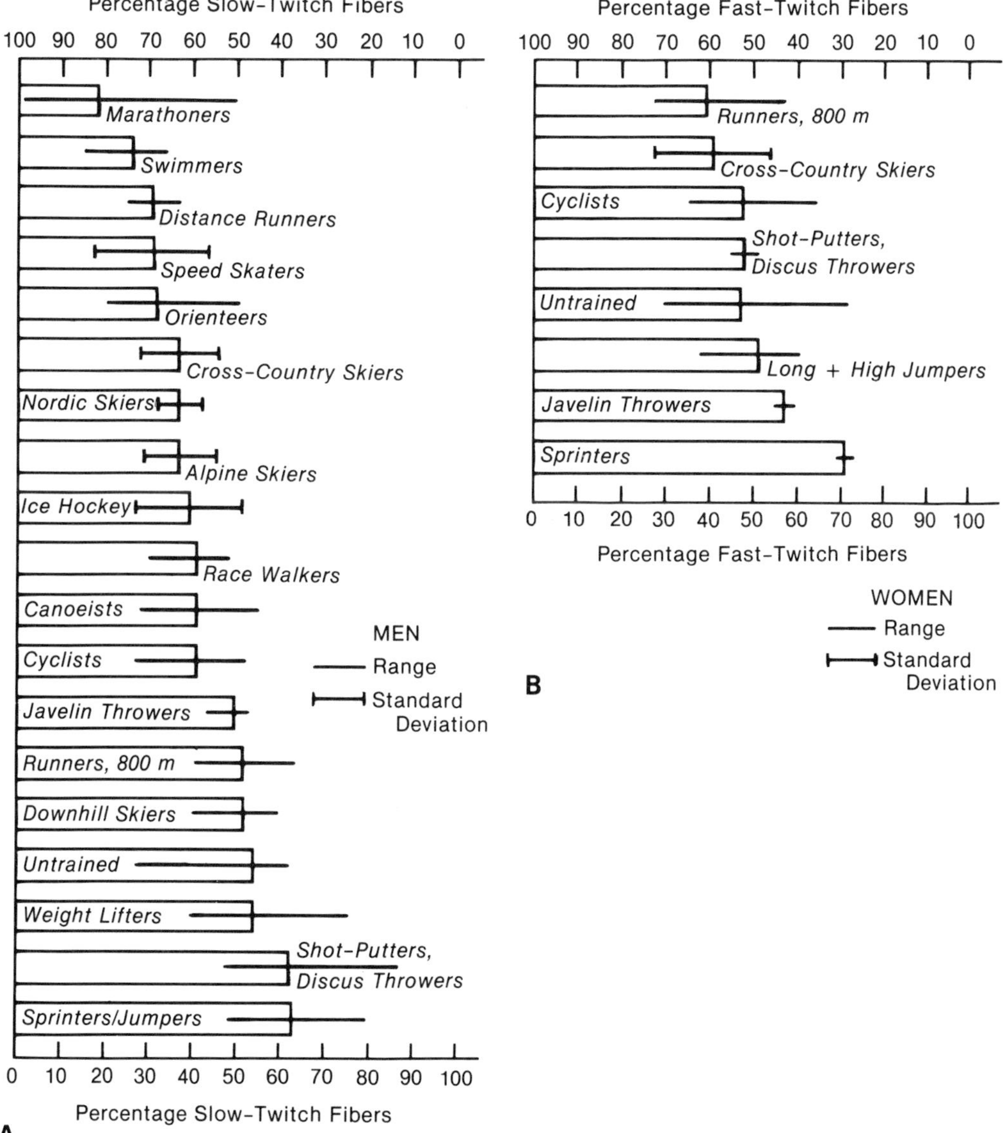

Figure 19–5. The distribution of fast-twitch (FT) and slow-twitch (ST) fibers in muscles of different groups of male **(A)** and female **(B)** athletes. Although there is some variation, endurance athletes tend to have greater percentages of ST fibers, whereas nonendurance athletes tend to have greater percentages of FT fibers as compared with their nonathletic counterparts. (Based on data from Burke et al,[8] Costill et al,[9] Gollnick et al.,[10] Komi et al,[11] and Thorstensson et al.[12] *From* Fox EL, Bowers RD, Foss ML: The Physiological Basis of Physical Education and Athletics, ed 4. Philadelphia, WB Saunders, 1988, p 108.)

the same person, different muscle groups have different proportions.[8–12] For example, ST fibers comprise 40% to 65% of the fibers in the gastrocnemius and 80% to 95% of those in the soleus. The reason for this difference should be clear when one remembers that the gastrocnemius is the larger muscle of the calf used for jumping, whereas the soleus is the smaller muscle located closer to the bone and used for walking.

It is known that the energy required to do a given PO does not change, unless there is a change in mechanical efficiency or work done while performing that activity. In addition, intensity is a relative term and is usually expressed as a percentage of $\dot{V}O_{2max}$, that is, the energy required for a given activity compared with the maximal amount of energy that a person can provide aerobically. Thus, it is obvious that the relative intensity of a given absolute PO (eg, 100 W on a cycle ergometer requiring a $\dot{V}O_2$ of about 1.5 L/min) will vary from one person to another and within the same person over time if the $\dot{V}O_{2max}$ is different. As a result, the relative importance of the various energy systems must be determined for each activity and for each person to comprehend better what the acute effects of that activity might be for a given person or what chronic adaptations (training) might occur with repeated bouts of that activity.

RESPONSES AND ADAPTATIONS IN AEROBIC ENERGY PRODUCTION

Given the limited ATP and PC reserves and the problems associated with anaerobic glycolysis (accumulation of LA and H^+), it is logical to assume that the body's main method for supplying energy is the aerobic breakdown of fats and CHO. This production of aerobic energy can be limited by either the *transport* of oxygen (eg, as might occur at altitude, with cardiovascular or pulmonary disease, or with anemia) or its *utilization* by muscle.

To comprehend better the acute responses and chronic adaptations by the aerobic system to exercise and training, respectively, a molecule of oxygen will be followed from its entry into the lungs from ambient air to its use within the muscle cell. Knowing what is required of each body system involved in the transport and utilization of oxygen, the reader can logically decide which functional and structural adaptations are needed to provide more aerobic energy. A summary of the chronic adaptations to endurance training is given in Table 19–1.

Oxygen Transport System

RESPIRATORY SYSTEM

Gas exchange in the lungs is accomplished by diffusion, which is controlled by the partial pressure gradients existing between the alveolar air and the blood passing by. This exchange can be improved in several ways: (1) by increasing alveolar ventilation (depth of breathing more than frequency), which reflects the actual amount of air reaching the alveoli where exchange can occur; (2) by improving the alveolar ventilation/perfusion ratio so that more blood is shunted to those regions of the lungs that are well ventilated; and (3) by increasing the speed of diffusion of oxygen across the alveolar-capillary membrane.

The body consumes only the oxygen needed to resynthesize the ATP and PC that have been used at a given PO. It is also able to store only a small amount of oxygen. This is not a problem at rest, as the need for oxygen is easily satisfied. During exercise, the frequency and depth of breathing increase (minute and alveolar ventilation rise), the ventilation/perfusion ratio improves, and oxygen perfusion across the alveolar-capillary membrane is faster. The most economical ventilation is one in which the rate and depth

Table 19–1. STRUCTURAL AND FUNCTIONAL ADAPTATIONS TO ENDURANCE TRAINING

System	Structural	Functional	R	S	M
General					
		Oxygen intake ($\dot{V}O_2$)	0	0	+
		Sympathetic nervous system			
		Drive	−	−	
		Sensitivity	+	+	+
		Liver glycogen and FFA			
		Speed of release	+	+	+
		Amount released	+	+	+
		Rate of rise and fall in $\dot{V}O_2$ and heart rate		+	+
		Blood lactate level	0	−	0
		Oxygen debt	0	0	+
Oxygen Transport					
Lungs	+ Number and size of alveoli	Diffusing capacity	+	+	+
	+ Total lung capacity	Frequency	−	−	0
		Depth (tidal volume)	+	+	+
		Ventilation ($\dot{V}E$)	−	−	+
		$\dot{V}E/\dot{V}O_2$	−	−	0
Blood	+ RBC; + Hb; + Blood volume				
Heart	+ Volume (+ cavity)	Vagal tone	+	+	
	+ Capillary density	Heart rate	−	−	0
	+ Glycogen stores	Strokevolume	+	+	+
		Cardiac output	0	0	+
		End-diastolic volume	+	+	+
		End-systolic volume	−	−	−
		Contractility	+	+	+
Blood vessels	+ Capillary density	Peripheral resistance	−	−	−
		Blood pressure			
		Systolic	0	−	0
		Diastolic	0	0	0
Oxygen Utilization					
Muscle cell	+ Glycogen	Enzyme activity			
	+ Triglycerides	Oxidative	+	+	+
	+ Myoglobin	Lipolytic	+	+	+
	+ Number and size of mitochondria	Oxygen extraction	+	+	+
		Muscle blood flow	−	−	0

Abbreviations: R = rest, S = submaximal (same absolute power output), M = maximal exercise, + = increase, 0 = no change, − = decrease, blank = not applicable or unknown, FFA = free fatty acids, RBC = red blood cells, Hb = hemoglobin.

of breathing are automatically adjusted. The rise in ventilation is linearly related to exercise intensity until about 50% to 60% $\dot{V}O_{2max}$, after which ventilation begins to rise exponentially as a result of the metabolic acidosis associated with elevated LA in extracellular fluid. With this excess ventilation, the partial pressure of alveolar CO_2 drops, permitting a faster CO_2 diffusion from the plasma and pushing the following reaction to the left:

$$H_2O + CO_2 \rightleftharpoons H_2CO_3 \rightleftharpoons HCO_3^- + H^+$$

In this way, a fair amount of CO_2 can be eliminated in expired air, helping to maintain the acid-base balance of extracellular fluid. As the exercise intensity increases, however, the excess ventilation cannot eliminate enough CO_2 to compensate for the marked rise in LA and H^+. This hyperventilation also increases the energy expenditure of the respiratory muscles, such that some of the rise in $\dot{V}O_2$ is needed for the extra work of breathing and is not available for other working muscles.

Repeated stimulation of the respiratory system produces a rise in total pulmonary capacity; this may be due to an increase in the number and/or size of alveoli. There is also a reduction in the functional residual capacity with training. Nevertheless, these structural adaptations are less important than the functional adaptations seen during exercise in trained persons, in whom pulmonary airway resistance is reduced and maximal voluntary ventilation is increased. For a given $\dot{V}O_2$, tidal volume is higher but is more than offset by a lower breathing frequency, such that minute ventilation is lower but alveolar ventilation is greater (Fig. 19–6). A better ventilation/perfusion ratio and a higher diffusion capacity (Fig. 19–7) facilitates the exchange of oxygen, while reducing the ventilatory requirements and the energy cost of breathing during submaximal exercise.[13] Finally, maximal ventilatory capacity is increased, partially explaining the higher $\dot{V}O_{2max}$ that occurs with endurance training.

BLOOD

The hemoglobin (Hb) in arterial blood is 98% saturated with oxygen at rest in both sedentary and trained persons and generally remains very high during exercise. To increase the amount of oxygen that can be transported, therefore, there must be an increase in total Hb. With endurance training, total blood volume increases about 10% to 15%, while Hb concentration drops 3%. The similar concentration in a larger blood volume actually means that there is an increased total Hb in a more dilute volume that is easier for the circulatory system to move.

HEART

Heart rate (HR) increases linearly with exercise intensity until $\dot{V}O_{2max}$. Cardiac output ($\dot{Q}$) is the product of HR and stroke volume (SV) and also increases linearly (Fig. 19–8). It

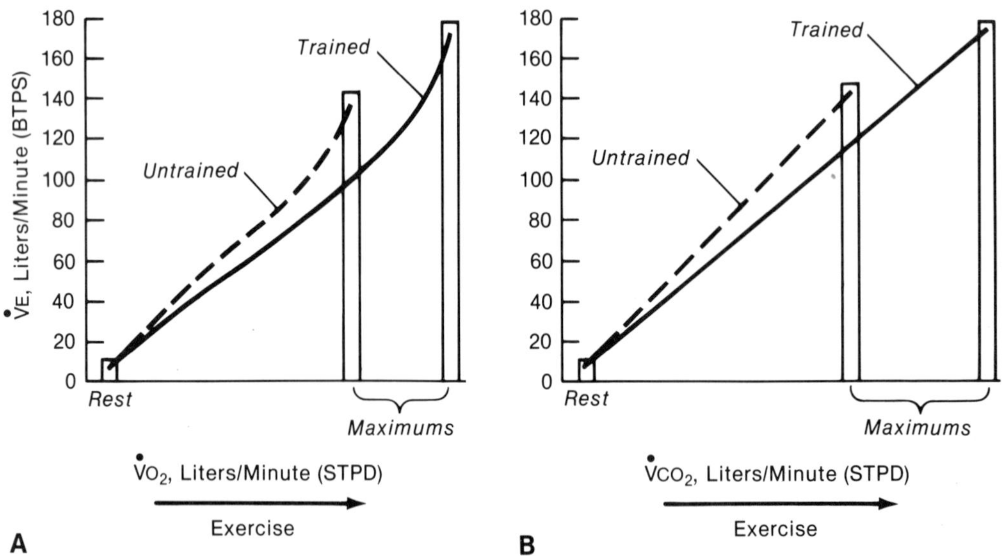

Figure 19–6. Effects of exercise on minute ventilation ($\dot{V}E_{BTPS}$) in trained and untrained subjects. **A:** The close relationship of $\dot{V}E$ to $\dot{V}O_2$. **B:** The close relationship of $\dot{V}E$ to $\dot{V}CO_2$. Note that $\dot{V}E$ is disproportional to $\dot{V}O_2$ but not to $\dot{V}CO_2$ at maximal and near-maximal levels. (*From* Fox EL, Bowers RD, Foss ML: The Physiological Basis of Physical Education and Athletics, ed 4. Philadelphia, WB Saunders, 1988, p 206.)

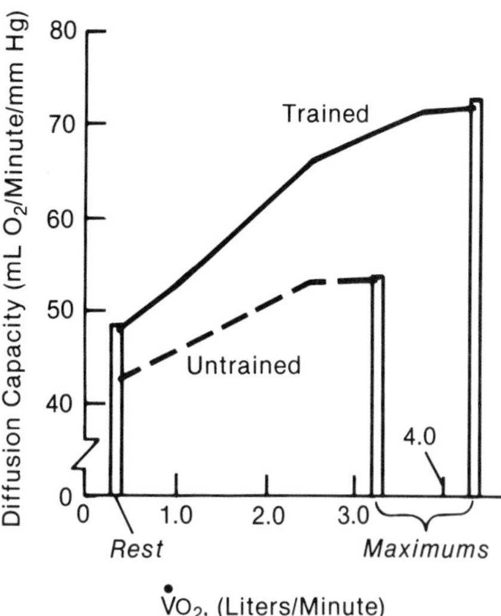

Figure 19–7. The pulmonary diffusing capacity for oxygen increases during exercise in trained and untrained subjects. (Based on data from Magel and Andersen.[13] *From* Fox EL, Bowers RD, Foss ML: The Physiological Basis of Physical Education and Athletics, ed 4. Philadelphia, WB Saunders, 1988, p 231.)

should be noted that in the supine position, where venous return is at its maximum, SV is also at its peak. Upon standing, hydrostatic pressure reduces venous return. As a result, SV drops and remains low until the muscle and respiratory pumps assist the return of blood to the heart during exercise, such that SV is at or close to its maximal level at about 40% to 50% $\dot{V}O_{2max}$.

With endurance training and its associated rise in blood volume, SV increases owing to more filling during diastole (greater end-diastolic volume, or EDV) and/or more complete emptying during systole (smaller end-systolic volume, or ESV). In addition to the structural adaptation of greater left ventricular mass and wall thickness, there are functional adaptations. At a given HR, systolic duration is shortened after training (resulting in a greater ejection velocity and smaller ESV), while ventricular relaxation is faster during diastole, which is now longer and part of the reason for the greater EDV. At rest, as well as at the same $\dot{V}O_2$ during submaximal exercise, SV rises and HR drops, such that $\dot{Q}$ remains essentially unchanged. During maximal exercise, HR remains unaltered, while SV and $\dot{Q}$ rise markedly. Thus, the system for transporting blood and oxygen improves and is a major reason why $\dot{V}O_{2max}$ rises.

BLOOD VESSELS

According to Laplace's law, $\dot{Q} = P/R$. Blood flow ($\dot{Q}$) during exercise is increased by raising the heart's systolic or driving pressure (P) and by lowering peripheral resistance (R). In addition, blood is shunted by vasoconstriction away from nonactive, splanchnic areas toward the active skeletal muscles by vasodilation and a lower resistance[14] (Fig. 19–9). The general redistribution is controlled by the autonomic nervous system, whereas blood flow to specific muscle fibers is controlled locally by conditions surrounding motor units (motor nerves and the muscle fibers they innervate). For example, active muscle fibers need more blood, oxygen, and nutrients. Blood flow to these active fibers is increased by local arteriolar vasodilation when there is a rise in temperature or partial pressure of CO_2, and a drop in pH or the partial pressure of O_2.

Oxygen carried to the skeletal muscle by blood diffuses toward muscle fibers according to the pressure gradient for oxygen. This gradient increases during exercise when more oxygen is removed by the muscles to produce ATP. Diffusion is facilitated by a shift to the right of the oxyhemoglobin dissociation curve; this shift is caused by a rise in tem-

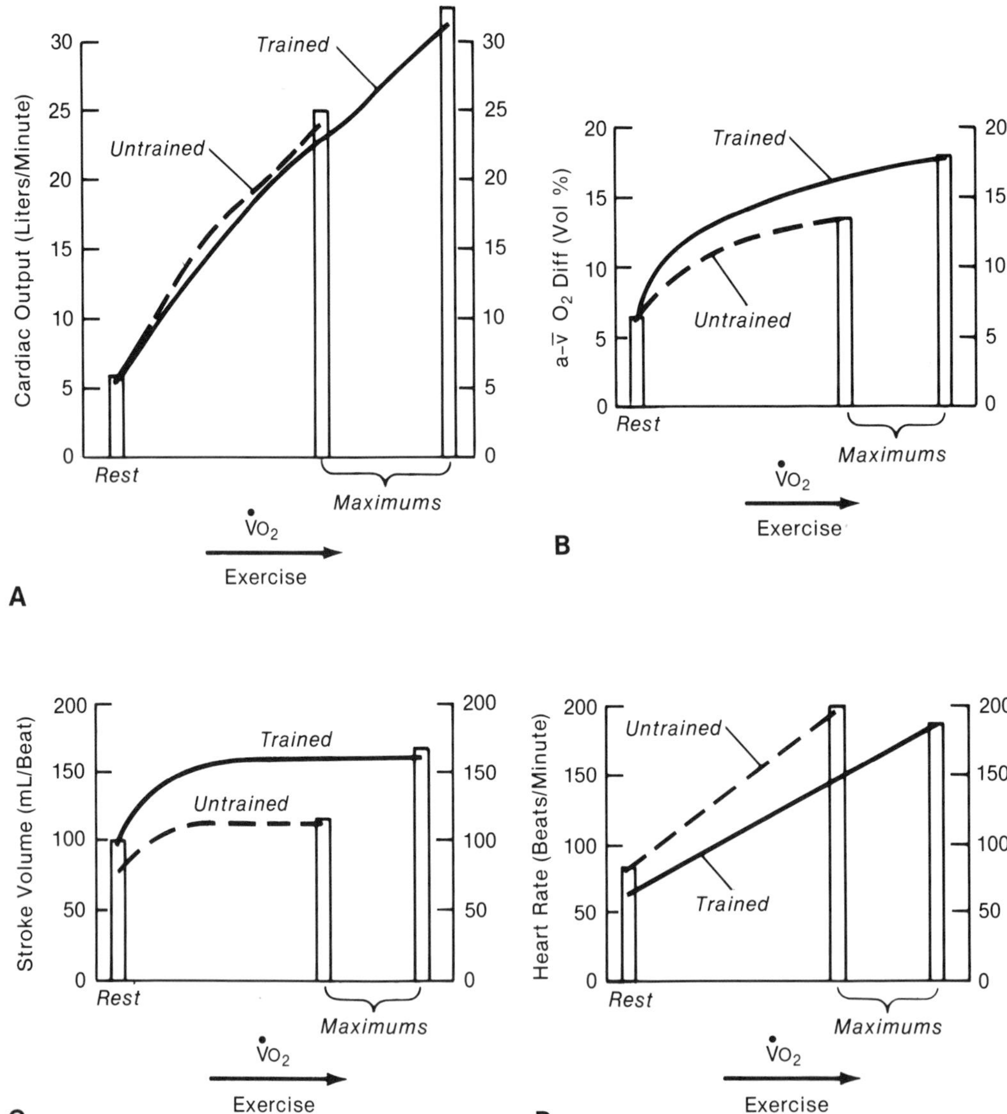

Figure 19–8. **(A)** Cardiac output, **(B)** arteriovenous oxygen difference, **(C)** stroke volume, and **(D)** heart rate during exercise in trained and untrained subjects. Cardiac output is the product of stroke volume times heart rate. Oxygen intake ($\dot{V}O_2$) is the product of cardiac output times arteriovenous oxygen difference. Cardiac output and heart rate are closely related to $\dot{V}O_2$ over the entire range from rest to maximal exercise in the upright position. Maximal stroke volume is usually reached at a submaximal exercise intensity of 40%–50% $\dot{V}O_{2max}$. During exercise, the muscles extract a greater amount of oxygen from a given quantity of arterial blood that is transported. (*From* Fox EL, Bowers RD, Foss ML: The Physiological Basis of Physical Education and Athletics, ed 4. Philadelphia, WB Saunders, 1988, pp 236, 250.)

Figure 19–9. Distribution pattern of cardiac output through the various organs of the body at rest and during exercise. Blood flow to each area is expressed in milliliters and as a percentage of the total blood flow. The insert illustrates the percentage of blood flow to the muscles versus that going to all other organs combined. (*Adapted from* Chapman CB, Mitchell JH: The physiology of exercise. Sci Am 212:88–96, 1965; Copyright © 1965 by Scientific American, Inc. All rights reserved. *From* Fox EL, Bowers RD, Foss ML: The Physiological Basis of Physical Education and Athletics, ed 4. Philadelphia, WB Saunders, 1988, p 256.)

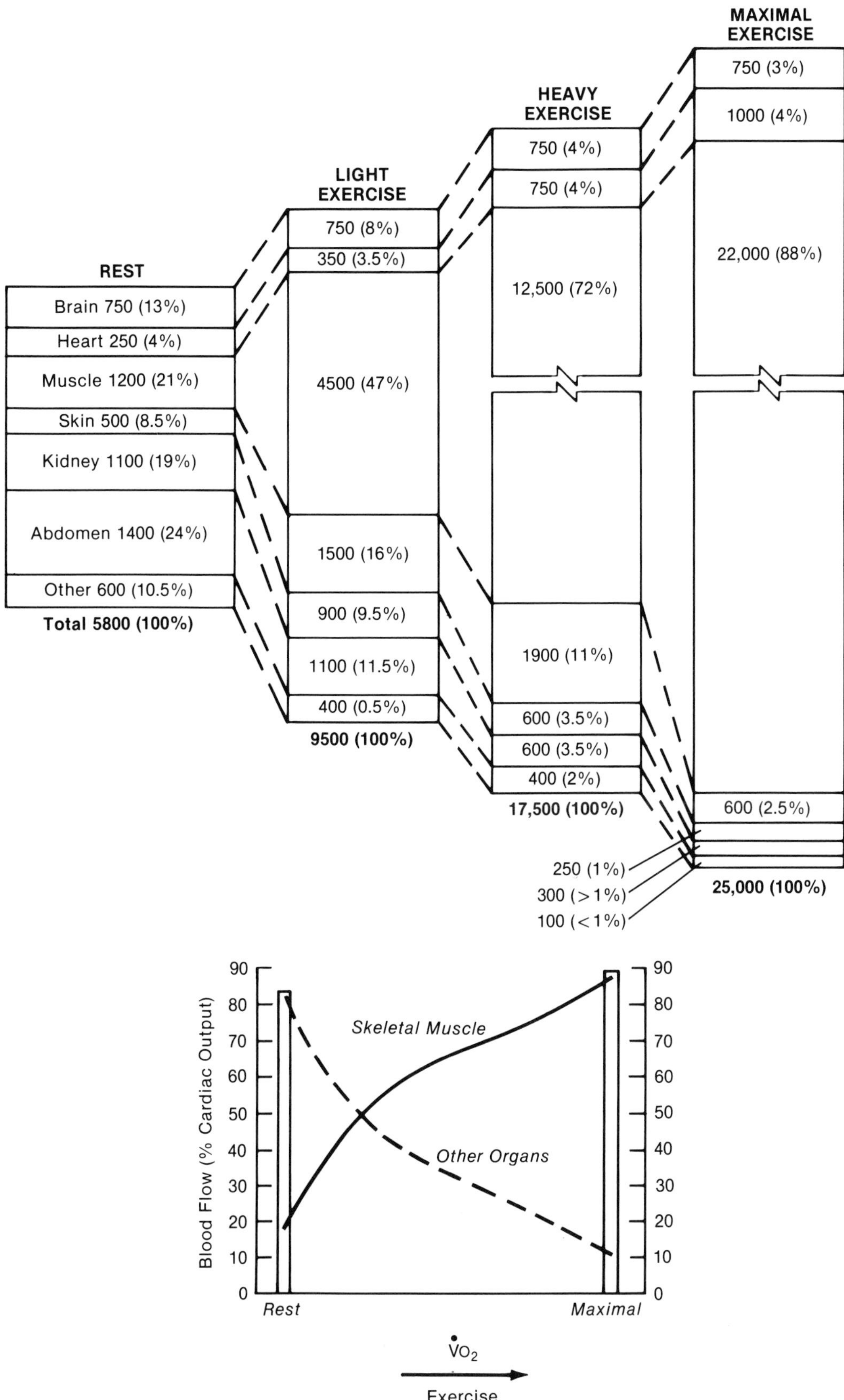
REST
Brain 750 (13%)
Heart 250 (4%)
Muscle 1200 (21%)
Skin 500 (8.5%)
Kidney 1100 (19%)
Abdomen 1400 (24%)
Other 600 (10.5%)
Total 5800 (100%)
LIGHT EXERCISE
750 (8%)
350 (3.5%)
4500 (47%)
1500 (16%)
900 (9.5%)
1100 (11.5%)
400 (0.5%)
9500 (100%)
HEAVY EXERCISE
750 (4%)
750 (4%)
12,500 (72%)
1900 (11%)
600 (3.5%)
600 (3.5%)
400 (2%)
17,500 (100%)
MAXIMAL EXERCISE
750 (3%)
1000 (4%)
22,000 (88%)
600 (2.5%)
250 (1%)
300 (>1%)
100 (<1%)
25,000 (100%)
Blood Flow (% Cardiac Output)
90
80
70
60
50
40
30
20
10
0
Skeletal Muscle
Other Organs
Rest
Maximal
VO2
Exercise

perature or partial pressure of CO_2, and by a drop in pH or partial pressure of O_2 in the blood. These are the same factors that increase local blood flow.

It is known that $\dot{V}O_2 = \dot{Q} \times$ arteriovenous oxygen difference (a-$\bar{v}$ O_2). Thus, oxygen consumed by the body is a product of the amount of oxygen transported in the blood and the amount the body extracts. Because there is no change in $\dot{V}O_2$ or in $\dot{Q}$ required for an absolute submaximal PO, it is obvious that the total oxygen extracted by the body will be similar (see Fig. 19–8). Given that there is a drop in systolic blood pressure at the same submaximal PO after endurance training, however, blood flow to active tissue will drop unless there is a bigger reduction in peripheral resistance. In fact, the peripheral circulation adapts to endurance training with a greater capillary density, facilitating the diffusion of oxygen to muscle fibers. As a result, blood flow to active muscles decreases and local extraction increases and less blood must be shunted away from inactive areas of the body at the same submaximal PO. At maximal exercise, on the other hand, a-$\bar{v}$ O_2 is much higher after training. This reflects an increase in mitochondria and oxidative enzymes of trained muscle and contributes to the rise in maximal $\dot{V}O_2$.

The result of all these changes is as follows. Untrained subjects can increase their $\dot{V}O_2$ ten times from rest to maximal exercise. This is accomplished by a 1.5-fold rise in SV, a 2.4-fold increase in HR (yielding a 3.6-fold higher $\dot{Q}$), and a 2.8-fold rise in a-$\bar{v}$ O_2. Endurance athletes, on the other hand, can have an 18.5-fold rise in $\dot{V}O_2$; this is produced by a 5.8-fold increase in $\dot{Q}$ (2.5 SV $\times$ 2.3 HR) and a 3.2-fold higher a-$\bar{v}$ O_2.

Oxygen Utilization System

OXYGEN EXTRACTION

The rate of oxygen extraction by muscle depends on its rate of utilization (ie, the intracellular metabolic activity), as well as the type of muscle fiber doing the work. As mentioned before, slow-twitch (ST) fibers are more adapted for aerobic metabolism, while fast-twitch (FT) fibers are better suited for anaerobic metabolism. As oxygen must diffuse across the membrane for processing into ATP by the mitochondria, endurance training causes an increase in (1) number and size of mitochondria; (2) activity of their oxidative enzymes; (3) myoglobin; and (4) ability to metabolize fats. That is, muscle fibers become more like an oxidative ST fiber. This type of adaptation is possible in both ST and FT muscle fibers and can produce a doubling of the total oxidative capacity and a faster rate of aerobic enzymatic reactions in skeletal muscle.

As can be observed in athletes, there is little or no increase in muscle mass with endurance training. While there is a net protein synthesis, it is associated with larger and more mitochondria and more enzymes and not with increased contractile proteins. Thus, even if there is no change in the intramuscular reserves of ATP and PC associated with muscle hypertrophy, energy production is increased in endurance-trained muscle.

SUBSTRATE UTILIZATION

After a meal, there is a surplus of CHO, amino acids, and FFA. Depending on the needs of each tissue, the approriate nutrients enter. However, for all practical purposes, amino acids are not used directly for energy. Excess protein is converted into fat or CHO (gluconeogenesis); surplus CHO are converted into fats and stored.

Glucose is the form CHO takes in blood (and all liquids), where it is transported to the liver, kidney, heart, and skeletal muscle for use or to be converted into glycogen for storage. Fats are generally absorbed and stored as triglycerides. They must be broken down into FFA and glycerol before they can diffuse across the membrane of fat cells.

When they enter the blood, they are recombined as triglycerides and transported to other tissues, where they are again degraded. Glycerol is liberated and recirculated, while FFA diffuse easily across the muscle membrane. Between meals, the liver liberates its glycogen to maintain a normal level of blood glucose and fat cells release FFA.

Given that the nervous system uses only glucose for energy, the body attempts to preserve its glycogen reserves but is able to store only a limited quantity. Each gram of glycogen contains 4 kilocalories (kcal) of energy and is stored in the presence of 3 g of water. Fat cells also represent a reservoir of *potential* energy but are not stored with water (fat cells contain only about 5% water). Thus, adipose tissue is a compact, dense energy reserve, with 1 g of fat containing 9 kcal. The 3500 kcal of energy in 1 lb of fat is enough for a 150-lb man to run a 26.2-mile marathon.

At rest, as well as during moderate-intensity exercise requiring less than 50% $\dot{V}O_{2max}$, both CHO and FFA provide equal amounts of energy. Given that the anaerobic system uses only CHO to produce ATP, it is obvious why the proportion of energy from CHO increases as exercise becomes more intense. With high-intensity exercise, intramuscular tension increases and blood flow may become insufficient, such that the main way to obtain energy is through the anaerobic degradation of CHO (especially muscle glycogen), the end result of which is an accumulation of blood LA. If the associated acidity rises too much (eg, at a blood LA level of 7 mmol/L), the efficiency of the aerobic enzymatic reactions is reduced and anaerobic glycolysis is needed even more.

Because there are limited quantities of glycogen and essentially unlimited quantities of energy stored as fat, and because fat can be metabolized only through aerobic processes, logical adaptations to aerobic, endurance training include increased storage of muscle glycogen and a greater capacity to use more FFA for energy, further conserving limited glycogen. A greater maximal aerobic power ($\dot{V}O_{2max}$) after endurance training means that any absolute PO is now at a lower relative intensity. As a result, more fat and less CHO will be used. In addition, endurance training delays the point where anaerobic glycolysis begins in *absolute* and in *relative* terms (Fig. 19–10). Thus, there will be a delay in the PO and intensity where limited muscle glycogen must be used, thereby increasing the dependence on the aerobic breakdown of FFA and of CHO stored in the liver.

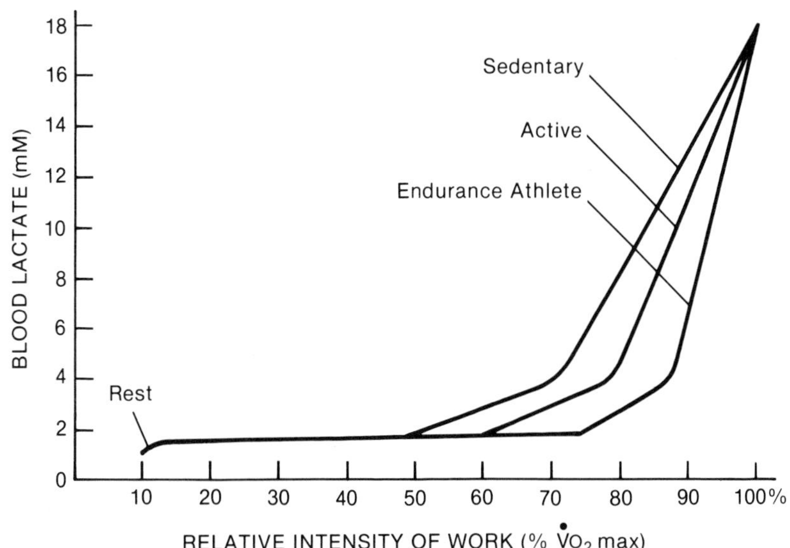

Figure 19–10. Blood lactate level in relation to exercise intensity (% $\dot{V}O_{2max}$) and level of training. (*From* Skinner, JS: Body Energy. Mountainview, CA, Anderson World, Inc., 1981; with permission.)

The result of all these adaptations is a higher $\dot{V}O_{2max}$. Endurance-trained persons can now do more exercise and the exercise they do is less intense. For example, for a sedentary man with a $\dot{V}O_{2max}$ of 2.5 L/min, a PO requiring 1.5 L/min was 60% $\dot{V}O_{2max}$ before training. If his $\dot{V}O_{2max}$ rose 20% to 3 L/min, the same PO requiring 1.5 L/min now would be only 50% $\dot{V}O_{2max}$. More important, however, is the fact that the point where LA begins to accumulate in the blood could be increased from 60% $\dot{V}O_{2max}$ (1.5 L/min before training) to 70% of the new $\dot{V}O_{2max}$ ($3.0 \times 0.70 = 2.1$ L/min). Thus, the net result of the 20% increase in $\dot{V}O_{2max}$ ($3.0/2.5 = 1.20$) is that he can now do 40% more exercise ($2.1/1.5 = 1.40$) before he begins to accumulate LA and use anaerobic glycolysis to replace the ATP being used. Recuperation after exercise also will be easier because the LA level in the blood and the oxygen debt are less. Thus, endurance-trained persons are capable of meeting the aerobic demands of exercise better, fatigue sets in at higher intensities of exercise, and they recover faster.

RESPONSES AND ADAPTATIONS IN ANAEROBIC ENERGY PRODUCTION

Given the principles of overload and specificity mentioned earlier, little or no change in anaerobic energy production should be expected to occur with endurance (aerobic) training, whereas one might expect more changes with anaerobic exercise (eg, brief, high-intensity activities involving strength and sprinting). Compared with the number and magnitude of adaptations associated with endurance training, however, changes in anaerobic energy production are not as impressive.

Part of the reason for this difference has to do with the duration of stimulation and the number of systems that are stimulated to adapt. For example, strength and sprinting activities mainly affect the neuromuscular system for brief periods, whereas endurance exercise requires responses from more systems (eg, neuromuscular, cardiovascular, respiratory, hormonal, and thermoregulatory systems) over a prolonged period. Some of the adaptations to strength and sprint training can be seen in Table 19–2.

Increased strength and speed come as a result of repeated stimulation of the neuromuscular system. A major structural adaptation is muscle hypertrophy (greater cross-sectional area) due to an increase in (1) the number and size of myofibrils per muscle fiber; (2) the amount of contractile proteins (myosin $>$ actin); and (3) the amount and strength of connective, tendinous, and ligamentous tissue. There is a greater hypertrophy of the FT muscle fibers, because they are the ones used during high-intensity muscular contractions. Mainly as a result of the larger size of muscle, there is also a greater storage of phosphagens (ATP and PC) but no change in concentration. In other words, the rise in amount is proportional to the increase in muscle mass.

Although the concentration of ATP and PC is not altered, the activity of the enzymes involved in their turnover is increased, that is, these phosphagens provide energy at a faster rate. If a high-intensity training program is of sufficient duration (eg, 30 to 120 sec) to stimulate the production of LA, then the activity of the glycolytic enzymes also increases; such would not be the case with a strength-training program, with its brief periods of intermittent exercise.

Some of the improvements seen in strength and speed are due to functional changes in the nervous system and can occur without muscle hypertrophy; this may be an important reason why women improve their strength without major increases in muscle size. Altering the pattern of motor unit recruitment, as well as having a better synchronization of their firing, permits a more effective and perhaps more skilled application of force.

An example of the interrelationship between structure and function can be seen in

TABLE 19–2. ADAPTATIONS TO STRENGTH AND SPRINT TRAINING

Structural
Muscle hypertrophy (especially fast-twitch fibers)
  Increased number and size of myofibrils per muscle fiber
  Increased amount of contractile proteins (actin and especially myosin)
  Increased amounts and strengths of connective, tendinous, and ligamentous tissue
Increased muscle stores
  ATP and PC (amount, not concentration)
Increased heart volume
  Normal ventricular cavity and thicker ventricular walls

Functional
Increased enzyme activity
  ATP-PC enzymes (ATPase, myokinase, CPK)
  Glycolytic enzymes (eg, PFK)
Decreased inhibition of the central nervous system
  Decreased sensitivity of Golgi tendon organs
Improved recruitment pattern
Better synchronization of motor units

Abbreviations: ATP = adenosine triphosphate, PC = phosphocreatine, CPK = creatine phosphokinase, PFK = phosphofructokinase.

the Golgi tendon organs, which have a protective, inhibitory effect on muscle force being applied to tendons. With the increased amount and strength of tendinous tissue after high-intensity training, the Golgi tendon organs are stretched less and become less sensitive, the result of which is a reduced inhibition of the central nervous system.

Although there is evidence that heart volume increases with both aerobic and anaerobic training, the stimuli and adaptations are quite different. With endurance training, venous return and stroke volume increase owing to a *volume* overload and remain elevated for prolonged periods. This supposedly produces a larger ventricular cavity with normal wall thickness. Athletes who train with brief, high-intensity activities, on the other hand, have elevated arterial blood pressures while they are attempting to push blood against a high peripheral resistance. Their *pressure* overload supposedly produces a normal cavity and a thicker ventricular wall.

CONCLUSION

There are many immediate responses to exercise and chronic adaptations to training, depending on the type and mode of activity and the metabolic system(s) being stimulated. These can be modified by the characteristics of the person doing the activity, as well as by the environment in which it is being done. The changes brought about by regular exercise respect the principles of overload and specificity and generally do not occur without a logical reason.

If the preceding description of events occurring with exercise appears to be logical and straightforward, then it has achieved its objectives of simplification, clarification, and education. However, if readers are left with the impression that the structural and functional responses and adaptations are simple and uncomplicated, then they should remember (1) that there are few activities which are purely aerobic or anaerobic, and (2) that the single and combined effects of many factors can modify the responses and adaptations. Nevertheless, readers are invited to look for these "logical responses and adaptations" for they are what make studying the physiology of exercise and training so simple, interesting, and challenging.

REFERENCES

1. Åstrand PO, Rodahl K: Textbook of Work Physiology, ed 3. New York, McGraw-Hill, 1986, pp 1–756.
2. Brooks GA, Fahey TD: Exercise Physiology: Human Bioenergetics and Its Applications. New York, John Wiley & Sons, 1984, pp 1–726.
3. Fox EL, Bowers RD, Foss ML: The Physiological Basis of Physical Education and Athletics, ed 4. Philadelphia, WB Saunders, 1988, pp 1–734.
4. Lamb DR: Physiology of Exercise: Responses & Adaptations, ed 2. New York, Macmillan, 1984, pp 1–489.
5. Skinner JS: Functional effects of physical activity. *In* Zeigler EF (ed): Physical Education and Sport: An Introduction. Philadelphia, Lea & Febiger, 1982, pp 69–93.
6. Wilmore JH, Costill DL: Training for Sport and Activity, ed 3. Dubuque, William C Brown, 1988, pp 1–420.
7. Skinner JS, Noeldner SP, O'Connor JS: The development and maintenance of physical fitness. *In* Ryan AJ, Allman FD (eds): Sports Medicine, ed 2. New York, Academic Press, 1989, pp 515–528.
8. Burke F, Cerny F, Costill D, et al: Characteristics of skeletal muscle in competitive cyclists. Med Sci Sports 9:109–112, 1977.
9. Costill D, Daniels J, Evans W, et al: Skeletal muscle enzymes and fiber composition in male and female track athletes. J Appl Physiol 40:149–154, 1976.
10. Gollnick P, Armstrong R, Saubert C, et al: Enzyme activity and fiber composition in skeletal muscle of untrained and trained men. J Appl Physiol 33:312–319, 1972.
11. Komi P, Rusko H, Vos J, et al: Anaerobic performance capacity in athletes. Acta Physiol Scand 100:107–114, 1977.
12. Thorstensson A, Larsson L, Tesch P, et al: Muscle strength and fiber composition in athletes and sedentary men. Med Sci Sports 9:26–30, 1977.
13. Magel J, Andersen KL: Pulmonary diffusing capacity and cardiac output in young trained Norwegian swimmers and untrained subjects. Med Sci Sports 1:131–139, 1969.
14. Chapman CB, Mitchell JH: The physiology of exercise. Sci Am 212(5):88–96, 1965.

20

PSYCHOLOGICAL ASPECTS OF EXERCISE AND SPORT

Kathleen A. Ellickson, PhD

Interest in the psychological aspects of exercise and sport can be traced to early work in philosophy and science. Although the field of sport psychology is relatively young, and the "founding father" of North American sport psychology is considered to be Coleman Griffith, who established a sport psychology laboratory in 1925, the history of sport psychology actually dates back to ancient times. Whereas sport psychologists have existed for less than three quarters of a century, the concerns of sport psychologists were previously studied by philosophers and scientists. For example, St. Augustine (354–430 AD), using introspection as a method for exploring self-consciousness, investigated participant and spectator behavior at chariot races. Throughout history, *mens sana in corpore sano* (ie, a strong mind in a strong body) has been promoted as a cultural ideal.[1]

The field of sport psychology, itself a subspecialty, includes individuals working in a variety of subareas, such as clinical, developmental, health, motivation, personality, and social psychology. Individuals from such diverse fields as biomechanics, exercise physiology, kinesiology, motor control, and motor learning have also contributed to research and applications in sport psychology.

Three areas of scientific investigation currently exist within exercise and sport psychology. One area is concerned with health issues, such as the effect of exercise on high blood pressure, affective disorders (anxiety and depression), and self-esteem. A second area is concerned with performance issues, such as motivation and the enhancement of athletic skills through psychological techniques. A third area, ergonomics, is concerned with the person-machine interaction. The focus here is the relationship of the exerciser with his or her equipment (eg, scuba diver). The purpose of this chapter is to review selected advances in sport psychology that a medical practitioner may find useful in his or her treatment of patients engaged in recreational exercise or competitive athletics.

Recreational exercisers and competitive athletes will be treated as two discrete groups for the purposes of this review. Exercisers are defined as individuals engaged in physical activity for the primary motivation of maintaining or improving their level of health and physical fitness. Competitive athletes are defined as individuals engaged in physical activity to prepare for performing in a specific sporting event. This commonly involves training regimens of an intense nature designed to improve or refine the athlete's skill, strength, or endurance levels.[2]

This distinction is necessary because the two areas of scientific investigation differ in terms of methodology. Research data generated in both areas contribute to the body of knowledge in exercise and sport psychology. However, care needs to be taken with regard to application because the training stimulus and subject populations are so discrete.

PSYCHOLOGICAL ASPECTS OF RECREATIONAL EXERCISE

Quality of Life: Coping with Daily Stressors

In 1987, the American Psychiatric Association published statistics on the prevalence of psychiatric disorders in the United States.[3] According to this report:

1. Twenty percent of all adults will experience at least one episode of clinical depression in the course of their lifetime.
2. Eight percent of all Americans suffer from anxiety disorders so severe that their daily lives (ie, ability to work, enjoy interpersonal relationships, or leave home) are disrupted.
3. It is estimated that only about 20% of all severely troubled Americans ever seek professional help.

Many of the psychosocial symptoms that result from modern day living appear to be a result of inadequate coping responses to the stresses of daily existence. Individuals attempt to cope with stress through a variety of methods such as pharmacologic therapy, alcohol ingestion, and binge eating, to name a few. Although these methods may be effective in alleviating negative emotions for a brief period, they do not enhance the individual's adaptive qualities in any lasting way. In order to modify stress responses, an individual must understand the precipitants of their emotional reactions.

Spielberger[4] has challenged the view that stress and anxiety are synonomous states or emotions. Rather, he suggests that stress is a complex psychobiologic process, which includes three elements:

1. A stimulus variable (stressor).
2. A cognitive appraisal of the stimulus variable (perception).
3. A response.

The stressor may be either an external situation as diverse as weather conditions or interpersonal relationships or an internal stimulus, such as worry. Following exposure to the stressor, a cognitive appraisal is made by the individual. If the stressor is viewed as harmful or threatening, the perception may be followed by an anxious response. A response to the stressor is based upon the individual's perception of the stressor as well as his or her perceived ability to cope with it. Spielberger's model[4] suggests that stressors can not always be "managed" because they often occur in the external environment. Also, stressors are not inherently "good" or "bad" and their meaning is influenced by an individual's aptitude, coping skills, and past experience as well as by the perceived danger of the situation. An advantageous point of attack for altering adverse responses to stress is to change the individual's perception of the stressor. An alternative strategy for stress management is to increase one's tolerance levels (ie, one's coping skills) for stressors.

Exercise and Affect

An extensive literature exists describing a positive correlation between exercise and improved levels of affective disorders and mood states. It should be noted, however, that a variety of conditions, such as owning a pet,[5] sitting quietly in a recliner-type chair,[6] meditating,[7] and eating lunch,[8] have also been found to positively influence mood states. Therefore, exercise is only one method to achieve higher states of well-being.

Individuals engaged in vigorous physical activity on a regular basis seem to experience a variety of changes as a result of their exercise involvement. Alterations in mood states, blood pressure, galvanic skin response, heart rate, metabolism, and muscular strength and endurance occur as sedentary individuals become increasingly physically fit. Scientists may be more interested in the quantifiable psychophysiologic measures that monitor the benefits of an individual's response to exercise. However, the exerciser may value more highly the improved quality of his or her life, which is also associated with exercise involvement. Despite an inability of empiric data to explain the state of "feeling better," those engaged in vigorous physical activity generally report this seemingly universal phenomena.[9] A number of hypotheses have been advanced to explain the altered states associated with exercise. These include being distracted from the cares and worries of the day, reregulation of brain monamine systems, and increases in endorphin levels. Excellent reviews of the pros and cons of these hypotheses can be found elsewhere.[9]

One of the more crucial studies has compared exercise to more traditional therapies in the treatment of depression. Greist and colleagues[10] found that running was as effective as time-limited psychotherapy and more effective than time-unlimited psychotherapy for reducing symptoms in a group of 28 mildly depressed men and women randomly assigned to treatment conditions. Exercise was found to be more effective than either therapy condition for keeping depressive symptoms down at 9-month follow-up. Because the majority of affected Americans do not seek psychiatric treatment for mood disorders, exercise may be a self-help method which physicians can prescribe to enable their patients to regulate psychopathology.

Some of the most consistent research findings have demonstrated improvements in self-concept with exercise training. Self-concept differs from self-esteem, and indeed, one hypothesis advanced to explain the increased self-concept associated with exercise of a vigorous physical nature involves enhanced levels of self-esteem.[11] Self-esteem is defined as the "degree to which individuals feel positive about themselves."[12] In other words, self-esteem is the evaluative component of self-concept. According to the self-esteem model proposed by Sonstroem and Morgan,[11] physical activity leads to increased beliefs (ie, self-efficacy) concerning one's ability to perform certain physical activities, such as a 12-minute walk. Higher levels of self-efficacy lead to increases in actual participation in the exercise and confirmation that the task is within the individual's capabilities. This increased sense of competence leads to increased self-esteem. As participation in physical activity continues, the individual becomes more satisfied with his or her physical appearance and this also has a positive effect on self-esteem. Furthermore, the increased self-esteem results in improved self-concept both at a specific and a global level.

Exercise Addiction

The American College of Sports Medicine (ACSM) recommends a prescription of 15 to 60 minutes of continuous aerobic exercise, 3 to 5 times a week for "developing and maintaining cardiorespiratory fitness and body composition in the healthy adult."[13] Most North Americans have difficulty exercising at the level suggested by the ACSM. However, clinical data suggest that some participants develop just the opposite problem: an unhealthy attachment to exercise. The etiology of exercise "addiction" is not well understood. However, excessive commitment to intense training for whatever reason may result in a form of dependence. Solomon's Opponent Process theory of acquired motivation has been used to explain alterations in motivational and mood responses to exercise.[14] According to this model, pain and pleasure comprise an internal feedback loop. When sedentary individuals begin to exercise, they often experience muscle soreness and a variety of aches and pains. If they continue the exercise program, the pain is replaced by tolerance. Eventually, pleasure will be associated with the training program as the individual experiences increased self-esteem resulting from his or her improved physical fitness.

It is often necessary with mood-altering substances, such as sedative-hypnotics, to steadily increase the dosage to obtain the same effect.[15] Exercisers who become dependent on the altered mood states associated with vigorous physical exercise may find that they must continually increase the exercise dose to achieve the desired effect. Failure to increase mileage, for instance, in the case of a runner, will result in the pain of not experiencing the needed euphoria. Devoting increasingly greater amounts of time to workouts results in compromises in the exerciser's vocational, social, and marital commitments.[16] As the addictive process develops, exercisers adopt an inward focus and become less concerned with environmental matters. External rewards, such as job promotions and monetary bonuses, may lose their importance as the exerciser measures his or her self-worth by gains made in the training regimen. Previously cherished family and friends may also lose their significance as the addict becomes increasingly devoted to exercise.

A true exercise addict will tend to demonstrate self-destructive behaviors when an injury requires cessation of the training regimen. Cognitive awareness of the need to rest an injured muscle or bone often does not prevent exercise behavior. It is possible that the need to achieve the desired mood state supercedes the need to properly rehabilitate an overused muscle or bone.

Exercise and Mental Health: The National Institute of Mental Health Consensus Statement

The Office of Prevention of the National Institute of Mental Health (NIMH) sponsored a state-of-the-art workshop in the spring of 1984. The purpose of the workshop was to establish guidelines for primary care physicians and mental health professionals concerning the potential and limits of exercise as a means of coping with stress.[12] The following consensus statements are a result of the state-of-the-art workshop regarding exercise and mental health, and the conclusions remain valid today:

1. Physical fitness is positively associated with mental health and well-being.
2. Exercise is associated with the reduction of stress emotions, such as state anxiety.
3. Anxiety and depression are common symptoms of failure to cope with mental stress, and exercise has been associated with a decreased level of mild-to-moderate depression and anxiety.
4. Long-term exercise is usually associated with reductions in traits such as neuroticism and anxiety.
5. Severe depression usually requires professional treatment, which may include medication, electroconvulsive therapy, and/or psychotherapy, with exercise as an adjunct.
6. Appropriate exercise results in reductions in various stress indices, such as neuromuscular tension, resting heart rate, and some stress hormones.
7. Current clinical opinion holds that exercise has beneficial emotional effects across all ages and in both sexes.
8. Physically healthy people who require psychotropic medication may safely exercise when exercise and medications are titrated under close medical supervision.

PSYCHOLOGICAL ASPECTS OF COMPETITIVE ATHLETES

Mental Health Model

Competitive athletes involved in endurance sports, such as distance running, rowing, swimming, and wrestling, are characterized by positive mental health.[17] Male and female athletes who participate at the college, national, and Olympic levels have been observed to score approximately one standard deviation below the population mean on standardized measures of anxiety and depression. These findings have led to the development of the "mental health model," which predicts that athletes who possess positive mental health are more likely to be successful than are individuals with elevated mood states, such as anxiety or depression. Although successful athletes are typically characterized by positive mental health, it has been demonstrated that approximately 10% of any given sample will experience anxiety states and depression of clinical significance.

Primary care or team physicians may employ an objective assessment measure, such as Zung's Self-Rating Depression Scale (SDS),[18] Beck Depression Inventory (BDI),[19] or Profile of Mood States (POMS),[20] to assist in the diagnosis of affective disorders. Assessment instruments quantify the level of mood states and can be used to monitor changes in clinical scales over time. A scale such as the POMS provides scores on six measures of mood (ie, tension, depression, anger, vigor, fatigue, and confusion) and could easily become part of the athlete's annual medical exam. This information could serve as a baseline point for further assessment data.

It should be noted that athletes may be reluctant to call attention to affective disturbances for fear that this information will negatively affect their selection or participation on the team. The physician may be in a position to act as an advocate for the athlete who needs to be referred for psychological counseling or treatment.[21] The physician and athletic coach should discuss the way in which to handle this situation before it occurs, keeping the welfare of the athlete and the confidential nature of the problem as the most important considerations.

Overtraining and Staleness

Athletes may reach a point in training where they experience a performance plateau or decrement. Despite intense training and high levels of motivation, the athlete is unable to maintain previously achieved levels of athletic performance. This state may occur in all sports, but it is a particular problem for athletes involved in endurance sports, such as cycling, distance running, rowing, skiing, and swimming. When athletes demonstrate a performance plateau or decrement in response to overtraining, they are usually diagnosed as being stale.[22]

Although some debate exists concerning the symptoms associated with staleness, the following sequelae routinely accompany the subpar athletic performance:

1. Sleep impairment (initial, middle insomnia).
2. Chronic fatigue.
3. Appetite disturbance (aphasia, hyperphasia).
4. Myopathy.
5. Elevated blood pressure.
6. Elevated blood levels of creatine kinase.
7. Increased effort sense.
8. Affective disturbance (elevated mood states, such as anxiety and depression).

Staleness is a complex psychophysiologic state. It is associated with cardiovascular, endocrine, metabolic, perceptual, and psychometric alterations. Prevention is of course the best solution to the problem of staleness. Athletes and coaches who are alert to the early warning signals may divert staleness from occurring through a reduction in the training load. However, this can be difficult because athletes train hard to achieve maximal performance. The symptoms used to diagnose staleness can be employed to avoid distress through daily or weekly monitoring.

If staleness occurs, the only known remedy is rest. The amount of time needed to recover from staleness is mediated by individual differences. Several weeks or months may be required before the athlete is able to return to his or her sport.

Team physicians are in an excellent position to monitor the symptoms of staleness and to make appropriate recommendations to coaches concerning tapers in the training load. Monitoring selected physiologic and psychological parameters to prevent staleness is clearly a potentially valuable service that the physician can contribute to the athletic team.

Motivation and Performance

It is widely accepted that preperformance "jitters" exist before a variety of participant activities. Individuals participating in sport may find this to be particularly true because the evaluative nature inherent in winning and losing increases the pressure to perform well. The effect of impending competition on anxiety often can be striking. The management of precompetition anxiety has received much attention in recent years as a potential means to enhance performance in part because the difference between a winning and losing performance has become so small. It is not uncommon for the margin of victory to be measured in milliseconds in events such as track. The challenge for researchers has become one of trying to understand the relationship between anxiety and performance so that performance can be enhanced rather than inhibited by one's arousal level.

Historically, a variety of theoretical views have been used in sport to explain the role that precompetition anxiety plays in performance. However, there is a lack of basic and applied research to substantiate these theories. A more complete review of this topic can be found elsewhere.[23] The following section will briefly review four theoretical views.

For many years, it was believed that increases in arousal lead to enhanced performance in sport settings. Drive theory maintains that increases in precompetition anxiety lead to improved performance. This theory results in coaches using a variety of psyching techniques, such as pep talks, prior to competition, in an effort to get athletes "ready" to play.

Drive theory was eventually rejected in favor of the inverted-U theory (Yerkes-Dodson law), which maintains that increases in anxiety lead to increases in performance, but only up to a certain point. Then, as anxiety continues to increase, performance actually decreases. Inverted-U theory suggests that a moderate level of arousal is necessary for performance to be successful.

More recently, it has been argued that decreases in arousal lead to enhanced performance. Quiescence theory is the antithesis of drive theory; it suggests that as arousal decreases, performance increases. Unfortunately, this theoretical view is not supported by a compelling body of basic or applied research. While it is true that various technologies exist to alter states of arousal (eg, relaxation, hypnosis, meditation), it is not clear what the optimal level of arousal is in terms of athletic performance.

Compelling research on motivation and performance has been carried out by the Soviet sport psychologist, Yuri Hanin.[24] Hanin has demonstrated that each athlete has an "arousal zone of optimal functioning" (ZOF). ZOF theory maintains that each individual has an optimal arousal zone of "useful" anxiety necessary for performance. If the individual is within that zone prior to competition, he or she will be more likely to experience success in athletics than if the anxiety level is either higher or lower than the "useful" amount.

Many contemporary sport psychologists in the United States have dismissed Hanin's theory on the basis that it is a reiteration of inverted-U theory. The two theories are very different, however, because the ZOF theory does not argue that a moderate level of precompetition anxiety is superior to low or high levels. The ZOF predicts that some athletes will be most successful when highly aroused, others when very relaxed, and others when moderately aroused. A significant observation made by ZOF, which earlier theories have not addressed, is individual variation. ZOF maintains that the appropriate level of arousal for a task is dependent on the individual performing it, rather than being inherent in the task itself.

Based on this theory, the challenge is to help each individual athlete reach his or her optimal level of "useful" anxiety. Interventions aimed at increasing or decreasing arousal levels in entire teams would not be appropriate because no single level of anxiety is desirable for all athletes.

Athletic Injuries

Injuries that disrupt the athlete's participation in sport often create a variety of difficulties for the individual. Expectations for rehabilitation and return to physical activity may be predicated more on the athlete's need for sport involvement or interpretation of the debilitating injury than on realistic rates of recovery.[25] An important factor to consider in determining the severity of an athletic injury is the emotional ability of the athlete to cope with the injury rather than the loss of physical functioning per se.

Intense training of a physical nature has been shown to reduce mild-to-moderate levels of anxiety and depression.[12] Individuals unable to complete their daily exercise regimen due to an injury may experience decreased abilities to cope with everyday stressors. Compensatory activities that provide outlets for discharging anxiety may help to alleviate uncomfortable negative emotion. However, it may be more difficult to find a compensatory activity to satisfy the athlete's psychological attachment to the sport.

Little[26] demonstrated that men who overvalued their physical strength, skill, or stamina were exquisitely more vulnerable to even minor injury (for example, sprained ankle) than men who showed little interest in sport or physical activities. Men who defined themselves as athletic displayed symptoms of anxiety and depression when threats were made to their physical abilities but were relatively impervious to work- or interpersonal-related stressors. Little defined the athlete's reaction to injury as a bereavement response to a loss of self requiring new ways of coping, which the athlete had not yet developed.

Athletic injuries, however temporary, that threaten an individual's identity-confirming roles and sense of adequacy may create significant emotional distress. Nicholas[27] suggests that "injuries result in punishment to the soul as well as to the body of the person" and recommends that "a comprehensive, scientific, multidisciplinary approach" be taken to hasten the athlete's recovery from injury. Although no empiric data currently exists demonstrating the need for all injured players to engage in psychotherapy, team physicians may hasten a player's recovery by monitoring mood states and referring the athlete to a mental health professional if a significant elevation in psychopathology occurs. An athlete suspected of malingering may be helped by a referral for psychological help because physical rehabilitation may not address the player's significant concerns.[28]

CONCLUSION

The field of sport psychology derives contributions to its knowledge base from a diverse field of exercise scientists and applied practitioners. Team physicians are encouraged to include psychological considerations in their sports medicine practices. Multidisciplinary referral networks and support systems aimed at conducting research and providing treatment will enhance the comprehensive care of exercising and competing sports medicine patients.

REFERENCES

1. Weiss P: Sport: A Philosophical Inquiry. Carbondale, IL, Southern University Press, 1983.
2. Brown D: Exercise and sport as elements in therapy. Clin Psychol 39(3):71–74, 1986.
3. American Psychiatric Association: Fact Sheet. Washington, DC, American Psychiatric Association, 1987.
4. Spielberger CD: Stress, emotions, and health. *In* Morgan WP, Goldston SE (eds): Exercise and Mental Health. Washington, DC, Hemisphere, 1987, pp 11–16.
5. Katcher A, Beck T: New Perspective on Our Lives with Companion Animals. Philadelphia, University of Pennsylvania Press, 1983.
6. Raglin JS, Morgan WP: Influence of acute exercise and distraction therapy on state anxiety and blood pressure (in preparation).
7. Michaels RR, Huber MJ, McCann DS: Evaluation of transcendental meditation as a method of reducing stress. Science 192:1242–1244, 1976.
8. Wilson VE, Berger BG, Bird EI: Effects of running and of an exercise class on anxiety. Percept Mot Skills 53:472–474, 1981.
9. Morgan WP: Affec e beneficience of vigorous physical activity. Med Sci Exerc Sport 17(1):94–100, 1985.
10. Greist JH, Klein MH, Eischens RR, et al: Running as treatment for depression. Compr Psychiatry 20:41–54, 1979.
11. Sonstroem J, Morgan WP: Exercise and self esteem: Rationale and model. Med Sci Exerc Sport 17(1):329–337, 1989.
12. Morgan WP, Goldston GE (eds): Exercise and Mental Health. Washington, DC, Hemisphere, 1985.
13. American College of Sports Medicine: Position statement on the recommended quantity and quality of exercise for developing and maintaining fitness in healthy adults. Med Sci Exerc Sport 8(2):xi–xiii, 1976.
14. Solomon RL: The opponent process theory of acquired motivation. Am Psychol 35:691–721, 1980.
15. Gerald MC: Pharmacology. Englewood Cliffs, NY, Prentice Hall, 1981, pp 186–188.
16. Morgan WP: Negative addiction in runners. Physician Sportsmed 7(2):57–69, 1979.
17. Morgan WP: Selected psychological factors limiting performance: A mental health model. *In* Clarke DH, Eckerts HM (eds): Limits of Human Performance. Champaign, IL, Human Kinetics Pub, 1985, pp 70–80.
18. Zung WW: The Measurement of Depression. Merrill National Laboratories, 1974.
19. Beck AT: Depression and Its Treatment. Philadelphia, University of Pennsylvania Press, 1972.
20. McNair DM, Lorr M, Droppleman LF: Profile of Mood States Manual. San Diego, CA, Educational and Industrial Testing Service, 1971.
21. Ogilvie BC: The orthopedist's role in children's sports. Orthop Clin North Am 14(2):361–372, 1983.
22. Morgan WP, Brown DR, Raglin JS, et al: Psychological monitoring of overtraining and staleness. Br J Sports Med 21(3):107–114, 1987.
23. Morgan WP, Ellickson KA: Health, anxiety, and physical exercise. *In* Spielberger CD, Hackbarth D (eds): Anxiety in Sport: An International Perspective. New York, Hemisphere, 1987.
24. Hanin Y: A study of anxiety in sports. *In* Straub WF (ed): Sport Psychology: An Analysis of Athlete Behavior. Ithaca, NY, Mouvement Publications, 1980, pp 236–249.
25. Eldridge WD: The importance of psychotherapy for athletic-related orthopedic injuries among adults. Compr Psychiatry 24(3):271–277, 1983.
26. Little JC: Neurotic illness in fitness fanatics. Psychiatr Ann 9(3):49–56, 1979.
27. Nicholas JA, Reilly JP: Orthopedic problems in athletes. Compr Ther 11(1):48–56, 1985.
28. Scott SG: Current concepts in the rehabilitation of the injured athlete. Mayo Clin Proc 59:83–90, 1984.

21

PREVENTION OF SPORTS INJURIES

Per Renstrom, MD, PhD
Pekka Kannus, MD, PhD

Interest in sporting activities has grown in recent decades because of the increase in leisure time as well as the belief that general health can be enhanced by improved physical fitness.[1–3] Regular aerobic exercise has been linked to decreased risk of cardiovascular diseases[4] and to assistance in weight reduction.[5] In addition, fitness and exercise have been claimed to decrease the morbidity and mortality of aging.[6] As a result, sporting activities are now described as beneficial for the society as well as for the individual. A certain amount of physical activity is considered an important element in health promotion, as has been stated by the American College of Sports Medicine (ACSM) in 1978 and the International Federation of Sports Medicine (FIMS) in 1989.[7,8]

With the resultant upsurge in sporting activity, there has been an increase in sports injuries, both from acute and from overuse trauma.[3,9–14] An *acute injury* is defined as a single-impact macrotrauma, which, for example, can be a blow to a leg resulting in a fracture, a rotational injury of a joint resulting in a ligament sprain, or a direct blow to the muscle resulting in a muscle strain.[15] An *overuse injury* is defined as a long-standing or recurring orthopedic problem and pain in the musculoskeletal system, which have started during training or performance due to repetitive tissue microtrauma.[10,15] Repetitive microtrauma, which is basically repeated exposure of the musculoskeletal tissue to low-magnitude forces, results in injury at the microscopic level, and no single acute trauma is normally involved in the pathogenesis of an overuse injury.

Numerous epidemiologic studies of sports injuries are available.[3,10,11,14,16–22] However, owing to the fact that the population at risk is extremely difficult to identify, the actual incidences of sports injuries in one society or more specific groups are still almost unknown. In addition, the fact that the population which takes part in physical activity does so at different levels and with considerably different intensity makes the evaluation even more difficult. Hence, studies analyzing sports injuries have not been able to identify athletes at risk or the real risk factors regarding injury, and the etiologic factors have not yet been fully assessed.[23] However, to develop preventive strategies, epidemiologically valid studies analyzing sports injuries must be performed.

Today, the number of acute sports injuries treated in hospitals is rather well known. Forty years ago, sports injuries formed 1.4% of all injuries seen at a casualty department.[24] During the 1970s, this figure varied between 5% and 7%,[19,22,25] and at the moment, about 10% of all traumatic injuries treated in the emergency rooms of hospitals in industrialized countries are sustained in sports.[14,26–28] These numbers, of course, do not represent any real incidence of these injuries, but rather only "the tip of an iceberg."

Regarding overuse injuries, exact incidence rates are even more difficult to establish. Their definition is less clear, the diagnosis is more difficult to establish, and the population at risk is almost always unknown. In addition, these injuries are treated independently in many different places (sports injury clinics, hospitals, primary care units, physical therapy departments, private clinics) by many different persons (specialized and nonspecialized physicians, podiatrists, chiropractors, osteopaths, physical therapists, athletic trainers). As a matter of fact, the only thing which is certain is that, owing to the general increase in sporting activities, the absolute number of overuse injuries has increased dramatically during the last decade.[2,10,29] The claim about relative increase (ie, increase in the incidence) remains without scientific evidence.

Both acute and overuse sports injuries are generally considered to be of relatively mild character.[10,14,20,30] It is estimated that up to 75% of all sports injuries can be classified as mild to moderate, requiring only short sick leave and absence from sports.[14,23] The number of patients requiring further treatment as inpatients because of sports injury appears to be about 10%.[14,22,24,25,27,31] Furthermore, the number of patients needing operative treatment of their acute or overuse injury varies from 5% to 10%.[10,11,14,20,29,30,32]

Despite the fact that most sports injuries are mild or moderate by character, the treatment of injured athletes often requires special judgment and experience. Physicians who treat need not only special knowledge in sports medicine, but they should also be familiar with the sport as such and with its rules and demands. A correct diagnosis, immediate treatment, and effective rehabilitation program are prerequisites for a comeback to the sports arena. Only 100% recovery from injury ensures successful return. In this respect, ordinary patient care must fulfill clearly minor demands.

Despite advanced knowledge, modern technology, and improved skills in sports medicine, many patients fail to return. Therefore, the prevention of injuries should be a major goal of every physician as well as staff working in the field of sports medicine.[33]

STRATEGIES IN SPORTS INJURY PREVENTION

By sports injury prevention, we mean all efforts to prevent injuries occurring in connection with physical activity. Efforts may be at individual, group, or society level. Injuries may, in turn, be acute or overuse by nature, and connections to sports may be direct or indirect. Furthermore, the level of physical activity may vary from mild recreational to strenuous professional.

The direct or indirect prevention of sports injury at the individual level can be called *primary prevention,* as is often the case in the prevention strategies in general medicine and health education. Medical preseason examination of a subject, warming up before the competition, and usage of protective equipment (eg, helmets, face guards, gum shields, different paddings, safety-release ski-bindings, braces, tape) are typical examples of primary prevention. In general medicine, a good example of primary prevention of lung cancer is the individual's decision to stop smoking.

Sports injury prevention at group level can be called *secondary prevention.* The most common method of secondary prevention is group information and education. Lectures to athletes and coaches about the importance of proper warm-up and cooling-down; careful following of the rules (fair play); the disadvantages of drugs, alcohol, and tobacco; and known risk factors of injuries are typical examples. Any decision within individual sport events making that particular sport safer can also be seen as secondary prevention. Regarding lung cancer, a public information campaign against smoking in mass media is an excellent way to accomplish secondary prevention.

All efforts undertaken at society level to prevent sports injuries can be called *tertiary prevention.* Normally, tertiary prevention means looking far ahead; consequences will not be seen until years after strategies were planned and put into effect. Society planning is often seen as a tool in tertiary prevention. Concerning sports injury prevention, an example might be a political decision to build new, safe biking routes that are completely separate from motor vehicle traffic. Also, a legislative decision of one state or country to deny in boxing all hits to the head can be seen as a tertiary effort of prevention. In prevention of lung cancer, a typical tertiary action is the decision to increase the price of the pack of cigarettes. Figure 21–1 summarizes the three different levels of sports injury prevention.

Sports injury prevention also can be seen from different views than those presented here. For example, all three levels can be applied to one individual.[2,34] In this strategy,

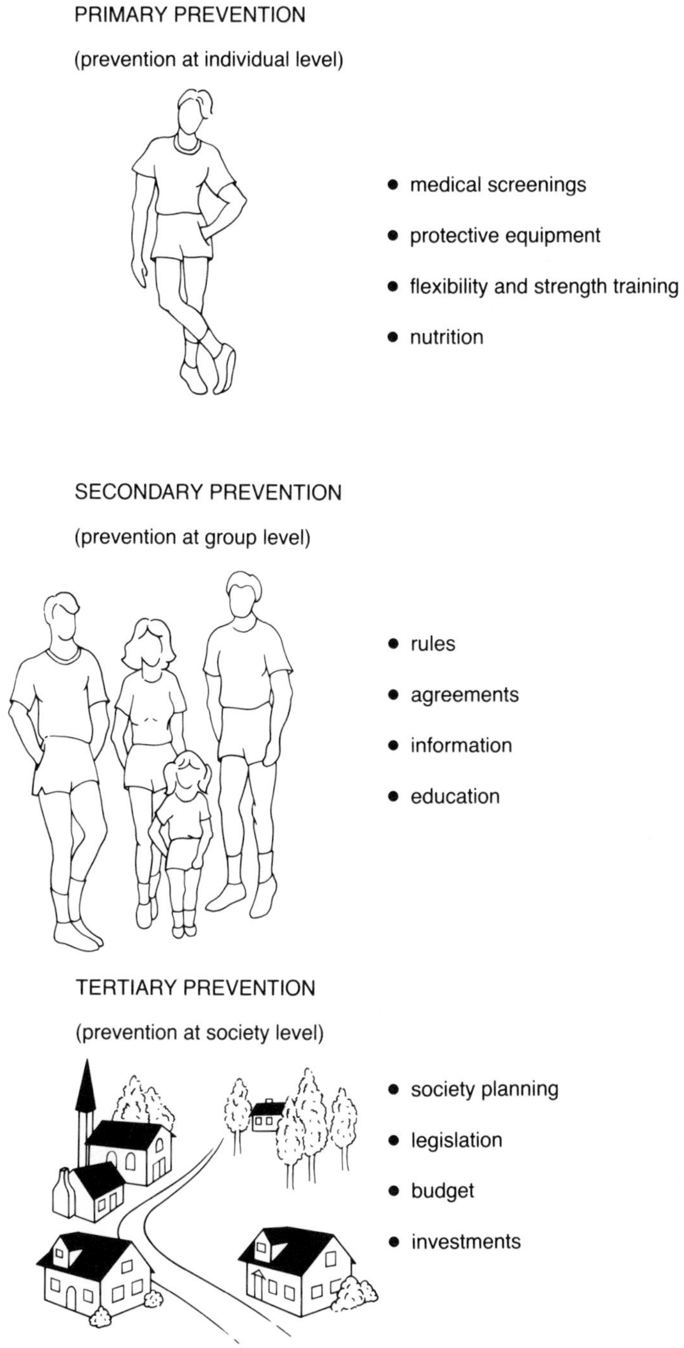

Figure 21–1. Strategies in sports injury prevention.

prevention of an injury before its occurrence can be called primary prevention. Efforts to prevent reinjuries or to keep existing injuries from becoming chronic can be called secondary prevention. Finally, preventing a chronic injury from becoming functionally irreversible can be called tertiary prevention.

Whatever view is taken, it is of great importance that the framework of the selected strategy is clear and that everyone involved understands the basic principles. If this basis of injury prevention rests on shaky grounds, only disappointing and frustrating results can be expected.

GENERAL PREVENTIVE METHODS

In practice, the strategies in primary, secondary, and tertiary prevention of sports injuries overlap. For example, medical screening before a marathon running competition can be directed to one individual by his or her personal examination, to many people by group examinations, or to the whole society by a legislative decision that every runner should have a medical screening before participation in a competition.

General prevention of sports injuries includes all the methods, which concern everyone involved in physical activity. Specific preventive methods are directed to affect the intrinsic and extrinsic predisposing factors of sports injuries.

Basic Physical Fitness

Physical fitness is of the utmost importance in avoiding sports injury. Those whose basic fitness level is below normal are more prone to injury, both from acute trauma and from overuse.[2,15]

After a period of inactivity, the ability of the body tissues to absorb oxygen decreases noticeably. Three weeks of bed rest leads to a 20% to 45% reduction in oxygen uptake capacity.[2,35] When the demands are reduced, there is a corresponding decrease in cardiac output, blood volume, and muscle mass and strength. As a result, the body is less efficient in transporting oxygen from the lungs to the tissues, and the energy supply of muscles and other peripheral tissues is reduced.

Inactivity and immobilization also have deleterious effects on the musculoskeletal tissues. Bones become decalcified, tendons and ligaments lose their tensile strength, muscle tissue atrophies and becomes weaker, and cartilages lose their elasticity.[36–42]

A basic level of physical fitness can be achieved by regular exercise and general physical activity throughout the year. General conditioning and training of large muscle groups are of great importance in most sports. Training should progress gradually; this applies above all to those who are no longer young. During the period of rehabilitation following illness or injury, or after a break in training, it is important that a reasonable level of physical fitness is reached before competition is resumed.

Warm-up and Cooling-down

Warm-up exercises are designed to prepare the body for the ensuing sporting activity (Fig. 21–2). They have two functions: to prevent injury and to enhance performance.

In a body at rest, the blood flow to the striated skeletal muscles is relatively low, and most of the small blood vessels (capillaries) supplying them are closed. When activity begins, the blood flow to these muscles increases as the vessels open. At rest, 15% to 20%

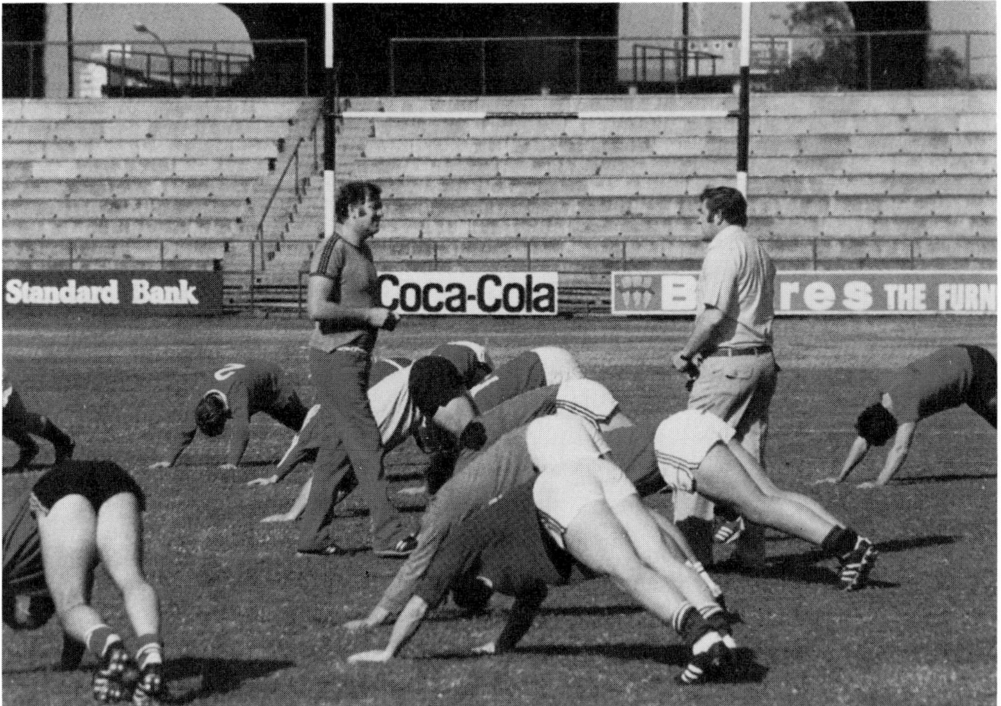

Figure 21–2. In injury prevention, warm-up exercises are essential before training and competition.

of the blood flow supplies the skeletal muscles, whereas the corresponding figure after 10 to 12 minutes of all-around exercise is 70% to 75%.[2] A muscle can achieve maximum endurance performance only when all its blood vessels are functional and maximally open.

Regarding injury prevention by warm-up exercise, the most common and important injuries to be prevented are not only muscle strains but also tendon, ligament, and other soft tissue injuries. Physical work increases the energy output and the temperature of the muscles. This, in turn, leads to improved brain-muscle coordination and cooperation with less likelihood of uncontrolled muscle activities and strain. At the same time, warm-up exercise increases general alertness, providing psychological preparation for the task to come.

Warm-up exercises should begin with movements of the large muscle groups as these are the main areas to which blood is redistributed. Jogging and stationary biking are often used for this purpose. After this general warm-up, more event-specific exercises can begin. Runners, for example, should concentrate their further warm-up on the muscles, tendons, joints, and ligaments of the lower extremities. Stretching is also essential, but heavy loads at the outer limits of joint movement should be avoided.

The final stage of warm-up concentrates on technique, perhaps checking a run-up or practicing event-specific movements. The pace of the exercises can be gradually increased, and the whole warm-up session should last for at least 15 to 20 minutes, depending on the sport involved. After the warm-up period, the effect of the warm-up soon starts to wear off; therefore, mild exercises should be continued. Ideally, the time delay before competition should be no longer than 10 minutes. During this time, the athletes also prepare themselves psychologically.

After training or competition, cooling-down exercises are desirable. Cooling-down enhances the washout of the waste products of muscle metabolism (eg, lactic acid), thus shortening the recovery time. It also offers a good opportunity for stretching exercises, since the muscle temperature is still high and stretching can be performed safely and easily.

Cooling-down is normally carried out in two phases. The first phase is event-specific, including sport-specific movements with 50% to 70% of maximal capacity. This phase should be aerobic by nature. For example, after cross-country skiing competition, the athlete should ski an additional 1 to 3 km at mild or moderate speed. The second phase consists of general large-muscle exercises, such as gentle jogging, performed after the first phase with 30% to 50% of maximal capacity. Stretching for 5 to 15 minutes (depending on the sport) is included in this phase.

Slow Progression

Slow progression principle in injury prevention means that we allow the musculoskeletal system to adapt gradually to increasing loads. It is well known that at least 50% of all overuse injuries are caused by training errors.[43,44] The majority of these errors are, in turn, due to failure to follow the slow progression principle.

A male competitive runner, who has increased his weekly mileage slowly but steadily every year, is able to run after 10 years' progression more than 130 miles (200 km) per week without musculoskeletal problems. At the same time, his colleague, who has increased his mileage faster, is much more prone to overuse troubles while running the same amount per week.

Musculoskeletal adaptation to stress is a slow but effective process. Therefore, to avoid injuries in muscles (eg, pain, soreness, strain, and compartment syndromes), tendons (tendinitis, peritendinitis, tendinosus, and partial or complete ruptures), joints (cartilage softening or avulsion, meniscal ruptures, ligament sprains, synovitis, and osteoarthritis), and bones (stress fractures, osteoporotic fractures, and apophysitis), special attention is required from athletes and their coaches to the importance of slow progression. This especially concerns children and adolescents.[15]

Preventive Training

Training of the musculoskeletal system is the key to both the prevention of injuries and successful recovery after an injury. Repeated, slowly progressive exercises will improve the mechanical and structural properties of the muscles, tendons, joints, ligaments, and bones by increasing their mass and tensile strength. Preventive training includes muscle training, mobility and flexibility training, coordination and proprioceptive training, and sports-specific training.[2]

Muscle Training. Muscle training can be isometric (static work), concentric (positive work), or eccentric (negative work). Isometric training means muscular contractions against a load that is not moved or is too much to overcome. The muscle can develop maximum tension, but its length remains constant.[2,15,45] For example, a weight can be held in the hand with the arm outstretched. Isometric exercise is an effective method for increasing strength, but only around the angle at which the training is carried out. In addition, long periods of isometric training impair speed and power capabilities, indicating that it has limitations with regard to injury preventive training.

Concentric muscle work means that a muscle is activated and shortens in length simultaneously so that its attachments are drawn closer together.[2,15] For example, bending an elbow with a weight in the hand is a concentric, isotonic action. Isotonic means that the load is constant throughout the range of motion; thus, the muscle tension (tonus) is also constant. Isotonic exercises are the most frequently used training methods in injury prevention. If a concentric training is performed with an accommodated load at a con-

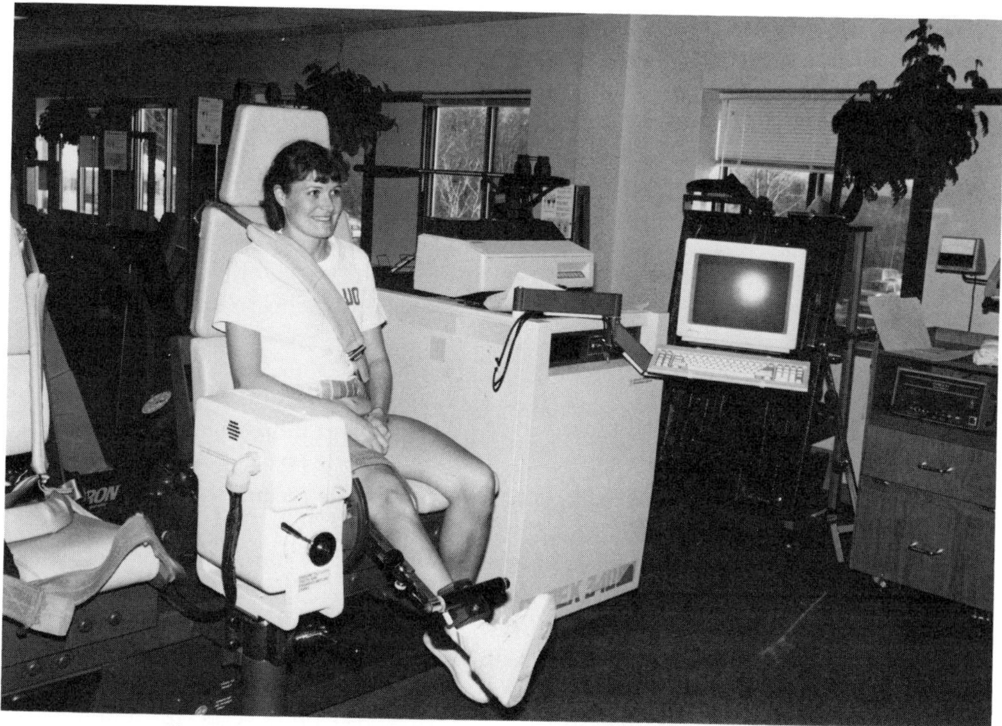

Figure 21–3. A modern device for concentric isokinetic muscle training.

stant angular velocity throughout the range of motion, the muscle contraction is isokinetic. Isokinetic exercise needs, however, a special apparatus (Fig. 21–3). If carried out through different speeds of movement, from 0 to 300 degrees per second, isokinetic training is a very effective method for increasing muscle strength, power, and endurance.[46] Top-level athletes sometimes need to exercise at higher speeds, too, but most of the devices can not exceed the speed of 300 degrees per second.

Eccentric exercise implies that the muscle is activated and increases its length simultaneously so that its attachments are drawn apart (eg, lowering the arm with a weight in the hand).[15,47,48] Eccentric action is common to many preloaded situations in sports (eg, kneeling before jumping). It should, however, be emphasized that the "normal" function of human skeletal muscle is not isometric, concentric, or eccentric action, but the stretch-shortening cycle, in which the stretch (eccentric action) precedes the shortening (concentric) action.[49] Eccentric exercises combined with stretching can be used in the preventive as well as rehabilitative phases of overuse injuries.[47] However, it is important to realize that eccentric actions may sometimes be involved in the production of chronic tendon problems as a part of deceleration. Therefore, eccentric exercises are not recommended to elderly athletes as a part of their regular training until more scientific evidence of their value and safety is available.

Mobility and Flexibility Training. Strength training alone has a negative effect on joint mobility and flexibility.[50] This can be counteracted by flexibility training. The flexibility of a particular joint is primarily limited by the tightness of the connective tissue—that is, flexibility is elasticity.[15] Flexibility exercises should be started after the growth spurt (ie, at the age of 15 to 17 years), when there is a rapid increase in muscle volume and power. Flexibility then decreases with age; therefore, flexibility training should be emphasized in older age groups.

The aims of flexibility training in injury prevention are to maintain and/or improve joint mobility, to reduce the risk of joint overloading at extreme joint angles, to increase muscle and tendon strength, to enhance coordination between the various parts of the musculoskeletal system, and to adapt the musculoskeletal system to the specific demands of a particular sport.

Stretching is one of the most important methods of flexibility training. It should be preceded by a 3- to 5-min warm-up period. There are different types of stretching. Dynamic (ballistic, spring, bounce, or rebound) stretching means repeated muscle extension to its limit followed by immediate relaxation. This type of stretching is not considered effective as it activates protective reflexes; therefore, it is nowadays seldom used.

Static (hold or prolonged) stretching involves slowly stretching the muscle as far as possible and then holding that position for 20 to 60 seconds. This technique is commonly used.

Static contract-relax-hold stretching includes first a slow stretch to the limit of motion, and then a maximum isometric contraction at that position for 4 to 6 seconds. This is then followed by a relaxation for 2 to 3 seconds, and thereafter, a passive stretch to the extreme position and maintenance of that position for 10 to 60 seconds. This technique is a modification of the proprioceptive neuromuscular facilitation (PNF) technique frequently used by physical therapists.

The 3S system (scientific stretching for sport) is a fourth type of stretching. It means that a muscle is passively stretched and then exposed to an isometric contraction. This technique is effective but requires a partner to hold and stretch the leg.

Coordination and Proprioceptive Training. This involves training of the interaction between the nervous system and muscles, tendons, joints, and ligaments. Especially after an injury, it takes a long time, usually months, to learn how to perform movements in an economic but effective way. Even after the injury itself has healed, it usually takes some time before the interaction returns to a satisfactory level.

In many sports events, good technique and coordination are essential in prevention of acute and overuse injuries. Baseball pitching or javelin throwing can be mentioned as examples. For example, following an ankle ligament injury during which the nerves in the joint capsule are often injured, proprioceptive training performed on a tilt board is encouraged (Fig. 21–4).[51,52] This should be carried out periodically for at least 2 months to regain full function, then continued to prevent recurrent injuries.

Sport-specific Training. This type of training is important in injury prevention. It involves training of those muscles, tendons, and joints involved in the specific sports event. Sport-specific conditioning can usually be achieved by training within the sport itself. For example, many soccer and tennis coaches prefer training carried out in the soccer field or tennis court, respectively. If the sports event is, however, very dangerous by nature (eg, boxing, motor sports, aerials in freestyle skiing) or involves a high risk for injuries (eg, gymnastics), simulating exercises should be performed before taking part in the sport itself. In freestyle skiing, this involves training and jumping into a water pool.

Sport-specific training very often includes all the other parts of preventive training; therefore, it is one of the most effective parts in the primary prevention of sports injuries. After an injury, the sport-specific exercise program should be the final step in the rehabilitation process before going back to the sports arena.

Medical Examinations

Routine physical examinations of recreational or competitive athletes are time-consuming and may be costly, and their efficacy in injury or health hazard prevention is questionable.[53] If such examinations are to be performed, there must be good reasons for doing so. In addition, planning and preparation for such examinations should be done far in advance.

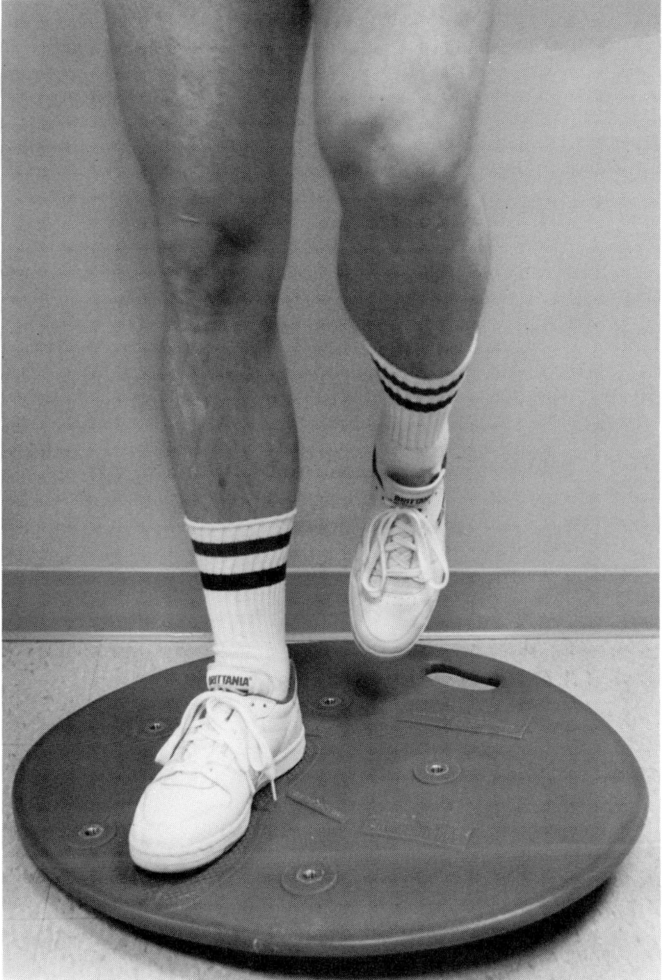

Figure 21–4. Tilt board training is an excellent way to increase ankle proprioception after a ligament injury.

Generally, the task of the medical examination of athletes is straightforward. It must be determined if there is any physical defect or condition that would jeopardize an athlete playing a particular sport. The question is how effective these examinations can be in injury prevention.

Concerning sports injury prevention, there are several ways to do the medical examination. Traditionally, in the United States, any athlete who is to play athletics on an organized level in a high school, college, national, or professional team, should have a physical screening examination and a complete medical history upon entry to that particular team. The following yearly examinations do not have to be as complete, but do require a check for any new illnesses or injuries. If so-called preseason examinations are performed, they usually concentrate more on the musculoskeletal system (joint flexibility and muscle strength).

Some sports events require medical examination just before competition (boxing, ultramarathon running) to prevent injuries or general medical complications. The risk for sudden death during physical activity is very small[54] and usually concerns persons with a previous, recognized cardiovascular disease. This group of people should be subjected to a careful medical examination before participating in sports. For middle-aged and older people (eg, 35 and over) who have decided to start a regular exercise program, a medical screening examination is recommended.[2,8]

Regarding injury prevention, such screenings should include a complete orthopedic evaluation to discover possible risk factors: overweight; previous musculoskeletal diseases like osteoarthritis, osteoporosis, and chondromalacia; malalignments, such as leg length discrepancy, scoliosis, joint hyperlaxity, and foot hyperpronation; muscle weakness and imbalance; and decreased flexibility. In most screenings, a precise medical history and a physical examination are enough. Further diagnostic tools (radiographs, bone scans, ultrasound, and laboratory tests) should be reserved for special cases, or performed only as a further examination of one individual.

Nutrition and Diet

In injury prevention, nutrition becomes important in those long-lasting training and competition situations during which the body's carbohydrate (muscle glycogen) stores are emptying. Under normal circumstances, the muscle and liver glycogen stores are sufficient to supply energy for exercises lasting up to 1.5 hours, but after that their capability for that task decreases quickly. The performance level, reactions, and coordination of the subject impair respectively, and the athlete is then prone to injury.

To avoid complete emptying of the glycogen stores, a carbohydrate-loading technique can be used. Before competitions or exercises that last for up to 1.5 hours, no particular dietary adjustment is necessary, as the body's normal glucogen stores are sufficient. Before competitions that last for more than this, in the 3 days leading to it, meals should include foods that are rich in carbohydrates (cereals, vegetables, fruits, and berries). As it takes about 48 hours for glycogen stores to be built up, no prolonged or hard training, which would deplete the stores, should take place in the 2 days prior to the performance.

Previously, 3 to 4 days before this carbohydrate-loading phase, competitive athletes performed hard exercises and followed a low-carbohydrate diet to deplete their glycogen stores completely. It was believed that, by this method, the glycogen stores would be filled better during the loading phase, and that exhaustion would be put off until later in the competition. However, recent studies have shown that a pure carbohydrate-rich diet with a decreased amount of training during the last 3 days before the competition produces exactly the same effect, but without any risks of overtraining or unpleasant feelings of fluid retention in the body.[55]

In injury prevention, other nutritional elements of food (fat, proteins, vitamins, and minerals) are of secondary value. Of course, they have a tremendous effect on general well-being; therefore, a well-balanced diet is recommended for every active individual.

Drugs, Medication, and Doping

The therapeutic uses of drugs in sports and exercise, as well as the effects of several classes of drugs on both athletic performance and health, are covered elsewhere in this book. Therefore, in this chapter, drugs and doping are dealt with only in their connection with injury prevention.

Basically, all athletes taking part in competitions should be healthy and not taking medication of any kind. However, if the medication used is really needed, is not under the banned substances list of the International Olympic Committee (IOC), and is prescribed by athlete's own physician, it obviously enhances the athlete's general well-being and allows him or her to take part in sports and enjoy it. Drugs like those for asthma or diabetes can be seen only in a positive light, and also as tools of injury prevention in these individuals.

The doping substances are, however, a real problem. The word "doping" implies all attempts to improve sporting performance in artificial ways, usually with the help of drugs.[2] Doping is dishonest; it is a form of cheating. The IOC Medical Commission gave the following doping classes for the 1988 Olympic Games in its list of "Doping Classes and Methods": stimulants; narcotics; anabolic steroids; beta-blockers; diuretics; and different doping methods, such as blood doping, and pharmacologic, chemical, and physical sample manipulation. In addition, some drugs are subjected to certain restrictions (alcohol, local injections of anesthetics and corticosteroids).[56]

From the point of view of injury prevention, stimulants, narcotics, anabolic steroids, diuretics, alcohol, and local anesthetics and corticosteroids are dangerous. Clinically, stimulants give the athlete a feeling of reduced fatigue, increased aggressiveness, hostility and, therefore, competitiveness. As a group, these symptoms produce a false sense of ability and may cause a loss of judgment. This may result in injuries to the doped athletes themselves and others within the sport. Narcotics also act in a way that gives athletes a higher threshold of pain and a sudden rush of euphoria. Alcohol, in turn, increases aggressiveness, hostility, and self-confidence, but at the same time, decreases the accuracy of movements (coordination). As a result, the risk for injuries increases considerably. Poor balance and coordination can be seen during the next 1 to 2 days; therefore, sporting activities during the "hangover" should be avoided.

Pain inhibition of all kinds is extremely dangerous concerning sports injuries. Pain is a warning signal and a guide for a correct diagnosis and treatment. If pain is reduced by chemical (local anesthetics or corticosteroids) or technical (current therapies like transcutaneous neural stimulation) manipulation, the athlete should not participate. The athlete cannot then evaluate the extent of the injury, which usually becomes worse. Treatment with local corticosteroids in an area of tendon inflammation may lead to serious consequences, like tendon ruptures. Corticosteroids, on the one hand, dampen inflammation and pain very effectively, allowing hard efforts; on the other hand, they may cause hypoxia, and degenerative and necrotic alterations in the tendon tissue, weakening the tensile strength of the tendon.[57,58]

The effects of anabolic steroids on muscle strength are not completely known. Even though it is accepted that they can increase muscle mass through increased intracellular protein synthesis, their effect on muscle performance is still controversial. What is known for sure is that athletes use anabolic steroids a lot. It is also known that large muscles produced by anabolic steroids contain a higher concentration of water and salt, weakening the muscle. This may lead to muscle ruptures. Also tendinitis or tendon ruptures may be a problem.[59] Even pathologic bone fractures have been described.

Diuretics have been used to decrease weight in sports, such as wrestling, boxing, judo, and weight lifting. Because they act on the kidneys to excrete potassium into the urine, levels of potassium in the blood may become low; this may cause muscle fatigue and cramps.

Hygiene

The skin secretes sweat and grease in which dust and dirt may adhere. If the dirt is allowed to accumulate, it becomes a breeding ground for bacteria, which break down the dirt and produce unpleasant odors. Rashes, irritation, and pimples can occur as a result, which, in turn, may expose one to infection or inflammation.

In sports, foot hygiene needs special attention. Inadequate foot care allows dirt to collect between the toes and the cuticles and become a breeding ground for bacteria and fungi. Fungal foot infection is so common among athletes that it has been named "athlete's foot." Prevention of athlete's foot is simple: daily washing of the feet with soap and water followed by a change of socks, use of proper shoes, and avoidance of visits to public swimming pools and showers barefoot or when having fungal infection.

General Preparation for Sport

In the general preparation is included a rather well-regulated daily life with regular food habits, enough sleep, and avoidance of drug abuse. The importance of regular, sound living habits cannot be overemphasized for an athlete with aspiration.

The athlete needs to be both physically and mentally well prepared for training and competitions. Mental preparation means that the athlete should be aware of the requirements of the sport and what it takes to fulfill a race or competition. The degree of mental tension varies from sport to sport. Increased mental tension can cause reactions such as lack of appetite, headaches, and occasionally defect coordination, which can lead to an increased risk of injury.

If mental tension is too great, it is the responsibility of the coach to explore ways to reduce it. Confidential discussions with the athlete and an increased number of competitive elements included in the training program have often been used for this purpose. In addition, by increasing the frequency of participation in competitive events, an athlete usually learns quickly what is his or her optimal level of mental tension for maximal performance.

Information, Education, Rules, and Society Planning

These topics have already been discussed earlier. They form the basis of secondary and tertiary prevention of sports injuries. Without these efforts, the previously mentioned methods of primary prevention are less effective.

SPECIFIC PREVENTIVE METHODS

Any sports injury can be caused by intrinsic or extrinsic factors, either alone or in combination.[60] In acute traumas, extrinsic factors are dominant, whereas in overuse injuries, the reasons are more multifactorial. In overuse injuries, an interaction between these two categories is common. In order to achieve an effective injury prevention, it is vital to be able to affect these predisposing (risk) factors.

Intrinsic Factors

The most common intrinsic factors related to overuse injuries are alignment abnormalities, leg length discrepancy, muscle weakness and imbalance, decreased flexibility, joint laxity, female sex, young or old age, overweight, and some predisposing diseases (Table 21–1). In a recent study of running injuries, Lysholm and Wiklander[61] found that in 40% of the cases, intrinsic predisposing factors were present, but in only 10% were they the only demonstrable factor. However, it should be kept in mind that this area is highly conjectural and many plausible hypotheses at present lack substantiating evidence.[60]

Malalignments. The most common malalignment of the foot is hyperpronation. In 1978, James and colleagues[43] noticed that increased pronation was present in 60% of a group of injured runners. Hyperpronation means that during the stance (support) phase of walking or running, the pronation of the subtalar joints occurs too excessively or is too prolonged, creating increased or unusual stress on the structures of the foot.

TABLE 21–1. INTRINSIC FACTORS RELATED TO OVERUSE INJURIES IN SPORTS

Malalignments	Leg length discrepancy
Foot hyperpronation/hypopronation	Muscle weakness/imbalance
Pes planus/cavus	Decreased flexibility
Forefoot varus/valgus	Joint laxity
Hindfoot varus/valgus	Female sex
Tibia vara	Young/old age
Genu valgum/varum	Overweight
Patella alta/baja	Predisposing diseases
Femoral neck anteversion	

Hyperpronation of the foot is often physiologic but may occur owing to anatomic reasons (forefoot varus, leg length discrepancy, or ligamentous laxity), or to muscular weakness or tightness in gastrocnemius and soleus muscles. Hyperpronation may, in turn, cause secondary effects to the lower extremities, resulting in lower leg and knee problems.[58] Several overuse injuries have been proposed to be caused by or associated with this foot malalignment: medial tibial stress syndrome, tibialis posterior tendinitis, Achilles bursitis or peritendinitis, plantar fasciitis, patellofemoral pain syndrome, iliotibial band friction syndrome, and lower extremity stress fractures (Fig. 21–5).[15,43,60]

If excessive or prolonged pronation occurs in an athlete complaining of pain in the lower extremity, foot orthotics to be used in the shoes may be indicated. Athletes most commonly use semiflexible loose sole orthotics. In hyperpronation, shoe correction is usually performed by elevating the medial side of the sole and forefoot. If hyperpronation is found in an asymptomatic person, shoe corrections are seldom necessary. The same principles can be followed in the prevention and treatment of other injuries associated with malalignments.

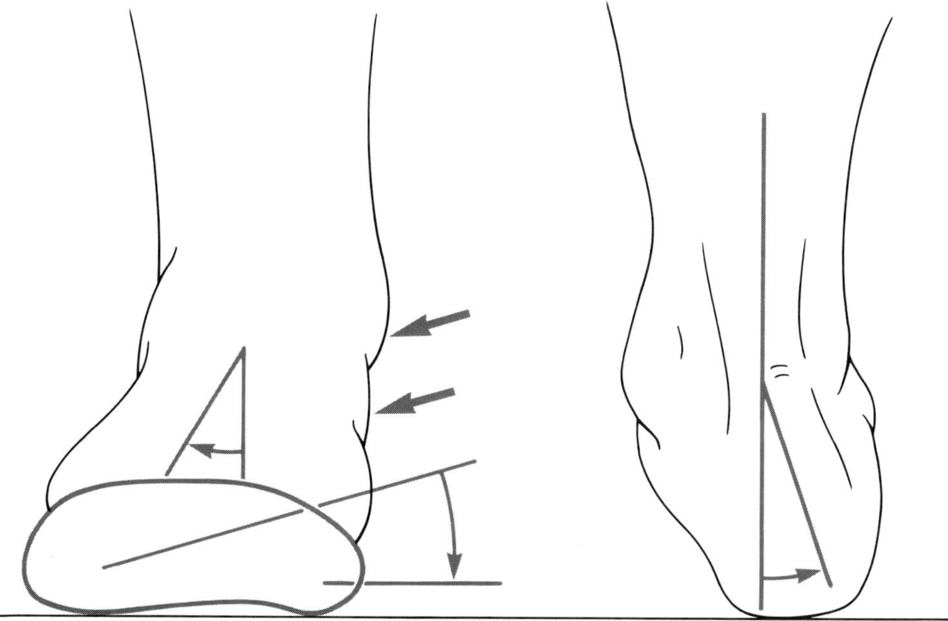

Figure 21–5. Hyperpronation of the foot will result in increased medial stress and angulated traction of the Achilles tendon.

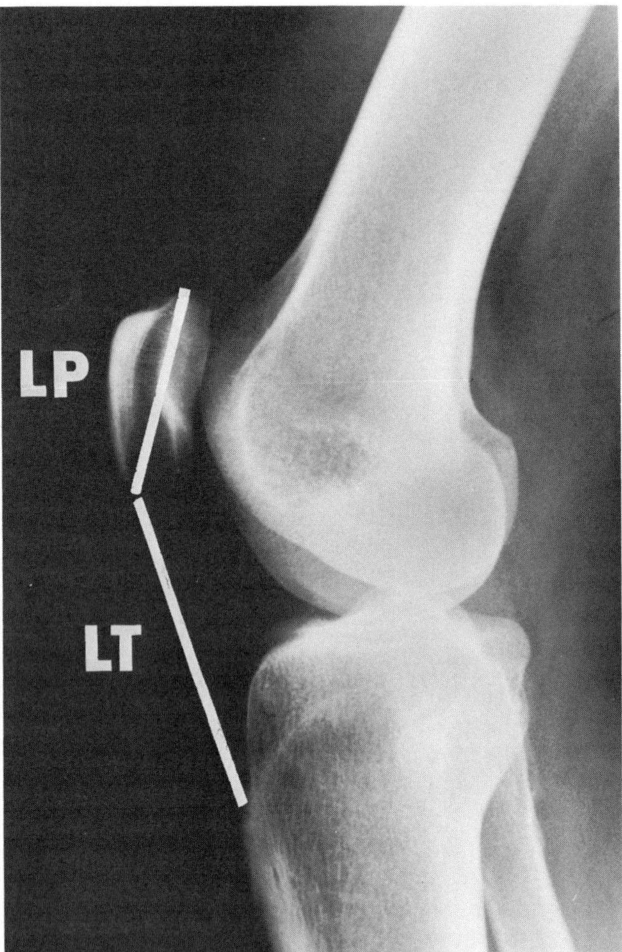

Figure 21–6. Patella alta (a high-riding patella) may be a predisposing factor for patellofemoral pain. In this patient, the LT/LP ratio (length of the patellar tendon/length of the patella) is 1.6, exceeding the normal range (0.8–1.2) considerably.

In the development of patellofemoral pain syndromes, some additional predisposing (risk) factors may be present, such as patella alta (Fig. 21–6) and excessive lateral displacement of the patella. In those individuals, patellar bracing or taping may be beneficial in prevention of reinjuries. Quadriceps muscle training is, however, the most common route to success.

Leg Length Discrepancy. In addition to foot hyperpronation, the importance of leg length discrepancy (LLD) is one of the most discussed and argued topics in orthopedic and sports medicine.[62] The orthopedic view has been that discrepancies of less than 20 mm are mostly cosmetic.[60,63] In elite athletes, however, a discrepancy of more than 5 to 6 mm may be symptomatic; for a discrepancy of 10 mm or more, a built-up shoe or insert-type of orthotics may be used.[62,64]

As in foot hyperpronation, many biomechanical alterations have been proposed to occur as a result of LLD: pelvic tilt to the shorter side followed by compensatory lumbar scoliosis and compression of the intervertebral disc on the concave (inner) side of the curve, increased abduction of the hip (longer leg), excessive pronation of the foot (on the longer or shorter side), secondary increased knee valgus, and outward rotation of the leg.[63,65] As a result, LLD has been suggested to be a causative factor in the development of lower back pain, hip osteoarthritis, trochanteric bursitis, patellar tendinitis, iliotibial band friction syndrome, and stress fractures (Fig. 21–7).

Concerning injury prevention, we must realize that the real occurrence of these proposed biomechanical alterations, their magnitude, and above all, their clinical significance

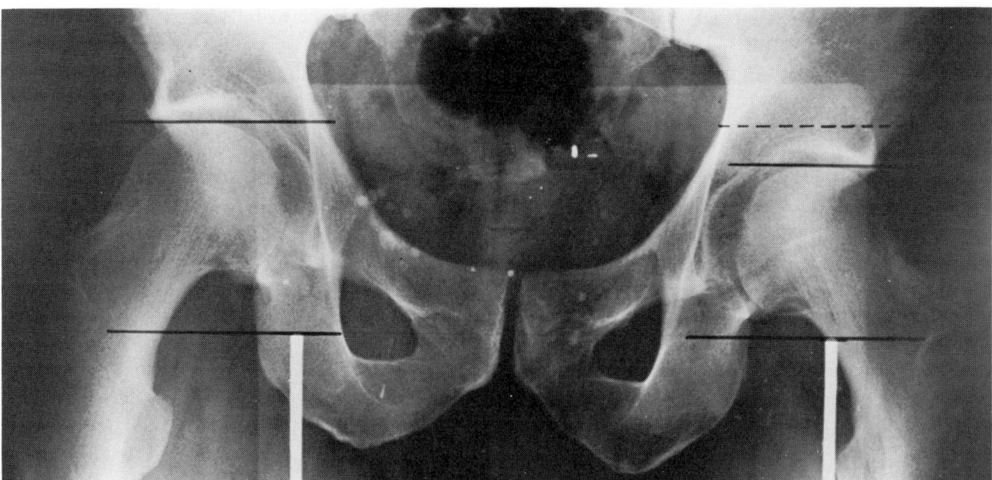

Figure 21–7. A 39-year-old marathon runner had suffered from lower back pain and exercise-induced pain in his right knee, ankle, and Achilles tendon for years. A biomechanical examination revealed leg length discrepancy confirmed to be 12 mm in weight-bearing radiographs of the pelvis (right side 12 mm longer). A 10-mm thick, insert-type shoe orthotic on the left side led to considerable pain relief within 2 weeks.

are not well known. There are some indirect clinical associations between malalignments and injuries, but so far little direct scientific evidence exists. Therefore, correction of training errors may be warranted more often than orthotics.[60]

Muscle Weakness and Imbalance. The significance of muscle weakness and imbalance in injury prevention is also a matter of debate. Muscle imbalance means that there is an asymmetry between the agonist and antagonist muscles in one extremity, asymmetry between the extremities, or a differential with an anticipated normal value.[66,67]

It is well documented that athletes with previous joint injuries have persistent and long-lasting muscular strength, power, and endurance deficits in their affected extremity[45,60,68] and that those joints are in greater danger for reinjury than are uninjured joints.[45] However, it is not clear how important muscle imbalance per se is as a causative factor for reinjury, because persistent joint instability, pain, swelling, and impairment of neuromuscular coordination are also involved.

There is some evidence that multifactorial conditioning programs can lessen the injury rate,[69] whereas other studies have not found any direct relationship between muscle weakness or imbalance, and injury.[23,67] Thus, the question of any relationship between these variables remains open. However, rehabilitation after an injury is not only a tool to increase muscle strength, but also a tool to improve dynamic stability of the joint and coordination of the whole extremity. Therefore, it should always be the most important step in the athlete's way back to sports.

Decreased Flexibility. The techniques of mobility and flexibility training have already been discussed. In sports, musculotendinous flexibility is an important part of physical performance,[70] and it is most likely also important in the prevention of certain sports injuries, such as muscle spasm, muscle rupture, tendinitis, apophysitis, and patellofemoral pain syndrome.[45,60]

The field is, however, open to speculations. The studies do not allow any conclusion on whether musculotendinous tightness is the cause or the consequence of injuries. Furthermore, prospective follow-up studies are needed. Meanwhile, flexibility training must be seen as an important tool in prevention of muscle and tendon injuries.

When discussing flexibility training, it should be stressed that a steady-state value of the stretched musculotendinous tissue will ultimately be achieved. In other words, there is an optimal length of that tissue over which further stretch is of no anatomic or physiologic value.[60] It is, however, important to preserve this optimal length with regular stretching.

Joint Laxity. In some persons, especially in some women, joints can be hypermobile. This means that the range of motion of the joint may be excessive in normal physiologic directions of movement, in abnormal directions, or in both. Joint hypermobility is often genetic, and as a rule, it does not require any special attention in injury prevention.

However, a ligamentous injury may lead to an excessive joint laxity (usually called instability) causing many residual problems, especially in the knee, ankle, and shoulder joints. In posttraumatic instability, the patient often complains about fear of "giving way," recurrent sprains, and pain or swelling during activity. Also, serious long-term consequences, like posttraumatic osteoarthritis, have been described to occur after ligament injuries provided that the joint has become unstable.[71,72]

In prevention of reinjuries to these unstable joints, specific muscle strengthening exercises are of great value. Good muscle function can to some extent compensate ligamentous instability. Also, joint braces, which can be custom-made or off-the-shelf models, may be useful in prevention of abnormal movements and reinjuries.[73] In the ankle joint, taping has been shown to be of value, too.[23]

Female Sex. During the past decade, the proportion of women in sports injury surveys has shown a clear increase.[3,10,20,30] In the 1970s, the proportion of women was between 10% and 18%.[3,10,20] A recent prospective study from an outpatient sports medicine clinic in Finland showed that 31% of injured athletes were women.[30] The proposed reasons for the increase were an increased female interest in sport and physical activity in general, and an increased female interest in sports events with high risk of injury, such as gymnastics, soccer, and team handball.

Studies of sports injuries have reported a higher incidence of overuse injuries among women.[30,74] The reason for the higher incidence may be that the repetitive impact loads of the body weight will be absorbed by a weaker musculoskeletal system in women compared with that of men of equal body weight.[60] In conditioned women, the average percentage of body fat is 10% to 15% of body weight, whereas conditioned men generally have less than 7% body fat. Women have less muscle mass per unit body weight (20% to 25%) than equally trained men (40%), and their overall muscle strength averages about two thirds that of men.[74] Men also have greater bone mass than do women. Theoretically, these factors together with the well-known female risk factors in body anatomy and biomechanics (wider hips and more mobile joints) may predispose to overuse injuries in women.

Menstrual irregularities, which are much more common among female athletes than among nonathletes,[74] constitute a clear risk factor for certain overuse injuries. Several studies have reported an increased incidence of stress fractures among amenorrheic athletes compared with eumenorrheic athletes in the same sport.[74–76] A prolonged hypoestrogenic state may also result in a loss of bone mass (especially in trabecular bone areas), and may, therefore, increase the risk for osteoporotic acute fractures.[74]

Regarding injury prevention, it is of great importance that, before entering "the sports world," girls and women have an effective physical conditioning period including muscle strength, power, and endurance as well as motor skills. If expressed as percent improvement, the trainability of women is almost the same as for men.[74] In endurance sports, continuous registration of menstrual cycles and follow-up of dietary habits (food with enough proteins, calcium, and vitamin D) are compulsory. In sport events including lots of jumping and running movements, a biomechanical screening of a female athlete may be necessary before intensive participation.

Young Age. Regular training of children and young adults is becoming more common in sports. Competitive sports are carried out with increasing intensity at lower ages. In some sports, such as figure skating, swimming, and gymnastics, children start regular training at 4 to 5 years of age, and training from 2 to 4 hours, 5 to 6 days a week is not unusual.[62] As a result, risk for acute or overuse injury increases.

Before puberty, a child's body seems to stand repeated voluntary stress very well. During the growth spurt (and especially towards the end of it), into which most girls enter between 10 and 13 years and boys between 12 and 15 years, there is, however, a great imbalance between muscle strength, tightness, joint mobility, and coordination. In addition, during that phase the growth plates are extremely vulnerable to external forces. Thus, in this phase of children's development, there is an increased risk for acute and overuse injuries.[62]

Well-known examples of injuries during growth spurt are traumatic epiphysiolyses of different joints, patella alta associated with traction apophysitis of the tibial tubercle (Osgood-Schlatter disease), and traction apophysitis of the humeral medial epicondyle in young pitchers (Little Leaguer's elbow). Adaptation as a result of prolonged one-sided training in childhood can cause permanent asymmetric changes. An example of this is the so-called tennis shoulder, in which the end result is an increased laxity in the joint capsule, ligaments, and tendons, an increased bone growth, a dropping of the shoulder, and a relative lengthening of the racquet arm. In gymnasts, intensive training over a long period of time may produce hypermobility of the vertebral column and other joints, and the end result may be premature osteoarthritis in middle age.

It is therefore essential that regular hard training in children and adolescents is carried out under supervision. One-sided and repetitive training should be avoided, especially during the growth spurt.[62] In this respect, secondary and tertiary preventive methods, such as protective rules, information, and education, are of the utmost importance.

Old Age. With aging, various functions of a living body gradually deteriorate. This also includes the musculoskeletal system, even if not so extensively as cardiovascular functions.[77] Regarding musculoskeletal problems, Lane and associates[78] showed in a controlled study in 1987 that musculoskeletal disability appeared to develop with age at a lower rate in long-distance runners aged 50 to 72 years than in nonrunning community control subjects. Runners had less physical disability, maintained more functional capacity, and had fewer physician visits per year. However, 40% had suffered from a running-related injury over the preceding year, and one third of their physician visits were attributable to this.

The sports injury profile of elderly athletes varies from that of their younger colleagues. Recently Kannus and co-workers[32] showed in a 3-year prospective, controlled study that, in elderly athletes, the sports injuries are more frequently overuse-related than acute, and that they more commonly have a degenerative basis (osteoarthritis, or ligamentous and musculotendinous degeneration). In a study of the veteran elite athletes competing in the world master championships, it was found that the most common injuries were muscle and tendon strains in the lower leg.[79]

Prevention of sports injuries in master athletes should, therefore, be concentrated on these areas. Maintenance of flexibility and neuromuscular coordination through daily stretching and calisthenics is recommended. Long warm-up and cooling-down periods should be the rule. The slow progression principle is especially suitable for elderly people. Regular medical examinations are much more important than in younger athletes. Finally, in master sports, special attention and caution should be paid to sports events in which the lower extremities are fully weight bearing (running and ball games including repeated jumpings), because rapid progression of preosteoarthritic changes may occur in hip and knee joints. In this respect, participation in sports like swimming, cycling, or rowing, in which the whole body weight is not on the lower extremities, is more recommendable. Racquet sports like tennis are also low-risk sports and, therefore, suitable for the elderly, too.

Overweight. Overweight or obesity is one of the greatest problems in modern Western societies. The prevalence of obesity increases with age. In Finland, for example,

34% of women and 16% of men over 50 years of age are obese (overweight by $\geq$20%).[80] Overweight or obesity, in turn, has been associated with many of the general diseases (diabetes, hypertension, stroke, ischemic heart disease, heart failure, lung emphysema, gall stones, and osteoarthritis), either as a direct causal factor, or as an indirect cofactor in the disease progress.

Regarding sports injury prevention, overweight may be a problem in full weight-bearing recreational physical activities, because the development of knee and hip osteoarthritis is associated with overweight,[80–84] and physical activity may accelerate the osteoarthritis process. A low-energy diet and participation in sports events in which the whole body weight does not stress the lower extremities are, therefore, recommended for overweight people.

Predisposing Diseases. In injury prevention, we should always take into account that a subject may have a predisposing disease making him or her prone to injury. For example, diabetic patients in long-distance running competition need special care because patients with low blood glucose levels may lose their concentration and coordination capability. Children who have had Perthes' disease may have lost the rotatory functions of the hip and may, therefore, secondarily develop hip or knee swelling and irritation in strenuous physical activities. Accordingly, children with Osgood-Schlatter disease in the knees have an increased risk for patella alta in adulthood. The presence of patella alta has been linked to recurrent patellofemoral subluxation and to chondromalacia problems during physical activity.[60]

Extrinsic Factors

By extrinsic predisposing factors, we mean all the factors acting externally on the human body.[85] The most common extrinsic factors related to sports injuries are excessive loads on the body, training errors, environmental malconditions, poor equipment, and ineffective rules (Table 21–2). Extrinsic factors are mainly excessive loads on the body due to training errors. In runners, they are involved in 60% to 80% of reported injuries.[43]

Excessive Load on the Body. Repeated overload in running and jumping activities is often associated with overuse injuries. In the running gait, a force in the range of three to five times the body weight ascends the lower extremity at heel strike. This force behaves like a sound wave with a short duration (20 to 40 msec) and rapid dissipation. Considering an impact of 250% of body weight, a runner absorbs at ground contact 110 Mg (110 tons) on each foot per 1 mile (1.6 km).[86] The forces for longer distances can be imagined, considering that a long-distance runner who runs 100 miles (160 km) per week plants each foot about 3 million times a year.[15]

TABLE 21–2. EXTRINSIC FACTORS RELATED TO INJURIES IN SPORTS

Excessive load on the body	Training errors (*continued*)
Type of movement	Poor technique
Speed of movement	Fatigue
Number of repetitions	Environmental malconditions
Footwear	Dark
Surface	Heat/cold
Training errors	Humidity
Over distance	Altitude
Fast progression	Wind
High intensity	Poor equipment
Hill work	Ineffective rules

Once it is realized how large these forces can be, it is not surprising that they may be causal factors for injuries. Accordingly, it is possible that a reduction of forces may be connected to a reduction in injuries.

In injury prevention, one possible way to decrease the load on the body is to change the type of movement. For example, in running, one can land on the heel or on the forefoot. In landing on the heel, the point of application of the ground reaction force and the line of action of the force are both behind the ankle joint.[85] Therefore, the structures on the anterior part of the leg are loaded on first contact and the Achilles tendon is unloaded. Heel landing, therefore, can be used to unload the Achilles tendon (eg, during the recovery period of Achilles peritendinitis).

A second way to reduce the load on the body is to decrease the speed of the movement. By decreasing the speed of heel-toe running from 6 m/sec to 3 m/sec, the decreases in vertical impact and active forces are 40% and 20%, respectively.[85] Change in the speed of movement also changes the speed of the involved limbs and, therefore, has an influence on the forces acting on the athlete's body.

Theoretically, little is known about the number of repetitions and their effects with respect to load on the living body. Steel, for instance, loses its particular resistance against bending during a repeated loading process. However, living biologic materials can have a significant response to the applied stress provided that the stress increase is slow enough. As a matter of fact, if the response effect is stronger than the mechanical fatigue effect, the tissue is strengthened. Generally, bones and muscles have a high and fast response, whereas cartilage and tendon show a smaller and slower response because of low nutrition flow. In sports medicine practice, fatigue injuries like stress fractures occur frequently, and in prevention, the only choice is to increase the number of repetitions slowly (the slow progression principle).

During each contact of the foot with the ground, the ground acts on the foot with a ground reaction force and the foot acts on the ground with a force of the same magnitude but in an opposite direction. These forces during landing and takeoff can be quite different on different surfaces. The impact force (the force at first contact) is much higher for running on asphalt than for running on grass or sand.[85] However, the active part of the ground reaction force remains about the same when comparing running on grass with running on asphalt. It is speculated that these high-impact forces are one of the causes of many running injuries as well as other sports injuries.[85] In tennis, adolescents often sustain more overuse injuries, such as medial tibial stress syndrome and Achilles tendinitis, on surfaces with high friction. These problems are rarely seen on clay courts.[62] Therefore, it is very important that people who are responsible in the development of sports facilities know the possibilities of reducing forces through the appropriate selection of sports surfaces (tertiary prevention of injuries).

In reduction of impact forces, shoes are also of great importance. A good running shoe should absorb and/or reduce impact forces, and should provide mediolateral stability, avoiding excessive pronation, as well as guidance at takeoff, avoiding oversupination of the foot. In other words, it is the question of cushioning, support, and friction.[85] Today, an acceptable sports shoe should have a relatively high and hard heel counter, good shock-absorbing characteristics, and good flexibility in the forefoot. In addition, an ideal shoe should not wear out within the first months of use. It is more important to buy good shoes than expensive clothing.

To protect the athlete from excessive load on the body, we must keep in mind acute injuries, too. In many sports, protective equipment for the legs, knees, genital organs, face, shoulders, and elbows is essential in prevention of acute traumas. Their key role has been already emphasized in this chapter.

Training Errors. Training errors are present in 60% to 80% of reported injuries to runners.[43] The most common errors are too long distance, too high intensity, too fast progression, and too much hill work. Monotonous, asymmetric and specialized training (running only) is a great risk factor for overuse problems. Running on the edge of the road means running with one leg short and one long, resulting in overuse injuries like trochanteric bursitis and iliotibial band friction syndrome. By varying the exercise method (biking, swimming, and cross-country skiing in addition to running), a much larger amount of total work can be carried out with less risk for injuries.

In addition, poor technique and fatigue play a role. Even minor technical faults, which are continually repeated, can cause overuse injuries. A minor fault in the throwing technique of a javelin may cause medial epicondylitis after 1000 repetitions. The same problem applies to baseball pitching. Fatigued muscles have a decreased ability to absorb repetitive shock or stress and may result in overuse injuries, such as stress fractures, tennis elbow, and medial tibial stress syndrome.

Environmental Malconditions. Weather may have an effect on injury frequency during sports activities. Darkness, too high or too low temperature and humidity, high altitude, and hard wind may play a key role in injury pathogenesis. Darkness has to be taken into account when planning orienteering competitions. High temperature and humidity without wind may block the heat transportation system of marathon runners with potentially serious consequences (heat exhaustion, heatstroke, or death). Low temperatures with hard wind may produce frostbites, hypothermia, and other cold injuries in sports like downhill or crosscountry skiing, ski jumping, and mountain climbing.

In injury prevention, it is essential to have clear rules concerning when training or competition must be cancelled because of these environmental malconditions. Not only the temperature but also other weather factors should be taken into consideration. For example, the windchill factor is critical in many winter sports because the wind has a marked effect on heat loss. If the thermometer reads 20°F (−7°C) and the wind velocity is 20 mph (32 km/hour), the real exposure is comparable to −10°F (−23°C).[87]

Poor Equipment. The importance of protective equipment, proper shoes, and corrective orthotics has already been discussed in this chapter. They do form the basic strategy for primary prevention in all kind of sports injuries. In addition, the efficacy of equipment can be increased significantly by secondary and tertiary preventive efforts, such as information, education, legislation, and planning.

Ineffective Rules. The last extrinsic predisposing factor to be mentioned is the inefficacy of many of the rules in sports. Changing the rules to make the sport safer is a key factor in the reduction of the number of sports injuries. Good examples are easy to give: making it compulsory to use safety helmets in amateur boxing and ice hockey to avoid head injuries, restriction in the amount of pitching per season in junior baseball to avoid "Little Leaguer's elbow," cancellation of a cross-country skiing competition if the temperature is below −4°F (−20°C) to avoid cold injuries, and prohibition of stepping on the net line in volleyball to avoid ankle sprains. In junior ice hockey, for example, a mandatory use of face masks has almost eliminated facial and dental injuries in that sport.

In the future, rules may be a very important way to reduce the number of sports injuries because both the number of new (often high-risk) sports events and the number of participants seem to increase exponentially.

CONCLUSION

The battle against the increasing number of acute and overuse sports injuries should be concentrated on injury prevention. Preventive work needs a clear strategy, which should include individual, group, and society level activities. Accordingly, prevention is wisely divided into primary, secondary, and tertiary preventive efforts, as well as general and specific preventive methods. General efforts should reach everyone involved in physical activity. Specific methods are directed to specific groups of people in an attempt to affect the intrinsic and extrinsic predisposing factors of sports injuries.

Only through well-organized preventive work can we expect encouraging results.

REFERENCES

1. Ryan AJ: Sports medicine today. Science 200:919–924, 1978.
2. Peterson L, Renstrom P: Sports Injuries: Their Prevention and Treatment. London, Martin Dunitz, 1986, p 488.
3. Devereaux MD, Lachmann SM: Athletes attending a sports injury clinic—a review. Br J Sports Med 17:137–142, 1983.
4. Paffenbarger RS, Wing AL, Hyder T: Physical activity as an index of heart attack risk in college alumni. Am J Epidemiol 108:161–175, 1978.
5. Lewis S, Haskell WL, Wood PH, et al: Effects of physical activity on weight reduction in middle-aged women. Am J Clin Nutr 29:151–156, 1976.
6. Bortz WM: Disuse and aging. JAMA 248:1203, 1982.
7. American College of Sports Medicine: Position statement on the recommended quantity and quality of exercise for developing and maintaining fitness in healthy adults. Med Sci Sports 10:vii, 1978.
8. International Federation of Sports Medicine: Physical exercise—an important factor for health: a position statement. Int J Sports Med 10:460–461, 1989.
9. Fasler S: Sportunfalle: Statistik 1963–1973. Soz Praventivmed 21:296–301, 1976.
10. Orava S: Exertion injuries due to sports and physical exercise [academic dissertation]. Kokkola, Finland, Osterbottningen Press, 1980.
11. Maehlum S, Dahljord OA: Acute sports injuries in Oslo: A one-year study. Br J Sports Med 18:181–185, 1984.
12. Koplan J, Siscovick D, Goldbaum G: The risk of exercise: A public health view of injuries and hazards. Public Health Rep 100:189, 1985.
13. Walter S, Sutton J, McIntosh J, et al: The aetiology of sports injuries: A review of methodologies. Sports Med 2:47–58, 1985.
14. Sandelin J: Acute sports injuries: A clinical and epidemiological study [academic dissertation]. Helsinki, Yliopistopaino, 1988.
15. Renstrom P: Diagnosis and management of overuse injuries. *In* Dirix A, Knuttgen HG, Tittel K (eds): The Olympic Book of Sports Medicine. Oxford, Blackwell Scientific Publications, 1988, pp 446–468.
16. Robey JM, Blyth CS, Mueller FO: Athletic injuries—application of epidemiologic methods. JAMA 217:184–189, 1971.
17. Sperryn PN: Athletic injuries. Rheumatol Phys Med 11:246–249, 1972.
18. Weightman D, Browne RC: Injuries in eleven selected sports. Br J Sports Med 9:136–141, 1975.
19. Crompton B, Tubbs N: A survey of sports injuries in Birmingham. Br J Sports Med 11:12–15, 1977.
20. Kvist M, Jarvinen M: Typical injuries at an outpatient sports clinic. Duodecim 94:1335–1345, 1978.
21. Devereaux MD, Lachmann M: Athletes attending a sports injury clinic. Br J Sports Med 17:137–142, 1983.
22. Axelsson R, Renstrom P, Svenson H-O: Akuta idrottsskador pa ett centrallasarett. Lakartidningen 77:3615–3617, 1980.
23. Ekstrand J: Soccer injuries and their prevention [academic dissertation]. Linkoping, Sweden, Linkoping University, 1982.
24. Perasalo O, Vapaavouri M, Louhimo I: Uber die Sportverletzungen. Ann Chir Gynaecol Fenn 44:256–269, 1955.
25. Vuori I, Aho AJ, Karakorpi T: Injuries sustained in sports and exercise. Duodecim 88:700–711, 1972.
26. Franke K: Traumatologie des Sports. Stuttgart, Georg Thieme Verlag, 1980.
27. Lorentzon R, Johansson C, Bjornstig U: Fotballen orsakar flest skador men badmintonskador ar dyrast. Lakartidningen 81:340–343, 1984.
28. Korhonen K: Sports injuries [academic dissertation]. Kuopio, Finland, University of Kuopio, 1986.
29. Kannus P, Niittymaki S, Jarvinen M: Athletic overuse injuries in children: A 30-month prospective follow-up study at an outpatient sports clinic. Clin Pediatr 27:333–337, 1988.
30. Kannus P, Niittymaki S, Jarvinen M: Sports injuries in women: A one-year prospective follow-up study at an outpatient sports clinic. Br J Sports Med 21:37–39, 1987.
31. Watters D, Brooks S, Elton R, et al: Sports injuries in an accident and emergency department. Arch Emerg Med 2:105–112, 1984.

32. Kannus P, Niittymaki S, Jarvinen M, et al: Sports injuries in elderly athletes: A three-year prospective, controlled study. Age Ageing 18:263–270, 1989.
33. O'Donoghue DH: Treatment of Injuries to Athletes. Philadelphia, WB Saunders, 1984.
34. Hlobil H, van Mechelen W, Kemper HCG: How can sports injuries be prevented? Oosterbeek, NISGZ publication no 25E, 1987, pp 1–136.
35. Saltin B, Blomqvist G, Mitchell JH, et al: Response to exercise after bed rest and after training. Circulation 38(suppl 7):1–78, 1968.
36. Akeson WH, Amiel D, Woo SL-Y: Immobility effects on synovial joints: The pathomechanics of joint contracture. Biorheology 17:95–100, 1980.
37. Jarvinen M: Healing of a crush injury in rat striated muscle with special reference to treatment of early mobilization and immobilization [academic dissertation]. Turku, Finland, University of Turku, 1976.
38. Jozsa L, Jarvinen M, Kannus P, et al: Fine structural changes in the articular cartilage of the rat's knee following short-term immobilization in various positions: A scanning electron microscopical study. Int Orthop 11:137–140, 1987.
39. Jozsa L, Reffy A, Jarvinen M, et al: Cortical and trabecular osteopenia after immobilization: A quantitative histological study of the rat knee. Int Orthop 12:169–172, 1988.
40. Jozsa L, Thoring J, Jarvinen M, et al: Quantitative alterations in intramuscular connective tissue following immobilization: An experimental study in the rat calf muscles. Exp Mol Pathol 49:267–278, 1988.
41. Noyes FR: Functional properties of knee ligaments and alterations induced by immobilization. Clin Orthop 123:210–242, 1977.
42. Woo SL-Y, Inoue M, McGurk-Burleson E, et al: Treatment of the medial collateral ligament injury: II. Structure and function of canine knees in response to different treatment regimens. Am J Sports Med 15:22–29, 1987.
43. James SL, Bates BT, Osternig LR: Injuries to runners. Am J Sports Med 6:40–50, 1978.
44. Clement DB, Taunton JE, Smart GW, et al: Survey of overuse running injuries. Physician Sportsmed 9:47–58, 1981.
45. Kannus P: Conservative treatment of acute knee distortions—long-term results and their evaluation methods [academic dissertation]. Tampere, Finland, Vammalan Kirjapaino OY, 1988, pp 1–110.
46. Lesmes GR, Costill DL, Coyle EF, et al: Muscle strength and power changes during maximal isokinetic training. Med Sci Sports 10:266–269, 1978.
47. Curwin S, Stanish WD: Tendinitis: Its etiology and treatment. Lexington, Collamore Press, 1984, p 189.
48. Komi PV, Buskirk LR: Effect of eccentric and concentric muscle conditioning on tension and electrical activity of human muscle. Ergonomics 15:417–434, 1972.
49. Komi PV: Physiological and biomechanical correlates of muscle function: Effects of muscle structure and stretch-shortening cycle on force and speed. Exerc Sports Sci Rev (ACSM) 12:81–121, 1984.
50. Moller M: Athletic training and flexibility: A study on range of motion in the lower extremity [dissertation no 182]. Linkoping, Sweden, Linkoping University, 1984.
51. Freeman MAR: The etiology and prevention of functional instability of the foot. J Bone Joint Surg 47B:678–685, 1965.
52. Tropp H: Functional instability of the ankle joint [dissertation no 202]. Linkoping, Sweden, Linkoping University, VTT-Grafiska, 1985, pp 1–92.
53. Leach R: Medical examination of athletes. *In* Dirix A. Knuttgen HG, Tittel K (eds): The Olympic Book of Sports Medicine. Oxford, Blackwell Scientific Publications, 1988, pp 572–582.
54. Vuori I: The cardiovascular risks of physical activity. Acta Med Scand [Suppl] 711:205–214, 1986.
55. Costill DL: Carbohydrates for exercise: Dietary demands for optimal performance. Int J Sports Med 9:1–18, 1988.
56. Dirix A: Classes and methods of doping and doping control. *In* Dirix A, Knuttgen HG, Tittel K (eds): The Olympic Book of Sports Medicine. Oxford, Blackwell Scientific Publications, 1988, pp 669–675.
57. Jozsa L, Reffy A, Kannus P, et al: Pathological alterations in human tendons. Arch Orthop Trauma Surg 1990, in press.
58. Renstrom P, Johnson RJ: Overuse injuries in sports: A review. Sports Med 2:316–333, 1985.
59. Voy RO: Clinical aspects of the doping classes. *In* Dirix A, Knuttgen HG, Tittel K (eds): The Olympic Book of Sports Medicine. Oxford, Blackwell Scientific Publications, 1988, pp 659–668.
60. Lorentzon R: Causes of injuries: Intrinsic factors. *In* Dirix A, Knuttgen HG, Tittel K (eds): The Olympic Book of Sports Medicine. Oxford, Blackwell Scientific Publications, 1988, pp 376–390.
61. Lysholm J, Wiklander J: Injuries in runners. Am J Sports Med 15:168–171, 1987.
62. Renstrom P, Roux C: Clinical implications of youth participation in sports. *In* Dirix A, Knuttgen HG, Tittel K (eds): The Olympic Book of Sports Medicine. Oxford, Blackwell Scientific Publications, 1988, pp 469–488.
63. Friberg O: Clinical symptoms and biomechanics of lumbar spine and hip joint in leg length inequality. Spine 8:643–651, 1983.

64. Micheli LJ: Overuse injuries in children sports: The growth factor. Orthop Clin North Am 14:337–360, 1983.
65. Friberg O, Kvist M, Aalto T, et al: Leg length inequality in the etiology of low back pain and low limb overuse injuries in young athletes. Idrotts Med 5:5–7, 1985.
66. Grace TG: Muscle imbalance and extremity injury: A perplexing relationship. Sports Med 2:77–82, 1985.
67. Grace TG, Sweetser ER, Nelson MA, et al: Isokinetic muscle imbalance and knee-joint injuries. J Bone Joint Surg 66A:734–740, 1984.
68. Kannus P, Latvala K, Jarvinen M: Thigh muscle strengths in the anterior cruciate ligament deficient knee: Isokinetic and isometric long-term results. J Orthop Sports Phys Ther 9:223–227, 1987.
69. Heiser TM, Weber J, Sullivan G, et al: Prophylaxis and management of hamstring muscle injuries in intercollegiate football players. Am J Sports Med 12:368–370, 1984.
70. Corbin CB: Flexibility. Clin Sports Med 3:101–117, 1984.
71. Kannus P, Jarvinen M: Posttraumatic anterior cruciate ligament insufficiency as a cause of osteoarthritis in a knee joint. Clin Rheumatol 8:251–260, 1989.
72. Harrington KD: Degenerative arthritis of the ankle secondary to long-standing lateral ligament instability. J Bone Joint Surg 61A:354–361, 1979.
73. American Academy of Orthopaedic Surgeons: Knee braces, seminar report. Chicago, August 18–19, 1984.
74. Drinkwater B: Training of female athletes. *In* Dirix A, Knuttgen HG, Tittel K (eds): The Olympic Book of Sports Medicine. Oxford, Blackwell Scientific Publications, 1988, pp 309–327.
75. Lloyd T, Traintafyllou SJ, Baker ER, et al: Women athletes with menstrual irregularity have increased musculoskeletal injuries. Med Sci Sports 18:374–379, 1986.
76. Marcus R, Cann C, Madvig P, et al: Menstrual function and bone mass in elite women distance runners. Ann Intern Med 102:158–163, 1985.
77. Kuroda Y: Sport and physical activities in older people: Maintenance of physical fitness. *In* Dirix A, Knuttgen HG, Tittel K (eds): The Olympic Book of Sports Medicine. Oxford, Blackwell Scientific Publications, 1988, pp 331–339.
78. Lane NE, Bloch DA, Wood PD, et al: Aging, long-distance running, and the development of musculoskeletal disability: A controlled study. Am J Med 82:772–780, 1987.
79. Peterson L, Renstrom P: Varldsmasterskapen for veteraner—en medicinsk utmaning. (Championships for veterans—a medical challenge.) Lakartidningen 77:3618, 1980.
80. Takala J, Sievers K, Klaukka T: Rheumatic symptoms in the middle-aged population in southwestern Finland. Scand J Rheumatol [Suppl]47:15–29, 1982.
81. Kannus P, Jarvinen M, Kontiala H, et al: Occurrence of symptomatic knee osteoarthritis in rural Finland: A prospective follow-up study. Ann Rheum Dis 46:804–808, 1987.
82. Leach RE, Baumgard S, Broom J: Obesity: Its relationship to osteoarthritis of the knee. Clin Orthop 93:271–273, 1973.
83. Hinz G, Pohl W: Die Bedeutung des Korpergewichtes bei degenerativen Skeletterkrankungen. (Importance of bodyweight in degenerative musculoskeletal diseases.) Z Orthop 115:12–18, 1977.
84. Hartz AJ, Fischer ME, Bril G, et al: The association of obesity with joint pain and osteoarthritis in the HANES data. J Chronic Dis 39:311–319, 1986.
85. Nigg B: Causes of injuries: Extrinsic factors. *In* Dirix A, Knuttgen HG, Tittel K (eds): The Olympic Book of Sports Medicine. Oxford, Blackwell Scientific Publications, 1988, pp 363–375.
86. Mann RA: Biomechanics of running. *In* Mack RP (ed): Symposium on Foot and Leg in Running Sports. St. Louis, CV Mosby, 1982, pp 1–29.
87. Boswick JA Jr, Danzl DF, Hamlet MP, et al: Helping the frostbitten patient. Patient Care 17:90–115, 1983.

22

MANAGEMENT OF EMERGENCIES

Douglas A. Rund, MD

Accidents and life-threatening events can occur at any time to anyone. Athletes are no exception. Physicians, trainers, and even participants are best prepared to deal with emergencies when they understand basic principles of emergency management and how and when to utilize the community's emergency medical services system.

There are several general principles of emergency medical management: rapid assessment of the patient and the situation; a call for help; protection of vital structures, such as the cervical spine; patient stabilization; and preparation for transfer to another level of care. In mass casualty situations, triage becomes fundamental activity.

Emergency life support skills required of medical providers include assessment and management of the airway, relief of factors interfering with adequate ventilation, provision of circulatory support, control of hemorrhage, management of cardiac arrest, and an approach to trauma based on management priorities.

GENERAL PRINCIPLES

Rapid Patient Assessment

In most conscious patients, assessment begins with a 10-second inquiry, during which the physician evaluates general appearance and mental status. In cases where the initial impression suggests the need for life support or immediate hospital treatment, the physician should proceed to rapid mobilization of resources, primarily the summoning of paramedics or emergency medical technicians (EMTs). Assessment and treatment can then continue as the paramedic team heads to the scene. For example, when a 56-year-old spectator complains of chest pain and appears pale, ashen, or cyanotic, the treating physician must first think about stabilizing the patient with oxygen, intravenous access, and cardiac monitoring; and then think about safely transporting the patient to another level of care. Such activities inevitably require the resources of a paramedic unit.

In the unconscious or semiconscious patient, immediate assessment must begin with evaluation of the airway. When the loss of consciousness follows an injury, one must protect the cervical spine while such assessment proceeds. This is usually accomplished by having an assistant apply gentle "in-line" traction to the head. The second step involves making sure that the patient is breathing. Breathing assessment and airway assessment go hand in hand: air moves in and out of the mouth and nose, and the chest rises and falls symmetrically. The third basic kind of assessment involves evaluation of circulation as determined by pulse, skin color, and mental activity. The radial pulse can usually be palpitated until the systolic blood pressure falls below 80 mm Hg, the femoral pulse can be

Airway

Breathing

Circulation

Disability (neurologic)

Exposure/**E**xamination

Fracture

Gross instability or deformity of a joint

Hemorrhage

Figure 22–1. Elements of brief evaluation of a patient with an acute medical event or injury.

palpated above 70 mm Hg, and the carotid pulse remains palpable to a systolic pressure of about 60 mm Hg. The carotid pulse is the most sensitive indicator of presence or absence of cardiac function in the emergency setting. With the spine and back immobilized, the physician can briefly assess distal motor and sensory function by testing for movement response to a painful stimulus; expose certain injured areas; look for major extremity deformity, fractures, or unstable joints; and detect sites of major bleeding or hemorrhage and apply direct pressure on the area. A rapid emergency evaluation, sometimes termed a "primary survey," can follow the alphabetic mnemonic, "ABCDEFGH," as outlined in Figure 22–1.

Stabilization

One of the most important concepts in the management of clinical emergencies is patient stabilization. The concept, in essence, is that *the patient's vital signs, life-sustaining processes, and neurologic function must be preserved if they are in jeopardy even before complete examination or a definitive diagnosis is made.* Such support should be in place as early as possible if a subsequent collapse of vital signs is even remotely suspected. For example, in the middle-aged patient with severe chest pain and shortness of breath, supplemental oxygen treats hypoxemia and "preoxygenates" the patient in the event that intubation is required. An intravenous line allows administration of fluids to combat hypotension and drugs to treat cardiac dysrhythmias or pulmonary edema.

The trauma victim who has head injury, suspected neck injury, or loss of consciousness requires protection of neurologic function using cervical spine immobilization and backboard prior to transport. Cervical spine immobilization includes a rigid cervical collar, sandbags, and head secured to backboard with tape across the forehead. The patient's body must also be secured to the backboard. The backboard protects the entire spine including the neck. The patient must be "log rolled" onto the board to prevent any bending of the vertebral column.

Mobilization of Support Services

The emergency medical services system (EMSS) exists to respond immediately to medical emergencies. Designed originally to provide mobile coronary care unit treatment to victims of heart attack, paramedic units are now summoned for virtually any serious medical event or injury. In most communities, an EMS unit can be on scene within minutes after being called.

If there is any question at all that they may be needed, the paramedics should be notified as soon as possible. Appropriate calls for immediate help include severe chest pain, fainting, shortness of breath, abrupt onset of headache, severe abdominal pain, or apparent serious injury. A false alarm in notifying the EMS system inappropriately is always preferable to a delay in lifesaving treatment.

Decision-making and Standardized Approaches

Decision-making in an emergency situation is difficult and stressful because physicians must base decisions on small fragments of data. The pressure to decide quickly is so insistent and so inescapable that the decision-making process hardly resembles the thoughtful investigation and reflection one gives to nonurgent patient complaints in the office or hospital.

Recognizing these difficulties, certain standardized approaches to emergencies have been developed by organizations such as the American Heart Association and the Committee on Trauma or the American College of Surgeons. The Advanced Cardiac Life Support course, for instance, simulates cardiac arrest and conditions leading to cardiac arrest. The approach to eaoh condition is standardized. Because the guidelines are well known by the entire team, the resuscitation runs smoothly. The Advanced Trauma Life Support course provides similar guidelines for the management of trauma. In the simulated presentation, there is opportunity for feedback and teaching at each step of the process. Rehearsal of approaches to cardiac and traumatic events, well in advance of the actual emergency, streamline the entire process.

OBSTRUCTED AIRWAY

Although the cause of airway obstruction may vary from patient to patient, the urgency does not. Maintenance of an adequate airway constitutes the "A" in the ABCs of basic life support because without ventilation the patient can suffer irreversible central nervous system (CNS) damage in 4 to 6 minutes. When the airway is completely blocked, the rescuer cannot hear or feel airflow at the nose or mouth despite respiratory retractions of sternal, supraclavicular, and intercostal areas during spontaneous breathing attempts, and one cannot ventilate the lungs with mouth-to-mouth or mouth-to-mask ventilatory techniques.

In cases of partial airway obstruction, certain characteristic sounds suggest the cause of obstruction: snoring suggests that the tongue obstructs the hypopharynx; stridor (crowing) suggests that edema, tumor, or foreign body obstructs the larynx; and gurgling suggests the presence of liquid material (e.g., vomitus or blood) in the airway. Wheezing is prominent when smaller airways are obstructed in cases of endobronchial foreign body or bronchospasm.[1]

If unrelieved, complete airway obstruction results in asphyxia. Hypoxemia and hypercarbia develop rapidly to produce the characteristic picture of acute respiratory distress: a desperate struggle that progresses from violent agitation and aphonia to eventual exhaustion, loss of consciousness, and cardiac arrest.

In many cases of partial airway obstruction, hypoxemia causes agitation, restlessness, and confusion. Early recognition that such behavior can result from inadequate ventilation especially in the injured, allows one to proceed with lifesaving therapy including opening the airway, providing ventilation, and administering supplemental oxygen.

In cases of trauma, airway management must always proceed in a way that protects the cervical spine from motion. The mandibular lift, chin lift, and triple airway maneuver must be accomplished while someone else prevents neck flexion, or after a rigid cervical collar has been placed around the neck. Management of airway obstruction depends, of course, on the cause, but certain immediate treatment procedures, such as mandibular lift, are nearly always appropriate.

Mandibular Lift

The mandibular lift method of bringing the jaw forward and lifting the tongue away from the hypopharynx is particularly effective in patients with good muscle relaxation. To lift the mandible, one usually places the fingers behind the vertical rami of the mandible and thrusts the jaw forward. The technique can be used with or without a cervical collar in place. As the obstruction is relieved, a snoring sound changes to one of free-flowing air in and out of the hypopharynx.

Chin Lift

The airway can often be opened by lifting the chin forward. To do so the rescuer grasps the chin and pulls the mandible forward. When the mandibular symphysis is fractured, the tongue's anterior attachments may be disrupted. This is particularly true when the mandible is fractured in two places adjacent to the chin producing a "flail mandible." In such cases, the tongue itself must be grasped with gauze or cloth and pulled forward. In extreme cases, especially when the patient is unconscious, the tongue can be grasped with a towel clip or similar tool or pliers and pulled forward to provide temporary relief until tracheal intubation can be accomplished.

Triple Airway Maneuver

With the stipulation that the head cannot be tilted backward in cases of suspected neck injury, the triple airway maneuver may be useful in opening the airway to provide cardiopulmonary resuscitation. The triple airway maneuver's three components include tilting the head backward, opening the mouth, and displacing the mandible forward. With the person performing the maneuver standing at the patient's head, the ascending rami are grasped with fingers two through five. The mouth is opened with the thumbs, and the head is gently tilted backward.

Repeated Attempts to Ventilate

After each maneuver to open the airway, one should attempt to ventilate the patient. Mouth-to-mouth, mouth-to-nose, mouth-to-mask or bag and mask ventilation are all appropriate techniques. Special masks with one-way valve arrangements that direct secretions and vomitus away from the rescuer have been developed in response to fears of contacting the AIDS virus and other infectious diseases. Although not yet widely available, such devices permit the early ventilation of a victim without fear of exposure to infectious material.

Manual Clearing

Solid particles may occlude the mouth or hypopharynx to create airway obstruction. If such an obstruction is apparent or if one cannot provide ventilation following the jaw thrust or chin lift maneuver, manual clearing may be required. To accomplish this, the patient should be rolled to one side and the mouth forced open. The crossed-finger technique can be used when jaw muscles are relaxed. The thumb is placed on the upper teeth and the index or middle finger placed on the lower teeth in a crossed fashion to open the jaw. A bite block can be placed between the teeth if there is any danger of the teeth clenching together. One or two fingers covered with gauze or cloth, when possible, can then be swept deeply through the mouth and pharynx to remove any solid material. With the finger sweep completed, one again attempts to ventilate the patient. Additional sweeps deep into the throat may be required to remove obstructing debris.

The Heimlich Maneuvers

In 1974, Heimlich described a lifesaving maneuver to prevent deaths associated with choking on food. Observing during open chest surgery that the diaphragm rises several centimeters into the thorax when the fist is pressed upward into the epigastrium, Heimlich postulated that such a maneuver would be valuable in dislodging food from the throat in the choking victim. He noted that a food bolus or other foreign body was often drawn against the larynx during inspiration. Despite air-filled lungs, the victim could not inhale or exhale and typically died from asphyxia. He postulated that a sudden forceful compression of the upper abdomen would decrease intrathoracic volume, increase the air pressure within the trachea and larynx, and thus, "eject the offending bolus like the cork from a champagne bottle."[2] Heimlich proposed that we adopt a universal sign for choking as an indication to others that the problem is related to choking and not heart attack. The signal for "I'm choking on food" is demonstrated when the victim grasps his neck between the thumb and index finger of one hand to signal that he or she is choking.

For a standing victim, the rescuer stands behind the victim and puts both arms around the abdomen just above the beltline allowing head, arms, and upper torso to hang forward. Then, grasping his own right fist with his left hand, the rescuer rapidly and strongly presses into the victim's abdomen forcing the diaphragm upward, compressing the lungs, and expelling the obstructing bolus.

For the victim lying face down, the rescuer sits astride the body, encircles the victim's torso, and performs the maneuver. For a victim lying on his back, the rescuer sits astride the pelvis and presses both hands, one on top of the other, forcefully upward into the subdiaphragmatic region of the abdomen. It is important that the maneuver be performed correctly. Variations from the procedure can result in fractured ribs or injury of intra-abdominal organs, such as liver or spleen. The position for the hand on the abdomen is an area in the midline midway between the umbilicus and xiphoid process. The other hand is then cupped around the first and provides the actual pressure for the inward thrust. The maneuver can be repeated as often as necessary until the foreign body is removed. Following each maneuver, the mouth or hypopharynx can be swept with the gauze-covered fingers for removal of the foreign body.

The maneuver allows a minimally trained rescuer to remove particles from the hypopharynx or larynx that create a choking episode. When such episodes occur during eating, the pattern of rapid loss of consciousness and pulse can resemble myocardial infarction, which led historically to the term "cafe coronary." In typical cases, edentulous or intoxicated patients swallow a large bolus of meat or other food product which obstructs the larynx producing asphyxia and death. The Heimlich maneuver is the treatment of choice in such instances.

Although it was initially thought that the maneuver would work only in cases of total obstruction, case reports have indicated that the maneuver is clearly helpful in removing hard objects that only partially obstruct the trachea. Such objects include hard candy, pills, or cough drops. In addition, near-drowning victims have been treated successfully by the maneuver. When applied to victims of a near-drowning, large amounts of water have been expelled from the lungs. Several patients have successfully performed the maneuver on themselves by falling against a kitchen chair or the edge of the sink.

Suction

Liquid material that gathers in the mouth and pharynx can include blood, vomitus, or mucus. Adequate suctioning of such secretions is essential in maintaining the airway. The rigid tonsil-tipped suction device is most effective in removing pharyngeal secretions rapidly. Portable, battery-operated suction devices are available and should be part of basic resuscitation equipment. Adequate suctioning of the hypopharynx involves opening the mouth as wide as possible and inserting the suction device deep in the pharynx to remove liquid and small particles. Rubber flexible suction catheters are more appropriate for suctioning deeply in the trachea and bronchi. They are more appropriate in the hospital setting when passed through a properly positioned endotracheal tube.

Oral and Nasal Airway

The oral airway lifts the tongue from the hypopharynx, but also may stimulate the gag reflex. The oral airway has usefulness in the out-of-hospital setting, especially to prevent the teeth from clamping together, thus allowing bag-mask ventilation. The major disadvantage of bag-mask ventilation becomes apparent when the stomach distends with air and vomiting occurs. The unprotected larynx allows gastric secretions and food particles to enter the trachea and lungs resulting in the problems of aspiration. A shortened oral airway extending only to the posterior teeth may be useful following intubation to prevent the patient from biting the endotracheal tube. Biting the tube can lead to obstruction, perforation, or complete division, all of which are to be avoided. Soft nasal airways are somewhat more comfortable than oral airways and are easily positioned. When lubricated with an anesthetic gel, the soft nasal airway may be placed prior to nasotracheal intubation and thus, provide some topical anesthesia for the nasopharynx.[3]

Esophageal Airway

Two types of esophageal airways (EA) are in current use: the esophageal obturator airway (EOA); and the esophageal gastric tube airway (EGTA). Both the EOA and EGTA consist of a face mask and esophageal tube. The esophageal tube, 34 cm long, is inserted into the mouth and passed into the esophagus. A soft cuff, which can be inflated through a one-way valve, lies just above the distal portion of the tube. The proximal end of the esophageal tube connects to a face mask that can be inflated by a one-way valve. The inflated mask helps form a tight seal around the mouth. The EOA has a blind esophageal end, whereas the EGTA has a lumen through which a nasogastric tube can be passed. With the EOA, ventilation is accomplished by administration of air or oxygen through the tube itself. The tube has perforations which allow air to enter the hypopharynx. With the esophagus occluded and the mask tightly sealed on the face, air should pass into the tube, through the perforations, and into the lungs. The EGTA tube, in contrast, has a separate ventilation port above the esophageal tube. The esophageal tube then serves as the conduit for the passage of a nasogastric tube. It is unusual that a physician would ever place an EA in preference to an endotracheal tube (ET), but certain circumstances might dictate such a procedure: the EA might be the only airway available. Once placed, the EA must be *left in place* until the patient is successfully intubated and the ET cuff inflates. Only then, should the EA be removed. Suction apparatus should be used when removing the EA. because emesis often occurs when the esophageal balloon deflates and the tube is removed.

Endotracheal Intubation

Endotracheal intubation is the preferred way to ensure a protected airway. Intubation is indicated in the following situations: cardiac arrest, patients who require mechanical ventilation, patients with severe maxillofacial trauma interfering with breathing, and patients with copious secretions or risk of aspiration. The unconscious patient generally requires intubation, a procedure often performed when the patient arrives in an emergency department. Orotracheal or nasotracheal intubation are rather straightforward techniques, but successful performance is not always easy, especially in the emergency setting. Procedure is outlined as follows:

1. Select, prepare, and check all equipment, including the light source on the laryngoscope.
2. Identify proper-sized endotracheal tube based on patient's age, size, and sex; set aside a spare tube one size smaller. Adults usually require tubes sized 7.5, 8.0, or 8.5 mm internal diameter.
3. Check the cuff by inflating and deflating it with air, making sure no air leaks are present. Lubricate the tube with sterile lubricant.
4. Position the patient with the occiput elevated and the head tilted backward ("sniffing position") unless there is a possibility of neck injury.
5. When possible, oxygenate the patient with 100% oxygen for at least 2 minutes.
6. Interrupt ventilation, open the patient's mouth, and pass the laryngoscope blade along the right side of the tongue to the vallecula. Elevate the epiglottis by pulling the handle upward and forward perpendicular to the blade.
7. Visualize the arytenoid cartilages and, if possible, the vocal cords.
8. Pass the endotracheal tube through the larynx into the trachea and inflate the cuff.
9. Check for tube placement by inflating the lungs several times while listening to the chest with the stethoscope. The thorax should expand with inflation, and breath sounds should be heard equally on both sides. Listen over the epigastrium to make sure that air does not enter the stomach.
10. A bite block may be placed between the teeth and the tube securely taped to the face.

Cricothyrotomy

Cricothyrotomy is indicated if the airway cannot be established by intubation as, for instance, in laryngeal edema or laryngeal spasm. The method has the advantage of being relatively easy to perform, with small likelihood of immediate complication, such as laceration of a major blood vessel. The technique of cricothyrotomy is outlined as follows:

1. Locate the cricothyroid membrane at the bottom of the thyroid cartilage and just above the cricoid cartilage.
2. Make a 2-cm longitudinal incision over the cricoid cartilage and spread the incision with a blunt hemostat.
3. Incise the cricothyroid membrane and insert a 15-mm cannula with an inside diameter of at least 5 mm.
4. Ventilate the patient with 100% oxygen.

CARDIAC ARREST

Although typically the result of an arrhythmia associated with acute myocardial ischemia in older persons, cardiac arrest can occur in patients of all ages and has many different causes. Arteriosclerosis of the coronary vessels can occur in younger persons, especially when there is a strong family history of early myocardial infarction, diabetes, hypertension, heavy smoking, or elevation of cholesterol. The use of cocaine, now considered a positive risk factor in the emergency evaluation of patients with chest pain, is also a cause of coronary spasm, cardiac arrest, and sudden death in younger persons. Although a rare event, cardiac arrest has also occurred in athletes without evident coronary pathology. In addition, various conditions that deprive the heart of oxygen or blood flow eventually cause cardiac arrest. Such conditions include severe respiratory distress (as in exercise-induced asthma), severe anemia, shock, or certain poisons, such as carbon monoxide or cyanide.

Cardiac arrest may be defined as the cessation of effective cardiac output. While the causes of cardiac arrest are varied, the final common pathway is one of the following cardiac arrhythmias: ventricular tachycardia, ventricular fibrillation, asystole, electromechanical dissociation, or pulseless idioventricular rhythm. These five conditions cause ineffective contraction of the cardiac ventricles. Ineffective contraction leads to a cessation of cardiac output and hence to the cessation of blood flow to the most vital organs: the heart and central nervous system. The clinical recognition of cardiac arrest is straightforward; the patient is unconscious, with an absent pulse and agonal or absent respirations.

Cardiopulmonary Resuscitation

In cardiac arrest, cardiopulmonary resuscitation (CPR) provides ventilation and circulation to the victim who has sustained cessation of such vital functions. The goal of CPR is to maintain cerebral and myocardial viability while the underlying cause of the arrest is determined and corrected. *Basic* life support (BLS) continues until *advanced* life support (ALS) measures are available, usually from a paramedic or ACLS mobile unit responding to the scene of the arrest. Although some components of standard CPR, such as chest compression, have been questioned as to their effectiveness, the technique is widely taught, and probably most effective if instituted immediately on the scene.

Although some of the current controversial areas in CPR will be highlighted in this discussion, the three major components of cardiopulmonary resuscitation include opening the airway, ventilation, and closed chest cardiac massage.

Immediately after the clinical recognition of a patient in cardiac arrest, the first priority of CPR is the establishment of an open airway. This can be accomplished by the mandibular lift, chin lift, or triple airway maneuver. Such maneuvers lift the tongue away from the back of the throat to open the airway. One must always provide in-line traction to the head to protect the cervical spine in cases of cardiac arrest associated with severe trauma and possible neck injury.

Ventilation

If spontaneous breathing does not resume after a patent airway has been established, artificial methods of breathing for the patient should be initiated immediately. Mouth-to-mouth or mouth-to-nose methods are both acceptable alternatives. The well-equipped athletic facility might have a pocket mask or even a bag-valve-mask and oxygen supply for ventilation. Upper airway obstruction from a foreign body should be determined and treated. Following two initial ventilations, the rescuer should check the carotid pulse.

If no pulse is palpated, current guidelines call for closed chest cardiac massage. Chest compressions (external cardiac massage) are performed by first locating the midpoint of the sternum. One palpates the xiphoid-sternal junction and then identifies a point two finger breadths upward, toward the head. The heel of the left hand is placed over this point, and the heel of the right hand is placed directly over the left hand; the fingers should interlock. The appropriate depth of compression in an adult is 1.5 to 2 in. The compression should account for 50% of the cycle. An acceptable sequence for both one- and two-person CPR starts with two to four initial ventilations over 3 to 4 sec, followed by 15 chest compressions and two more ventilations, and so on. Two-person CPR can be performed in a sequence of five chest compressions and one ventilation.

The sequence is then repeated in this pattern until spontaneous circulation is restored or the resuscitation is discontinued. If restoration of spontaneous breathing and circulation do not occur after several cycles of artificial breathing and circulation, "advanced" life support techniques, such as intubation, defibrillation, and drug therapy, will be required. The institution of such techniques often depends on the arrival of a paramedic unit. Some paramedic units operate under a set of standing orders approved by a physician medical director. Others receive direct orders from a hospital-based physician via radio. In either case, medic teams are usually well practiced in working as a team during cardiopulmonary resuscitation. Most emergency physicians prefer to allow paramedics to proceed with their well-rehearsed resuscitation technique under their supervision.

The effectiveness of closed chest massage has been the subject of debate for the past several years. It has been taught for years that irreversible cerebral anoxic injury developed after 4 to 6 minutes of ischemic anoxia. However, evidence suggests that cerebral neurons may be more tolerant to complete ischemic anoxia than previously thought.[4] Neurologic injuries seen in patients following resuscitation from cardiac arrest may be due to the relatively low level of cerebral blood flow produced during closed chest massage ("trickle flow").[5] Because closed chest massage produces cerebral blood flow that is less than 10% of normal, the amount of oxygen and glucose delivered to cerebral tissues is insufficient to maintain normal cerebral energy metabolism. The delivery of substrates during trickle flow actually leads to lactic acid production and neuronal injury.[6] Experimental approaches toward the protection of cerebral tissues during cardiac arrest include attempts to lower cerebral vascular resistance to flow and to scavenge destructive free radicals or block their production.[7]

As currently practiced, the chances of neurologic recovery after CPR decrease dramatically beyond 5 to 10 minutes. To effectively alter ultimate outcome in cardiac arrest defibrillation, intubation and intravenous access need to be in place as soon as possible. When initial defibrillation, fluid challenge, epinephrine, and oxygenation are unsuccessful, other causes for arrest, such as tension pneumothorax, internal hemorrhage, or cardiac tamponade, should be considered.

Electrical and Pharmacologic Therapy

Specific pharmacologic and/or electrical therapy depends on the underlying dysrhythmia. The treatments outlined here are essentially those contained in the American Heart Association's Advanced Cardiac Life Support course, which is highly recommended for all physicians who might be called upon to manage cardiac arrest.

Ventricular tachycardia usually causes weakness, palpitations, and perhaps, chest pain. Under some instances, there may be loss of pulse and loss of consciousness. This degree of pump failure is treated as cardiac arrest. A precordial thump may be administered first. A precordial thump consists of a sharp blow with the fleshy portion of the closed fist delivered to the midsternum from a height of 8 to 10 in. This will generate an electric current of approximately 30 to 40 joules within the heart, which may be sufficient to convert the dysrhythmia. If ventricular tachycardia persists in the pulseless, unconscious patient, one must initiate immediate therapy as one would treat ventricular fibrillation, the most common cause of cardiac arrest in the emergency setting.

Electrical Defibrillation

A defibrillator should be available to sports medicine personnel from the local EMS unit designated to respond in case of emergency. Large sports programs may wish to have a defibrillator on site along with other advanced life support equipment. The unsynchronized mode is used to convert ventricular fibrillation. A dose of 200 to 300 joules may be given initially. If fibrillation persists, a second 200- to 300-joule dose is repeated immediately. Persistence of ventricular fibrillation is treated with a third defibrillation at 360 delivered joules.

Each previous countershock lowers the transthoracic resistance and increases the delivered current to the heart. Between defibrillations, basic airway management, breathing, and external cardiac massage should proceed. The current recommended approach to paddle placement is to position one defibrillating paddle over the apex of the heart and the second paddle anteriorly over the second intercostal space, just to the right of the sternum. Failure to defibrillate may be caused by high transthoracic resistance. The transthoracic resistance can be reduced by (1) defibrillating at the end-expiratory phase of respiration, (2) applying firm pressure (about 25 lb of force) to each paddle, (3) using low-impedance paste or gel, (4) using a shorter time interval between defibrillations, and (5) changing the paddle placement to an anterior-posterior location (so that a maximum amount of myocardium is included in the defibrillation field).

Pharmacologic Therapy

If ventricular fibrillation persists despite defibrillation, drug administration begins with epinephrine in doses ranging from 0.5 to 1.0 mg (5 to 10 mL of 1:10,000 solution). Epinephrine improves coronary blood flow and cerebral blood flow. Alpha-adrenergic vasoconstriction caused by epinephrine leads to an increase in aortic diastolic pressure, and hence, improved coronary perfusion. This makes the heart more amenable to subsequent defibrillation. Following epinephrine administration, defibrillation with 360 joules should be reattempted.

Persistent ventricular fibrillation must be treated with antidysrhythmic drug therapy. Lidocaine remains the most widely recommended first-line antidysrhythmic. Lidocaine is effective in raising the fibrillation threshold in myocardial tissue. The recommended loading dose is 1 mg/kg. The loading dose should always be followed by a constant lidocaine infusion of 1 to 4 mg/min. One half the loading dose is repeated in 10 minutes to ensure adequate blood levels. As a general rule, the total of two loading doses should not exceed 300 mg. Defibrillation at 360 joules should always follow antidysrhythmic therapy. Bretylium may be effective against ventricular fibrillation unresponsive to defibrillation and lidocaine. The recommended initial dose is 5 mg/kg. A second dose of 10 mg/kg can be administered and repeated every 15 to 30 minutes as needed.

Intravenous sodium bicarbonate therapy remains controversial. Current recommendations state that (1) sodium bicarbonate should not be used until 10 minutes into the resuscitation, (2) bicarbonate therapy should be dictated by arterial blood gases, (3) the initial dose in the absence of arterial blood gases is 1 mg/kg intravenously, and (4) bicarbonate therapy should only be administered when adequate control of ventilation has been achieved. This usually means that one has accomplished endotracheal intubation and provides a good bag-and-valve ventilation technique or controlled ventilation with a volume-cycled ventilator. Bicarbonate combines with water to form CO_2, which must be eliminated by adequate ventilation or acidosis will persist. Following administration of bicarbonate, any remaining bicarbonate solution should be flushed from the line because the alkaline bicarbonate solution precipitates calcium chloride and partially inactivates epinephrine.

Other Arrhythmias

Asystole is absence of any discernible cardiac rhythm. Its presence on a cardiac monitor strip is a "flat line." Asystole may be the initial dysrhythmia, may follow defibrillation of ventricular fibrillation/tachycardia, or may be seen following degeneration of ventricular fibrillation over time. The specific initial management of asystole is with epinephrine and sodium bicarbonate as outlined for the management of ventricular fibrillation. The role of the vagus nerve in asystole is not entirely clear, but atropine provides vagal blockade and is thus recommended for treatment of asystole. An initial dose of 1 mg is to be followed in a few minutes by another 1-mg dose. Two milligrams of atropine should be fully vagolytic. Proper overall evaluation of asystole should include consideration of many causes, including hypothermia. Additionally, fine ventricular fibrillation may appear as asystole in certain ECG leads. Therefore, defibrillation may be attempted.

Electromechanical dissociation represents the ECG appearance of a narrow QRS rhythm (less than 0.12 msec) in the absence of palpable pulses. Pulseless idioventricular rhythm is similar except that the QRS complex is greater than 0.12 msec. Therapy for both entities includes epinephrine and sodium bicarbonate in doses used for the treatment of asystole. The treating physician should also consider other causes of these dysrhythmias, where electrical activity persists in the absence of effective cardiac output. Such causes include hypovolemia, tension pneumothorax, pericardial tamponade, and pulmonary embolism.

TRAUMA

As for all emergencies, the initial approach to the victim of an injury includes rapid assessment and stabilization. The fundamental initial considerations include protection of the cervical spine, assurance of an adequate airway, assessment of breathing, assessment of circulation, and control of hemorrhage by direct pressure. If a deficiency is found in one of these critical parameters, it must be corrected. Field stabilization, therefore, can include cervical collar with backboard and supplemental oxygen. Hypotension from external or internal blood loss usually requires intravenous volume infusion (2 large-bore IVs) and the MAST garment.

Current opinion about the field management of trauma tends toward minimal intervention at the scene and rapid transport to a properly equipped trauma center. This "scoop and run" philosophy has called into question the practice of starting intravenous fluids in the field (dubbed "stay and play" by those who favor "scoop and run"). A satisfactory strategy seems to be one which advocates immobilization of the spine and neck, transport from the scene, and initiation of intravenous fluids while en route to the hospital.[8]

The physician's role therefore requires rapid primary survey (airway, breathing, and circulation) with cervical spine immobilization and notification of the prehospital care system. Having opened the airway and noticing adequate breathing and circulation, the physician can begin a "secondary survey," which is essentially a head-to-toe examination searching for lacerations, contusions, fractures, dislocations, head injuries, eye or nose injuries, and chest and abdominal injuries.

The description of such injuries is relayed to the paramedic team and alternately to trauma center personnel where definitive care will be provided. Planning for rapid medical management of emergencies includes staff training, maintenance of some emergency equipment supplies, and rapid access to a paramedic system. Preparation by the team physician in advance of an emergency gives an unexpected victim the best chance for survival without handicap.

REFERENCES

1. Rund DA: Emergencies in sports: Airway obstruction: Recognition and immediate management. Physician Sportsmed 17(10):173–174, 1989.
2. Heimlich HJ: Pop goes the café coronary. Emerg Med 6(6):154, June 1974.
3. Rund DA: Emergencies in sports: Opening the airway: Equipment and techniques. Physician Sportsmed 17(11):145–148, 1989.
4. Ames A: Earlier irreversible changes during ischemia. Am J Emerg Med 2:139–146, 1983.
5. Rehncrona S, Mela L, Siesjo BK: Recovery of brain mitochondrial function in the rat after complete and incomplete cerebral ischemia. Stroke 10:437–446, 1979.
6. Rehncrona S, Mela L, Siesjo BK: Excessive cellular acidosis—an important mechanism of neuronal damage in the brain? Acta Physiol Scan 110:435–437, 1980.
7. White BC, Aust DS, Arfors KE, et al: "Brain injury by ischemic anoxia." Hypothesis extension—a tale of two ions. Ann Emerg Med 13(2):9, 1984.
8. Jones SE, Nesper TP, Alcouloumre E: Prehospital intravenous line placement: A prospective study. Ann Emerg Med 18:244–246, 1989.

SECTION IV

THE ENVIRONMENT

23

HEAT ILLNESS

John R. Sutton, MD

Heat illness is common in endurance sports and also is seen in football. Races like San Francisco's "Bay-to-Breakers" have been held for more than 70 years; however, it is only in the last decade that the numbers of participants have risen dramatically. The 1970s witnessed a worldwide surge in the number of "fun runners" as well as the number of "fun runs." Nor has the craze been limited to the shorter distance races. In the 1980s, it became common for marathons (26 miles, 385 yards) to be oversubscribed.

In my own experience over more than two decades of fun runs, I remember being amazed to find 2000 entrants in Sydney's inaugural fun run, the "City-to-Surf" race.[1] Nowadays, there are upward of 25,000 entrants annually (Fig. 23–1).[2–5] If these numbers seem excessive, consider the Auckland "Round the Bays" race, which now attracts about 70,000 runners per year.[6] Longer races are also extremely popular. London's marathon attracted over 80,000 applicants in 1982; the numbers accepted were naturally considerably fewer, although 16,350 started and 15,758 finished.[7]

Along with this exponential rise in the number of active people participating in fun runs, an increase in running-related injuries has also occurred. In fact, almost weekly in the medical press, we read of new complications associated with running, from simple muscle, joint, and skin problems, to penile frostbite, excoriated nipples, and jogger's amenorrhea.[8] However, the illnesses of heat exhaustion, heat syncope, and heat stroke are the most important, the last being potentially life-threatening. Furthermore, when one considers the numbers of runners and joggers exposed to such problems—more than 30 million in North America alone—the number of heat-related casualties resulting from fun runs could be astronomical.

When I described a minor epidemic of heat-related illnesses in the 1971 Sydney "City-to-Surf" race, the topic was virtually unknown in the jogging world.[1] However, thanks to further analysis and medical surveillance,[9–15] and particularly to the lay and running press,[16–19] there is now a much wider understanding of these problems. Today the average jogger probably has a better understanding of the pathophysiology of thermal illness occurring during fun runs than did the physician of the 1960s. This review emphasizes the heat problems related to fun runs and examines the topic in a way that should be most useful to the sports physician.

ASSESSMENT OF ENVIRONMENTAL HEAT STRESS

The ambient temperature is only one component of environmental heat stress and certainly not the most important. The other components are humidity, air movement, and radiant heat. Because evaporation is the most important means of heat loss and depends on relative humidity, it follows that a measurement of relative humidity by the wet bulb thermometer (WBT) is the most important single index of environmental heat stress. The wet bulb temperature is obtained by wrapping a wet wick around the bulb of a thermom-

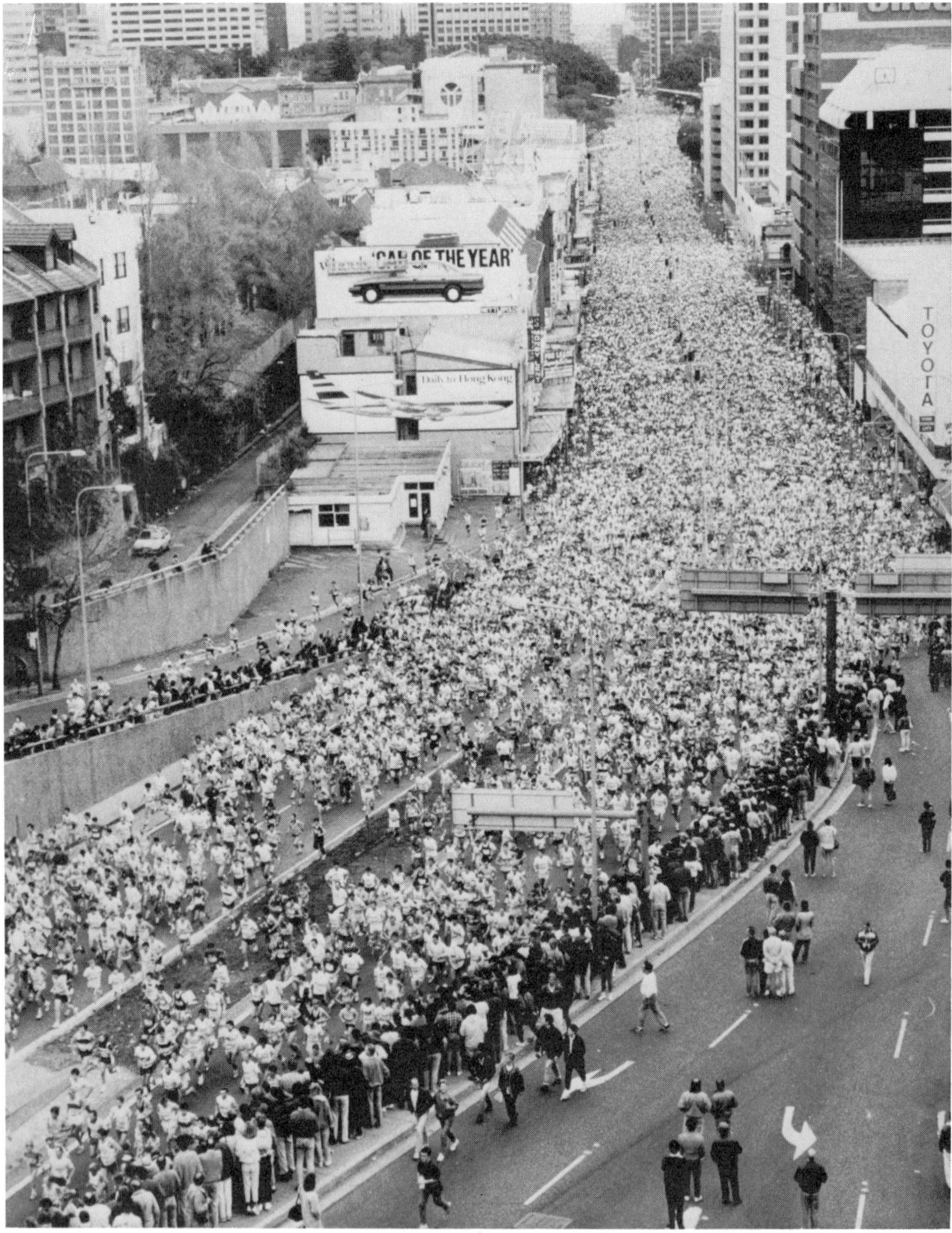

Figure 23–1. "City-to-Surf" race—from a humble beginning in 1971 with about 2000 runners to the present in which more than 30,000 runners compete annually. (Courtesy of Dr. R. Richards.)

eter and examining the effect of evaporation on the recorded temperature. The evaporation will depend on wind velocity and on the amount of water vapor in the air. Thus, a high wet bulb temperature—one that approaches or is equal to that of the dry bulb (it can never exceed the dry bulb temperature)—represents a great amount of water vapor present, and little evaporation will be possible. By contrast, a low wet bulb temperature indicates that there is little water vapor present and that a high rate of evaporative heat loss is possible. Relative humidity is the wet bulb/dry bulb comparison.

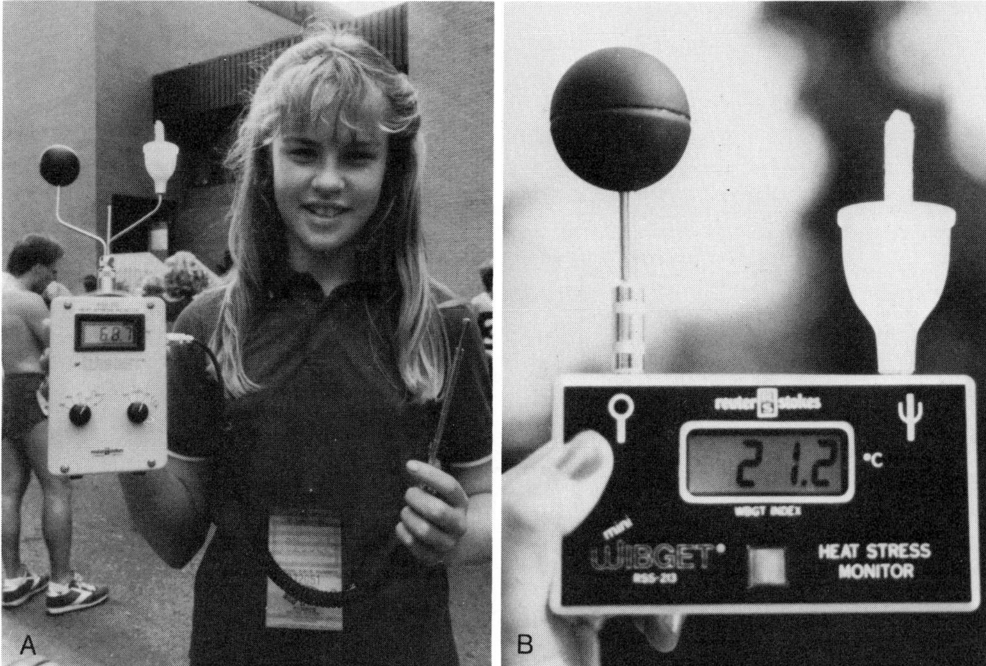

Figure 23–2. A: A "heat stress monitor" measures each variable of dry bulb, wet bulb, and globe temperature in addition to wind speed. It will also compute the web bulb globe temperature (WBGT) index and is simple to operate. **B:** The cheaper and simpler model of "Heat Stress Monitor" gives direct digital readout of WBGT. It is available from Reuter Stokes, Cambridge, Ontario, Canada.

There have been many attempts to assess environmental heat stress, for example, by *effective temperature,* which gives the humidity, air temperature, and wind velocity. Perhaps an even more comprehensive and widely applicable approach is that developed by the U.S. armed forces—the wet bulb globe temperature (WBGT) (Fig. 23–2). In this approach, ambient temperature is measured using a dry bulb thermometer, humidity is assessed with a wet bulb thermometer, and radiant heat is measured with a black globe thermometer. From this, a WBGT index (in units of °C) is calculated using the following formula:

$$\text{WBGT} = 0.7\text{T}_{wb} + 0.2\text{T}_{g} + 0.1\text{T}_{db}$$

where T_{wb} = temperature wet bulb thermometer, T_{g} = temperature black globe thermometer, and T_{db} = temperature dry bulb thermometer.

The importance of wet bulb temperature can be immediately appreciated because it accounts for 70% of the index, whereas dry bulb temperature accounts for only 10%. Thus, a mild, humid day can represent more of a heat stress than a hot, dry day.

For a WBGT of less than 18°C (64°F), the risk of heat injury is slight (but still exists), whereas above 28°C (82°F), races should not be conducted. Specific guidelines are detailed later in the discussion of race organization.

THERMOREGULATION

With efficient protection, humans are able to tolerate great environmental temperature variations, from about −100°C to +100°C. Obviously, the thermal range of cellular viability is much less, extending from about −1°C when ice crystals form and disrupt the cells, to about 45°C (113°F) when heat denaturation of vital proteins occurs. Optimal

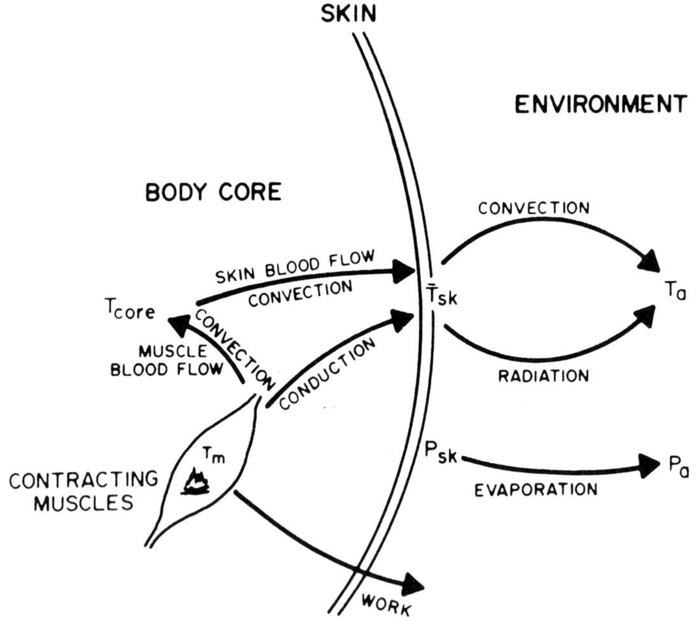

Figure 23–3. Avenues for thermal exchange between the body and the environment during exercise. (*From* Nadel E: Control of sweating rate while exercising in the heat. Med Sci Sports 11:31, 1979; with permission.)

biologic function requires a much smaller thermal range, and an increase or decrease of more than 2°C in normal body core temperature will result in a significant impairment of mental and physical function. Although the coagulation and denaturation of cellular proteins does not occur until a temperature of about 45°C (113°F) is reached, the body can tolerate a core temperature in excess of 41°C (106°F) for only a short time. We are able to tolerate significant increases in core temperature much less than decreases; thus, we live our entire lives within a few degrees of our thermal nemesis. It is not surprising, therefore, that elaborate temperature-regulating mechanisms have evolved to prevent overheating (Fig. 23–3). These adaptations involve complex integrations between the circulatory, neurologic, endocrine, and exocrine functions, which operate maximally during exercise in hot, humid environments.

Body core temperature increases during exercise, and the mean body temperature is the result of the dynamic balance between those processes producing heat and those responsible for heat loss. This is embodied in the equation of Winslow and others[20]:

$$S = M \pm R \pm C_d \pm C_v - E$$

where S = the amount of stored heat, M = the metabolic heat production, R = the heat gained or lost by radiation, C_d = the conductive heat lost or gained, C_v = the convective heat lost or gained, and E = the evaporative heat loss.

Heat Production

The rate of metabolic heat production increases linearly with running speed and is the most important source of body heat during exercise (Fig. 23–4). Because the body is only about 25% efficient, 75% of all the energy will be converted into heat; thus, the faster the running pace, the greater the rate of heat production. For example, over a 10-km run, the average athlete will produce about 1500 kilocalories per hour (kcal/hr).[21] In contrast, the average runner (70 kg) will produce about 800 to 1000 kcal/hr and the slower ones, about 400 to 500 kcal/hr.

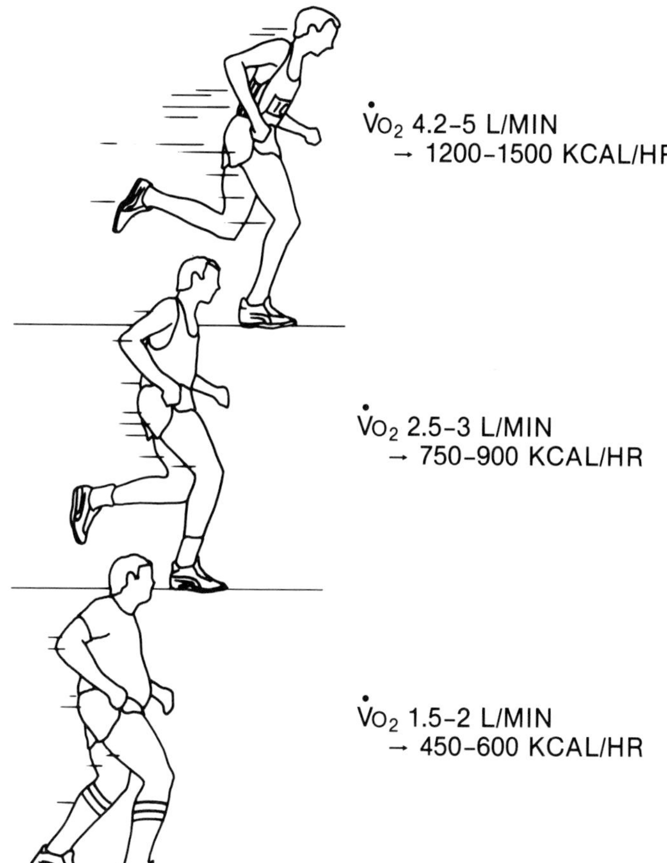

Figure 23–4. Effect of running speed on heat production.

Another source of heat comes from solar radiation. On bright, cloudless days this may represent an extra heat load of more than 150 kcal/hr. Thus, in a fun run of 10 km, an average runner might incur a heat load of between 1000 and 1200 kcal/hr. In the absence of elaborate heat-loading mechanisms, this would result in an increase in body core temperature from 37°C (99°F) to nearly 50°C (122°F).

Heat Loss

By far, the quantitatively most important process for losing heat during a run is through evaporation of sweat. Blood is transported to the body surface, where heat is lost by conduction and convection. If the heat load is great enough, sweat glands will be activated; with the evaporation of the sweat, the skin and then the body will be cooled. About 500 to 600 kcal are needed for evaporation of 1 L of sweat; although a certain amount of sweat drips from the body and is lost in the cooling process, this still represents the most efficient heat-dissipating mechanism. Thus, in an average fun run with the runner sweating about 1 L/hr, about 400 to 500 kcal/hr would be lost, assuming that only 80% of the sweat is likely to be available for the heat loss. By contrast, the heat-acclimatized athlete may lose up to 2 L of sweat per hour, thus being able to dissipate 800 to 1000 kcal/hr. The ability to lose heat effectively will also depend on the air temperature, relative humidity, and wind. While there is a temperature gradient from the skin to the air, heat will also be lost by convection and conduction. However, with increasing air temperature, these avenues of heat loss diminish.

When the heat elimination processes are outstripped by the rate of heat gain, body temperature rises and thermal illness follows. The importance of efficient heat-dissipating mechanisms to prevent heat injury during exercise is demonstrated by the relatively few heat illnesses in trained athletes as compared with fun runners. In athletes, metabolic heat production may be twice that of the jogger who collapses from heat injury, thus underlining the importance of efficient heat-dissipating mechanisms. Athletes also begin to sweat sooner than nonathletes.

HEAT-RELATED DISORDERS

Heat Syncope

Heat syncope is the abrupt loss of consciousness usually observed in unacclimatized people in the upright position.[22] Usually, it results from venous pooling of blood in the vasodilated periphery. In turn, this results in a diminished venous return, reduced cardiac output, and impaired cerebral perfusion with loss of consciousness. Heat syncope is more commonly found in the following settings:

1. Prolonged standing in the heat (eg, a soldier on guard duty).
2. Standing suddenly from a lying down or sitting position.
3. Stopping at the end of a race. The muscle pump is then no longer working to enhance venous return.
4. Clinical settings involving patients with autonomic neuropathy, such as diabetes or the Shy-Drager syndrome; dehydration—salt, water, or both; and drugs such as ganglion-blocking agents, diuretics, peripheral vasodilators, beta-blockers, and calcium-channel antagonists.

Heat Cramps

Heat cramps most commonly affect the legs, arms, or abdominal wall, and occur several hours after exercise. They are due to spasms of skeletal muscle and classically, subjects sweat profusely and then consume large amounts of fluid without replacing the lost sodium. The diagnosis is usually obvious. However, when the muscles of the abdominal wall are involved, the differential diagnosis may include an acute surgical abdomen, acute gastroenteritis, or exercise-induced peritonitis.[23] Knochel and Reed[24] have suggested that heat-acclimatized individuals are more susceptible to heat, but the Israeli soldiers[25] and the Indian army[26] would disagree. Furthermore, this was not the experience of Talbot with the workers on the Boulder Dam[27] or the Youngstown, Ohio steelworkers.[28]

Precise mechanisms responsible for heat-induced cramps are not understood. However, there seems to be general agreement that a relative sodium depletion and/or a dilutional hyponatremia is almost universal.[28–30]

Heat Stroke and Heat Exhaustion

These two conditions are part of a continuum with relatively minor changes in heat exhaustion but with loss of consciousness, possibly leading to death, in heat stroke.

Exertional heat stroke appears more frequently during fun runs and marathons when

TABLE 23–1. FACTORS THAT PREDISPOSE TO HEAT STROKE

Personal	Environmental
Young	Heat
Old	Humid
Dehydrated	Windless
Ill—febrile illness	Polluted
Obese	Unseasonably hot
Unfit	
Unacclimatized to heat	
Predisposed to malignant hyperthermia	

the environmental conditions are not particularly hot.[1] During severe heat stress, skin blood flow begins to fall[31]; this is rather similar to the situation found when central venous pressure is reduced by lower-body negative pressure.[32] Rowell,[33] in a study of exercise in the heat, concluded that a hierarchy of homeostatic mechanisms favored the maintenance of arterial pressure in the circulation to vital organs at the expense of skin vasodilatation and thermoregulation, a hypothesis supported by the observation of a marked reduction in skin blood flow in collapsed fun runners.[34] Factors that predispose to heat stroke are listed in Table 23–1.

Central nervous system impairments, such as epilepsy, delirium, and coma, are the main distinguishing features of heat stroke, which differentiate it from heat exhaustion. Unlike hypothermia, there is no one temperature that defines heat stroke. A rectal temperature of 41°C or by some 40.6°C (105°F) and a hot, dry skin were once considered essential components for the diagnosis of heat stroke.[25,35] Nowadays, to regard the presence of these features as essential may mislead the physician and delay diagnosis and treatment.[36]

A distinction should be made between exertional heat stroke and classic heat stroke (Table 23–2). The latter is usually observed after several days when the ambient temperature was particularly high (above 37.9°C, 100°F). Classic heat stroke occurs in the very young and the old, the unwell, and the sedentary. Many of the elderly patients suffering classic heat stroke also use medications that impair thermoregulation.

Exertion-associated heat stroke occurs when the heat produced by an exercising individual outstrips the ability to lose heat to the environment and the body temperature

TABLE 23–2. CHARACTERISTICS OF CLASSIC AND EXERTION-INDUCED HEAT STROKE

Characteristics	Classic	Exertional
Age	Older	Young
Occurrence	Epidemic form	Isolated cases
Pyrexia	Very high	High
Predisposing illness	Frequent	Rare
Sweating	Often absent	Usually present
Acid-base disturbance	Respiratory alkalosis	Lactic acidosis
Rhabdomyolysis	Rare	Common
Disseminated intravascular coagulation	Rare	Common
Acute renal failure	Rare	Common
Hyperuricemia	Mild	Marked
Enzyme level elevations	Mild	Marked

Data from Khogali M, Hales JRS (eds): Heat Stroke and Temperature Regulation. Sydney, Academic Press Australia, 1983, p 3; with permission.

continues to rise. This is well known in endurance events, such as the marathon,[21,37] and among cyclists.[38] These observations were extended to fun runners by Sutton and coworkers[1] in 1972 and have since been confirmed many times in fun runners in short races,[3,9,10,39] in military recruits,[25,40–43] and in football players.[44,45] In events, such as rowing or wrestling, where there is a need to "make weight," dehydrating practices can be disastrous. Sometimes athletes run in track suits, impervious plastic, such as garbage bags, or in one instance resulting in death, a wet suit.[41] There is sometimes a misconception that water denial accelerates physical conditioning; worse still is the situation in which fluid retention is used as a disciplinary measure in the military.[24]

Pathophysiology of Heat Stroke. At a comparable rectal temperature, tissue damage to various organs is greater in exertional heat stroke rather than in classic heat stroke.[24] There is considerable interindividual variation in the temperature required to produce tissue damage. Some people have survived with temperatures of 46.5°C (115.7°F),[46] whereas others have died of exertional heat stroke with a temperature not above 40.6°C.[24] Although absolute core temperature is important, its duration and rate of change may be more important. However, the most crucial determinant of organ damage is the state of circulation. Once the circulation fails, heat and waste products accumulate and ischemic injury is likely. A variety of legitimate drugs, which may be prescribed by the athlete's physician, may also increase the risk of heat stroke.

Cardiovascular Effects. Sinus tachycardia is common. There may be transient hypertension and, less commonly, hypotension with clinical shock. Rarely, acute left heart failure may occur. Electrocardiographic changes include sinus tachycardia, nonspecific flattening and inversion of the T-waves, various transient conduction disturbances, and prolonged or borderline QT intervals. Cardiac pathology in heat stroke includes dilatation of the right heart, particularly the atrium, and subendocardial, subpericardial, and myocardial hemorrhages, which are most common in the intraventricular septum and on the posterior wall of the left ventricle.[47,48] Fragmentation and ruptured muscle fibers are also common with the presence of interstitial edema. A recent report of a football player who died of heat stroke noted a hemorrhagic infarction in the anterior papillary muscle (Barschenas and associates as quoted in Knochel and Reed[24]).

Renal Impairment. Up to 25% of patients with heat stroke may have oliguria, anuria, and acute renal insufficiency with acute tubular necrosis.[10,24,49–52]

Acute renal failure is much more common in exercise-related heat stroke than in classic heat stroke probably because of the much higher incidence of rhabdomyolysis. Most patients recover well although they may require a prolonged period of peritoneal dialysis and/or hemodialysis.[10,52] However, a few patients develop a progressive renal impairment following recovery from heat stroke. Kew and colleagues[53] have demonstrated interstitial nephritis in renal biopsies of such patients.

Liver Function. Herman and Sullivan[54] showed a frequent occurrence of jaundice in patients who survived heat stroke after more than 2 days. Increased bilirubin levels (direct and indirect) and marked increases in liver enzymes (aspartate aminotransferase, alanine aminotransferase, gamma glutamyl transpeptidase), indicating hepatocellular damage, together with elevations of serum alkaline phosphatase levels, indicating impairment of the liver's excretory function, are usually found. Following this, impairment of the liver's synthetic function may occur, with decreases in serum albumin and coagulation factors. Pathologic findings in the liver include perisinusoidal edema and a centrilobular necrosis. Desquamation of sinusoidal and lining cells and ballooning and flattening of the microvilli as well as changes in the mitochondria have been described.[53,55]

Central Nervous System Effects. A transient loss of consciousness is common in heat stroke. Other central nervous system (CNS) changes include delirium, hallucinations, status epilepticus, oculogyric crisis, opisthotonos, coma, cerebellar syndromes, and hemiplegia. There may also be decerebrate posturing.[10,24,49]

Pathologic changes documented by Malamud and colleagues[47] consist of edema, patchy congestion, and diffuse petechial hemorrhages. It is the presence of disseminated intravascular coagulation that persists in the unconscious patient which is most worrisome as this often results in cerebral hemorrhage and death.

Hematologic Effects. In 1967, Meikle and Graybill[57] demonstrated fibrinolysis and hemorrhage in a fatal case of heat stroke. Disseminated intravascular coagulation (DIC), a consumption coagulopathy characterized by consumption of fibrinogen factor VIII and factor V, is seen and is usually due to circulating thrombin; thrombocytopenia is usually seen within 24 hours of the onset of heat stroke but nowadays is also seen in patients treated with heparin for their DIC. Laboratory determinations of fibrinogen and fibrin split products, and assays of factors V and VIII will discriminate DIC from fibrinolysis. Clinical manifestations of DIC include petechial hemorrhages and ecchymoses.

Pulmonary Effects. Alveolar hyperventilation and tachypnea are common in heat stroke. Pulmonary edema, usually of an adult respiratory distress syndrome (ARDS) type, occurs especially in those who develop a DIC. In this state, pulmonary artery wedge pressure is low, distinguishing it from cardiogenic pulmonary edema. Such patients have a reduced lung compliance with severe arterial hypoxemia and a low P_{CO_2}. Usually, P_{CO_2} is low, but as ventilation becomes more difficult, P_{CO_2} may rise. If patients are also in circulatory failure, they may develop lactic acidosis. With both respiratory and metabolic acidosis, the prognosis is poor. At postmortem, pulmonary edema and hemorrhages are often noted.[58]

Case Reports. Some characteristic presentations follow which illustrate the conditions of such patients after fun runs, marathons, and football games.

CASE 1

A 17-year-old male athlete ran in a 14-km race when the WBGT was 12°C (54°F) accompanied by a cool breeze and a bright clear sky. He had trained for several months in preparation for the race and was in good health. He was trying for his best time and ran faster than his usual pace. He collapsed after crossing the finish line and subsequently was unable to recall this period of the race. When examined at the sports medicine center located at the finish line, he was deeply unconscious, responding only to painful stimuli. He was sweating freely and had cold skin, generalized pallor, and cyanosis of the lips and ears. Pulse rate was 160 beats/min and blood pressure was 60 mm Hg systolic. Oral temperature was 35.5°C (96°F), but rectal temperature was 42°C (108°F) (Fig. 23–5). He vomited copious amounts of bile-stained fluid and was resuscitated by elevation of the legs, intravenous fluids, and cooling with ice wrapped in towels. He regained consciousness rapidly, although he was still disoriented, and was transferred to a hospital where his recovery continued. He was discharged 8 hours after admission and was well to follow-up.

CASE 2

A 21-year-old woman competed in a 10-km fun run in the autumn in a black woolen track suit when the WBGT was 21°C (70°F). She collapsed near the finish line. Her rectal temperature was 41.5°C (107°F). She was rapidly cooled with ice and fans, and she made an uneventful recovery.

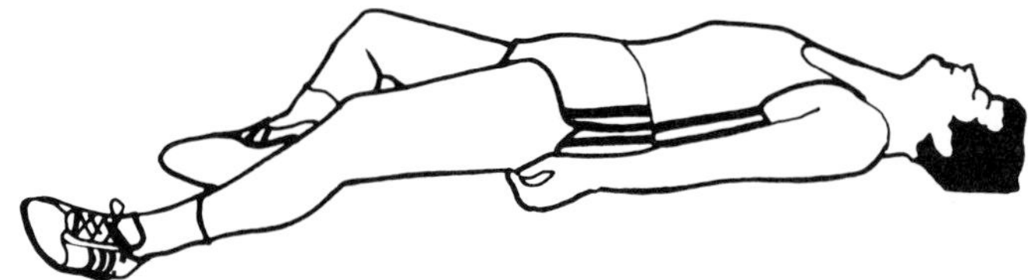

Figure 23–5. The importance of measuring rectal temperature in fun runners who "collapse." Axillary or even oral temperature may be low, especially if the runner has peripheral circulatory collapse; thus, the presence of life-threatening hyperthermia may be overlooked. In one patient, the oral temperature was 35.5°C (96°F), but the rectal temperature was 42°C (108°F).

CASE 3

A 41-year-old man collapsed after 9 km of a 10-km fun run held in the spring in southern Ontario. He was an athlete, but his training had been restricted to early morning and evenings; therefore, he had no opportunity for heat acclimatization. He had previously competed successfully in the Ottawa marathon in 3 hours 17 minutes. This race commenced at 1345 hours (1:45 PM) when the weather conditions were as follows: ambient temperature, 31.6°C (89°F); relative humidity, 80%; and humindex, 40.5°C (105°F).

He reported no premonitory symptoms but at the 9-km mark was seen to increase his speed; shortly thereafter, he veered off the track and collapsed. Bystanders doused him with water and called an ambulance, which took him to hospital. At the time of admission, the man was found to be comatose, unresponsive to painful stimuli, and sweating profusely. Pulse rate was 180 beats/min with regular rhythm, and blood pressure was 140/90. Respiratory rate was 36 breaths/min. Rectal temperature was recorded in the hospital at 40.3°C (105°F). He remained unconscious for 6 hours and required intravenous administration of diazepam to control early signs of convulsions and decerebrate posturing of one arm. Over the ensuing 24 hours, he vomited and became anuric. Investigations on admission revealed mild elevations in levels of blood urea nitrogen (BUN), creatinine, bilirubin, aspartate aminotransferase, creatine phosphokinase, and lactate dehydrogenase. His platelet count fell, and prothrombin and partial thromboplastin times became prolonged. Serum enzyme levels became grossly elevated, as did the BUN and creatinine levels. Diagnosis was made of heat-induced acute renal failure, rhabdomyolysis, disseminated intravascular coagulation, and hepatic necrosis. He was transferred to a renal dialysis center, where he was placed on peritoneal dialysis on alternate days. An elevated serum uric acid level of 20.7 mg/dL (1.23 mmol/L) was recorded 60 hours after admission.

Renal function was slow to recover, and the first indication of a diuretic phase occurred 3 weeks after admission. However, it was 22 weeks before the serum creatinine level returned to normal.

CASE 4

A 29-year-old first-grade Rugby League footballer sustained several hard tackles and was removed from the game in a confused state. Ambient temperature was 23°C with high humidity and no wind. He had a seizure in the dressing room and was transferred to a nearby hospital with a diagnosis of head injury. He remained deeply unconscious and required assisted ventilation. A rectal temperature of 40.8°C was recorded. He subsequently developed acute renal failure, liver failure, and disseminated intravascular coagulation. He commenced hemodialysis and after 10 days regained consciousness. He is still recovering as this chapter goes to press.

In reviewing these presentations, it is important to remember that entrants in an 8- to 12-km fun run who develop heat stroke are in very different circumstances than those we have considered in the past to be particularly predisposed to heat stroke, such as explorers and soldiers in deserts, or pilgrims making their way to Mecca. In these instances, heat exposure is prolonged for days, even weeks, and marked dehydration is universal. In contrast, particularly in the shorter fun runs of less than 10 km, dehydration is unlikely to be particularly significant. In longer races, especially the marathon, dehydration is important. In football games and other contact sports, there is always the dilemma of making a diagnosis in a patient with altered consciousness—could it be head injury or could it be something else (eg, heat stroke)?

Prevention and Management of Exertional Heat Stroke. "I am of the opinion that in healthy subjects the only serious potential risk to life from violent exercise is heat stroke—a danger well exhibited by examples I have seen of alarming collapse and, on one occasion, death. The correct precaution would be to prohibit the race in circumstances in which an occurrence might be expected—a moisture laden atmosphere, a following wind and the early afternoon of a day with a shade temperature of 85°F (29.5°C) or higher."—*Sir Adolphe Abrahams, British Encyclopaedia of Medical Practice, 1950.* This comment is as relevant today as it was 40 years ago. Heat stroke is a medical emergency and the sooner the diagnosis is made and treatment commenced, the better. Treatment must begin immediately *on site.*[1,3,4,59,60] With the advent of mass participation events, such as marathons that attract 20,000 participants and fun runs with 30,000 to 50,000 participants, the potential for large-scale disaster is very real and perhaps should be approached as a disaster exercise.[61–63] However, many organizers of such events fail to take even elementary precautions to prevent and treat possible victims of heat stroke.

In 1971, following the first "City-to-Surf" race, an analysis of the predisposing factors enabled us to suggest improvement in three general areas:

1. Race organization.
2. Medical support.
3. Competitor education.

These recommendations have been refined over the years with further experience.[64] Staging a fun run also requires an enormous amount of logistic and medical support. It is now not acceptable to simply advertise a "fun run for charity" and see who turns up to run. There ideally should be a medical director who is responsible for the coordination of all the preventive and therapeutic aspects related to the fun run. This person should work closely with the race director and be involved in many aspects of the race planning.

Organization of the Race. Races and most endurance sporting events should be organized to avoid the hottest summer months and the hottest part of the day. Unseasonably hot days in the early spring are particularly hazardous as it is unlikely that entrants will be heat acclimatized.

Athlete Education. The education of athletes has increased greatly in recent years, owing largely to the popular scientific articles on running, football, cycling, and rowing, which appear in magazines. Distributing guidelines to athletes at the time of registration (if preregistration occurs) and holding clinics before runs can be valuable. In fun runs, all athletes should be advised of the following:

1. Training and fitness are important for full enjoyment of the run and will also help to prevent heat stroke.

2. Heat acclimatization will also reduce the risk of heat injury in all sports. Train at the time of day at which the race will be held.

3. Fluid consumption before and during the race will also reduce the risk of heat injury, particularly in the longer runs, such as the marathon.

4. Don't run if you are ill. This applies especially to any febrile conditions where temperature control is already impaired and dehydration may be present (eg, gastroenteritis or upper respiratory tract infection).

5. Athletes should know the early symptoms of heat injury. These include headache, nausea, dizziness, ataxia, incoordination, and any gradual impairment of consciousness.

6. Athletes should choose a comfortable pace and not run faster than the maximum pace they have achieved during training.

7. Athletes would be wise to run with a partner, each being responsible for the other's well-being.

Medical Organization and Medical Facilities. Full scale resuscitation and cooling should be available at the race site or at the football stadium. In addition to the routine resuscitation equipment, ice packs and fans for cooling are required. First aid officers should be stationed along the course with the right to stop runners who exhibit signs of impending heat stroke or other abnormalities. One or more ambulances or vans with accompanying medical personnel should follow the competitors at intervals.

In many sporting events, athletes will be cold and will require "space blankets" and warm drinks to prevent hypothermia on cold, wet, and windy days.[1,65] The slower athletes are especially vulnerable when lightly clad and will lose heat faster than their rate of metabolic heat production.

The importance of measurement of core rectal temperature to an accurate diagnosis cannot be overemphasized. In the past, problems have occurred when oral or axillary temperatures were taken and found to be misleading. Also, the cold and clammy skin of more than 80% of heat stroke victims of fun runs suggests that they may not be suffering heat stroke when indeed they are. The initial assessment should include full CNS and cardiovascular measurements, together with the measurement of rectal temperature. The insertion of an intravenous catheter and care of the airway, if appropriate, must also be instituted.

Treatment is better begun on site and since instituting this approach in fun runs, there has been little need for subsequent hospitalization. In an experience extending to several hundreds of thousands of runners, no serious sequelae have resulted when resuscitation and cooling were begun at the race site. This has not been the case in other circumstances.

TABLE 23–3. EFFICACIES OF DIFFERENT BODY COOLING PROCEDURES RELATIVE TO PASSIVE COOLING

	Cooling Rate	
Method of Cooling	***Relative***	***°C·min^{-1}***
Passive	—	0.054
Ice packs on six major arteries	−9	0.049
Body covered with ice packs	+35	0.074
Evaporative cooling	+50	0.081
Evaporative cooling plus six ice packs	+59	0.086
Whole body immersion (25°C)	+39	0.075
Whole body immersion (12°C)	+385	0.262

Cooling and rehydration are the cornerstones of treatment. Whole body immersion in water at 12°C produced the most rapid cooling at 0.262°C/min compared with evaporative cooling (the "Mecca" cooling method) at 0.081°C/min (Table 23–3).

Thus, complications from heat stroke usually are preventable if a diagnosis is made immediately and cooling commenced forthwith. Should complications arise, the patient will require transfer to a critical care unit of a hospital. Here, the management of the unconscious, seizing, ventilated patient in pulmonary edema with DIC, liver failure, dehydration, and acute renal failure is routine. Management of the patient in the intensive care unit is beyond the scope of this discussion.

REFERENCES

1. Sutton J, Coleman MK, Millar AP, et al: The medical problems of mass participation in athletic competition: The "City-to-Surf" race. Med J Aust 2:127, 1972.
2. Richards R, Richards D, Schofield PJ, et al: Reducing the hazards in Sydney's The Sun City-to-Surf runs—1971 to 1979. Med J Aust 2:453, 1979.
3. Richards D, Richards R, Schofield PJ, et al: Management of heat exhaustion in Sydney's The Sun City-to-Surf fun runners. Med J Aust 2:457, 1979.
4. Richards R, Richards D, Schofield PJ, et al: Organization of The Sun City-to-Surf fun run, Sydney, 1979. Med J Aust 2:470, 1979.
5. Sutton JR: 43°C in fun runners! Med J Aust 2:463–464, 1979.
6. Roydhouse N: Personal communication, 1981.
7. Sutton JR: Community participation in long distance athletic events—The London Marathon. *In* Sergeant AJ, Young A: Proceedings of the Conference on Community Health and Fitness. The London Polytechnic Institute, 1982.
8. Sutton JR, Bar-Or O: Thermal illness in fun running. Am Heart J 100:778, 1980.
9. Hughson RL, Green HJ, Houston ME, et al: Heat injuries in Canadian mass participation runs. Can Med Assoc J 122:1141, 1980.
10. Hart LE, Egier BP, Shimizu AG, et al: Exertional heat stroke: The runner's nemesis. Can Med Assoc J 122:1144, 1980.
11. Nicholson RN, Somerville KW: Heatstroke in a "run for fun." Br Med J 1:525, 1976.
12. Roydhouse N, Karn H, Johnson L: "Round the Bays" 17.92 km fun run for 25,000 entrants. N Z J Sports Med 6:4, 1978.
13. Hanson PG, Zimmerman SW: Exertional heatstroke in novice runners. JAMA 242:154, 1979.
14. Noble HB, Bachman D: Medical aspects of distance race planning. Physician Sportsmed 7:78, 1979.
15. England AC III, Fraser DW, Hightower AW, et al: Preventing severe heat injury in runners: Suggestions from the 1979 Peachtree Road Race experience. Ann Intern Med 97:196, 1982.
16. Greene T, Collins V, Laney R: Risks in the heat of battle. Runner's World 12:38, 1977.
17. Braatz JH, Mahurin J, Davies GJ: Heat. Jogger 10:11, 1978.
18. Cockrill M: Heat adaptation. Runner's World 14:74, 1979.
19. Landwer GE, Glover ED: Heat. Runner's World 15:73, 1980.
20. Winslow CEA, Herrington LP, Gagge AP: Physiological reactions of the human body to various atmospheric humidities. Am J Physiol 120:288, 1937.
21. Pugh LGCE, Corbett JC, Johnson RH: Rectal temperature, weight losses and sweat rate in marathon running. J Appl Physiol 23:347, 1967.
22. Weiner JS, Horne GO: A classification of heat illness. Br Med J 1:1533, 1958.
23. Sutton JR, Sauder DN: Fever and abdominal pain following exercise. Med Sci Sports Exerc 21:S103, 1989.
24. Knochel JP, Reed G: Disorders of heat regulation. *In* Kleeman CR, Maxwell MH, Narin RG (eds): Clinical Disorders, Fluid and Electrolyte Metabolism. New York, McGraw-Hill, 1987, pp 1197–1232.
25. Shibolet S, Lancaster MC, Danon Y: Heatstroke: A review. Aviat Space Environ Med 47:280–301, 1976.
26. Malhotra MS, Venkataswamy Y: Heat casualties in the Indian Armed Forces. Indian J Med Res 62:1293–1302, 1974.
27. Talbot JH, Michelsen J: Heat cramps. J Clin Invest 12:533–535, 1933.
28. Talbot JH: Heat cramps. *In* Medicine. Baltimore, Williams & Wilkins, 1935, pp 323–376.
29. Ladell WSS: Heat cramps. Lancet 2:836–839, 1949.
30. Leithead CS, Gunn ER: The aetiology of cane cutter's cramps in British Guiana. *In* Environmental Physiology and Psychology in Arid Conditions. Liege, Belgium, UNESCO, 1964, pp 13–17.

31. Hales JRS: A case supporting the proposal that cardiac filling pressure is the limiting factor in adjusting to heat stress. Yale J Biol Med 59:237–245, 1986.
32. Nadel ER, Mack GW, Nose H, et al: Tolerance to severe heat and exercise: Peripheral vascular responses to body fluid changes. *In* Hales JRS, Richards D (eds): Heat Stress. Amsterdam, Elsevier, 1988, pp 117–131.
33. Rowell LB: Human cardiovascular adjustments to exercise and thermal stress. Physiol Rev 54:75–159, 1974.
34. Hales JRS, Stephens FRN, Fawcett AA, et al: Lowered skin blood flow and erythrocyte sphering in collapsed fun-runners. Lancet 1:1494–1495, 1986.
35. O'Donnell TF: The hemodynamic and metabolic alterations associated with acute heat stress injury in marathon runners. Ann NY Acad Sci 301:262–269, 1977.
36. Hart LE, Sutton JR: Environmental considerations for exercise. Cardiol Clin 5:245–258, 1987.
37. McKechnie JK, Leary WP, Joubert OM: Some electrocardiographic and biochemical changes in marathon runners. S Afr Med J 41:722–725, 1967.
38. Bernheim IT, Cox JN: Cours de chaleur et intoxication amphetamine chez un sportif. Schweiz Med Wochensch 90:322–331, 1960.
39. Hanson PG, Zimmerman SW: Exertional heatstroke in novice runners. JAMA 242:154–157, 1979.
40. Beller GA, Boyd AE: Heatstroke: A report of 13 consecutive cases without mortality despite severe hyperpyrexia and neurologic dysfunction. Milit Med 140:464–467, 1975.
41. Brahams D: Death of a soldier: Accident or neglect? Lancet 1:485, 1988.
42. Costrini AM, Pitt HA, Gustafson AB, et al: Cardiovascular and metabolic manifestations of heat stroke and severe heat exhaustion. Am J Med 66:296–302, 1979.
43. O'Donnell TF, Clowes GH: The circulatory abnormalities of heat stroke. N Engl J Med 287:734–737, 1972.
44. Knochel JP: Dog days and siriasis: How to kill a football player. JAMA 233:513–515, 1975.
45. Savdie E, Sutton JR: Heatstroke in a football player. Med J Aust, in press.
46. Slovis CM, Anderson GF, Solightly DP: Survival in a heatstroke victim with a core temperature in excess of 46.5°C. Ann Emerg Med 11:269–271, 1982.
47. Malamud N, Haymaker W, Custer RP: Heatstroke: A clinico-pathologic study of 125 fatal cases. Milit Surg 99:397–449, 1946.
48. Wilson G: The cardiopathology of heatstroke. JAMA 114:557–567, 1940.
49. Clowes GHA, O'Donnell TF: Heat stroke. N Engl J Med 291:564–567, 1974.
50. Schiff HB, MacSearraigh ET, Kallmeyer JC: Myoglobinuria, rhabdomyolysis and marathon runners. Q J Med 47:463–472, 1978.
51. Schrier RW, Henderson HS, Ticher CC, et al: Nephropathy associated with heat stress and exercise. Ann Intern Med 67:356–376, 1967.
52. Vertel RM, Knochel JP: Acute renal failure due to heat injury: An analysis of ten cases associated with a high incidence of myoglobinuria. Am J Med 43:435–451, 1967.
53. Kew MC, Abrahams C, Seftel HC: Chronic interstitial nephritis as a consequence of heatstroke. Q J Med 39:189–199, 1970.
54. Herman RH, Sullivan BH Jr: Heatstroke and jaundice. Am J Med 27:154–166, 1959.
55. Kew MC, Minick OT, Bahu RM, et al: Ultrastructural changes in the liver in heatstroke. Am J Pathol 90:609–618, 1978.
56. Kew MC, Bersohn I, Seftel HC, et al: Liver damage in heat stroke. Am J Med 49:192–202, 1970.
57. Meikle AW, Graybill JR: Fibrinolysis and hemorrhage in a fatal case of heat stroke. N Engl J Med 276:911–913, 1967.
58. Chao TC: Post-mortem findings of heat stroke. *In* Hales JRS, Richards DAB (eds): Heat Stress. Amsterdam, Elsevier, 1987, pp 297–301.
59. American College of Sports Medicine: Position stand on prevention of thermal injuries during distance running. Med Sci Sports Exerc 16:ix–xiv, 1984.
60. Sutton JR: Heat illness. *In* Strauss RH (ed): Sports Medicine. Philadelphia, WB Saunders, 1984, pp 307–322.
61. Richards CR, Richards D: Prevention of exercise-induced heat stroke. *In* Sutton JR, Brock RM (eds): Sports Medicine for the Mature Athlete. Indianapolis, Benchmark Press, 1986, pp 151–166.
62. Richards CR, Richards D: Providing medical care in fun runs and marathons in Australasia. *In* Sutton JR, Brock RM (eds): Sports Medicine for the Mature Athlete. Indianapolis, Benchmark Press, 1986, pp 167–180.
63. Dobbin SW: Providing medical services for fun runs and marathons in North America. *In* Sutton JR, Brock RM (eds): Sports Medicine for the Mature Athlete. Indianapolis, Benchmark Press, 1986, pp 193–203.
64. Sutton JR, Harrison HC: Health hazards in community jogs and fun runs. Med J Aust 1:193, 1977.
65. Maughan RJ, Light IM, Whiting PH, et al: Hypothermia, hyperkalemia and marathon running. Lancet II:1336, 1982.

24

COLD INJURIES

Bruce C. Paton, MD, FRCP (Ed)

HYPOTHERMIA

Humans, warm-blooded, thin-skinned, hairless bipeds, are ill suited to resist the cold, and it is only through the exertion of their intelligence and ingenuity that they have kept from freezing to death long since. Through the centuries, cold has played a major part in determining the outcome of human events. From Xenophon (and probably from the cavemen) to twentieth-century wars, cold has halted armies, turned victory into defeat, and resulted in thousands of deaths and injuries. In many major disasters at sea, more deaths have been caused by hypothermia than by drowning. When the SS Titanic sank, there were more than enough lifebelts available. However, when the rescuing ship, SS Carpathia, arrived on the scene only 1 hour and 50 minutes after the disaster, 1489 victims were found floating in the calm sea—all dead, and all with their heads above water supported by life belts. There were icebergs nearby and sea temperature must have been very low. Yet the official cause of death of all the victims was listed as drowning.

On a less lethal scale, cold affects our behavior, our clothing, our recreation, our industries, and the design of our homes and public buildings. Outdoor magazines are filled with glossy pictures of well-protected, beautiful, healthy-looking people skiing, climbing, and running in specially designed clothes. Vast industries have been developed to protect us from the cold.

In spite of all this effort, 7450 people died from cold in the United States between 1976 and 1985,[1] and in 1985, 1010 deaths were ascribed to excessive cold.[2] In Great Britain, about 500 people die every winter directly from hypothermia, with another 40,000 deaths from cold-related illnesses.[3] Deaths from cold have been reported from tropical countries. In a multicenter study[4] from the USA, the state contributing the most cases to the study was Florida. On only the very hottest of days does ambient temperature equal body temperature; so, on most days, the human problem is to conserve body heat, not to lose it.

Temperature Control

The body only works efficiently within a very narrow temperature range of 3 to 4°C. We all know that an elevated temperature of a degree and a half makes us feel ill and unable to work at maximum efficiency. Similarly, if core temperature falls below certain levels, the systems of the body cannot accomplish their tasks.

Central, or core, temperature is regulated by a control center in the hypothalamus, which responds both to changes in the temperature of circulating blood and to neurologic impulses from the periphery. Sensors in the internal carotid artery and, possibly, in peripheral veins[5] as well as in the brain provide signals that trigger the regulatory mechanisms. The preservation of normal termperature is a constant balance between heat production, conservation, and loss.

HEAT LOSS

Heat is lost by four routes: radiation, evaporation, conduction, and convection (Fig. 24–1).

Radiation. Heat is transferred by long-wave radiation in proportion to the fourth power difference between the heat of the body and the heat of surrounding objects. Radiation is not affected by air movement, wetness, or other factors, and is greater at night than during the day because dark sky absorbs more heat than the light sky of day. More heat is lost on a clear cloudless night than on a cloudy night. Radiation heat loss is greatest when large areas of bare skin are exposed. Loss is diminished by protective clothing and covering, not because clothes reflect radiation, but because the inner layers are warmed by other means (conduction). The temperature gradient between the skin and the inner layer of clothing is then quite small and radiation loss is proportionately low. Reflective layers, popularized in "survival blankets" and other clothing, have not experimentally been shown to reduce radiation loss greatly. (Their impervious layers may significantly reduce convective heat loss.)

Conduction. Direct contact between the body and a colder object results in the loss of heat until the temperatures are equalized. Reduction of loss by this route can be almost eliminated by good insulation. Thermal conductivity of clothing depends on the material from which it is made and is increased by wetness because thermal conductivity through water is 10 to 25 times as great as through air. Clothes made wet by sweat or soaked with

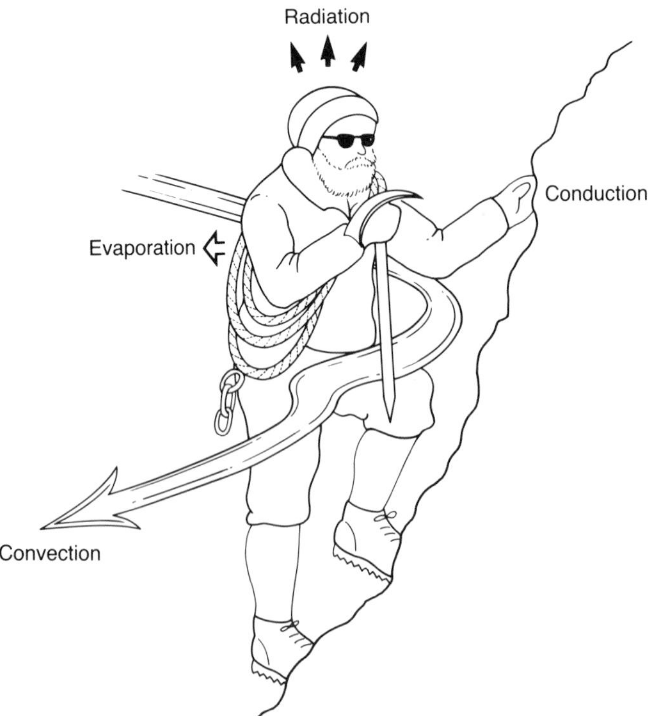

Figure 24–1. The four routes by which heat is lost: radiation, evaporation, conduction, and convection.

water may lose as much as 80% of their insulating capacity. Heat loss through wet clothes is 2 to 5 times as rapid as through dry clothes.

Convection. Convective heat loss is a combination of conduction and convection. In calm air, a microlayer of air next to the skin is warmed by conduction. Wind circulating over the body blows this heated layer away (convection), which then is rewarmed by conduction, only to be blown away again. Convective heat loss depends upon air movement, air viscosity and density, and thermal conductivity.

The wind-chill factor is a measure of the additional heat lost by wind flowing over the body. If ambient temperature remains constant, heat loss varies with the speed of the wind. A strong wind carries a greater wind-chill factor than a weak one because of increased convective heat loss. For instance, if the actual thermometer reading is −4°C and there is a 10-mph wind, heat loss will be equivalent to exposure to −12°C without a wind. The wind-chill table can be used to calculate the potential cooling effect of wind if the ambient temperature and windspeed are known (Table 24–1).

Convection is a major source of heat loss in water; therefore, people who fall into water conserve heat best if they do not thrash around (increasing convection) but remain quiet and assume the smallest possible surface area, the fetal position.[6]

Evaporation. Energy is consumed to convert liquid to gas in proportion to the volume of liquid evaporated and the heat of vaporization of the liquid. The volume evaporated, and therefore, the heat lost, depends on the humidity of the surrounding air. In a hot, humid climate you feel wet but there is little evaporation or cooling from the sweat running down under your shirt. In the dry desert, you may not seem to be sweating, but evaporation is rapid; you stay dry and heat loss is great. The heat lost by evaporation of 1 liter of sweat is 580 kcal.

Sweat is not the only source of evaporative heat loss. As air moves in and out of the respiratory tract, it is warmed and humidified, and dries the tracheal and bronchial mucosa. These processes consume energy. At high altitudes, the combination of cold and dry air requires a great expenditure of energy, with commensurate heat loss, to humidify and warm the inspired air. Water loss at altitude may amount to several liters a day with the consumption of 1500 to 2000 kcals. About 33% of evaporative heat loss is through the respiratory tract and the remainder from the evaporation of sweat. Evaporation accounts for 9% to 25% of total body heat loss.

TABLE 24–1. EFFECTS OF WINDCHILL

Wind Speed (mph)	Actual Thermometer Reading (°C)								
0	+4	−1	−7	−12	−18	−23	−29	−34	−40
	Equivalent Temperature								
10	+2	−4	−9	−15	−21	−26	−32	−37	−43
15	−1	−9	−15	−23	−29	−37	−40	−46	−57
20	−7	−15	−23	−32	−37	−46	−54	−62	−71
25	−9	−18	−26	−34	−43	−51	−60	−68	−76
30	−12	−18	−29	−34	−46	−54	−62	−71	−79
35	−12	−21	−29	−37	−46	−54	−62	−73	−81
40	−12	−21	−29	−37	−48	−57	−65	−73	−81
		Zone A			*Zone B*			*Zone C*	

Zone A Little danger if proper protective clothes are worn
Zone B Exposed skin may freeze in 1 minute
Zone C *Danger:* exposed skin freezes in 30 seconds

HEAT GAIN

Heat is produced by the basal metabolic activities of the body. Most heat is produced in the large central organs—liver, kidneys, and heart. Additional heat is produced by shivering and voluntary exercise.

Shivering is the first metabolic response to a falling temperature and can produce heat equal to five times basal metabolic rate. The production of this energy is not without its price. Oxygen consumption is increased in proportion to the vigor of shivering, and energy reserves may be reduced at the very moment they are needed most. Shivering is initiated by central and peripheral stimuli. Cooling of the skin stimulates shivering; warming of the skin may stop shivering without a change in central temperature. Shivering is inhibited by alcohol, sedative drugs, and hypoglycemia.

Nonshivering thermogenesis, triggered by noradrenalin, which is excreted in response to cold, refers to a specific process in which there is lipolysis of brown fat, a thermogenic fat found in hibernating animals, infants, and to a small extent, adults. Under circumstances of chronic and acute cold, brown fat produces energy not otherwise available. Cold also stimulates more usual metabolic pathways to produce heat (ie, pathways which depend on the nutrition and energy reserves of the body).

Radiation is an important source of heat for the body. We have all experienced the sudden warmth felt when passing from shadow into sunlight. Bright surfaces, such as snow, reflect radiation and the combination of snow and altitude may cause so much heat to be reflected and absorbed that climbers and polar travelers are spared the consumption of a great deal of energy in maintaining body temperature. The color of clothing is important in the absorption of heat: black clothes absorb 80% of radiated heat; khaki, about 60%; and white, only 30%.

Responses to Cold

INVOLUNTARY RESPONSES

When the thermoregulatory center first senses peripheral cold or a falling blood temperature, several involuntary conservative mechanisms are initiated. Vasoconstriction reduces the volume of blood exposed to the cold, and changes the insulative properties of subcutaneous tissue. With vasoconstriction, the skin becomes cooler, the temperature gradient between the skin and the air narrows and, therefore, heat loss is reduced.

Most areas of the body have a capacity for vasoconstriction; some more than others. The fingers, toes, nose, and ears have very reactive beds, but the scalp and face have little or no ability to vasoconstrict and are, therefore, sites of considerable heat loss in cold weather. Lloyd[7] reported the case of a Scottish woman who became unconscious from hypothermia because she had been smuggling frozen chickens under her bonnet and the resultant heat loss caused near-fatal hypothermia.

Shivering (see above) is the major involuntary source of increased heat production augmented by increases in other metabolic pathways.

VOLUNTARY RESPONSES

Passive insulation, whether by subcutaneous fat or clothing, greatly reduces heat loss. The thickness of the natural shell (subcutaneous fat and skin) cannot be changed from moment to moment in humans, although vasoconstriction changes the insulative properties of subcutaneous tissue. Animals can fluff up their fur or feathers. The best humans can do is to don or shed their clothes as comfort demands.

A natural reaction to cold is to exercise; metabolism can be increased tenfold by energetic activity. Under some circumstances, this may be sufficient to rewarm a mildly hypothermic person. However, an exhausted person may not be able to summon the energy necessary to rewarm themselves in the face of increasing heat loss to the environment.

Measurement of Temperature

At a given moment, the temperature in the body may range from 5 to 10°C in the skin to 37°C in the heart. Body temperature is constantly changing. Even within organs, such as the heart, there are temperature gradients between the endocardium and the epicardium. Temperature measurements, therefore, must be interpreted with caution.

Many different thermometers are available. Clinical mercury thermometers do not usually read below 34°C, but special low-reading thermometers are made. In the hospital, electronic probes, which can measure a wide range of temperatures, are the best. This is not only because of the ease of taking the temperature, but also because the probe can be left in the esophagus or rectum for continuous measurements. Battery-driven electronic probes are available, but the efficiency of batteries is reduced by cold and the thermometer must be kept warm if it is to work accurately. Heat-sensitive liquid crystal pads have little application in the field, where skin temperature is likely to be very cold and not close to core temperature.

Core temperature is much more important than peripheral temperature and can be measured at several sites: rectum, esophagus, bladder, eardrum, posterior pharynx. All have advantages and disadvantages. Rectal temperature is commonly taken in hospital but is impractical in the field; a thermometer intruded into a cold stool does not reflect a true temperature. Esophageal temperature if taken at a site that is too high is influenced by the temperature of the ventilating gas in the trachea. If the probe is in the middle third of the esophagus, it lies directly behind the left atrium and the temperature is that of the heart—a valuable reading. Temperatures taken in the external auditory canal may damage the tympanic membrane. The simplest, most accurate site is the bladder, using an indwelling catheter with a built-in temperature probe.[8] If a bladder catheter has to be inserted to collect urine, two purposes are served at the same time.

In the field, the mouth may be the only accessible site. If the oral temperature is greater than 34°C, then it can be assumed that the patient is not severely hypothermic because core temperature is always higher than oral temperature. A hand placed under the clothes on the abdomen or the chest wall may indicate body temperature, and taken in conjunction with other signs, can give a clue as to the severity of the situation.

Definition of Hypothermia

Hypothermia is a generalized physiologic state in which core (central) temperature is below 35°C. It is frequently classified as mild, moderate, severe, and profound, depending upon the core temperature. A simpler classification is "mild" if the temperature is >32°C, and "severe" if the temperature is <32°C.

Etiology

Hypothermia neither is a problem of winter or cold climates, nor is it restricted to certain age groups. The public may think of hypothermia when reading of a skier stranded in a wilderness, and while this situation occurs, it is not the most common one. More hypothermia is found in elderly, urban patients than in young healthy athletes in winter. The

TABLE 24–2. HYPOTHERMIA IN SEVERE INJURY

1. Incidental hypothermia is common: >60%.
2. Severe hypothermia has 75% to 100% mortality.
3. Hypothermia is related to severity of injury.
4. Consider need to warm the severely injured.

elderly are less able to accommodate to cold than the young, and in cool, poorly heated apartments may become hypothermic, especially if they have an accident, such as falling and breaking a hip.

Associated diseases influence both onset and outcome. Endocrine diseases—hypothyroidism, diabetes, hypopituitarism—can set the stage for hypothermia. Myocardial infarction or stroke in elderly persons living by themselves may so reduce metabolism and cardiac output that hypothermia ensues, compounding the underlying problem.

Drugs and alcohol, especially if sufficient to induce somnolence or coma, overcome normal mechanisms for maintaining thermal equilibrium. Those who overdose are frequently cold and a common street method of reviving an overdosed person is to leave them in a tub of cold water—with inevitable results!

Hypothermia may result from any severe accident in which there is a combination of blood loss and shock (Table 24–2). Mortality from trauma is greatly increased by secondary hypothermia.[9]

Exposure of marathon runners to cold can induce severe and occasionally fatal hypothermia,[10] and men have developed frostbitten genitalia while running on cold windy days. The exact incidence of cold injury in marathon runners is not known because rectal temperatures are seldom taken unless the runner is clearly ill. In one survey of injuries in a marathon run in Boston when the ambient temperature was 7 to 10°C, "hypothermia" was listed as the most common complaint, and was manifested by intense shivering and feeling of cold by the runner; rectal temperatures were not taken, but all runners seemed to have only mild hypothermia.

Hypothermia is a danger in all water sports, whether inland or in the ocean—kayaking, canoeing, small boat sailing, windsurfing. The danger is greater if the sport involves repeated wetting. A wet suit is good protection if it is dry, or if the wearer is fully in the water. Protection is less if the wearer is frequently in and out of the water and repetitively cooled by evaporation.

Hypothermia is a danger in all jobs that demand prolonged exposure to severe cold, such as fishing off Alaska and in the North Sea, working in refrigerated plants or trucks, and deep sea diving.[11]

Physiologic Changes

In general, hypothermia is a physiologic decelerator, slowing enzymatic reactions. If there is doubt about the physiologic effects of cold on a reaction, it is safe to assume that it will be reduced in intensity and slowed.

OXYGEN AVAILABILITY

Oxygen consumption is reduced about 7% per degree Celsius, so that it is about 50% at 30°C, 20% at 20°C, and 10% or less at 10°C. Because hypothermia reduces oxygen consumption, it is protective and has been used clinically for this reason. Whereas reduced oxygen consumption is a general rule, some tissues and organs need more oxygen than can be supplied by cold blood and become acidotic, even with the protection of reduced oxygen demand.

The oxyhemoglobin curve moves to the left and upward, and oxygen becomes less able to dissociate from hemoglobin; but, at the same time, the ability of oxygen to dissolve in plasma is increased, providing increased oxygen availability from this source.

CARDIOVASCULAR SYSTEM

On sudden exposure to cold, such as immersion in freezing water, the heart rate and cardiac output increase and blood pressure rises. As cooling continues, heart rate, blood pressure, and cardiac output fall. Myocardial irritability increases, evidenced in part by the sensitivity of the heart to mechanical stimulation, and conduction slows. Atrial fibrillation frequently develops when the temperature is <30°C. When the temperature drops below 28°C, there is an increasing likelihood of ventricular fibrillation.

Ventricular fibrillation has been ascribed to rough handling, endotracheal intubation, and the insertion of central venous and pulmonary artery catheters. In addition, electrolyte imbalances including K^+ and Ca^{2+} may play a part in inducing arrhythmias. Several large studies have failed to show a connection between endotracheal intubation and fibrillation, and intubation should not be avoided for fear of causing fibrillation.

The mode of death in many hypothermic victims, however, is bradycardia progressing to asystole.

The peripheral circulation reacts by vasoconstriction, which may be followed by a phase of vasodilatation. This reaction, on a larger scale, may be why some victims remove their clothes although profoundly hypothermic, are found naked, and immediately become the object of police investigation.

The responses of the elderly are blunted; vasoconstriction may be absent, the perception of cold is not as great as in the young, and shivering frequently does not develop.[12]

RESPIRATORY SYSTEM

Initially with sudden exposure there is frantic hyperventilation, the blowing off of CO_2, and rapid changes in pH, which are sometimes sufficient to induce ventricular fibrillation. Below 32°C, respiratory rate slows and respiration stops somewhere around 25°C; but the response is variable from person to person. As the muscles of the chest wall cool and stiffen, ventilation decreases and becomes increasingly difficult. One of the reasons that people drown rapidly in very cold water is deterioration in ventilatory capacity because of poor respiratory muscle function.

Pneumonia and pulmonary edema are common complications of hypothermia. Edema develops because of intercompartmental fluid shifts, also apparent as peripheral and facial edema. The likelihood of pneumonia is enhanced because cold paralyzes the bronchial cilia.

NERVOUS SYSTEM

Confusion, lethargy, incoordination, and speech difficulties are among the earliest manifestations of hypothermia. As cerebral function becomes impaired, so does neuromuscular function. Muscles become stiff and difficult to move; but, in addition, nerve impulses become slow, the periphery becomes anesthetic, and confusion lapses into unconsciousness. Reflexes disappear, the pupils become dilated and fixed, and patients are sometimes thought to be dead. Electroencephalogram (EEG) "silence" occurs at about 20°C.

The unconscious patient needs special evaluation because unconsciousness may be due to hypothermia, an illness, or injury. If the temperature is >33°C and the patient is unconscious, it is very unlikely that unconsciousness is due solely to hypothermia.

BLOOD

Blood viscosity increases as temperature decreases, impeding capillary flow and increasing cardiac work. The increase in viscosity is due to dehydration, an increase in hematocrit, and physical changes in plasma proteins. Coagulation is slowed but otherwise unchanged. Normality returns with rewarming and rehydration.

KIDNEY

The initial reaction to cold is a diuresis induced by peripheral vasoconstriction and an increase in central blood volume. Diuresis stops after core temperature has dropped more than 2 to 3°C, but may be prolonged or increased by a high blood alcohol level. Renal blood flow decreases in proportion to the fall in cardiac output and is only 50% of normal at 28°C. If exposure is prolonged, dehydration and poor fluid intake increase the chance of renal failure. While the patient is cold, urine output is low. Only after the patient has been rewarmed may renal failure become apparent when there is no urine output in spite of a normal core temperature.

LABORATORY DATA

The overall extent of biochemical and hematologic changes depends on the etiology and duration of hypothermia. Acute immersion hypothermia may produce few biochemical changes; accidental hypothermia protracted over many hours or days, even without associated diseases, may induce severe metabolic disturbances. The need for frequent monitoring of these changes during treatment is paramount.

Alterations in biochemical values may be nonexistent or severe depending on the etiology of the hypothermia and the presence of associated diseases. Owing to a shift of potassium from intra- and extracellular compartments, elevations in K^+ occur when hypothermia has been severe and prolonged. An elevation of the K^+ level is a bad prognostic sign, and a K^+ level >10 mEq/L is an almost certain sign that the patient is beyond resuscitation. Potassium levels may be only moderately elevated on admission, but may rise sharply during rewarming. This is a sign of diffuse ischemic cellular damage, possibly fatal.

Glucose levels may be elevated or decreased. Insulin does not function below 30°C and, therefore, glucose levels are more frequently high than low. Low glucose levels occur in patients with hypothermia secondary to diabetic hypoglycemia, alcohol intoxication, or exhaustion.

Blood urea nitrogen (BUN) and creatinine levels are elevated in severe cases; a persistently high BUN level is a bad prognostic sign.

Serum enzyme (creatine phosphokinase, lactate dehydrogenase, aspartate aminotransferase) levels are elevated if there has been significant cellular damage or associated myocardial infarction.

Adrenal function as measured by cortisol levels is usually normal, but in patients who have been exposed and stressed for a long time, there may be mild adrenal insufficiency.

Clinical Assessment

HISTORY

Obtaining a history from the patient or others is very important, especially in patients discovered unconscious. The critical information to obtain is time and place of discovery;

how the patient was discovered; possible duration of hypothermia; and evidence of medications, drugs, alcohol, or a preexisting disease or injury. Find out what treatment has already been given, if the patient has responded in any way, and if the first aid personnel were able to obtain any history from neighbors or others.

CASE 1

An 85-year-old man was found unconscious behind his trailer home. Rectal temperature was 28°C. Only after relatives appeared at the hospital was it possible to discover when he was last known to be normal, and that he was receiving certain medications. The information helped in deciding that his condition was probably purely accidental without associated factors. He had fallen while feeding his dog. Unable to rise from the icy ground, he had lain outside for 6 hours. Recovery was complete.

SYMPTOMS

The classic story of impending hypothermia is of a young hiker in the summer, dressed only in a T-shirt and jeans, caught in a hail storm without a rain jacket. He starts to shiver, then becomes mildly disoriented and lethargic and wants to lie down and rest until the storm passes. He cannot remember the right direction to camp, and is unusually argumentative over trivial matters. Next his muscular coordination is affected: he cannot do up his buttons, stumbles on the trail, and spills the water bottle he is offered. This is the moment for the group to act to prevent increasing hypothermia and possible unconsciousness.

CASE 2

An 18-year-old boy on an outdoor adventure course became very cold in a rainstorm. The group camped and the boy crawled into his sleeping bag with all his wet clothes on. He was shivering hard. Thirty minutes later, he could not be roused. The group leader was informed. Appropriate measures were taken and he was back to normal in an hour.

The progression of symptoms is seen in Figure 24–2. The rate at which the victim moves from one stage to the next varies, depending on weather, wind, clothing, food and fluid intake, and many other factors.

APPEARANCE

In mild cases, the patient is talking and conscious but shivering, and core temperature is only down 1 to 2°C. Skin color may be normal, or even redder than normal because of vasodilatation. In more severe cases, facial edema is common, the skin is pale, speech is garbled, and movements are clumsy.

In the most severe cases, the patient may appear to be dead, with stiff limbs; ashen gray, cold skin; dilated pupils; impalpable pulses; and no apparent respirations.

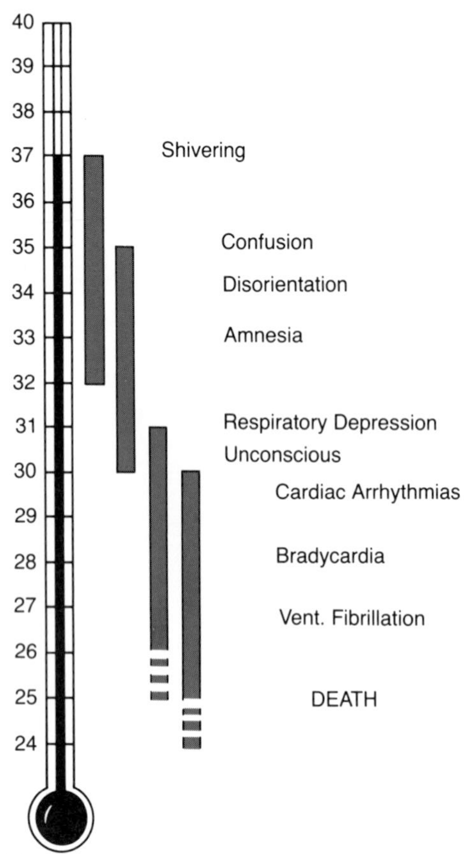

Figure 24–2. Symptoms of hypothermia related to temperature at which they occur.

Management

The first objectives of management are (1) prevention of further heat loss, and (2) rewarming.

AFTERDROP

Core temperature may continue to fall even after rewarming has started. There are two explanations for this phenomenon. First, conductive dissipation of heat equalizes the temperature between the cold extremities and the warmer core. Second, venous blood cooled by its passage through the cold periphery cools the core.

There is evidence that rapid external and airway rewarming can either abort or shorten the afterdrop. The most important practical matter is to realize that afterdrop is an important reality and that it can be detected by frequent temperature monitoring at multiple sites.

IN THE FIELD

The prime task in the field is to protect the victim from the environment and to prevent further heat loss (Table 24–3). The management of hypothermia in the field is necessarily different from that in the hospital. An appropriate plan helps in the organization of help and the care of the patient. Remove wet clothes, pitch a tent or shelter for protection from wind, insulate the person from the cold ground (it is of little use to pile blankets on

TABLE 24–3. MANAGEMENT OF HYPOTHERMIA IN THE FIELD

Assessment
- Victim
  - Conscious or unconscious?
  - General condition
  - Temperature
  - Shivering: coordination
  - Other injuries
- Party
  - Number
  - Strength
  - Experience
- Circumstances
  - Communications
  - Time
  - Weather
  - Supplies
  - Transportation
  - Distance
  - Protection

Plan
- Help
  - Source
  - How to get
- Use of group
  - Skills
  - Strength
- Disposition of victim
  - Evacuate?
  - Warm?
- What to do until help/transportation arrives

Treatment
- Shelter
- Insulation: clothes
- Food, drink
- Rewarming
- Treat other injuries
- Keep records of progress

top of the victim if he or she is still lying directly on the earth), build a fire, make a hot drink, and give the person food. Some measures will be more effective than others, but if the four routes of heat loss are clearly remembered, rational steps can be taken to block the loss of heat.

Rewarming in the field is difficult, often impossible. Some techniques are available (see below, Rewarming Techniques), but most of them require special equipment. In cases of moderate or severe hypothermia, the patient will receive greater benefit from being transported as quickly as possible to a hospital than from being rewarmed or resuscitated under less than ideal circumstances.

IN HOSPITAL

Mild Hypothermia. If the patient is conscious and core temperature is >32°C, management should be conservative and concerned with confirming the temperature, and watching the vital signs and the state of consciousness. Laboratory tests are unnecessary unless otherwise indicated. Radiographs should only be taken to demonstrate known or suspected injuries. The patient should be kept under observation until the temperature is normal and then can usually be discharged.

Severe Hypothermia. Patients with a core temperature <32°C, and especially <30°C, must be admitted to an intensive care unit and managed as though they have a serious illness with a potential for dying. Monitor temperature, continuously, by an indwelling bladder catheter temperature probe; ECG; fluid intake and urine output; blood gases and acid-base status; standard 22 test biochemical survey; complete blood count; coagulation factors including prothrombin time (PT), partial thromboplastin time (PTT), platelets, and fibrinogen; and drug screen, if indicated.

Insert a large-bore central venous line, an arterial line, and possibly a pulmonary artery catheter, for complete monitoring of pressures and arterial gases. A pulmonary artery catheter permits the measurement of cardiac output, which may be very valuable in the most severe cases. A bladder catheter is needed to measure urine output.

A chest radiograph is required because of the high incidence of pneumonia and pulmonary edema. If necessary, intubate and ventilate the patient. The risk of inducing ventricular fibrillation is small and far outweighed by the benefit of ventilation (Fig. 24–3).

Rewarming Techniques

PRINCIPLES

The technique chosen must be suitable to the severity of the problem and sufficient to warm the patient without doing harm. A noninvasive method is better than an invasive method, but if an invasive method is indicated it must be used. Slow rewarming is best for mild and moderate cases. If the heart has stopped, the most efficient, rapid, controlled methods must be used. Access to the patient should be maintained not only by intravenous lines, but also so that cardiac resuscitation can be started. A warm tub is an efficient means of rewarming, but makes access difficult and defibrillation impossible without taking the patient out of the tub.

METHODS

Passive. The patient is removed from the cold environment, dried and put into a warm place, fed warm food and drink, and allowed to rewarm spontaneously. This method is suitable for all mild cases.

Active, External. These methods of rewarming include water baths, warm blankets, radiant heaters, water-filled heating blankets, and hot-water bottles. The heat obtainable by various methods varies from about 17 kcal/L from warm IV fluids to more than 1000 kcal/hr from immersion in a hot bath. A hot water bath is the most efficient noninvasive method of rewarming. Water temperature should not exceed 45°C. These methods are suitable for most moderately and for some severely hypothermic patients. Care should be taken in applying heat directly to the skin, because cold skin is easily burned.

Active, Internal. These methods include warm humidified air or oxygen; warmed intravenous fluids; peritoneal dialysis; lavage of the pleural cavity, stomach, bladder, or mediastinum; and partial or complete extracorporeal circulation.

Warm Humidified Air/Oxygen. The inhalation of warm humidified air or oxygen diminishes heat loss and rewarms the body to about 0.5 to 1.5°C per hour. This technique is the simplest available for internal rewarming; it can be started rapidly and should be used in all patients. It is essential that the gas be 100% humidified so that energy is not expended in humidification.

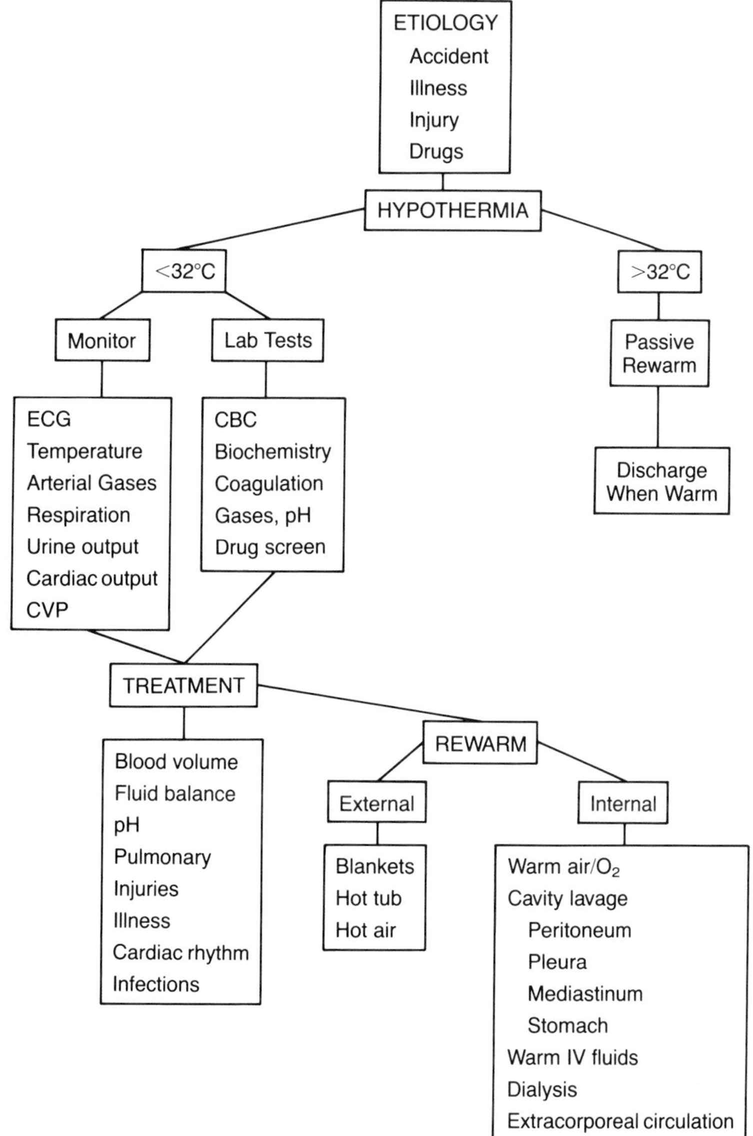

Figure 24–3. Algorithm for the management of hypothermia in the hospital.

If air inhaled at 17°C is warmed to 37°C and humidified, the loss of heat is 13 to 15 kcal/hr. In a hypothermic patient with a core temperature of 30°C, the loss may be 17 to 20 kcal/hr—about 30% to 50% of heat production at that temperature. Inhalation of fully humidified air/oxygen at 45°C converts the energy balance from negative to positive with a small gain of 2 to 23 kcal/hr.[7]

There are several portable field systems for warming air or oxygen. In the hospital, standard anesthesia humidifiers can be used if the patient is mask breathing. Administration is easier and more efficient if the patient is intubated.

Warmed IV Fluids. It is not possible to rewarm a patient with the volumes that can be infused, but all IV fluids and blood should be passed through a warmer to prevent additional heat loss. Severely injured patients may already be hypothermic before admission, and giving them cold bank blood makes the hypothermia worse. A single channel, countercurrent blood warmer is the only type efficient enough to meet the needs of flow and heat-exchange under these circumstances.[13]

Body Cavity Lavage. The peritoneum, pleural cavity, bladder, stomach, and mediastinum all present surfaces of varying sizes which can be used as heat-exchangers.

Peritoneal Dialysis. Standard peritoneal dialysis catheters are inserted into the peritoneal cavity in both lower quadrants and warmed physiologic dialysis fluid at 42 to 44°C is infused and allowed to flow out under gravity. A cycle of infusion and drainage should take about 15 min. This is an effective method. Although invasive, it does not require specialized technique beyond that available in many small hospitals. It is suitable for the treatment of moderate and severe hypothermia and, when necessary, can simultaneously remove intoxicating drugs. Hemodialysis has also been used for warming and drug removal.

Lavage of the Pleura, Mediastinum, Stomach, Bladder, or Bowel. Lavage of the pleura requires insertion of one or two chest tubes. The surface area is not large and warming is slow. The mediastinum can be used if the chest has to be opened for other reasons. Lavage of the stomach should only be done with a closed irrigation system to prevent excessive infusion of fluids. The bladder is too small to be worth irrigating. Warm enemas have been used. No results are available to assess the usefulness of this method.

Extracorporeal Circulation. Partial and total extracorporeal circulation have been used effectively and may be the only techniques that will retrieve a patient with profound hypothermia and cardiac arrest. This method can only be used in a center with facilities for cardiac surgery. The possible need to use the method should be considered in deciding where to send a patient. Newer methods for the percutaneous insertion of perfusion catheters may make this technique available in the future.

Control of pH

Acidosis occurs in most hypothermic patients and, therefore, the correct control of pH and acid-base balance is important. For many years, the method used was to "correct" the pH measured to the pH at the temperature of the body, and attempt to keep the corrected pH at 7.40 and the Pco_2 at 40 mm Hg.

There are, theoretically, three ways to control pH: (1) keep corrected pH at 7.40; (2) keep Pco_2 at 40 mm Hg; and (3) keep CO_2 content constant. The last method is the basis of the "ectothermic" principle (Fig. 24–4).

It is now recognized that the most physiologic method is to use the ectothermic principle: read the pH at 37°C and keep the uncorrected pH at 7.40 and the Pco_2 at 40 mm Hg. This technique maintains changes in pH parallel with the changes in pH of neutral water.[14]

Fluid Replacement

The need for fluid replacement should be judged by the usual criteria. Because central blood volume is contracted and vasodilatation will occur with rewarming, a boosting volume of up to 500 mL physiologic crystalloid solution should be given before rewarming is started. The need for additional volume may be determined by the changes in filling pressures, and the need for electrolyte modification depends on the results of biochemical tests.

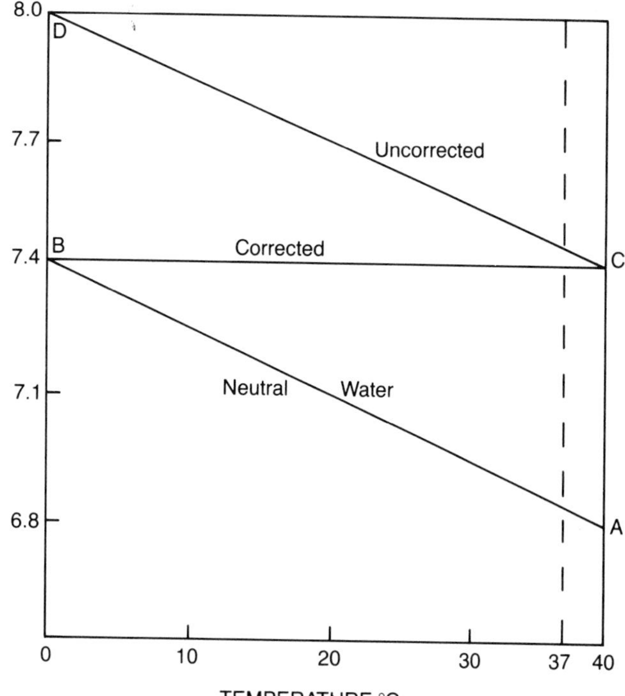

Figure 24–4. The pH increases with decreasing temperature. The pH of neutral water (A–B) and the "uncorrected" pH of blood (C–D) run parallel courses. The "corrected" pH of blood maintains pH at 7.4 (C–B).

Use of Medications

Medications lose effectiveness and are slowly metabolized in cold patients because their actions are temperature-dependent.

ANTIARRHYTHMICS

Most arrhythmias, with the exception of ventricular fibrillation, revert to normal sinus rhythm when the patient rewarms. Bretylium tosylate is useful in refractory ventricular arrhythmias, but the best way to restore normal rhythm is to raise core temperature above 30°C as quickly as possible. Lidocaine can be tried. Neither digitalis nor the calcium-channel blockers are effective during hypothermia.

Resuscitation

If the patient shows any signs of life—breathing or movement—there is obviously no need to start cardiopulmonary resuscitation (CPR). The difficult decision comes when there is no sign of life, but the means are not present to detect and monitor cardiac action. The best response is to start CPR, recognizing that there may be a very slow heart beat which could be converted into ventricular fibrillation by the stimulus. The chest wall may be very stiff and effective compression may be difficult. Because the patient is cold, minimal blood flow may be sufficient to provide cerebral protection. Once started, CPR must be maintained until a definitive diagnosis of life or death can be made.

In the field, the decision to start CPR depends on many factors, such as time, place, weather, and distance to help, which do not apply in an urban setting.

Paramedics should be trained not to waste time trying to insert IVs and endotracheal tubes in very cold, apparently dead victims if the hospital is only a short distance away. The best management is to get the victim to the emergency room as quickly as possible.

Prevention

CLOTHING

The insulating ability of clothing is measured in units of Clo; one Clo is roughly the insulation afforded by a business suit. The basis of clothing insulation is to trap warm air between layers. If several layers of clothing, all trapping warm air, are surrounded by a windproof outer coat to prevent convective loss, heat can be well conserved. The insulating ability of down is greater than that of synthetics. However, if down becomes wet, it loses much of its insulating ability. In a dry but cold climate, down is unsurpassed. During a Biomedical Antarctic Expedition, experiments were done to test the loss of heat from heavily down-clothed subjects. When the temperature on the outer layer of clothing was −16.15°C, the temperature in the middle layers was 4.65°C, skin temperature was 31°C, and rectal temperature was 36.8°C.[15]

The torso should be kept warm with maximum insulation, but less insulation is needed towards the periphery. If hands and feet are insulated more than the trunk, the trunk may cool partly because of a warm, vasodilated periphery. If the trunk is kept warm, reflex vasodilatation of the periphery warms the hands and feet. Conductive heat loss through the feet is great if there is inadequate insulation in shoes or boots, especially the soles. Well-insulated, felt-lined boots can reduce heat loss by 60%. (It should be noted that a wet felt liner which freezes can cause disastrous frostbite.) A wool liner inside a windproof mitten keeps hands warmer than a pair of gloves.

Insulation should be correlated with the level of activity. Smolander and colleagues[16] measured body temperature, oxygen consumption, sweating, and heart rate in a 48-year-old man taking part in a 90-km ski race. Clothing insulation was 1 Clo. Sweat loss was 4000 mL; air temperature, −7 to −15°C; skin temperature, 21 to 24°C; and rectal temperature, 37.5 to 38°C. The man was comfortable while the exercise level was maintained. The danger would have come had he stopped; cooling then would have been rapid.

Special Problems

IMMERSION HYPOTHERMIA

There are about 140,000 drowning deaths per year, worldwide; in 1987, there were 5300 drowning deaths in the United States.[2] The number of victims who also became hypothermic is not known; but it can be assumed that many unprepared victims became cold, adding both to morbidity and mortality.

There are significant differences between "dry land" and immersion hypothermia. In most cases, immersion is sudden and cooling is rapid after the victim is thrown or falls into cold water. The duration of exposure is frequently quite short.

Prolonged exposure in very cold water is usually fatal unless the victim is very well protected by an insulated dry suit. The perfect suit does not exist. It must have watertight seals at the neck, ankles, and wrists, but they should not restrict venous return or chafe. A face mask is needed in rough water. The suits should not be hard to don in a hurry and they should not have protruding straps, which could catch on an escape hatch.

Hayward and Eckerson[17] calculated that in water at 0°C, 50% of people dressed in thin clothing will reach a core temperature of 30°C in 60 to 90 min. On the other hand, a well-protected person could last 24 hours in water of the same temperature.

Occasionally, a person will survive much longer than anticipated. In 1984, an Icelandic fisherman swam for 5 to 6 hours in water at 5 to 6°C dressed only in a shirt, sweater, and jeans. He remained conscious throughout. When he made his first landfall, the coast was too rough to climb, and he reentered the water and swam another half-mile before landing. He was very thirsty and drank from a water tub for sheep. When he was first examined, no pulse could be found.[18] Later testing under controlled conditions confirmed this individual's unique ability to maintain his body temperature under frigid conditions.[19]

Body habitus is important in determining the ability to withstand cold. This is one of the few situations in which fat is better than thin. Even if heavy clothing is worn, the thickness of subcutaneous fat affects heat loss.[20] Computer calculations indicate that with good insulation in water at 5°C, it would take 14 hours for core temperature to drop to 34°C; with poor insulation, that temperature would be reached in only 1 hour.

There have been many remarkable incidents in which young children have been totally submerged for up to 40 min in ice-water and have made a complete recovery.[21] The protective mechanisms involved are not clear but appear to be rapid cooling combined with a modified "diving reflex" response. The diving reflex is present in seals and other diving mammals and is triggered by stimulation of the trigeminal nerve. There is intense vasoconstriction, which concentrates blood volume centrally, and, at the same time, marked bradycardia, which reduces cardiac output and prevents an excessive rise in blood pressure. Vasoconstriction might be expected to slow heat loss, but heat loss seems to be accelerated in those children who survive, which would be a better explanation for the protection they receive than a diminution in the rate of heat loss. The best explanation for these remarkable cases seems to be that they suffered from acute, rapid submersion hypothermia.[22]

The variables that affect heat loss in water include (1) water temperature, (2) percent body fat, (3) state of the water (heat loss is greater in rough than in calm water), (4) type of protective clothing, (5) behavior (it is better to keep still than to attempt to swim to shore), and (6) the extent of body exposed (it is better to be out of the water on an upturned boat, even if there is wind, rather than be fully immersed in water).

Some factors are beyond the control of the victim, but others can be controlled. If time permits, and frequently it does not, as many clothes as possible should be donned, as well as a life jacket (personal flotation device, PFD).

During a 20-year period, there were 595 major accidents involving air crews in the Canadian Forces, of which 37 were water entry. In 92% of the accidents, there was less than 1-minute warning of impending water entry, and in 78%, there was no warning.[23] In air accidents, therefore, the chances of being able to don special clothing after there is awareness of the impending crash are nil. The clothing must already be on.

A PFD should keep the persons as high out of the water as possible to minimize immersion of the trunk in water and to keep the mouth and face out of the water. After entering the water, the victim should stay still, adopt a fetal position to reduce the body surface area, and hold on to other people. If victims can stay close together, hugging each other, heat loss may be reduced, and they can also afford each other some protection from waves and wind.

The U.S. Coast Guard policy for the management of victims of sea accidents is rescue, examine, stabilize, and transport. The principal objectives in immediate handling are (1) prevent cardiac arrest, and (2) prevent further cooling.

Water exerts a hydrostatic squeeze on the swimmer, which, in turn, affects venous return. When a victim is removed from the water, this pressure is removed, and the resulting fall in venous pressure may be sufficient to drop the blood pressure. After rescue, the victim should be kept horizontal to increase venous return. Prolonged immersion causes dehydration, further reducing blood volume and venous return. A cold, exhausted victim pulled rapidly from the water may immediately develop hypovolemic shock, and care should, therefore, be taken in handling such people.

Immediate activity of victims should be limited after they are pulled from the water, because exercise increases blood flow and may accelerate temperature afterdrop. Because "afterdrop" is a definite threat, temperature must be measured frequently. The victim's wet clothes should be removed, and he or she should be wrapped in warm, dry blankets or in a special rescue bag. Protection from the elements is essential and may be difficult if the rescuing boat does not have a sheltered cabin. If rescue is by helicopter, continued cooling may be difficult to avoid unless the patient is enclosed in a protective wind- and waterproof bag.

Respiratory heat loss continues after rescue, and the administration of warmed air or oxygen may prevent further heat loss, even if it does not add greatly to heat gain. If exposure has been prolonged, give IV fluids, 300 to 500 mL, before rewarming.

The principles of triage and the management of trauma are the same after immersion accidents as for dry land accidents, although it has been said that the "thinnest, quietest, and youngest" should be rewarmed first, because they will most likely also be the coldest.

DIVING

Deep underwater diving is becoming a worldwide activity for exploration, industrial development, and pleasure. In the North Sea, 11% of diving deaths have been due to cold.[24] Not all deaths occur in cold waters, and death from hypothermia in scuba divers is not unknown in California.

One hundred meters below the surface of the sea, the temperature is 4°C all over the world, except in arctic regions, where it is −2°C. Protective clothing is essential at that depth.

Heat loss increases in proportion to the depth of the dive, for several reasons. Pressure increases the thermal transport capacity of gases and decreases the thermal protection of neoprene wet suits. Respiratory heat loss increases, and may exceed metabolic heat production; heat loss is further accentuated if helium is used in the gas mixture because it has much greater capacity to transport heat than air. To counteract these factors for diving at extreme depths, suits through which warm water circulates are sometimes necessary. If helium is used, it has to be heated. Elaborate methods have been devised to conserve heat in diving bells which become lost. Rescue services need about 24 hours to find and retrieve a bell, but in order for the occupants to remain warm that long, it is necessary for them to remain in high-insulation sleeping bags, to breath through CO_2 scrubbers which retain heat from the soda lime, and even to use the heat from their urine.[25]

MOUNTAINS

Accidental hypothermia is not restricted to the great mountain ranges of the world, although the combination of extreme altitude, cold, and the exertion needed for climbing is an ideal setup for the development of hypothermia. Heat loss is high, the energy requirements to keep warm are great, appetite is diminished, and caloric and fluid intake are less than optimal. Discomfort from the cold is an accepted part of climbing, but the relative infrequency of clinical hypothermia, in the absence of an accident, is due to excellent equipment, experience, and care.

Hypothermia is, however, not uncommon under less rigorous conditions and is frequently the result of a combination of exhaustion, poor clothing, unexpected changes in the weather, inexperience, and lack of foresight. A recent example, which contained many of these factors, was the tragedy on Mount Hood in 1986, which resulted in the deaths of nine people, most of them schoolchildren.[26] Unfortunately, many similar examples have been published. In Colorado, the search-and-rescue groups report more evacuations for hypothermia in summer than in winter. All these examples emphasize the need for education of climbers and hikers about the dangers, and the need for adequate preparations for even an apparently benign outing.

SKIING

Hypothermia in downhill skiers at established ski areas is almost always due to improper clothing, especially skiing in cotton denim jeans. As soon as these garments become wet, heat loss by evaporation is rapid. The National Ski Patrol reports that the injury rate among cross-country skiers is about 0.5 per 1000 skier days, of which about 20% are due to cold. In pre-Olympic trials in 1979 at Lake Placid, New York, there were 76 cases of mild frostbite in skiers, most of whom were also hypothermic. Thin competition clothing and very cold weather contributed to the high incidence.[27]

The choice of suitable clothing and common sense will prevent most hypothermia from developing. An occasional well-protected skier may become marooned in backcountry because of weather, equipment failure, or accident; but even under these circumstances, good preparation and experience will avert trouble.

HYPOTHERMIA IN THE HOSPITAL

Iatrogenic hypothermia occurs in the hospital during prolonged operations as a result of anesthesia and the exposure of large raw surfaces to the cool environment of the operating room, during the transfusion of large volumes of cold bank blood, and in newborn premature infants. The maintenance of normothermia is important for the control of pH and cardiovascular stability, reduces postoperative oxygen consumption, and ensures an appropriate metabolic response to surgery.[28]

HYPOTHERMIA IN THE ELDERLY

The elderly are particularly susceptible to hypothermia because of both physiologic and social conditions. Their responses to cold are neither as brisk nor as well organized as those in the young: vasoconstriction may not develop, so heat is not conserved; cardiac output does not respond to metabolic needs; the sensing of changes in ambient temperature may be blunted so that a falling room temperature may not be recognized; and, as many elderly live by themselves, they may become ill or have an accident and remain without help for several days during which they become hypothermic.[29]

Results and Prognosis

Mortality varies greatly, depending on the circumstances; the etiology, duration, and severity of hypothermia; and the general condition of the patient when discovered and when treatment starts. Mortality increases with age according to some statistics, but not according to others. National statistics in the United States indicate a death rate from 0.021 per 100,000 for ages 15 to 24 to 1.067 per 100,000 for ages 75 to 84. In all age groups, the highest mortality was in nonwhite males.[30] In a 13-center retrospective study of accidental hypothermia, Danzl and associates[4] did not find that age was a significant prognostic factor.

Mortality rates from numerous studies have varied between 15% and 90%, depending on treatment and other factors. It is difficult to come to firm conclusions from published

TABLE 24–4. RESULTS OF TREATMENT OF HYPOTHERMIA

Method of Warming	Total Number of Patients	Survived	
		No.	%
Active, external	202	131	65
Active core	162	129	80
Peritoneal dialysis	26	20	77
Cardiopulmonary bypass	70	35	50

studies and be able to give definite mortality statistics. In general, the mortality for mild hypothermia should be low. If core temperature is <30°C, mortality increases; if there has been cardiac arrest, mortality is high.

Bad prognostic factors include (1) the need for preadmission resuscitation, (2) high BUN and serum K^+ levels with evidence of renal failure, (3) the need for endotracheal intubation, and (4) evidence of disseminated intravascular coagulation (DIC). Data collected from the literature concerning the results of treatment with various methods are shown in Table 24–4.

Although preadmission CPR is a bad prognostic sign, over 60 patients have been reported[31] who have survived CPR during hypothermia, with the duration of CPR varying between 1 and 240 min.[24]

There are numerous complications (some only apparent at autopsy) associated with

TABLE 24–5. COMPLICATIONS OF HYPOTHERMIA

Cardiovascular
- Hypovolemic shock
- Atrial arrhythmias
- Ventricular fibrillation
- Thrombosis: myocardial infarction

Respiratory
- Pneumonia
- Pulmonary edema
- Intrapulmonary hemorrhage

Gastrointestinal
- Gastric hemorrhage
- Pancreatitis

Neurologic
- Cerebral edema
- Seizures

Hematologic
- Disseminated intravascular coagulation
- Depression of bone marrow

Renal
- Acute renal necrosis
- Hematuria
- Increased potassium excretion

Miscellaneous
- Rhabdomyolysis
- Increased epinephrine secretion
- Adrenal insufficiency
- Peripheral edema

hypothermia, all of which should be kept in mind when dealing with a severe case (Table 24–5). In most mild cases, there are no complications specifically related to the lowering of temperature.

Hypothermia as an incidental complication of trauma increases the risk of death (see Table 24–2).

FROSTBITE

Hypothermia is frequently a generalized injury unassociated with frostbite, and frostbite may be an isolated injury without hypothermia: but whenever one occurs, the other should be regarded as a possibility.

The greatest number of frostbite cases has occurred in military campaigns. During the Russian campaign in World War II, it was reported that there were 10,000 cases in one night. Frostbite is not uncommon in civilian practice and usually occurs in the unprepared or the homeless. Severe frostbite is also a constant threat to high-altitude climbers. The combination of cold, dehydration, and hypoxia seems to increase the possibility of its occurrence.

Predisposing Factors

The essential requirement for the development of frostbite is that tissue temperature be reduced to −2 to −3°C. This requirement can only be met if ambient temperature is sufficiently cold, often with accentuation of heat loss by contact with moisture or metal, severe windchill, altitude and hypoxia, dehydration and poor caloric intake, inadequate insulation from clothing, or lost clothing.

Pathogenesis

There are three theories of the pathogenesis of frostbite: (1) tissue freezing (direct damage), (2) vascular injury (hypoxia and ischemia), and (3) rewarming injury (action of vasoactive substances). They are not mutually exclusive and all may play a part in any given case.

Ice crystals form in the intercellular free water, resulting in alterations in the osmotic environment of the cells, which become dehydrated and damaged. The ice crystals may damage cells directly, but these changes are reversible during rewarming without leaving significant damage.

Arterial spasm is the first vascular reaction to cold, followed by a brief period of vasodilatation. As cooling proceeds, there is slowing of capillary flow, increased viscosity, sludging and aggregation of cells, and, finally, thrombosis.

Experimental evidence[31] has shown that if frozen skin on a rabbit's ear is transplanted to a healthy ear, and healthy skin is simultaneously transplanted to the frozen ear, the frozen skin placed on a healthy ear survives, while the healthy skin on a frozen ear becomes necrotic (Fig. 24–5). The interpretation of these results was that freezing so damaged the vascular bed that even healthy skin could not survive if placed on a frozen area.

Clinical experience has confirmed the vascular aspects of frostbite. Pathologic specimens, measurements of blood flow, and plethysmography confirm the reduction in blood flow. In spite of the cold, catabolic activity continues until tissue temperature is −10°C to −25°C. During rewarming, there may be a discrepancy between the increasing oxygen

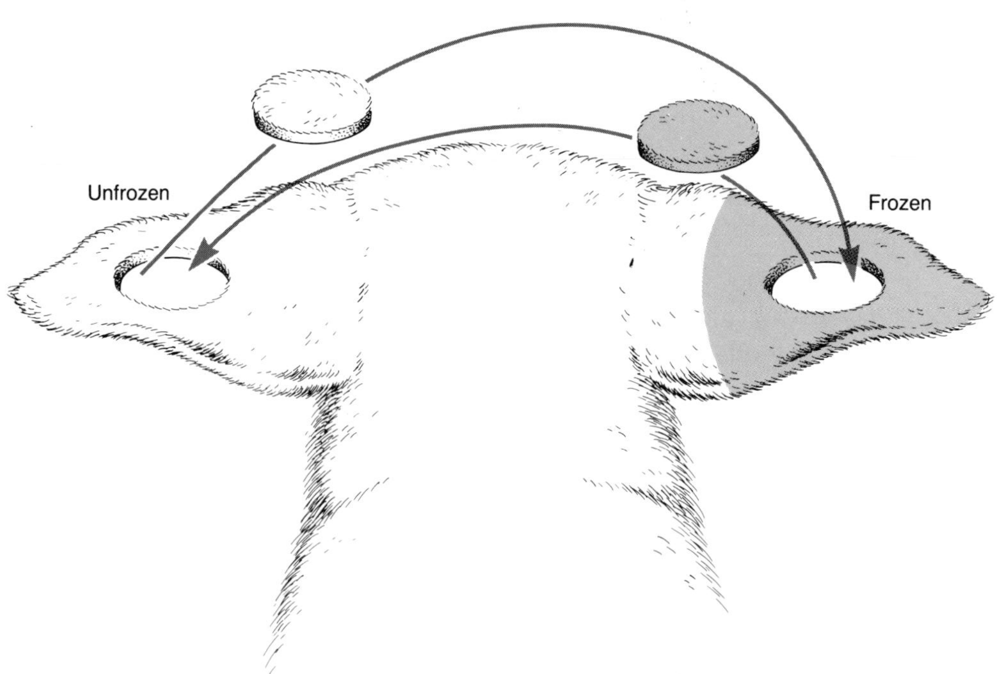

Figure 24–5. Crossover transplantation of frostbitten and healthy skin between rabbit ears. At first believed to demonstrate the vascular basis for necrosis, it is now thought that the results may have been due to the presence of toxic byproducts of reperfusion.

needs of the warming tissue and the availability of oxygen from cold blood. Ischemic injury could then occur during rewarming and not during cooling.

During the past decade, there has been an increasing accumulation of data on the importance of reperfusion injury in bowel necrosis, myocardial infarction, and other circumstances in which an ischemic area is revascularized.[32] Frostbite appears, in part, to be a postischemic reperfusion injury.

The biochemical markers of reperfusion injury are the accumulation of superoxide radicals and end products of the arachidonic acid cascade. Cell phospholipid breaks down into arachidonic acid and the process continues with the final release of prostacyclin, thromboxane, and leucotrienes. Superoxide is produced when oxygen becomes available during reperfusion. These end products contain powerful vasoconstrictors, vasodilators, and compounds that increase vascular permeability and attract leucocytes. Thromboxane A_2, for instance, constricts vessels and aggregates platelets.

The work on transplantation of rabbit ear skin may now be open to a different interpretation. It is possible that the frozen skin was placed in an area without vasoactive enzymes and survived, whereas the normal skin was placed in an area saturated with toxic by-products and became necrotic.

All the enzymes and radicals mentioned above have been identified in blister fluid from both experimental and clinical frostbite.[33,34] The pathogenesis of frostbite may not be postulated to consist of a series of events. During cooling and freezing, the vascular endothelium and smooth muscle is damaged. While the tissue is cold, there is little metabolic activity. As rewarming starts and oxygen becomes available, superoxide radicals are produced; chemotaxis attracts white cells, which produce leucotrienes; thromboxane and prostacyclins induce thrombosis and vasoconstriction, which potentiates ischemia. The part becomes swollen, vessels thrombose, tissue pressure increases, ischemia worsens, and a recurring cycle of damage starts.[35]

Clinical Features

Frostbite may be classified in a manner similar to burns (Fig. 24–6), but the simplest classification is "superficial" or "deep." Superficial frostbite involves only skin; deep frostbite involves all tissues beneath skin (Figs. 24–7 and 24–8). Superficial damage is generally mild and does not leave residual defects. Deep injury may result in everything from minor skin loss to limb loss.

"Frostnip" occurs on the nose, cheeks, or ears and appears as white, anesthetic patches, which disappear quickly with rewarming. There may be minor swelling with blistering, but there is no residual injury.

Moderate-to-severe frostbite causes the part to be white or mottled, anesthetic, and firm, even rock hard. It may not be possible for the patient to move the fingers or toes, but digits may be movable by unfrozen muscles originating higher up the limb although the digits themselves are seriously damaged. Blisters appear within a few hours. Damage is usually superficial if the blister fluid is clear. If the fluid is bloody, damage is almost always deep and severe.

The first symptoms are variable and may not be recognized as the start of frostbite. If toes become numb, is that the start of frostbite, or just cold feet? Frostbite will not occur until tissue temperature is below O°C and this temperature takes time to be reached. Generally, feet should not be allowed to stay numb for longer than an hour before an attempt is made to warm them.[36]

During the first few hours and days, the part swells. In severe frostbite, as the swelling

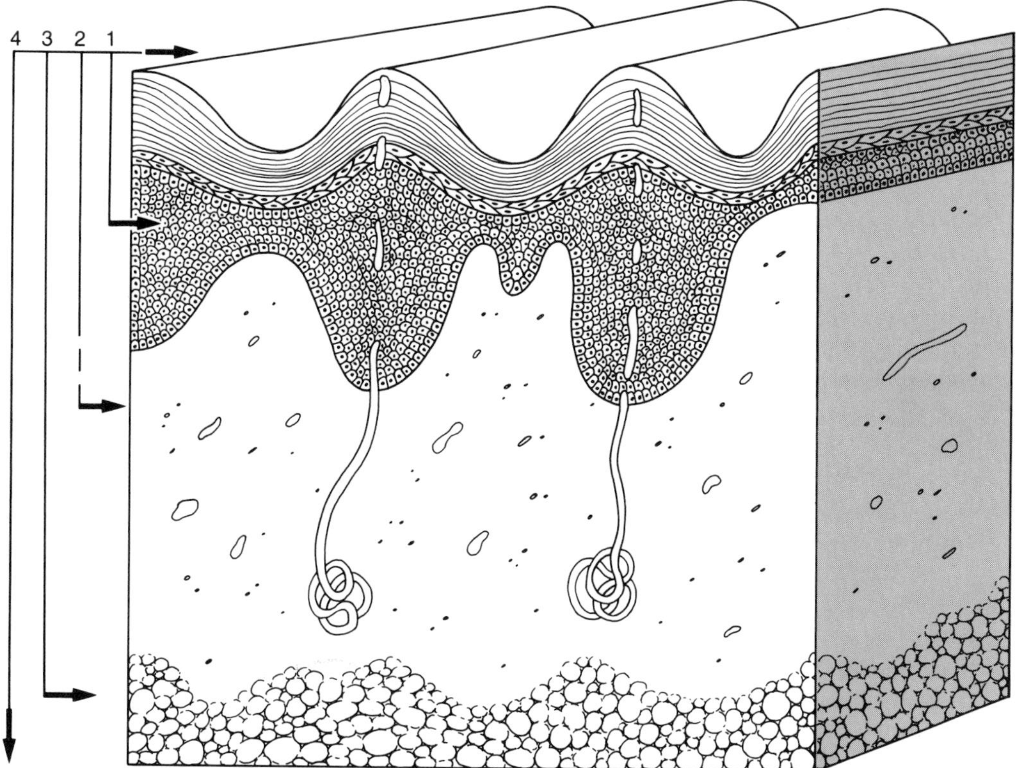

Figure 24–6. Diagram illustrating depths of frostbite as classically described, now better classified as superficial (1 & 2) or deep (3 & 4).

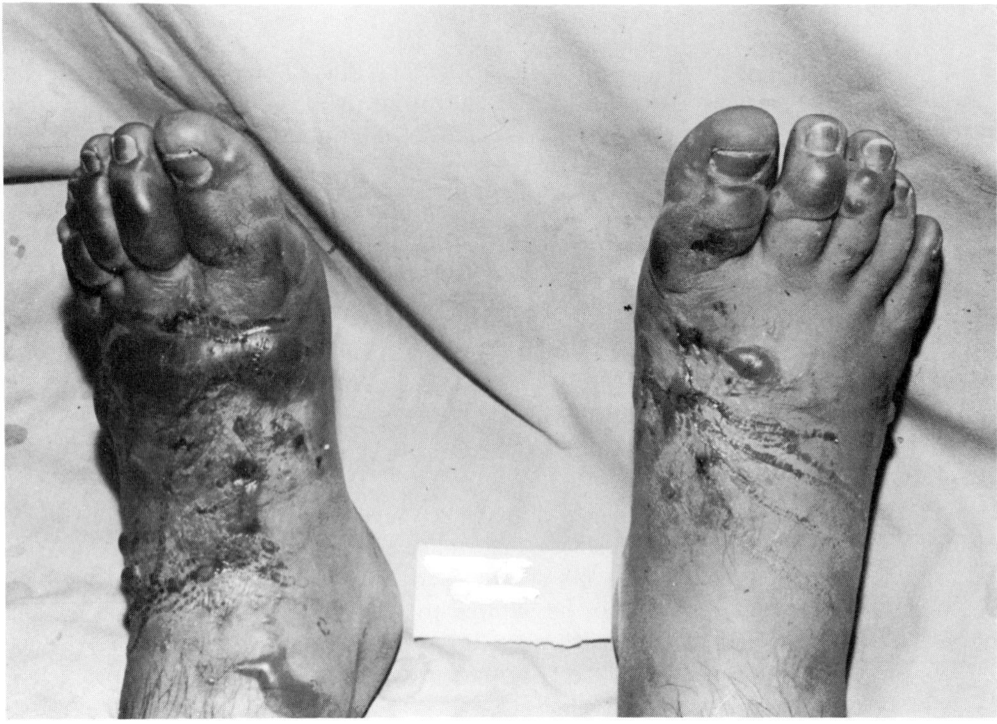

Figure 24–7. Superficial but alarming-looking frostbite with swelling and blisters 2 days after exposure. The patient recovered without loss of tissue.

disappears, the skin darkens and becomes black and mummified, and a clear line of demarcation eventually develops between healthy and necrotic tissue.

Prognosis

Prognosis at the time of first examination may be extremely difficult. The patient is anxious to know what the outcome may be, and the doctor wants to plan a course of treatment. Infrared thermography, radioactive scintiscanning, Doppler ultrasound, and plethysmography have all been tried. Mills[37] found scintiscanning to be more accurate than Doppler blood-flow measurements in determining the level of amputation. A potential disadvantage of Doppler measurements is that they not only measure acute, recent changes, but also reflect preexisting disease. In an elderly person, they may give an inaccurate prognostic picture.

Knowledge of the temperature and duration of exposure is important and useful in making a prognosis. The colder the temperature and the greater the duration of exposure, the greater the likelihood of tissue loss. The addition of wetness or contact with metal further increases the chances of severe damage.[38]

Treatment

Rapid rewarming was first suggested by Fuhrman and Crismon in 1947.[39] Since then, many other methods have been suggested—all directed towards the improvement of blood flow. Anticoagulants, antisludging agents, fibrinolytics, sympathetic blockade

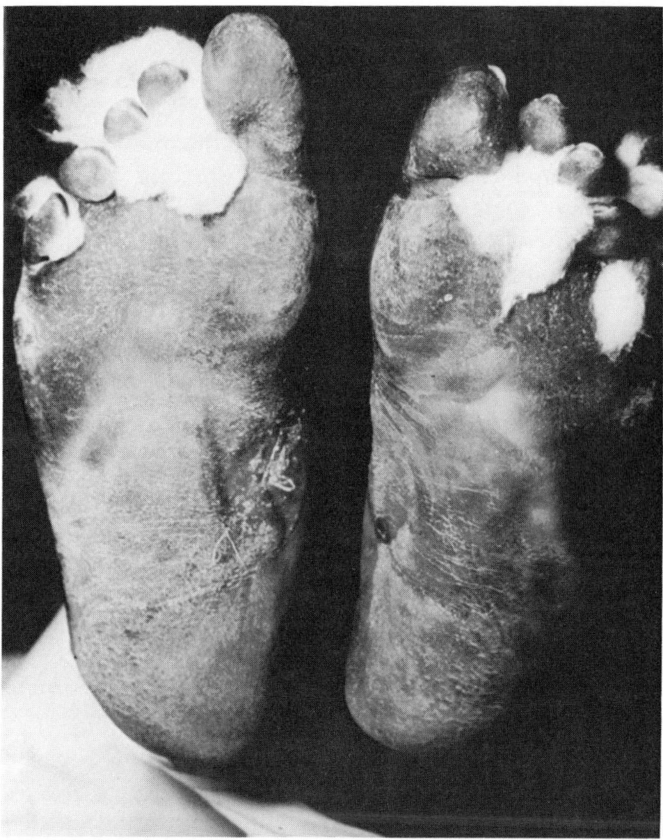

Figure 24–8. Severe frostbite with mummification and black necrotic eschars, worse on the left foot. The wool between the toes is to keep the area dry.

(either medical or surgical), vasodilators, and fasciotomy have been used to dissolve thrombi, dilate arteries, and relieve pressure in vascular spaces. Rapid rewarming remains the mainstay of treatment.

IN THE FIELD

There is nothing worse for a frozen part than to be thawed, then refrozen. This sequence guarantees severe damage.

> *Woe to the man benumbed with cold . . . if he entered suddenly into a too warm room, or came too near the great fire of a bivouac. The benumbed or frozen extremities . . . were struck with gangrene, which manifested itself at the very instant, and developed itself with such rapidity that its progress was perceptible to the eyes.*
>
> Baron Larrey on his experience in the retreat from Moscow

Treatment in the field, therefore, has to be very cautious and conservative. The frozen part should be treated gently. The old advice to rub the part with snow is totally wrong. There should be no attempts to warm the part in front of a camp fire or with additional external heat.

If it is possible for the victim to be transported in warmth and safety, rewarming may be feasible in a base camp. However, if this is impossible, it may be better for the part to remain frozen until it can be definitively rewarmed, provided the delay is hours rather than days.

The practicality of managing severe frostbite on a long mountain climb is that rewarming will take place spontaneously unless freezing continues or the climber becomes hypothermic and, therefore, cannot rewarm. Hackett,[36] at the University of Alaska High Latitude Research Station on Mount McKinley, where approximately 30 cases of severe frostbite are seen every year, has found that most frostbitten digits rewarm spontaneously either from the activity of climbing or when the climber gets into a sleeping bag. He does not believe, therefore, that it is possible to keep a limb frozen until a definitive treatment center can be reached. If the duration and severity of frostbite are great enough, there is no treatment, either in the field or in the hospital, which can prevent necrosis; it is probably impossible to say that damage would have been less or more had warming been delayed.

In prolonged expeditions, the best treatment—which may be the only available treatment—is to provide a dry, clean, protected environment, give an antitetanus booster and antibiotics as indicated, and permit natural rewarming and demarcation. It is important to keep the frozen part dry, because if gangrene is going to develop, the chances of infection are much less with dry, mummified gangrene than with swollen, wet gangrene. Narcotics should be given to control pain, but at high altitude, excessive use of narcotics should be avoided for fear of reducing the respiratory drive.

IN THE HOSPITAL

An initial evaluation must be made to assess the importance of the frostbite in relation to other problems, such as hypthermia, dehydration, respiratory problems, underlying illness, or other injuries. Frostbite may not be the most urgent problem affecting the patient.

Rewarming is done by placing the frozen part in water at 43°C, and allowing it to remain there until no further change in color is noted or until whatever line of demarcation has developed will progress no more (Fig. 24–9). This takes 30 to 45 min, and because the treatment may be painful, narcotics may have to be given. The part is dried carefully and the patient is nursed in a clean, light, airy, and dry environment (ie, exposure treatment).

The traditional advice concerning blisters has been to leave them intact for fear of introducing infection. In view of the recent evidence that blisters contain vasoactive substance which may increase damage, there is a basis for removing the roof of clear blisters under sterile conditions and dressing the exposed area with an aloe vera or steroid ointment. There have not been any controlled studies to substantiate this method, but there is considerable clinical experience which indicates that it is effective.[40] Nonsteroidal anti-inflammatory agents may also be added to the regimen.

Treatment for severe frostbite is prolonged and involves daily physical and occupational therapy, surgery, and rehabilitation. Daily baths in a Hubbard tank help to debride loose tissue, but surgical debridement is frequently necessary. The decision to amputate should be delayed until demarcation is complete and clear. There may be more skin necrosis than deeper damage, and as much tissue as possible should be preserved.

Apart from amputation, other surgical measures that may be needed are fasciotomy for relief of muscle compartment pressure, sympathectomy for late relief of causalgic pain, and late reconstructive plastic surgery for restoration of function after amputation.

Late Sequelae

There are many late effects of frostbite: sensitivity to cold, hyperhidrosis, skin changes, osteoporosis, and deformity of joints. The complications of frostbite are immediate and

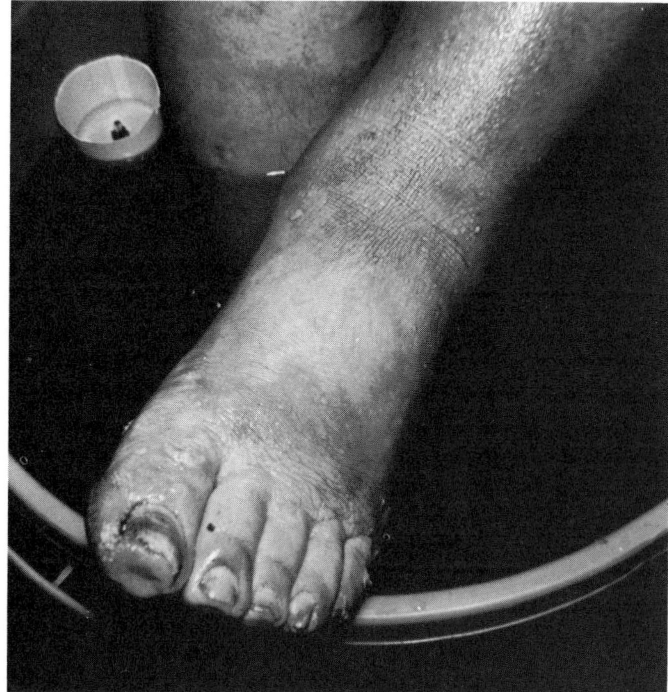

Figure 24–9. Simple technique for rewarming using a large container (clean garbage can) for water, and a thermometer floating in a paper cup to assure a constant water temperature.

chronic or long-term. Severe frostbite almost always leaves permanent or long-term ill effects (Table 24–6). Abnormal bone growth has been reported in children in whom there was freezing of the epiphyses.

Sensitivity to cold is very common and may last for many years. If the sensitivity amounts to pain, sympathectomy may be considered. For most people, all that is necessary is to take extra precautions against exposure to cold, including the use of heated socks. Loose boots with several layers of woolen socks are better than a single sock layer. Keeping the trunk warm reflexly heats the periphery.

TABLE 24–6. COMPLICATIONS OF FROSTBITE

Immediate Effects
- Infection
- Tissue necrosis
  - Superficial
  - Deep
- Muscle compartment swelling
- Blisters
- Causalgic pain
- Anesthesia

Late Effects
- Hyperhidrosis
- Abnormal nail growth
- Sensitivity to cold, cold feet or fingers
- Abnormal bone growth, arthritis, osteoporosis
- Abnormal color
- Scars, results of reconstructive surgery

Prevention

Frostbite cannot be "cured" in the same sense that many other lesions can be restored to normal. Prevention is the only way to avoid damage. Boots and clothes should be warm, dry, loose, and well insulated. The sole of a boot is the most important part to insulate, to reduce conductive heat loss. Vermiculite pads placed in the boot add extra warmth for 6 to 8 hours and provide additional protection during periods of extreme exposure. Good nutrition and hydration are essential for maintenance of good circulation, as the maintenance of good circulation is essential in the prevention of frostbite.

Contact with metal and moisture must be avoided. Special care must be taken to avoid contact with supercooled fluids and stove fuels. If a foot becomes wet by stepping into a half-frozen stream, or even with excessive sweating, dry the foot and change socks as soon as possible.

An alternative strategy is to wear vapor barrier socks or boots. The foot is then surrounded by a layer of warm moisture. If this technique is used for a long time, however, fungal infections between the toes may flare up and affect the whole foot.

Trench Foot

Trench foot is a nonfreezing cold injury sustained by prolonged soaking of the feet in cold, but not freezing, water. In World War I, the British Army had more than 115,000 cases. Many of the effects are similar to those of frostbite.

CASE 3

Ten people were on a rafting trip in the Brooks Range in Alaska in late August. The weather was unexpectedly cold with a mixture of rain and snow. The group spent 8 days on the river. Several members did not have waterproof boots, or had waterproof boots that were too low so that their feet became wet and stayed wet for most of the trip. By the end of the trip, four people had swollen, painful feet. Two lost toe nails and had anesthesia of the tips of the toes. A year later, several still had mild symptoms with cold sensitivity and abnormal nail growth.

The worst cases of trench foot may develop gangrene; but the big difference between the gangrene of trench foot and that of frostbite is that gangrene in trench foot almost always becomes infected because of the wet, soggy conditions under which the problem starts. The feet become swollen, blistered, soft, sensitive then anesthetic, and, finally, gangrenous. The treatment is to expose the feet to a dry, light environment, give antibiotics, and debride as necessary. If amputation is necessary, it must be done much sooner than with frostbite because of the presence of infection and "wet" gangrene. The long-term effects are similar to those of frostbite.

BIBLIOGRAPHY

Danzl DF, Pozos RS, Hamlet MP: Accidental hypothermia. *In* Auerbach P, Geehr EC (eds): Management of Wilderness and Environmental Emergencies, ed 2. St Louis, CV Mosby, 1989, pp 35–76.

Paton BC: Accidental hypothermia. Pharmacol Ther 22:331–337, 1983.

REFERENCES

1. Hypothermia prevention [editorial]. JAMA 261:513, 1989.
2. National Safety Council: Accident Facts, 1988 edition. Chicago, IL, National Safety Council, 1988, p 12.
3. Deaths in winter [editorial]. Lancet ii:987–988, 1985.
4. Danzl DF, Pozos RS, Hamlet JP: Multicenter hypothermia survey. Ann Emerg Med 16:1042–1055, 1987.
5. Lloyd EL: Temperature sensations in veins. Anaesthesia 34:919, 1979.
6. Hayward JS, Eckerson JD, Collis MD: Effect of behavioral variables on cooling rate of man in cold water. J Appl Physiol 1975;38:1074.
7. Lloyd EL: Hypothermia and Cold Stress. Rockville, MD, Aspen Publications, 1986, pp 28, 204–205.
8. Lilly JK, Boland JP, Zekan S: Urinary bladder temperature monitoring: A new index of body core temperature. Crit Care Med 8:742, 1980.
9. Jurkovich GJ, Greiser WB, Luterman A, et al: Hypothermia in trauma victims: An ominous predictor of survival. J Trauma 27:1019–1024, 1987.
10. Sutton JR: Hypothermia in joggers and marathon runners. *In* Sutton JR, Houston CS, Coates G (eds): Hypoxia and Cold. New York, Praeger, 1987, pp 257–263.
11. Rey L: Arctic Underwater Operations. London, Grahan and Trotman, 1985.
12. Cooper KE, Ferguson AV: Thermoregulation and hypothermia in the elderly. *In* Pozos RS, Wittmers RL (eds): The Nature and Treatment of Hypothermia. London, Croom Helm/Minneapolis, University of Minnesota Press, 1983, pp 37–46.
13. Flancbaum L, Trooskin S, Pedersen H: Evaluation of blood-warming devices with the apparent thermal clearance. Ann Emerg Med 18:355–359, 1989.
14. Delaney KA, Howland MA, Vassallo S, et al: Assessment of acid-base disturbances in hypothermia and their physiologic consequences. Ann Emerg Med 18:72–82, 1989.
15. Rivolier J, Goldsmith R, Lugg DJ, et al: Man in the Antarctic. London, Taylor and Francis, 1988, pp 25–27.
16. Smolander J, Louhevaara V, Ahonen M: Clothing, hypothermia, and long-distance skiing. Lancet ii:226, 1986.
17. Hayward JS, Eckerson JD: Physiological responses and survival time prediction for humans in ice-water. Aviat Space Environ Med 55:206–12, 1984.
18. McPhee J: The Control of Nature. New York, Farrar, Straus, Giroux, 1989, pp 126–128.
19. Keatinge WR, Coleshaw SRK, Millard CE: Exceptional case of survival in cold water. Br Med J 292:171–172, 1986.
20. Nunneley SA, Wissler EH, Allan JR: Immerson cooling: Effect of clothing and skinfold thickness. Aviat Space Environ Med 56:1177–1182, 1985.
21. Bolte RG, Black PG, Bowers RS, et al: The use of extracorporeal rewarming in a child submerged for 66 minutes. JAMA 260:377–379, 1988.
22. Conn AW, Barker GA, Edmonds JF, et al: Submersion hypothermia and near-drowning. *In* Pozos RS, Wittmers LE (eds): The Nature and Treatment of Hypothermia. Minneapolis, Croom Helm/University of Minnesota Press, 1983, pp 152–164.
23. Brooks CJ, Rowe KW: Water survival: 20 years Canadian Forces aircrew experience. Aviat Space Environ Med 55:41–51, 1984.
24. Bradley ME: Commercial diving fatalities. Aviat Space Environ Med 55:721–724, 1984.
25. Lloyd EL: Diving and hypothermia. Br Med J ii:68, 1979.
26. Hauty MG, Esrig BC, Hill JG, et al: Prognostic factors in severe accidental hypothermia: experience from the Mt. Hood Tragedy. J Trauma 27:1107–1112, 1987.
27. Hixson EG: Injury patterns in cross-country skiing. Physician Sportsmed 9(12):45–53, 1983.
28. Zwischenberger JB, Kirsh MM, Dechert RRT, et al: Suppression of shivering decreases oxygen consumption and improves hemodynamic stability during postoperative rewarming. Ann Thorac Surg 43:428–431, 1987.
29. Collins KJ, Dore C, Exton-Smith AN, et al: Accidental hypothermia and impaired temperature homeostasis in the elderly. Br Med J i:353–356, 1977.
30. Rango N: Exposure-related hypothermia mortality in the United States, 1970–79. Am J Public Health 74:1159–1160, 1984.
31. Weatherley-White RCA, Sjostrom B, Paton BC: Experimental studies in cold injury: II. The pathogenesis of frostbite. Surgery 66:208–214, 1969.
32. McCord JM: Oxygen-derived free radicals in post-ischemic injury. N Engl J Med 312:159–163, 1985.
33. Ehrlich HP, Needle AL, Rajaratnam J, et al: The role of prostacyclin and thromboxane in rat burn and freeze injuries. Mol Pathol 38:357–367, 1983.
34. Robson MC, Heggers JP: Evaluation of hand frostbite blister fluid as a clue to pathogenesis. J Hand Surg 6:43–46, 1981.

35. Paton BC: Pathophysiology of frostbite. *In* Sutton JR, Houston CS, Coates G (eds): Hypoxia and Cold. New York, Praeger, 1987, pp 329–339.
36. Hackett P: Personal communication, 1990.
37. Mills WJ: The initial management of frostbite injuries. Presented at The Conference on Initial Management of Thermal Injuries. University of Alaska and Providence Hospital, March 11–13, 1983.
38. Knize DM, Weatherley-White RCA, Paton BC, et al: Prognostic factors in the management of frostbite. J Trauma 9:749–759, 1969.
39. Fuhrman FA, Crismon JM: Studies on gangrene following cold injury: VII: Treatment of cold injury by means of immediate rapid rewarming. J Clin Invest 26:476–485, 1947.
40. Heggers JP, Robson MC, Manavalen K, et al: Experimental and clinical observations on frostbite. Ann Emerg Med 16:1056–1062, 1987.

25

ALTITUDE SICKNESS

Charles S. Houston, MD

During the last four decades, there has been a tremendous increase in activities of all kinds on high mountains. Skiing, mountain climbing, and trekking have become more and more popular. Military campaigns and extensive mining and construction have taken place at altitudes where, in de Saussure's day (1770–1790), death was considered certain if one spent a night above 12,000 feet, the same being held of 20,000 feet as late as 1906. Yet today, more than 50 persons have reached the summit of Everest (29,028 feet above sea level) breathing only the thin cold air about them. Hundreds more have come close to such heights and many millions go to elevations high enough to cause illness and even death due to hypobaric hypoxia.

This increase in activity at altitude has led to a parallel expansion of research and understanding of how oxygen lack affects us.

HISTORICAL BACKGROUND

Man's venturous sallies into the earth's atmosphere make a fascinating story of exploration and discovery advancing by leaps and bounds, especially in the last 100 years. From prehistoric times until the sixteenth century, few ventured high enough to feel adverse effects, and the physics of the atmosphere were dormant secrets under the spell of Aristotle's dicta on air. The Renaissance was accompanied by a burst of scientific discovery and innovative thought and experiment; air was shown to have weight, to be compressible and, conversely, a vacuum was proved to be possible. Berti's first crude barometer was improved by Torricelli, and Perier carried one to the summit of a small mountain and proved that atmospheric pressure decreased with increasing height.

A few years later, Mayow showed that something in air was essential to combustion and to life and he and his peers groped for a concept of metabolism. Harvey showed that blood was pumped by the heart through lungs and throughout the body, correcting Galen's age-old error (as Ibn-al-Nafis had almost done two centuries earlier). The stage was set, the physical laws had been clarified, and great advances in physiology could begin.

The bad effects of altitude were recognized by Chinese traders crossing the Hindu Kush, which they called the Greater and Lesser Headache Mountains, on their way to Europe two millennia ago. Mirza Muhammad Haidar vividly described a sickness which killed men and horses during his campaigns in high central Asia early in the sixteenth century. A Jesuit priest, Jose Acosta, deserves credit for his vivid description of altitude illness, which he experienced while he accompanied the Conquistadores in the conquest of the Incas a few decades after Haidar, and which he imaginatively blamed on "thinne aire."

Appreciation that hot air was lighter than cold air led to the invention of balloons, which soon carried men high enough to cause severe illness and death. The exact composition of air was resolved; oxygen was generated and shown to be the component of air which sustained life. Mayow and Scheele took the first steps; Lavoisier and Priestley brought their efforts to fruition. All that remained was to explain how food could be "burned" in the body to release energy without destroying tissue, and that took another hundred years.

By the early nineteenth century, balloons were a commonplace, and exploration of high mountains began. Within 50 years, men described mountain sickness and some died from it on Alpine, Andean, and Himalayan peaks, though few came closer than Acosta to understanding why. Some doctors and travelers advanced curious explanations: a Royal Navy surgeon believed that the difference in electrical polarity between northern and southern hemispheres explained different symptoms, which could be prevented by insulation from the earth's magnetic field—as by riding a horse; he claimed the best treatment was to lie flat on the ground with head toward the pole. Others contended that vapors from certain shrubs, or emanations from mineral deposits were responsible. A prominent physician argued that as atmospheric pressure decreased, the expansion of gases throughout the body caused symptoms. Not until the end of the century was it recognized that lack of oxygen alone was responsible.

Paul Bert is usually called the father of altitude physiology, though his great book, *Barometric Pressure,* was unappreciated for 50 years. Based on hundreds of travelers' tales and scores of experiments in decompression chambers, Bert conclusively showed that the decreased atmospheric pressure at higher altitudes caused increasingly severe symptoms, not from lack of atmospheric pressure but because oxygen partial pressure was decreased. He then showed that by breathing oxygen, these symptoms could be prevented or relieved. Unfortunately, his advice was not heeded by the passengers in the famous flight of the balloon *Zenith,* two of whom died when they ascended to nearly 30,000 feet. Bert's impressive data were challenged by a pioneering Italian physiologist, Angelo Mosso, who suggested that loss of carbon dioxide due to the overbreathing that is natural at higher altitude was as important as oxygen lack, but few accepted the acapnia theory.

In 1913, Ravenhill, then doctor to a mining company high in the Andes, described three forms of illness: ordinary mountain sickness, *"puna"*; pulmonary edema, *"cardiac puna"*; and brain edema, *"nervous puna."* These are the earliest clinical descriptions we have of altitude illness, and by then, insufficient oxygen had been acknowledged as the cause.

World War I saw the first combat between heavier-than-air craft, and victory went to the flier who could get above his foe. This greatly stimulated studies of altitude, primarily because of what happened after very rapid ascent rather than during the slower pace of climbing. Between World Wars I and II, mountaineers went higher and higher, aircraft were perfected, together with oxygen equipment for their crews, and basic research advanced. But the major developments occurred under the desperate spur of the Second World War when many fundamental physiologic principles were understood, and soon some were tested on ever higher mountain ascents. The great increase in climbing, fighting, and exploring on the highest mountains has led in the last 20 years to a rich inventory of knowledge about altitude illness. In the years ahead, these lessons from high altitude are certain to be applied to a wide range of illnesses and injuries causing lack of oxygen at sea level.

CAUSES OF ALTITUDE SICKNESS

Three factors affect man's response to altitude: the speed of ascent, the altitude reached, and the length of stay (Table 25–1). Minor, though frequently critical, factors include age, sex, general health, previous experience at altitude, and genetic inheritance. Others, only dimly understood, are diet, level of hydration, presence of even a mild respiratory or viral

TABLE 25–1. FACTORS AFFECTING INCIDENCE OF ALTITUDE ILLNESS

Major Factors
Speed of ascent
Altitude reached
Length of stay
Minor Factors
Weather
Physical fitness
Nutrition
Hydration
General health
Obesity
Individual Factors
Fresh respiratory infection
Genetic predisposition
Mutant hemoglobin
Cardiopulmonary status
Previous episodes of altitude illness

infection, emotional state, climate, and latitude. From a practical viewpoint, the variables of speed, altitude, and duration of exposure determine whether the individual will be well or ill. These same factors—speed of onset, and severity and duration of oxygen lack—also influence the course of illnesses that cause hypoxia at sea level.

DEFINITIONS

We may consider those who stay at altitude for several days or weeks as *visitors* or sojourners, those who live there for months or years as *residents,* and those born at altitude as *natives.* Speed of ascent can be called *rapid* if in minutes or hours, *fast* if in a day or two, and *slow* if over many days or weeks. For the sake of this discussion, we can define *moderate* altitudes as up to 10,000 feet; *high,* up to 18,000 feet; and *very high,* above 20,000 feet.

Rather than discrete clinical entities, the forms of altitude illness are a spectrum or continuum of signs and symptoms in which now one, now another, may predominate. This is important in diagnosis and especially for treatment because a mild case may develop rapidly into a severe, even life-threatening, problem (Case 1) (Table 25–2).

CASE 1

Rick drove from Oklahoma to a resort at 9000 feet and began skiing the next morning despite mild headache and slight nausea. He quit early, went to bed but slept poorly, and went to a doctor next morning. He was told he had mild altitude illness and to take it easy, but he did not want to lose a day and skied hard. By evening, he was weak and very short of breath. The doctor said he had fluid in his lungs and advised him to go immediately to lower altitude, which he did. By the time he arrived he was much better.

How likely to develop mountain sickness is the recreational skier, climber, or tourist who often drives or flies from low to moderate altitude in a day? Data defining the inci-

TABLE 25–2. FORMS OF ALTITUDE ILLNESS

Condition	Symptoms
Acute hypoxia	Mental impairment and usually collapse after rapid exposure; above 18,000 feet; rare on mountains
Acute mountain sickness	Headache, nausea, vomiting, sleep disturbance, dyspnea; above 7000 to 8000 feet; self-limited; common
High-altitude pulmonary edema (HAPE)	Dyspnea, cough, weakness, headache, stupor, and rarely, death; above 9000 to 10,000 feet; requires rapid descent or treatment early
High-altitude cerebral edema (HACE)	Severe headache, hallucinations, ataxia, weakness, impaired mentation, stupor, and death; above 10,000 to 12,000 feet; uncommon; descent mandatory
Chronic mountain sickness (CMS)	After months of residence at a moderate altitude, plethora, weakness, and congestive heart failure develop in some persons
Adult subacute mountain sickness	After weeks at a very high altitude, acute congestive heart failure occurs in a few individuals, necessitating descent
Subacute infantile mountain sickness	Some Chinese children born at a moderate altitude develop signs and symptoms similar to CMS

dence of altitude-related problems differ widely (Table 25–3), which perhaps is not surprising in view of the many variables that could not be well controlled in these surveys.

INCIDENCE AND SYMPTOMATOLOGY

On the average, about one out of five visitors going in a day from near sea level to 8500–9000 feet will probably experience symptoms for a few days. We lump these together under the name *acute mountain sickness (AMS).* The manifestations are unpleasant, generally brief, and seldom dangerous. Headache, nausea and vomiting, weakness, sleep disturbance, and lethargy are typical. Some few unfortunates become so dehydrated that they need medical care, but for most, AMS is like a bad hangover—to be endured for a short time. Some people are sick every time they go to a moderate altitude, no matter how slowly. Others are never affected. Age seems to be a minor factor.

More serious, but fortunately less common, is the accumulation of fluid in the lungs, a condition known as *high-altitude pulmonary edema (HAPE),* which affects 0.01% to 0.05% of visitors (Fig. 25–1). We know that most individuals going to altitude accumulate some

TABLE 25–3. REPORTED INCIDENCE OF ACUTE MOUNTAIN SICKNESS

Author (Year)	Location	Altitude (feet)	Incidence (%)
Montgomery (1989)	Colorado	6765	20
		6900	25
		8900	40
Houston (1985)	Colorado	8500	12
		9500	17
Honigman (1990)	Colorado	9300	23
Yip (1989)	Colorado	9800	42
Maggiorini (1989)	Alps	6700	9
		10,000	13
		12,000	34
		15,000	54
Hackett (1976)	Nepal	14,000	42

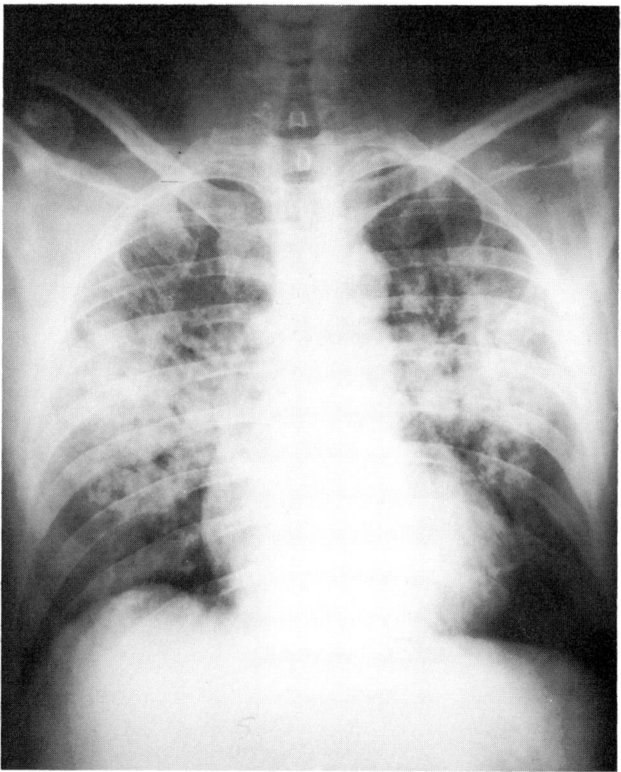

Figure 25–1. Chest radiograph showing high-altitude pulmonary edema.

small amount of excess fluid in the loose interstitial space between capillaries and alveolar walls, but usually this fluid is quickly reabsorbed. In some, this fluid continues to accumulate, leaks into the alveoli, and results in full-blown pulmonary edema (Fig. 25–2). HAPE generally takes a day or two to become clinically obvious. The initial shortness of breath increases, and a dry cough becomes productive of clear watery sputum, which often becomes profuse and bloody, until the victim is literally drowning in his or her own juices. Weakness and lethargy progress to drowsiness, coma, and death, sometimes within 10 or 12 hours. HAPE is a desperate, dramatic problem; it is fatal if not promptly and adequately tended (Case 2). But it is reversible if action is taken early.

CASE 2

Warren, a 45-year-old airline pilot, flew to Denver and drove to an altitude of 9500 feet with his wife and friends. They skied together the next day, feeling fine. On the second day, Warren had a bad headache and fell frequently; by afternoon he had trouble standing and his wife persuaded him to go home. Late in the afternoon, she found him asleep. Early the next morning, she heard him gasp, realized he was unconscious, and rushed him to a doctor. His heart arrested but cardiopulmonary resuscitation (CPR) restored cardiac function. He was airlifted to lower altitude, where he remained comatose until he died 11 days later with extensive hypoxic brain damage and pulmonary edema.

There are many puzzling aspects to HAPE. The resident who returns to altitude after a short stay lower down appears to be more vulnerable. Although most cases strike visitors

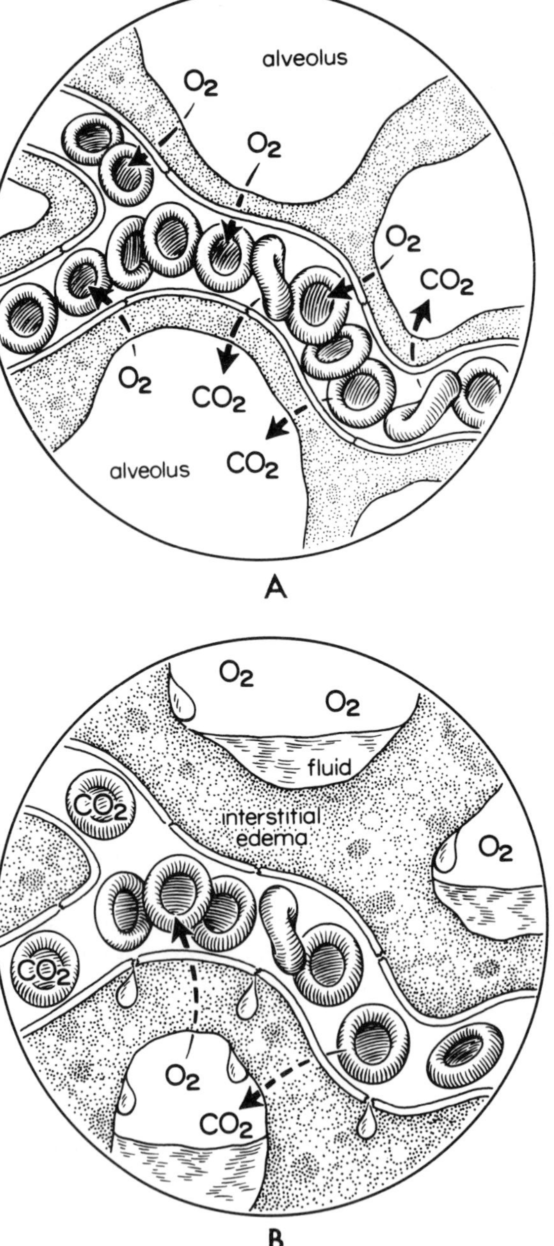

Figure 25–2. High-altitude pulmonary edema. **A:** Normal alveolus, alveolar walls, and capillaries. **B:** Interstitial and alveolar edema.

at altitudes above 9000 feet, veteran climbers have been affected at altitudes as high as 25,000 feet, even after weeks of acclimatization. HAPE usually develops within 24 to 48 hours after arrival, but rare cases have been described weeks later. A few individuals are very susceptible and may have three or ten attacks of classic HAPE at even moderate elevations. We know that the very rare individual who lacks normal circulation to one lung due to congenital absence of a pulmonary artery is prone to HAPE, even at 5000 feet. By extension, it seems likely, though not proven, that a person who acquires a deficit in pulmonary circulation from emboli or thromboses may also be more vulnerable to HAPE.

The third portion of the spectrum of altitude illnesses, known as *high-altitude cerebral edema (HACE),* is the most dangerous. Manifestations include staggering gait (ataxia), which occurs early and is a good warning sign; hallucinations; severe headache; disorientation; and stupor. Hand, trunk, and even head motions may also be ataxic. Curious psychotic reactions have occurred. HACE usually becomes obvious 24 to 72 hours after reaching altitude, and, like HAPE, may progress rapidly to coma and death. As more and more climbers go very high, unusual forms of HACE are being reported (Case 3).

CASE 3

Bob, an experienced mountain guide, was leading a party near the top of 21,000 foot Aconcagua; they had climbed slowly and were feeling great. Bob suddenly became weak, stopped to rest, and noticed his vision was dimming. In half an hour, he was completely blind and paranoid. His companions tied his hands and feet because he fought them so violently, and in 40 hours managed to drag him down to 14,000 feet, where he lapsed into quiet sleep. Eight hours later he roused. He regained his vision and his senses and, the next day, walked out, fully recovered.

Other less severe cases of partial or total transient blindness, usually above 14,000 feet, have been described. We assume that these are due to transient ischemia of the visual cortex or, less often, to a migraine equivalent.

High-altitude retinal hemorrhages (HARH) occur in half of all persons going above 17,000 feet but are seldom symptomatic. Some are small, typically flame-shaped (Fig. 25–3), but others may be large frightening pools or blobs. Only when the macula is affected does the individual notice a scotoma. Cotton-wool spots (Fig. 25–4), representing retinal edema, are rare but more serious. The ordinary hemorrhages resolve in a week or two leaving no residuals, but the cotton-wool spots and macular hemorrhages often leave scotomata which persist for years. HARH are not considered serious, but if the macula is involved or cotton-wool spots are present, prudence dictates descent. There is not enough data to tell whether HARH are more likely during subsequent visits to altitude, but today they are not seen as contraindications to going to altitude.

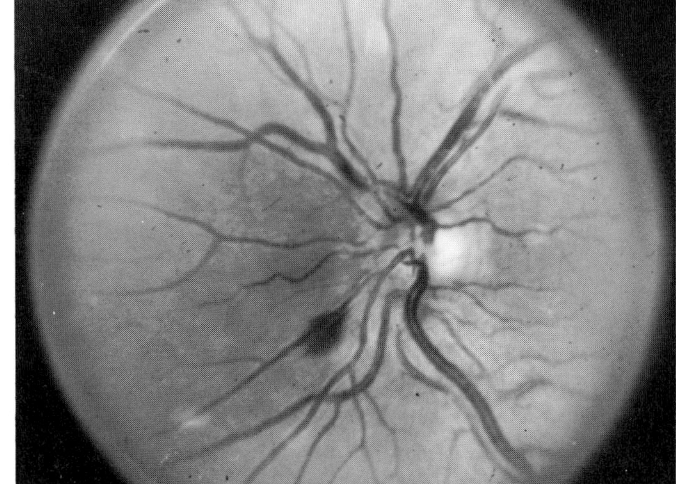

Figure 25–3. Retinal hemorrhage.

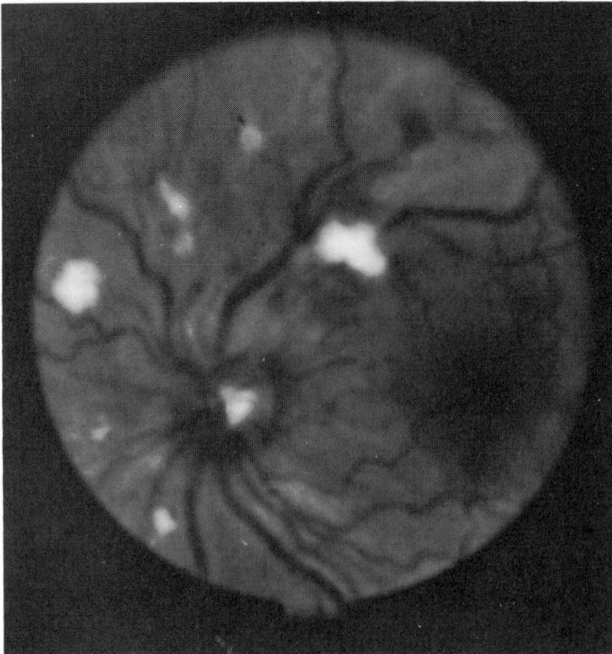

Figure 25–4. Retinal "cotton-wool" spots.

There is much debate over whether HARH may be evidence of hemorrhages elsewhere in the body, notably in the brain. However, there is little evidence to support this unattractive possibility. HARH have not been shown to indicate abnormal vascular fragility. They are probably due to the doubling of retina blood flow, which has been demonstrated at altitude, presumably accompanied by increased capillary pressure. They are uncommon below 14,000 feet but may be precipitated even there by strenuous exertion. No treatment is known—or apparently needed.

Three uncommon responses to long residence at altitude should be mentioned: chronic mountain sickness (CMS), subacute infantile mountain sickness (SIMS), and adult subacute mountain sickness (ASMS). The first (often called Monge's disease) develops in a healthy resident after many months or years at a moderate altitude and is characterized by weakness, plethoric cyanosis due to an unusually high hematocrit (often above 65%), multiple aches and pains, and eventually, congestive heart failure. Alveolar hypoventilation is present and assumed to be the root cause; in this respect CMS resembles the pickwickian syndrome. CMS leads to disability, heart failure, and death, but if the victim descends to sea level early in the progress of the disease, recovery occurs. SIMS is a recently defined syndrome, so far found only in Chinese children born on the high Tibetan plateau. The condition is similar to CMS. The most recently described form, ASMS, has been reported among East Indian troops occupying military posts at 20,000 to 21,000 feet for many weeks. The heart dilates and fails, and ASMS appears as acute congestive heart failure. It is not responsive to treatment at the altitude at which the onset occurred, but is slowly reversed after descent. These forms of subacute mountain sickness are not chronic, nor are they frequent or well understood. Also, it remains to be determined how these forms differ.

Periodic breathing, often called *Cheyne-Stokes respiration,* is common, indeed almost universal, above 9000 to 10,000 feet. Long apneic periods 10 to 20 seconds may be alarming. Periodic breathing is most evident and troublesome during sleep, and arterial oxygen saturation decreases during the apneic periods. This may explain the worsening of signs and symptoms on waking. Periodic breathing is eliminated by acetazolamide (Diamox; Lederle Laboratories, Wayne, NJ).

PATHOPHYSIOLOGY

The basic abnormality in altitude illness is believed to be a reversible breakdown in the "sodium pump"—the bioelectric mechanism by which each living cell pushes sodium out while holding potassium within its cytoplasm. The pump is highly oxygen-dependent and is impaired by any form of hypoxia, allowing sodium to accumulate within the cell; this in turn attracts water and the cell swells. Depending on the location and function and amount of swelling of affected cells, different signs and symptoms appear. One theory of the mechanism of AMS is that swelling of parts of the medulla affects the centers which cause nausea, vomiting, and disturbed sleep. The headache may be attributable to increased cerebrospinal fluid pressure (which has been measured only occasionally), to tension on the sensitive pia due to brain edema, or to distention of the arterioles, which have pain receptors as well.

Hypoxia from any cause increases the pressure in the pulmonary artery by increasing peripheral resistance in the lung. Since HAPE can be reversed by pulmonary vasodilators, it would seem to follow that pulmonary hypertension is a necessary contributor. However, other factors must be involved because primary pulmonary hypertension alone does not cause edema. Nor do altitude residents (who have chronically elevated pulmonary artery pressure) show pulmonary edema. Additional causative factors are necessary: one of these may be release of biologically active substances, such as fractions of the arachidonic acid cascade, thromboxanes, prostacyclins, and leukotrienes. Some of these dilate, others constrict vessels, some increase and others decrease platelet stickiness, so that their net effect varies between individuals and perhaps from time to time.

From these observations, we may logically conclude that HAPE is a high-pressure, high-permeability edema. The latter is confirmed by the observation that the alveolar fluid in HAPE contains a great deal of protein and few cells—it is typically a transudate. The presence of red blood cells, even gross bleeding, in the alveolar fluid suggests that the normally tight intercellular junctions in the walls of pulmonary capillaries are stretched by the increased flow and pressure, allowing leakage. Consequently, we hypothesize that when normal circulation is altered, the increase in pressure-flow at altitude will flood a lung beyond its capacity to absorb, and edema results. Some animals (pigs, ferrets, and certain strains of cattle) develop high pulmonary artery pressure when taken to altitude and are more susceptible to altitude edema than others. But there are still many gaps in our understanding.

HAPE differs importantly from adult respiratory distress syndrome (ARDS) because it is usually rapidly reversed by descent or by oxygen, which promptly decreases pulmonary artery pressure. In contrast, reversal of the edema by oxygen given to the ARDS patient takes days or even weeks, indicating that more lasting damage has been done to the capillaries.

The exact pathophysiology of HACE is unclear because blood flow (and presumably pressure) to the brain is sensitive (in opposite direction) to small variations in carbon dioxide and oxygen, which does not appear to be the case with the pulmonary vascular bed. Hypoxia from any cause produces generalized edema in the brain. One logical explanation for HACE is that the sodium pump fails in the brain cells as it does elsewhere, and the resulting patchy and variable edema causes a variety of signs and symptoms of central nervous system dysfunction. Similar symptoms and signs are seen in patients at sea level with either acute or chronic lack of oxygen due to disease.

TREATMENT

It is important to emphasize that when signs and symptoms are more than mild, getting down to lower altitude is the treatment of choice for all forms of altitude illness and is mandatory for HAPE and HACE.

AMS, though unpleasant, is usually brief and self-limited, requiring little more than symptomatic treatment. Oxygen relieves the headache almost at once, though the pain returns when oxygen is stopped. Bed rest is not as beneficial as being quietly up and about. Forcing fluids (partly to replace those lost by hyperventilating dry air and partly to "flush out" bicarbonate in the urine) is logical. Frequent small, high-carbohydrate meals are theoretically beneficial and seem to help. Because "one drink does the work of two" at altitude, alcohol is contraindicated.

From numerous anecdotes and a few well-controlled studies, it appears that acetazolamide (Diamox) in a dose of 250 mg every 6 or 8 hours will relieve AMS in most people; this is a safe and conservative treatment. Dexamethasone (4 mg every 6 hours) also relieves symptoms but seems to be an excessively strong treatment.

Addition of a small amount of carbon dioxide to inspired air has been shown to relieve the headache rapidly, and from this came the suggestion that patients breathe in and out of a paper bag. However, although it may increase carbon dioxide, this depletes oxygen and is not helpful. If feasible, breathing a mixture of 1% or 2% carbon dioxide in air may help. Descent is rarely necessary in AMS, but it relieves symptoms after going down only a few thousand feet, as does exposure to increased pressure in a hyperbaric bag.

When the increasing dyspnea, cough, and weakness are sufficient to make a diagnosis of HAPE likely, getting to lower altitude is rapidly and spectacularly curative. Within days or weeks, the patient can often return and resume activities. Oxygen is also helpful, but unless it is given through a well-fitted mask at a flow of 2 liters or more, it will not be as good as descent. On a high, remote mountain, oxygen often is logistically impractical. A diuretic (furosemide) has been used, but no controlled studies have proven its effectiveness, and there is the distinct risk of preciptating hypovolemic shock, thus converting the walking sick to a litter case. Morphine has been used in a few extreme situations and was helpful; digitalis is not. Nifedipine lowers pulmonary artery pressure rapidly and appears to improve early stages of HAPE, but the effect is transient and until a longer-acting form is available, nifedipine and its analogues are not recommended. Descent remains the best and safest management.

HACE, the least common but potentially most dangerous form of altitude illness, is an absolute indication for descent. Other treatments are not as effective. Based on the long-standing belief of neurosurgeons, hyperosmolar infusions have been recommended. Corticosteroids are also used, but they are slow to act and no adequate studies have been done to prove or disprove the clinical impression and anecdotal experience that they are helpful. A controlled study of cerebral edema caused by cerebral malaria showed that dexamethasone did more harm than good, but this special problem is quite different from the edema caused by altitude. Oxygen is helpful but as in HAPE, the best, the mandatory, and almost always curative treatment is descent—early descent before the problem has become far advanced.

Pressure treatment—in a hyperbaric bag—has been used frequently on mountain expeditions. Because descent is so effective, it seems logical that increasing the ambient pressure around the patient might be equally effective. For this purpose, a tough, lightweight plastic bag, 7 feet long and 3 feet in diameter, has been developed. The patient lies inside, the bag is tightly sealed by a strong zipper, and air is pumped into the bag by a powered or hand pump, until the pressure in the bag is about 2 lb per square inch above the outside pressure. Thereafter, pumping is continued to cause a steady flow of air into the bag and out through a spring-loaded relief valve, flushing out carbon dioxide. The bag has been used with striking benefit for severe cases of HAPE and HACE on high mountains. Recently, a controlled study showed that the hyperbaric bag relieved symptoms of mild to moderate AMS as well as did oxygen. On mountain expeditions it has been effective in treating severe cases of HAPE and HACE. Little information is available to define the longer lasting effects of hyperbaric bag treatment.

PREVENTION

Taking sufficient time to go from low to high altitude is the best way to avoid all of these problems. This is not always possible and, for a rare individual, even time is not a sufficient preventive. Acetazolamide (Diamox) has been used for almost 30 years to prevent or minimize altitude sickness. It acts as a carbonic anhydrase inhibitor in red blood cells and kidney, enabling larger ventilatory exchange with a lesser degree of alkalosis. It is often called "an artificial acclimatizer." The dose is still debated: consensus favors 80 mg (approximately one quarter of a 250 mg tablet) every 12 hours when starting the ascent and for 2 days after reaching altitude. Dexamethasone has been recommended as a preventive alone or in combination with Diamox and has been shown to be effective, but it seems a rather powerful agent to use for this purpose. Most authorities recommend taking only Diamox—when taking time is not practical. Older preventives (ammonium chloride, Rolaids, cytochrome, vitamin E) have no value. The analogues of Diamox are not superior. Nifedipine is risky.

Modifying the pattern of breathing has been suggested. In one form ("grunt breathing"), volume is not increased, but expiration is made against slight pressure of closed lips or glottis. The theory is that by increasing alveolar pressure slightly, transfer of oxygen into pulmonary capillaries will be enhanced. The only controlled studies (40 years ago) indicated that the slight accompanying hyperventilation rather than the increased pressure produced the benefit. More study is desirable. Also recommended by some is changing from primarily thoracic to diaphragmatic breathing; hard data are lacking here as well. Wearing a lightweight C-PAP mask with spring-loaded exhalation valves has been tried; here again controlled studies are lacking. Some mountain guides recommend exhaling against slightly pursed lips, as asthmatics have learned to do, though for a different reason.

A high-carbohydrate diet has been used on the basis that when the respiratory ratio approaches 1.0, oxygen is being most efficiently used. Frequent small feedings of easily assimilated, high-carbohydrate foods have seemed helpful to mountaineers, but much more work is needed to establish their benefit. Other considerations aside, taking only a small meal at bedtime would be beneficial by reducing the demand for oxygen for digestion during sleep, when periodic breathing and impaired ventilation exacerbate hypoxemia.

WHO SHOULD NOT GO HIGH

The increasing number of persons going to mountain resorts for skiing, or to higher mountains for other sports, and the growing number of older, or younger, or more handicapped persons seeking these recreational pleasures leads many persons to ask about their ability to tolerate altitude. Unfortunately, too few doctors can give informed opinions, most tending to be ultraconservative and warning against the hoped-for travel. In fact, there is not much hard data to support a veto!

Absolute contraindications to going to 9000 feet are few and debated. In general, the patient with heart or lung problems who is moderately active at sea level will tolerate light activity at altitude with little difficulty; prophylactic Diamox would be prudent. The individual who at sea level has poorly controlled angina, congestive failure or uncontrolled hypertension, or pulmonary insufficiency that causes dyspnea with even light activity, should probably not go above 6000 feet. Rare individuals with sickle cell trait have developed thrombotic infarcts at altitudes as low as 7500 feet. Though some have suggested that infants and young children, as well as the elderly, tolerate altitude less well, there is little solid data to support this. The rare congenital anomaly of absent pulmonary artery causes pulmonary edema at altitudes as low as 6000 feet. This is a strong reason for such an unfortunate person not to go to altitude and may even make an aircraft flight dangerous because, on most commercial flights, cabin pressures of 5000 to 6000 feet are maintained; occasionally, the cabin pressure is equivalent to an even higher altitude.

Relative contraindications to altitude are even less clearly defined. The mountain scene lures to a mountain resort or a Himalayan trek persons who would not have considered such an adventure a few decades ago. This presents the practitioner with challenges he or she may be poorly trained to accept. Individual consideration for each borderline patient is essential. For example, the experienced mountaineer who has had several bouts of HAPE or HACE must be advised differently than the neophyte who has never been to a mountain. Women in the first trimester of pregnancy probably should not go above 7000 to 8000 feet because of the very slight possibility of inducing a congenital defect in the fetus. Contraceptive pills are known to increase the risk of thromboembolic disease and pose an added risk factor at altitude, where blood tends to thicken and hematocrit to rise, even though the coagulation cascade may not be altered. Extreme obesity, by impairing pulmonary ventilation, increases the risk of altitude illness. Persons with latent psychoses, seizure disorders, or poorly defined neuromuscular problems must be individually advised.

More and more persons with known coronary artery disease, with or without angina, and with or without coronary artery bypass surgery are considering a visit to the mountains. Some persons have done things unthinkable a few years ago, as a prominent author wrote: "I had the [triple bypass] surgery in Cleveland on Monday, was home in California by Saturday, was skiing at 10,000 feet three months later, and a year later ascended Mount Everest to 22,000 feet without breathing supplementary oxygen."

A stress test may help to determine whether a visit to high mountains is prudent, but it does not replicate the cold, dry mountain environment or the type of exertion done there. Undoubtedly, the cardiovascular system is stressed above 6000 to 8000 feet, yet a large survey showed that the incidence of fatal or severe cardiac episodes at these and somewhat higher elevations is not increased. Few visitors have died from cardiac causes on the Alps or the lower Himalayas.

ACCLIMATIZATION

So much for the sojourner or visitor. We turn now to the physiologic changes which enable man to live for months or years at altitudes that cause dangerous problems for the new arrival. Approximately 40 million persons live above 8000 feet throughout the world, 12 million of them above 12,000 feet. Thousands of mountaineers have climbed above 20,000 feet, many spending many weeks there. How is this possible?

The visitor from sea level immediately uses *adjustments* or "struggle responses" to maintain oxygen supply near sea level values. After weeks and months at altitude, these adjustments have been integrated into changes that enable the body to function quite well despite the lower supply of oxygen; this is usually called *acclimatization.* After generations

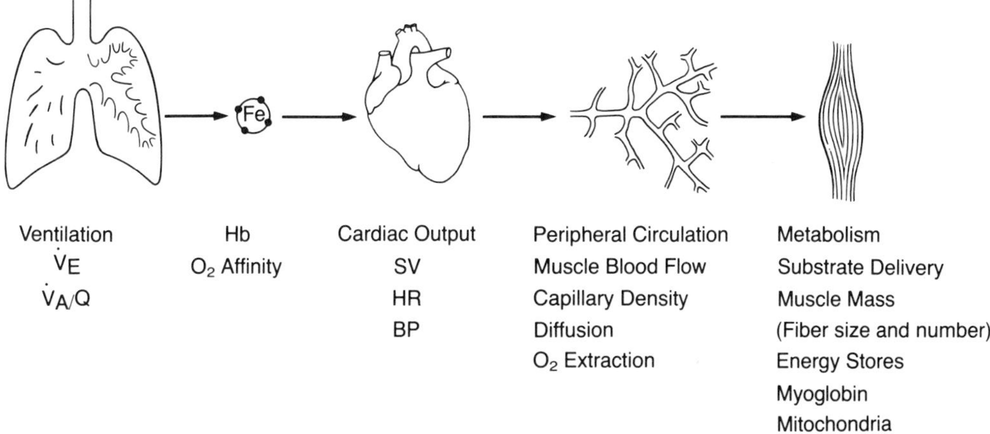

Figure 25–5. The oxygen transport system. (Courtesy of John Sutton, M.D.)

of life at altitude, the native develops genetic *adaptations* which make him somewhat different from the sea level native.

Adjustment, acclimatization, and adaptation involve (though in differing degrees) all stages of the oxygen transport system—the descriptor of how oxygen passes from ambient air to cellular mitochondria (Fig. 25–5).

First, pulmonary ventilation increases, bringing alveolar air closer to ambient air in both oxygen and carbon dioxide content. This is stimulated by the *hypoxic ventilatory response (HVR),* which is affected by many influences, among them inheritance, weight, fitness, starvation, fatigue, and probably others. The HVR appears to be "blunted" after prolonged hypoxia, but this is controversial. The stronger or brisker the HVR, the better the performance at altitude, and the less the likelihood of altitude illness, though the HVR is not an infallible predictor of success at extreme elevations because so many other factors are involved.

Passage of oxygen from pulmonary capillary to alveoli is probably by passive diffusion. No evidence supporting Haldane's theory of "oxygen secretion" in the lung has been produced thus far.

Movement of oxygen-enriched blood from lung to tissue capillaries is increased by an initial increase in cardiac output (both rate and stroke volume); this returns to normal (or even below) after a few weeks at altitude.

Both the number of red cells and their hemoglobin content increase. The immediate change is due to fluid shift from blood to interstitial tissue; later there is an absolute increase. Hypoxia is a powerful stimulus for erythropoietin formation, which stimulates the bone marrow to produce hemoglobin and red cells.

Tissue supply is improved by the opening of additional capillaries (recruitment), and perhaps by formation of new ones as well. Oxygen passes through the capillary wall into the interstitium and thence into the cell by passive diffusion. Within the cell, oxygen is used by the mitochondria, which increase in size and perhaps in number during prolonged hypoxia.

Each of these changes improves oxygen delivery, but each carries a price. Increased ventilation washes carbon dioxide out of the lungs and blood, producing a respiratory alkalosis, which is partially corrected over time by loss of base in urine. This slightly depletes the buffering power of blood (alkaline reserve), and results in a small additional increase in ventilation on exertion.

The increased red cell mass causes blood to flow more sluggishly through small vessels and may impair oxygen diffusion as the red cells form rouleaux. When the hematocrit rises excessively, as in CMS, thromboembolic problems occur. The coagulability of blood at altitude does not appear to be altered, but different studies have given different results.

These changes along the entire oxygen transport system are shown graphically in the "oxygen cascade" (Fig. 25–6). The newly arrived visitor uses the same changes in a "struggle" to sustain sea level oxygenation, but they are at first only partially compensated. The lifelong resident has integrated and modified the changes, adding to them enzymatic changes within the cell. After generations have lived at altitude, some anatomic changes evolve.

Studies of the high-altitude natives have been conducted longer and more intensively in the Andes than anywhere else in the world. From these studies emerged the concept that "Andean Man" has through the centuries acquired characteristics which sojourners and residents do not develop. Although this concept has been challenged, and although its advocates claimed more for Andean Man than could be demonstrated, it is now generally accepted that individuals born at altitude to parents whose ancestors have long been at altitude are different even from those born at sea level who stay for years at altitude.

Instead of one type of "altitude man," however, several have been identified. Sherpas in Nepal, genetically descended from Tibetans whose forebears have lived on the high Central Asian plateau for millennia, have made different adaptations than the Quechuas, whose ancestors have lived for a shorter period in the Andes. Both are born with a somewhat larger pulmonary diffusing surface than persons born at sea level, which gives them a greater area through which to absorb oxygen. Until recently, it was believed that the Sherpa does not have a higher than normal red cell count or hemoglobin, while the Quechua does; but recent studies show that there is wide variation between different groups in these people. The Sherpa does not have the large barrel-shaped chest typical of the Quechua. Anecdotal evidence suggests that the Sherpa can work harder at higher altitudes than the Quechua, but this may be a matter of experience, general health, motivation, or nutrition. One of the most impressive demonstrations of acclimatization is seen in the Andean miners who carry 100-lb bags of ore up out of mines at 16,000 feet for

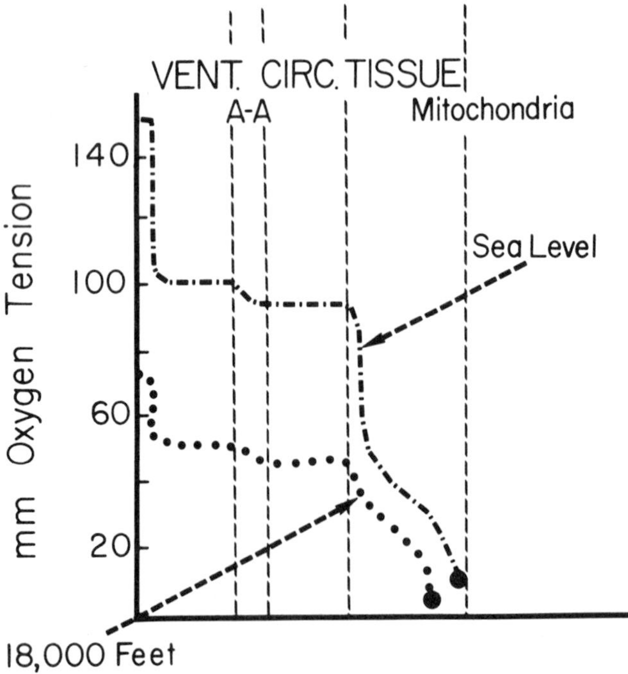

Figure 25–6. The pressure cascade, showing passage of oxygen from ambient air to mitochondria, the ultimate consumer. (VENT. = ventilation, CIRC. = circulation.)

many hours each day—and then go home to play soccer! Sherpas have done harder work high on Mount Everest than have Caucasians.

The child born at altitude acquires advantages in the womb, probably in the first weeks or months, and continues to improve them for a short time after birth. Infants brought from sea level to altitude a few weeks after birth adapt almost as well as those born at altitude, but when brought to altitude when older, do not. It seems likely that visitors and sojourners differ among themselves just as natives do, which may explain some of the peculiar differences in individual susceptibility to altitude sickness, and individual differences in performance at very great heights.

Although within a few weeks the visitor approaches sea-level well-being, not for a year or so does work capacity reach a maximum, and that is always less than at sea level. Even after years, the resident cannot match the native in capacity to work.

Can acclimatization be achieved by intermittent altitude exposure? This question has been asked for more than 50 years and is still being debated. During World War II, before pressurized aircraft and before military pilots were required to use oxygen above 10,000 feet, it was thought that repeated daily flights to moderate altitudes might produce some protection during even higher flights. In the United States, studies showed this to be untrue. However, the German air force claimed that repeated flights or "ascents" in decompression chambers did improve altitude tolerance. There is no doubt that living for weeks at moderate elevations does help fliers to tolerate higher altitudes. The issue became moot with the use of pressurized aircraft and the end of active combat. The increased interest in "alpine-style" climbing has revived the idea, and a number of experiments by Soviets and Japanese suggest that climbers can go higher faster after preliminary conditioning by daily decompression chamber ascents for several weeks or months prior to the expedition.

HOW FAST IS SLOW ENOUGH

Speed of ascent affects only the sojourner or visitor and after a few days or weeks has no effect on acclimatization.

For years, we have preached that too rapid a climb is a major contributor to altitude illness of all types. This is true—for most people most of the time—but there are important exceptions. For example, in the last 10 years, a few world-class mountaineers have made fantastically fast climbs at very great altitude—from base to summit of Mount Everest in 23 hours, and from base to summit of K-2 and return in 42 hours. Given good weather and absent a slip, these experts have emerged without serious results, but others have died. In most instances, the alpine-style climber spent considerable time living and working at 16,000 to 19,000 feet or higher before making the fast, long push. They have thus been partially acclimatized, enough apparently to protect them during the 24 to 60 hours of exposure. Others, by contrast, rushing from 11,000 to 21,000 feet without adequate preliminary acclimatization, have developed early but serious evidence of illness, which might have incapacitated or killed them should they have been delayed at altitude.

These experiences have shown that if one is to rush a very high mountain, one should be well acclimatized to a somewhat lower altitude before starting. Others have shown that rushing a high peak is possible even without acclimatization, *if and only if one can get up and down fast enough,* before altitude illness matures. For most people under most conditions, most of the time, going up slowly is wiser, safer, and more enjoyable.

Nonetheless, some people develop serious or even fatal altitude illness even though they follow the principles of going up only a thousand feet a day and "packing high but sleeping low." (This precept comes from the fact that respiration is irregular and less efficient, and thus, oxygen supply is reduced during sleep at altitude). In some cases, a respiratory infection, such as flu or the common cold, may account for the unexpected onset of HAPE or HACE. In other cases, some factor, such as illness, chilling, or extreme exertion, may be the precipitating cause.

Going up slowly is not an absolute guarantee of protection: speed must be determined by the state of well-being of the climber. If symptoms begin, the prudent climber slows down, stops, or even descends to return later and climb again. And this is equally true for the tourist visiting the mountains.

Going down to sea level after a long stay at altitude may expose the altitude resident or Himalayan climber to what has been called "reentry pulmonary edema." Several studies suggest that persons resident at altitude, or well acclimatized, may be at greater risk of HAPE when they go back up after a week or 10 days at low altitude. There is some evidence that the same is true on very high mountains.

ABILITY TO WORK AT ALTITUDE

The native is distinguished from the resident and the resident from the visitor not only by level of wellness but also by ability to do work. The better the degree of acclimatization, the more work can be done at altitude. However, even altitude natives cannot match the work possible at sea level.

Work can be described in terms of the maximal level of oxygen uptake that can be achieved by increasing the work load in stages over a short period (rarely more than 20 minutes) and is called $\dot{V}o_{2max}$ work. It is aerobic work accomplished using metabolic pathways dependent on oxygen. Aerobic work can only be done when the supply of oxygen is continuous and adequate and it often ends abruptly; runners speak of "hitting the wall." Thereafter, a short period of anaerobic work is possible, during which lactic acid accumulates, and a longer period of recovery is required to repay the "oxygen debt." Very little anaerobic work is possible at extreme heights.

What limits work at altitude? Despite a number of studies and theories, the answer is not completely clear. It seems likely that up to 10,000 to 15,000 feet, muscular fatigue is limiting. Between 15,000 and 20,000 feet, the inability to move enough air is an increasingly severe constraint. Above this, pulmonary diffusion is impaired and the lung may be the limiting organ. For persons with a normal cardiovascular system, the heart is not the limiting factor, even on top of Mount Everest. Always there is the will—the force that drives a person beyond his or her perceived limit; this may be the factor that keeps most of us from achieving the summit of Mount Everest.

$\dot{V}o_{2max}$ work is done by sprinters or in short-duration competitive games. Climbers at altitude are rarely called on for $\dot{V}o_{2max}$ effort, and then can perform only briefly and must take more time to recover.

Experienced climbers pace themselves so as to be able to perform aerobically for hours. The Andean miner and the Everest climber are each doing very different work than the experimental subject pedaling to exhaustion on a cycle ergometer. But the greater the ability to do $\dot{V}o_{2max}$ work, the greater the endurance; the two different capabilities run parallel.

Doctors knowledgeable about altitude physiology are frequently asked about the value of training at altitude. Will an individual acclimatized and trained at moderate altitude have an edge over his sea-level competitor? Where should competitors train for events held at moderate altitude? Much research and debate preceded—and followed—the 1968 Mexico City Olympics but led to only a few firm conclusions. The sprinter (who does not breathe during the race) gains nothing and may lose by training at altitude. Distance runners improve performance by many weeks of training at altitude but do not match the altitude native, born and working at moderate altitude, who consistently does better in distance events than do low-altitude natives. In shorter duration events demanding less extreme exertion, there is no clear evidence indicating that those trained at altitude do better or worse at low altitude. One factor may be that the athlete cannot train to the same extreme at altitude as at sea level and therefore is not as finely tuned.

As for training at altitude to improve performance at sea level, authorities have not made a final judgment. Many studies have been done but there is little consensus, probably because of the widely different conditions, subjects, and methods used in the studies. Anecdotal evidence suggests that training at moderate altitude (6000 feet) may improve performance in some events at sea level, but the evidence is far from conclusive and the subject needs more investigation.

HEALTH AND ILLNESS AT ALTITUDE

Does the altitude resident or native differ from his sea-level cohort in susceptibility to illness? Are there long-term benefits or risks to residence in mountainous country? For the native, life at altitude is usually rigorous: social, economic, sanitary, and educational advantages are lacking and the work is hard. On this account, one might expect the altitude native to have more illness than a sea-level cohort, but the reverse is true. Of many studies done, the most conclusive compared several hundred thousand Indian soldiers living for years at altitude with a matched group near sea level. Arteriosclerotic heart disease, hypertension, cancer (except skin cancer), and endocrine disorders were all significantly less common during altitude residence than at sea level. In fact, of 18 common diseases, only peptic ulcer, pneumonia, and goiter were more common at altitude. Other studies have shown that miscarriages, premature labor, and birth defects occur slightly more often at altitude. Term children tend to have lower birth weights, to develop more slowly, and to be smaller throughout life. Fertility is decreased during residence at altitude but is restored after descent to sea level. On the other hand, there is a tendency, shown in Colorado at least, for older persons to migrate downward. Whether this is because of health, social, or economic reasons is unclear.

A special problem involves persons of black heritage (and some of Mediterranean white heritage as well). Sickle cell anemia, sickle cell trait, and several other less common inheritable hemoglobinopathies alter oxygen transport. The sickling tendency is increased by hypoxia and the sickled red cell tends to obstruct capillaries, causing sickle cell crises. Consequently, persons with sickle cell anemia, sickle cell trait, thalassemia, and combinations of these are vulnerable to even moderate altitude. The deaths of several black recruits led the Air Force to ban blacks from flight training; the decision was later reversed. Blacks and others with sickle cell disease may have crises in mountainous country and should be advised to have the sickle screen test if planning to go high.

AVIATION

Much of our early knowledge about altitude came from balloon and later aircraft flights and decompression chamber "ascents." Flight involves very rapid ascent and responses that are quite different from those evoked in climbers, tourists, and others who generally reach altitude over a period of hours or days. Fliers show significant impairment in reflexes, judgment, and dim light vision above 10,000 feet. At 25,000 feet, the flier suddenly deprived of extra oxygen will be unconscious within minutes. Contrast this with the acclimatized mountaineer who can live and work hard at that height for days or weeks. The hypoxic experience in flight is not relevant to the subjects discussed here, except in one respect.

Modern aircraft cabins are pressurized to an altitude equivalent to 6000 or 7500 feet, which means that the passenger may go from sea level to 7500 feet in less than half an hour and remain there for hours. If the destination is a mountain resort at 9000 feet, the passenger may have approached that altitude in half an hour from sea level. Few people experience ill effects from this rapid ascent, probably because it is passive and does not demand the extra oxygen needed in strenuous exertion. But what of the patient whose activity is restricted by heart or lung disease at sea level? Few studies provide an answer, but in general, it may be said that the duration, more than the level of oxygen lack, dictates the reaction. Patients with acute illness or injury are at high risk in flight unless oxygen is given. Patients with chronic hypoxia are less likely to be affected.

SUMMARY

Three major variables—rate of ascent, altitude reached, and length of stay—determine susceptibility to altitude illness though other minor influences may also be involved. Altitude illness is a continuum or spectrum in which three forms are commingled in variable proportions: acute mountain sickness (headache, nausea, weakness); high-altitude pulmonary edema (dyspnea, cough, coma); and high-altitude cerebral edema (headache, ataxia, hallucinations, coma). High-altitutde retinal hemorrhages are frequent at higher altitude but rarely are clinically important. The visitor adjusts or accomodates and over weeks acclimatizes to altitudes as high as 19,000 to 20,000 feet. The visitor cannot achieve work capacity equal to the native and neither achieves sea-level capacity. Both deteriorate more rapidly than they acclimatize above 19,000 to 20,000 feet. Rate of ascent, if adjusted to the individual, is the best preventive; acetazolamide is the only chemical preventive of proven value. Descent at an early stage of illness is the best, indeed the only certain treatment and if delayed, death is not uncommon. Acetazolamide and dexamethasone are helpful in treatment when descent must be deferred. Simulating descent by placing the victim in a hyperbaric bag is as effective as oxygen in the treatment of AMS. There are few absolute contraindications to going to moderate altitude: uncontrollable angina, cardiac failure, pulmonary insufficiency, severe sickle cell disease, certain congenital defects, and many previous episodes of serious altitude illness.

BIBLIOGRAPHY

Anand IS, Malhotra RM, Chandrasekar Y, et al: Adult subacute mountain sickness: a syndrome of congestive heart failure in men at very high altitude. Lancet 335:561–565, 1990.

Bert P: Barometric Pressure. Bethesda, MD, Undersea Medical Society, 1978.

Cain SM, Dunn JE: Low doses of acetazolamide to aid accommodation of men to altitude. J Appl Physiol 21(2):1195–1200, 1965.

Cymerman A, Reeves JT, Sutton JR, et al: Operation Everest II: Maximal oxygen uptake at extreme altitude. J Appl Physiol 66(5):2446–2453, 1989.

Dean AG, Yip R, Hoffman RE: High incidence of mild acute mountain sickness in conference attendees at 10,000 foot altitude. Jour Wild Med 1:66–92, 1990.

DeJours P: Mount Everest and beyond: Breathing air. *In* Johansen K, Bolis L, Taylor CR (eds): A Companion to Animal Physiology. New York, Cambridge University Press, 1982, pp 17–30.

Douglas CG, Haldane JS: The causes of periodic or Cheyne-Stokes breathing. J Physiol 38:401–419, 1909.

Frayser R, Houston CS, Bryan AC, et al: Retinal hemorrhage at high altitude. N Engl J Med 282:1183–1184, 1970.

Gilbert DL: The first documented report of mountain sickness: The China or headache story. Respir Physiol 52:315–326, 1983.

Grover RF, Reeves JT: Oxygen transport in man during hypoxia: High altitude compared with chronic lung disease. Bull Eur Physiopathol Respir 15:121–128, 1979.

Hackett PH: Carbon dioxide breathing and acute mountain sickness [letter]. Lancet 1(8362):272, 1989.

Hackett PH, Bertmann J, Rodriguez G, et al: Pulmonary edema fluid protein in high-altitude pulmonary edema [letter]. JAMA 256(1):36, 1986.

Haidar M: The Tarikh-I-Rashida, a History of the Moguls of Central Asia. Elias N (Translator). London, Book Traders, 1896.

Heath D: The pathology of high altitude. Ann Sports Med 4(4):203–212, 1989.

Heath D, Williams DR: High-Altitude Medicine and Pathology. London, Butterworths, 1989.

Houston CS: Incidence of acute mountain sickness. Am Alpine J 27(59):162–165, 1985.

Houston CS: Going Higher. Boston, Little, Brown & Co, 1987.

Houston CS, Dickinson JG: Cerebral form of high altitude illness. Lancet 2(7938):758–761, 1975.

Houston CS, Sutton JR, Cymerman A: Operation Everest II: Man at high altitude. J Appl Physiol 63:877–882, 1987.

Hultgren HN: Coronary heart disease and trekking. Jour Wild Med 1:154–161, 1990.

King AB, Robinson SM: Ventilation response to hypoxia and acute mountain sickness. Aerospace Med 43(4):419–421, 1972.

Lane PA, Githens JH: Splenic syndrome at mountain altitudes in sickle cell trait: Its occurrence in nonblack persons. JAMA 253:2252–2254, 1985.

McGuire W, Spragg RG, Cohen AB, et al: Studies on the pathogenesis of the adult respiratory distress syndrome. J Clin Invest 69:543–553, 1982.

Milledge JS: The ventilatory response to hypoxia: How much is good for a mountaineer? Postgrad Med J 63:169–172, 1987.

Montgomery AB, Mills J, Luce JM: Incidence of acute mountain sickness at intermediate altitude. JAMA 261(5):732–734, 1989.

Moore LG, Harrison GL, McCullough RE, et al: Low acute hypoxic ventilatory response and hypoxic depression in acute altitude sickness. J Appl Physiol 60(4):1407–1412, 1986.

Mosso A: Life of Man in the High Alps. London, T Fisher Unwin, 1989.

Oelz O, Maggiorini M, Ritter M, et al: Nifedipine for high altitude pulmonary edema. Lancet 2:1241–1244, 1989.

Pugh LG, Gill MB, Lahiri S, et al: Muscular exercise at great altitude. J Appl Physiol 1964 19(3):431–440, 1964.

Ravenhill TH: Some experiences of mountain sickness in the Andes. J Trop Med Hyg 1620:313–320, 1913.

Reeves JT, Groves BM, Sutton JR, et al: Operation Everest II: Preservation of cardiac function at extreme altitude. J Appl Physiol 63(2):531–539, 1987.

Reeves JT, Groves BM, Sutton JR, et al: Oxygen transport during exercise at extreme altitude: Operation Everest II. Ann Emerg Med 16(9):993–998, 1987.

Reeves JT, Houston CS, Sutton JR: Operation Everest II: Resistance and susceptibility to chronic hypoxia in man. J R Soc Med 82:513–514, 1988.

Reeves JT, Jokl P, Cohn JE: Performance of Olympic runners at altitude of 7,350 and 5,350 feet. *In* Jokl E, Jokl P (eds): Exercise and Altitude. Baltimore, MD, University Park Press, 1968, pp 49–54.

Reeves JT, Stenmark KR, Voelkel NF: Possible role of leukotrienes in the pathogenesis of pulmonary hypertensive disorders. *In* Said SI (ed): The Pulmonary Circulation and Acute Lung Injury. Mt Kisco, NY, Futura Publishing, 1985, pp 337–356.

Rennie ID: Will mountain trekkers have heart attacks [editorial]? JAMA 261(7):1045–1046, 1989.

Santiago TV, Neubauer JA, Edelman NH: Correlation between ventilation and brain blood flow during hypoxic sleep. J Appl Physiol 60(2):295–298, 1986.

Schoene RB, Hackett PH, Henderson WR, et al: High altitude pulmonary edema: Characteristics of lung lavage fluid. JAMA 256(1):63–69, 1986.

Schoene RB, Lahiri S, Hackett PH, et al: The relationship of hypoxic ventilatory response to exercise performance on Mount Everest. J Appl Physiol 56(6):1478–1483, 1984.

Schoene RB, Roach RC, Harrison GL, et al: The effect of end positive airway pressure on subjects with high altitude pulmonary edema and normals during exercise at 4400 m on Mt. McKinley [abstract]. *In* Sutton JR, Houston CS, Coates G (eds): Hypoxia and Cold. New York, Praeger, 1987, p 543.

Schoene RB, Swenson ER, Pizzo C, et al: High altitude pulmonary edema (HAPE): A permeability leak [abstract]. *In* Sutton JR, Houston CS, Coates G (eds): Hypoxia: The Tolerable Limits. Indianapolis, IN, Benchmark Press, 1988, p 379.

Scoggin CH, Hyers TM, Reeves JT, et al: High-altitude pulmonary edema in the children and young adults of Leadville, Colorado. N Engl J Med 297:1269–1273, 1977.

Shlim DR, Houston R: Helicopter rescues and deaths among trekkers in Nepal. JAMA 261(7):1017–1019, 1989.

Singh I, Kapila CC, Khanna PK, et al: High-altitude pulmonary edema. *In* Jokl E, Jokl P (eds): Exercise and Altitude. Baltimore, MD, University Park Press, 1968, pp 165–181.

Singh I, Khanna PK, Srivastava MC, et al: Acute mountain sickness. N Engl J Med 280(4):175–218, 1969.

Strohl KP, Fouke JM: Periodic breathing at altitude. Semin Respir Med 5(2):169–174, 1983.

Sui GJ, Liu YH, Cheng XS, et al: Subacute infantile mountain sickness. J Pathol 155:161–170, 1988.
Sutton JR, Reeves JT, Wagner PD, et al: Operation Everest II: Oxygen transport during exercise at extreme simulated altitude. J Appl Physiol 64(4):1309–1321, 1988.
Ward MP: High altitude deterioration. Proc R Soc Lond (Series B) 143:40–42, 1954.
Ward MP, Milledge JS, West JB: High altitude medicine and physiology. Philadelphia, PA, University of Pennsylvania Press, 1989.
Webb P: Periodic breathing during sleep. J Appl Physiol 37(6):899–903, 1974.

26

MEDICAL ASPECTS OF SCUBA AND BREATH-HOLD DIVING

Eric P. Kindwall, MD
Richard H. Strauss, MD

Swimming underwater while using a self-contained underwater breathing apparatus (scuba) is a noncompetitive sport enjoyed by a large number of people. An astonishing 5.8 million divers have been certified by the national sport scuba diving accreditation associations. Of these, 2 to 2.8 million individuals make at least one dive a year. More than 400,000 Americans are trained to scuba dive each year and do so in inland bodies of water as well as in the oceans. Scuba diving, like driving a car, is not particularly dangerous when done carefully, but it does require training. The hazards involved, other than drowning, are not obvious, but they must be kept in mind so that they can be avoided. Breath-hold diving is simpler and less hazardous than scuba diving and is practiced by many persons who enjoy seeing shallower depths (where most of the sea life is) without the complexity and expense of scuba equipment.

Although the dangers of diving have been popularly associated with great depths, it is important to recognize that both shallow breath-hold and scuba diving—even in a swimming pool—present very real risks to the diver. The risks of scuba diving are due largely to the breathing of gases as ambient (surrounding) pressure increases during descent or decreases during ascent in water. Thus, it is helpful to review a few physical principles that govern the behavior of gases.

PHYSICAL PRINCIPLES

People normally live at the bottom of a sea of air. The weight of this air exerts a pressure on the body surface that is defined at sea level as 1 atmosphere (atm). Atmospheric pressure decreases relatively slowly with increasing altitude. In Denver, at an altitude of 5221 feet, ambient pressure is 0.83 atm. Under water, however, small changes in depth result in significant changes in pressure. A resident of Denver can return to 1 atm of pressure by diving 6 feet below the surface of a swimming pool.

A column of liquid exerts a pressure that is proportional to its height, its density, and the acceleration of gravity. At a depth of 33 feet, seawater exerts an additional pressure of 1 atm on the submerged diver—a total pressure twice that to which the diver is exposed at sea level. (A list of pressure equivalents is given in Table 26–1.)

TABLE 26–1. PRESSURE EQUIVALENTS

1 atmosphere	= 33 feet of seawater (fsw)
	= 34 feet of fresh water
	= 29.9 in Hg
	= 760 mm Hg
	= 14.7 pounds per square inch (psi)
	= 1 kg/cm^2

The tissues of the body are composed primarily of water, which is nearly incompressible and is thus unaffected by pressures within the usual diving range. Gases, however, are compressible. The behavior of gases is well described by the *ideal gas law:*

$$PV = nRT$$

where P is absolute pressure, V is volume, n is the number of moles of gas, R is the universal gas constant, and T is the absolute temperature. Several simpler gas laws originate from the ideal gas law and are commonly used under conditions associated with diving.

Boyle's law states that at a constant temperature, the volume of a given mass of gas is inversely proportional to its pressure. Stated mathematically:

$$PV = K$$

where K is a constant. Thus, if absolute pressure is doubled, the volume of a mass of gas is halved. Gas volume changes are particularly noticeable near the surface (Fig. 26–1).

In addition to the pressure and volume changes that affect gas spaces during submersion, there are also changes in the partial pressure of individual gases within these spaces. *Dalton's law* of partial pressure states that in a mixture of gases, the pressure exerted by each gas is the same as it would exert if it alone occupied the same volume; the total pressure is the sum of the partial pressures of the component gases. As ambient pressure increases, the total pressure of a gas mixture increases. The partial pressure of each gas within the mixture increases proportionally, although its percentage remains constant.

In general, the biologic effects of a gas depend on its partial pressure. This is because both diffusion and the amount of gas dissolved in a solvent are proportional to partial pressure. Thus, supplying the proper amount of oxygen to tissue depends on the partial

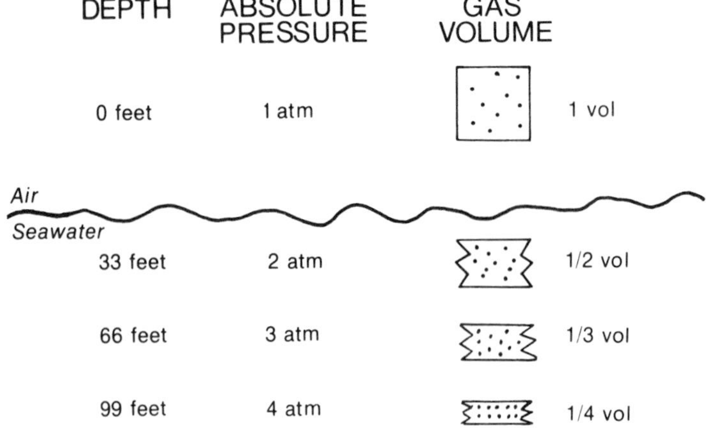

Figure 26–1. As depth increases, pressure increases and the volume of a mass of gas decreases. (*From* Strauss RH (ed): Sports Medicine and Physiology. Philadelphia, WB Saunders, 1979.)

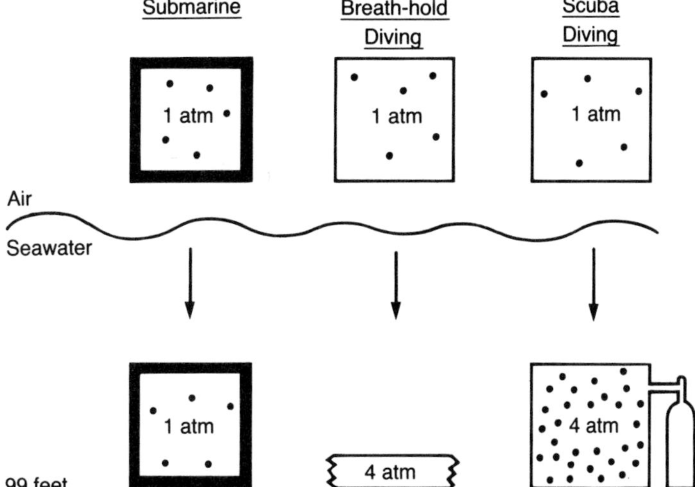

Figure 26–2. Within a submarine, pressure remains at 1 atm absolute (the pressure at sea level). In breath-hold diving, the lungs are compressed and the gas pressure within them is approximately the same as the surrounding (ambient) pressure. In scuba diving, gas is supplied at ambient pressure so that respiration can continue. (*From* Strauss RH (ed): Diving Medicine. New York, Grune & Stratton, 1976; with permission.)

pressure of oxygen (Po_2) and not merely on the total gas pressure or the percentage of oxygen. Similarly, the partial pressures of carbon dioxide and nitrogen determine their biologic effects.

Henry's law states that at a given temperature, the mass of a gas dissolved in a given volume of solvent is proportional to the pressure of the gas with which it is in equilibrium. Thus, as pressure increases during scuba diving, more and more nitrogen is dissolved in the body. During ascent, this nitrogen comes out of solution and, under certain circumstances, may cause *decompression sickness* (to be described later in this chapter).

Those who go underwater have several choices (Fig. 26–2):

1. They can ride in a submarine, the hull of which is designed to withstand hydrostatic pressure so that ambient pressure remains at 1 atm. Under these circumstances, there are no volume or pressure changes within the body.
2. They can hold their breath and dive. Gas pressure within the lungs approximates ambient pressure, and the volume within the thorax must decrease proportionally.
3. They can submerge while breathing compressed gas from scuba equipment. Under these circumstances, gas pressure within the lungs remains close to ambient pressure, but lung volumes remain normal because the person continues to breathe while underwater.

EQUIPMENT

At the surface, breathing generally is done through a snorkel (tube) that runs from the mouth to the surface (Fig. 26–3). This allows the diver to breathe without lifting the face from the water. The self-contained underwater breathing apparatus used by most sport divers consists of a tank containing compressed air and a regulator that delivers air through a mouthpiece when the diver inhales. Air entering the mouthpiece is automatically kept at about the same pressure as the surrounding water. Exhaled air is released into the water as bubbles.

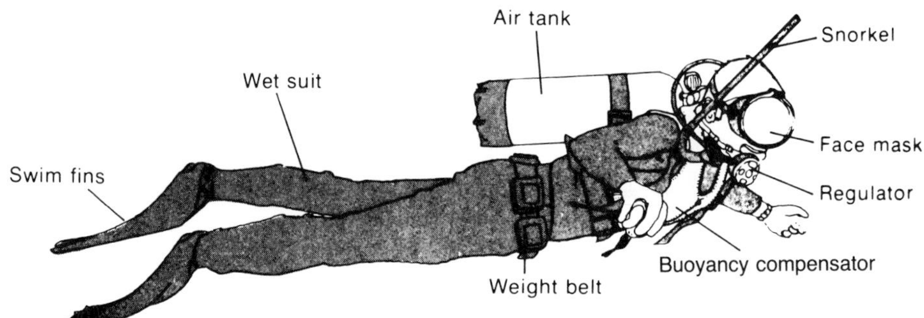

Figure 26–3. Equipment used in scuba diving. (*From* Strauss RH (ed): Sports Medicine and Physiology. Philadelphia, WB Saunders, 1979.)

Occasionally, during severe exercise, the demand for air volume may exceed the regulator's capacity. A subsequent feeling of dyspnea may contribute to panic. Furthermore, an air tank is exhausted more quickly as depth increases. A gauge indicating tank pressure is generally used by divers so that they do not run out of air under water, a dangerous situation for several reasons.

A face mask is worn for clear vision under water. In air, most of the refraction of light takes place at the front of the eye where the cornea meets air. When the eye is submerged in water, this refraction is lost and vision is out of focus. Wearing a face mask (Fig. 26–4) traps a pocket of air in front of the eye so that focusing can occur. Refraction at the front of the mask underwater makes objects appear closer or larger than they actually are—explaining, in part, why a fish that got away always seems bigger.

Persons who wear glasses can have special lenses attached to the inside of the mask. Contact lenses can be worn under a mask but may be lost if water comes in contact with the eye. On rare occasions, bubbles have formed under hard contact lenses during or following a dive, leading to transient edema of the cornea.

In cold water, a foam rubber wet suit is worn for insulation. Lead weights compensate for the buoyancy of the air trapped within the foam rubber. The most frequent cause of death among scuba divers is drowning. Many of these drownings could have been prevented if the diver had simply remembered to unbuckle and drop the weight belt in a time of emergency. The inflatable buoyancy compensator rarely should be used for rapid ascent to the surface. Rather, it is inflated at the surface for flotation, or air is added

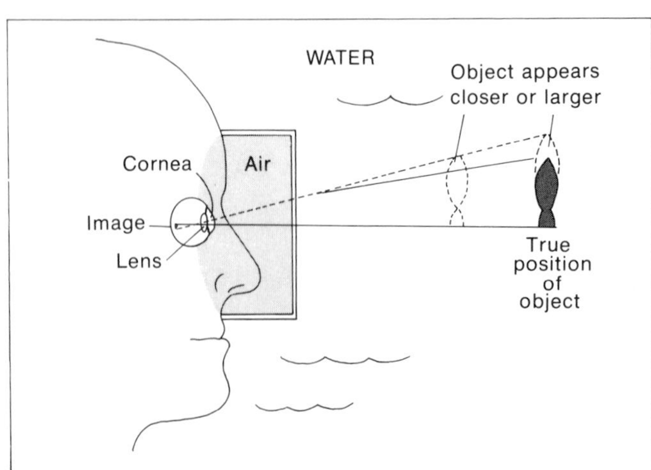

Figure 26–4. A face mask is worn for clear vision underwater. (*From* Strauss RH (ed): Sports Medicine and Physiology. Philadelphia, WB Saunders, 1979.)

underwater to adjust buoyancy. Rubber swim fins are worn on the feet for added propulsion.

BREATH-HOLD BLACKOUT

Many of the interesting forms of sea life that can be viewed by a scuba diver also can be seen by a breath-hold diver. The abundance of life decreases as water becomes deeper, because sunlight is the foundation of the food chain and water acts as a filter for light. Breath-hold diving is simpler, cheaper, and safer than scuba diving but often requires more exertion in the water. Basic equipment consists of a face mask, fins, and a snorkel. Persons who merely wish to swim at the surface and look at the bottom can do so with little expenditure of energy, given calm water conditions. Anyone who performs breath-hold dives should be aware of the danger associated with hyperventilation.

Each year, a number of persons die from loss of consciousness (blackout) underwater and from subsequent drowning. Breath-hold blackout occurs almost exclusively in young males who are demonstrating how far they can swim underwater or how long they can remain submerged.[1] Such incidents have occurred in guarded swimming pools. Swimmers often learn through experience that by hyperventilating immediately before submerging, they can extend their time underwater. However, unless alerted to the danger, they fail to realize that this maneuver can lead to loss of consciousness without warning as a result of hypoxia.

Figure 26–5 shows what happens to gases within the alveoli of the lung during breath holding: P_{CO_2} rises slowly, but P_{O_2} falls more rapidly. These changes are more pronounced during exericse.

When we try to hold our breath as long as possible, we are forced to terminate breath holding at a time (the breaking point) when the urge to breathe can no longer be suppressed. The breaking point is determined primarily by alveolar (arterial) P_{CO_2}, but other factors, such as arterial P_{O_2}, attention, motivation, and lung volume play a role.

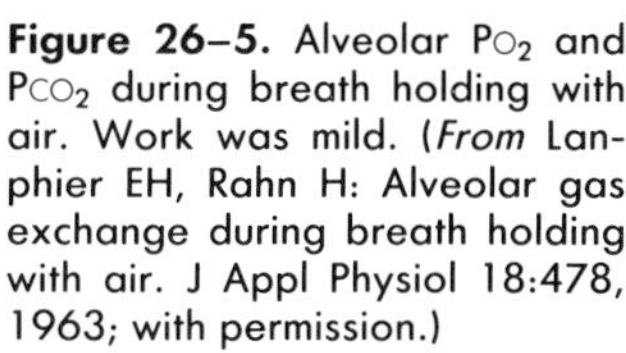

Figure 26–5. Alveolar P_{O_2} and P_{CO_2} during breath holding with air. Work was mild. (*From* Lanphier EH, Rahn H: Alveolar gas exchange during breath holding with air. J Appl Physiol 18:478, 1963; with permission.)

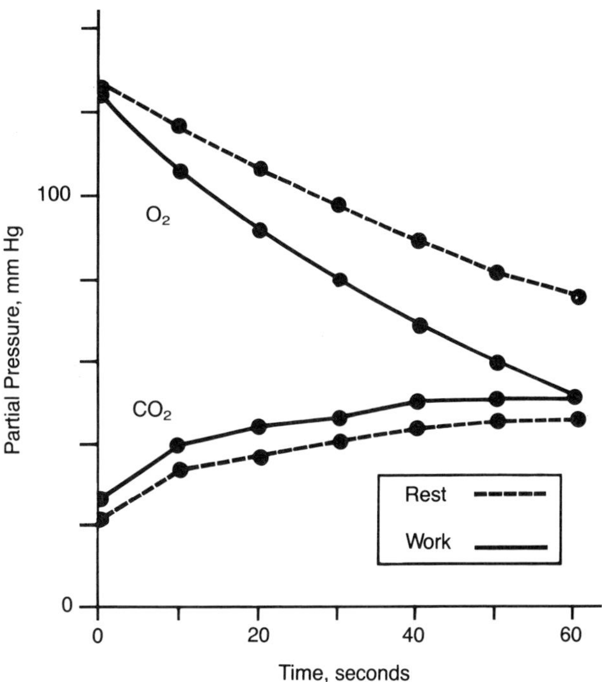

Greater lung volume permits longer breath holding, and sport divers usually inspire to nearly maximal lung volume before diving. Voluntary breath holding without hyperventilation (Fig. 26–5) is terminated even in highly motivated adults before alveolar Po_2 is sufficiently low to cause unconsciousness. (Small children may prolong breath holding to the point of cyanosis, unconsciousness, and convulsions.) However, hyperventilation can significantly decrease alveolar Pco_2 and body stores of carbon dioxide so that the urge to breathe is delayed during subsequent breath holding.

Unfortunately, hyperventilation increases body stores of oxygen only slightly; Po_2 may approach 140 mm Hg, but the quantity of oxygen in the blood is little increased because arterial hemoglobin is normally almost fully saturated with oxygen. As a result, after hyperventilation, arterial Po_2 may decrease to the point that consciousness is lost before arterial Pco_2 is sufficiently increased to result in a strong urge to breathe. The stimulus to breathing furnished by low arterial Po_2 is weak enough to be ignored by a highly motivated person. A practical guideline for divers is to take only one or two deep breaths before submerging.

Pressure changes during diving can increase further the chances for unconsciousness. During submergence, alveolar Po_2 may become quite low. Upon ascent, the ambient pressure decreases and gas within the lung expands. Alveolar Pco_2 also decreases, and the urge to breathe diminishes—a paradoxic event in terms of survival. Thus, it can be seen that there are really two types of shallow water blackout: the first involving a drop of arterial Po_2 caused by vigorous underwater swimming, and the second caused by the expansion of gas in the lungs (with a corresponding drop in alveolar and arterial Po_2) as the diver ascends from depth near the termination of his dive.

BAROTRAUMA OF DESCENT ("SQUEEZE")

During descent in water, ambient pressure increases but pressure within an unventilated gas space does not. The term "squeeze" is used to describe the result of such a process—usually hemorrhage. For squeeze to occur, a gas space must exist that is not entirely collapsible, and the gas within the space must not equilibrate fully with gas at ambient pressure.

Ears

Middle ear squeeze is a common problem among divers. As a scuba diver descends and water pressure increases, the diver normally opens the eustachian tubes every few feet so that air can flow into the middle ear cavity. By this method of "equalizing" pressure, the pressure across the tympanic membrane is kept small and no damage occurs. However, if pressure is not equalized during descent, as when the eustachian tube is edematous during an upper respiratory tract infection or allergy, damage may occur. Vessels within the lining of the middle ear contain blood at approximately ambient pressure. When the pressure within the middle ear is sufficiently less than ambient pressure, the walls of small vessels rupture and hemorrhage occurs.

The opening of the eustachian tube in the pharynx is slitlike and often functions as a check valve, permitting easy egress of air from the middle ear, but making entry of air difficult. If the diver descends more than about 4 feet without equalizing middle ear pressure, the slitlike opening of the eustachian tube is compressed shut. If this occurs, further descent will be impossible without danger. The diver must remember to descend no more than 4 feet without equalizing pressure.

In ear squeeze, the examining physician can see hemorrhage that occurs within the tympanic membrane. The degree of hemorrhage usually reflects the severity of the barotrauma, and sometimes blood accumulates within the middle ear. The tympanic membrane may itself be ruptured, and cold water that enters the middle ear can cause vertigo and disorientation under water—a hazardous state.

The treatment for ear squeeze is to avoid diving until the ear has healed and all symptoms have cleared. A decongestant may be used. Ear squeeze generally can be avoided if the diver simply heeds the warning of ear pain. On feeling any ear pain, the diver should stop the descent, ascend a few feet, and try to equalize ear pressure. If the ear pressure cannot be equalized, the dive should be terminated. Diving should be avoided when respiratory infection or allergy is present.

Many divers can equalize ear pressure without any conscious effort, but others use maneuvers such as trying to exhale forcefully against the pinched nose to force air through the eustachian tubes. This maneuver is occasionally associated with sudden deafness and tinnitus, usually in one ear. A probable mechanism is that increased pressure in the thorax and abdomen is transmitted to the cerebrospinal fluid as blood engorges veins within the spinal column. The increased pressure is in turn transmitted from the cerebrospinal fluid, by way of the endolymphatic and cochlear ducts, to the fluid of the inner ear. The increased perilymphatic pressure tends to rupture the round or oval window of the inner ear, with loss of fluid into the middle ear, which is at a lower pressure. The neural portion of the inner ear is damaged in the process. If a round or oval window rupture occurs, the diver should be put on complete bed rest with the head slightly elevated. Coughing should be suppressed (medically if necessary) and the diver should be cautioned against straining at the stool. If the symptoms do not disappear within 72 hours, surgical exploration and repair are mandatory.

Many experienced divers use a method of equalizing ear pressure that may well be safer (the Frenzel manuever). They increase pressure within the pharynx by occluding the nose, closing the glottis, and then contracting the pharyngeal muscles. Air is thus forced through the eustachian tubes without altering thoracic pressure. This can be performed with the mouth open or with a regulator in place, because the tongue and soft palate occlude the posterior oral cavity.

Barotrauma rarely affects the ears during ascent because, as noted before, the eustachian tube acts somewhat like a one-way valve. Air escapes from the middle ear with relative ease, although it may enter with difficulty. Still, occasional divers become vertiginous during ascent (alternobaric vertigo). It is believed that this occurs when the pressure within one middle ear slightly exceeds that in the other owing to a partially occluded eustachian tube. The pressure inequality, transmitted to the cochlea by way of the round and oval windows, sends unequal sensory stimulation to the brain, where it is interpreted as spinning. Similarly, if the eustachian tubes are equally patent, but one inner ear has old damage and is less sensitive, the same phenomenon results. Symptoms usually clear within the first few feet of ascent but, if severe, can disorient or panic a diver. Rarely, transient vertigo has also been observed in divers during descent.

Other Parts of the Head

Squeeze can affect any gas space that does not equilibrate with ambient pressure. Eye goggles are not worn because they can result in conjunctival hemorrhage. The diver's face mask encloses the nose as well as the eyes so that compressed air can reach the mask. Sinus squeeze causes pain over the affected sinus and sometimes results in extravasation of blood, which may be observed in the face mask on surfacing. Frontal sinus squeeze is the most painful, and sphenoid sinus pain is referred to the occiput or the vertex of the skull.

A gas pocket under the amalgam in a filled tooth can also cause excruciating pain when subjected to a change in pressure. If the tooth is in the upper jaw, it may be difficult to differentiate a tooth squeeze from a maxillary sinus squeeze.

BAROTRAUMA OF ASCENT

As ambient pressure decreases during ascent, gas within the lungs tends to expand in accordance with Boyle's law. This effect becomes especially important at shallow depths, where a relatively small change of depth can lead to a large change in gas volume. Thus, a 33-foot ascent from 99 feet (4 atmospheres absolute [ATA]) to 66 feet (3 ATA) changes gas volume by the ratio of 4 to 3, an increase of 33%. However, ascent from a depth of 33 feet (2 ATA) to the surface (1 ATA) leads to a 100% increase in gas volume.

Pulmonary Barotrauma

The ascending scuba diver must permit expanding gas to escape from the lungs either by breathing normally or, in case of an equipment problem, by exhaling continuously. Failure to do this can lead to overdistention of the lungs, tearing of lung tissue, and escape of air from the alveoli. The extra-alveolar air may travel to any of several locations:

1. Small amounts may dissect no further than the interstitial tissue of the lung.
2. Dissection may occur along vessels to the mediastinum and then to subcutaneous tissue or elsewhere.
3. Air may enter pulmonary vessels and be carried out to distant parts of the body as arterial emboli.
4. Pneumothorax may occur.

Air Embolism

Small vessels rupture as lung tissue is overstretched by expanding gas. Bubbles are carried quickly to the heart and then by the arterial system to various parts of the body. The bubbles lodge in small arterial vessels, occluding circulation beyond that point. They are stabilized by surface tension; loss of gas by diffusion is low.

Air embolism to the brain generally becomes apparent within seconds as a strokelike syndrome. A typical history is that of a scuba diver who ascends rapidly, often under emergency conditions, reaches the surface, gasps, and sinks unconscious into the water. If not rescued, the diver drowns. Almost any sign of cerebral damage may appear, including focal paralysis, paresthesias, or visual disturbances. Hemoptysis sometimes occurs.

Dog studies have demonstrated that the alveoli rupture at a transpulmonic pressure of 80 mm Hg.[2] This corresponds to a seawater depth of 3.47 feet. Thus, ascent to the surface from a depth of 4 feet while holding one's breath with fully expanded lungs can theoretically be fatal. Trainees should remember that cerebral air embolism has occurred on several occasions during scuba practice in a standard swimming pool. Decompression sickness does not occur under such shallow conditions.

Air embolism has occurred under conditions in which observers were sure that breath holding had not occurred. It is hypothesized that local obstruction to egress of air may be responsible for barotrauma to lung tissue. Potential causes of obstruction include broncholiths, gas-filled cysts, active asthma, and viscous secretions. It is possible for a diver wearing an inflated buoyancy compensator vest to surface from 50 feet in 7 seconds.

This would necessitate an unimpeded expansion of the air in the lungs to 2.5 times what its volume had been at depth during this short interval. For this reason, persons with obstruction to egress of air should not dive. Occasionally, a person may suffer from air embolism without any apparent cause.

Cerebral air embolism is a medical emergency, and treatment in a hyperbaric (high pressure) chamber should be initiated as soon as possible. Proper first aid is also important. Studies have shown that placing the patient in a steep Trendelenburg position lying on either side (to prevent aspiration) will cause the cerebral vessels to dilate, allowing bubbles to pass through the brain in the direction of arterial flow.[3,4] The Trendelenburg position, if used, should be at 30 to 60 degrees head down and maintained, if possible, for a maximum of 10 to 15 minutes. Prolonging the head-down position causes cerebral edema. Any benefits of increasing the hydrostatic pressure within the cerebral circulation should be maximized within that time. Obviously, if the patient is not breathing or is pulseless, cardiopulmonary resuscitation (CPR) would take precedence. The Trendelenburg maneuver should be used only when it will not otherwise compromise the patient. After the patient is returned to the horizontal position, it is important not to raise the head above the chest. The patient should be given oxygen continuously through a mask with a tight seal to insure a high inspired Po_2. The purpose of using oxygen is to denitrogenate the patient, not necessarily to oxygenate him. A good rule of thumb is that the mask should fit tightly enough so that the patient could breathe from it were he lying on his back underwater.

In the pressure chamber, the classic treatment schedule is similar to that used for decompression sickness except that initial pressurization is to 165 feet of seawater (fsw), or 6 ATA, with air breathing for 15 to 30 minutes. This initial high pressure is believed to decrease the size of bubbles sufficiently to permit them to be carried to smaller vessels, thus decreasing the size of the affected area. Bubble absorption also begins. In most civilian chambers, mixed gases are breathed while at 6 ATA: for example, 50% nitrogen/50% oxygen or 50% helium/50% oxygen. This immediately provides the patient with 3 atm of oxygen and decreases or eliminates iatrogenic nitrogen being introduced into the patient. Chamber pressure is subsequently decreased to 60 fsw so that 100% oxygen may be breathed with only a small risk of convulsions. Corticosteroids are no longer given because they have been shown in animal studies not to be effective unless given prior to embolization.[5] On the other hand, lidocaine, given in antiarrhythmic dosage, has been found to protect the brain following embolism.[6] Although massive cerebral edema leads to death within minutes, those victims who reach a hyperbaric chamber while still alive have an excellent chance for full recovery.

Dog experiments carried out by Leitch and associates[7] have shown that in experimental air embolism, increasing treatment pressure beyond an initial depth of 60 fsw offers no advantage. Once this threshold is reached, the mechanical effect of pressure will have maximally cleared bubbles within about 8 minutes. In their studies, they found no advantage in going initially to 165 fsw before oxygen breathing was started at 60 fsw. Similar results have been reported by Hart[8] in a series of patients with gas embolism who were all treated at depths no greater than 66 fsw in a monoplace chamber. His results were similar to those achieved by one of the authors (EPK), who treated 32 cases of air embolism using an initial pressure of 165 fsw.[9]

Cerebral air embolism is often accompanied by mediastinal emphysema sufficient to be visible on radiographs. Subcutaneous emphysema, palpable particularly in the supraclavicular fossae, may also be present. Mediastinal and subcutaneous emphysema do not require treatment in a pressure chamber if they occur without manifestations of air embolism and if they are asymptomatic or cause only mild symptoms, such as substernal discomfort or voice change. The breathing of oxygen by mask is usually sufficient treatment.

Pneumothorax occurs infrequently as a result of pulmonary overdistention in diving.

In contrast, during the use of positive-pressure breathing in patients, pneumothorax is well known and cerebral gas embolism is rare. Uncomplicated pneumothorax in a diver is treated in the usual manner. If it accompanies cerebral air embolism, the latter must be treated in a chamber. As ambient pressure increaes, additional air may enter the pneumothorax. When ambient pressure is subsequently decreased, a tension pneumothorax may result and require treatment. A chest tube may be inserted prophylactically before decompression.

DECOMPRESSION SICKNESS

Decompression sickness first became a problem in the 1800s when men began working in the compressed-air environment of tunnels and caissons, the closed underwater compartments used in the building of bridge foundations. Triger[10] reported the first human case of decompression sickness in 1845. While caissons and tunnels are being constructed below water level, air is maintained at a pressure slightly greater than that of the water to keep water out. After returning to the surface, these workers sometimes noticed steady, boring pains similar to a toothache, most often in the hip or knee joints. "One pays only on leaving," it was said of such work. The pains started within a few minutes or hours after surfacing and lasted several hours or longer. On the Brooklyn bridge project (1870), the afflicted men who limped were said by coworkers to be doing the "Grecian bend," a contortionist posture in walking assumed by fashionable ladies at that time.

The "bends" and "caisson disease" are synonymous with what we today call decompression sickness. The disease not only may affect the limbs directly but can also damage the central nervous system. Paraplegia is a particularly serious problem that occurs among sport divers today.

Decompression sickness is caused by the formation of gas bubbles in the blood and body tissues when ambient pressure is decreased. Gas absorption by the body is a critical factor in this illness. The quantity of a given gas dissolved in a tissue is proportional to the partial pressure of that gas within the tissue. As a scuba diver descends from the surface to a depth of 66 feet, the surrounding pressure increases from 1 ATA to 3 ATA and the partial pressure of nitrogen triples. As a result, a gradient exists for the net flow of nitrogen from the alveoli to the blood and finally into tissue. After some time at depth, equilibrium will be reached and all tissues will contain about three times as much nitrogen as before the dive.

When the cork is removed from a bottle of champagne, bubbles appear. During storage, the liquid is in equilibrium with the gas at its surface (mainly carbon dioxide) and is saturated with this gas at a pressure greater than 1 atm. When the bottle is uncorked, the ambient pressure is suddenly decreased. The champagne suddenly becomes supersaturated—that is, the surrounding pressure is less than the total gas pressure within the liquid. Supersaturation is a necessary condition for the type of bubble formation and growth discussed here. The formation of bubbles in divers on ascent is somewhat analogous to the formation of bubbles in champagne when the bottle is uncorked.

Pathogenesis

In severe cases of decompression sickness in which a diver or laboratory animal has died, bubbles have been reported everywhere: within blood vessels, presumably having impeded circulation; extravascularly, distorting tissues; and, possibly, within cells. In the more common, nonlethal form of decompression sickness, the location of bubbles is less clear. After some dives, bubbles can be detected in the venous circulation because they reflect ultrasonic signals of a Doppler flowmeter. even though decompression sickness has not occurred. There appears to be a correlation between increasing numbers of bubbles and the severity of some types of decompression sickness.

Numerous changes in the blood have been noted after decompression: clumping of red blood cells, formation of rouleaux, sludging of blood in small vessels, and a decrease in the number of platelets. Hematologic changes are believed to be largely a result of the gas-blood interface of bubbles. Hemoconcentration occurs, possibly from increased capillary permeability. Decompression sickness is association with release of numerous biologically active substances into blood.

Clinical Manifestations

Symptoms may appear during or immediately after decompression or, more usually, after a delay of minutes to hours. The delay may be due in part to the growth of bubbles and, perhaps more important, to the gradual progression of pathologic processes, such as swelling, after the original damage to tissue by bubbles.

SPINAL CORD AND BRAIN

Central nervous system "bends" is an especially serious type of decompression sickness because it can cause permanent nerve damage, such as paraplegia. According to the report of 1987 diving accidents compiled by the Diver's Alert Network based at Duke University, 75.6% of all cases of decompression sickness involved the central nervous system. Of these, 11.5% were "pain only" decompression sickness, and 12.6% carried the diagnosis of air embolism. Almost all of the victims were recreational divers. The high incidence of neurologic symptoms and signs among sport divers stands in stark contrast to a 25% incidence found in naval divers by Rivera.[11] Perhaps sport divers do more repetitive diving, dive closer to the edge of the tables, and are not in as good physical condition. It is also of interest that the vast majority of cases of decompression sickness involved "no decompression dives" (in which the diver spent all of his time at a single specific depth) and that the accident occurred after more than 1 day of repetitive diving. The reason most decompression sickness cases occur after 2 or 3 days of diving activity is not clear but could be secondary to retained nitrogen in the body, which builds up to a clinically significant level after more than 1 day. Fatigue and/or dehydration secondary to the use of alcohol may play a role. People on diving vacations may "party" extensively in the evenings. Decompression sickness on the second or third day may represent a cumulative effect.

Neurologic lesions often involve the spinal cord, particularly the thoracic segments, but also the upper lumbar and lower cervical segments. The white matter of the cord, rather than the gray matter, is generally affected. A primary cause of damage appears to be evolution of bubbles within the venous vertebral plexus, leading to stasis and obstruction of blood. Early lesions consist of small hemorrhages followed by degeneration of nerve fibers. Bubbles also may arise within the substance of the spinal cord itself. This is probably the case in situations in which there is an extremely rapid onset of paralysis following surfacing.

It is important that the diver and the physician recognize the early manifestations of spinal cord decompression sickness because immediate treatment in a pressure chamber may result in recovery, whereas delay significantly decreases the chances of a good outcome. Soon after surfacing, the diver's first symptom may be transient back pain radiating to the abdomen, which is often attributed to the lifting of air tanks. Therefore, the first manifestation to catch the diver's attention is usually a feeling of "pins and needles" in

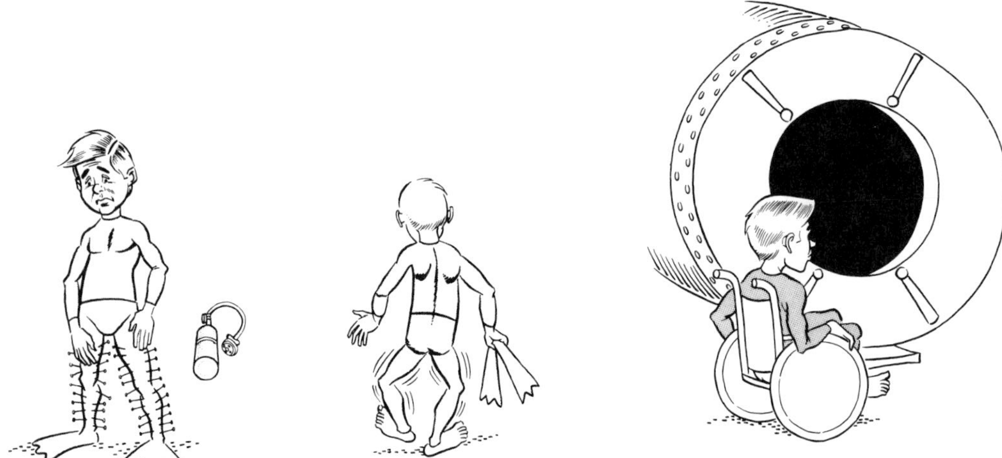

Figure 26–6. Decompression sickness of the spinal cord can progress, over a period of minutes or hours, from a feeling of "pins and needles" in the legs, to difficulty in walking, and finally, to paralysis. (*From* Strauss RH (ed): Sports Medicine and Physiology. Philadelphia, WB Saunders, 1979.)

the legs—that is, paresthesia and hypesthesia (Fig. 26–6). Next, the legs become weak and the walk unsteady; the diver often cannot initiate urination, although the bladder may be distended. Finally, paralysis below the waist or neck may ensue. The condition appears to be similar to that of a spinal fracture with cord injury; however, the diver is more fortunate because with prompt treatment, the chances for recovery are much better.

Clinically apparent brain damage is less frequent than spinal cord damage. Manifestations include visual disturbances. Vertigo ("the staggers") may result from damage to the inner ear and must be treated within about 45 minutes of the onset of symptoms if dramatic relief is to be achieved in the chamber.

Because clinically obvious brain involvement was rarely seen in divers, it was assumed that the brain was spared when other manifestations of decompression sickness occurred. However, Gorman and colleagues[12] reported that of ten divers presenting with "pain only" symptoms with completely negative neurologic examinations, six were found to have abnormal psychological testing when examined 1 week after successful treatment. Four divers had abnormal electroencephalograms (EEGs), and one had an abnormal computed tomographic (CT) scan. When the divers were reexamined a month later, the psychological test results had returned to normal in all of the divers and the number of divers with abnormal EEGs had dropped to two, but two divers showed abnormal CT scans indicating brain atrophy. Thus, all forms of decompression sickness must be taken seriously, even when treated successfully.

The maximal rate at which a diver can ascend safely to the surface or to a decompression stop is believed to be 60 feet per minute. Injury to the central nervous system is often associated with marginally adequate decompression and an unusually rapid rate of ascent in an emergency situation, such as running out of air during a dive. When decompression procedures have been violated badly, symptoms may appear immediately and may progress to paralysis within minutes. Even when standard practices are followed, decompression sickness occurs occasionally and may progress during several hours.

EXTREMITIES

Limb pain is another common symptom of decompression sickness. Although pain may occur at many locations in the extremities, shoulder and elbow joints are the most frequent sites in divers, as contrasted to the lower leg and knee joints in tunnel workers. The pain is usually steady, but occasionally it may be throbbing. It reaches a peak in minutes or hours and often subsides spontaneously several hours later even if left untreated. The mechanism of pain production is unclear. The arm or leg usually looks completely normal, there is little tenderness, and moderate joint motion is well tolerated. Treatment by recompression helps to relieve the pain and may decrease subsequent tissue damage. Pain in the extremities may also result from local injury unnoticed in the excitement of the dive. Such injuries bear characteristics of trauma (eg, swelling, discoloration, tenderness, and exacerbation of pain on motion). When in doubt, the patient should be given a "test of pressure" by letting him breathe oxygen at 60 feet for 20 minutes in a hyperbaric chamber. If, during that time, there is no *change* in the intensity, position, or character of the pain, one can safely decompress and treat the injury as simple trauma.

Osteonecrosis is a late consequence of inadequate decompression and was much more frequent in the past than at present. A single inadequate decompression can cause the disease. Its pathogenesis probably relates to sludging of blood in the veins draining the humeral or femoral head, with subsequent death of the osteocytes in the bone. It has been shown that if blockage exists for more than 6 to 12 hours, the bone cells will succumb. It is important to keep in mind that therapeutic recompression within 6 hours may help prevent dysbaric osteonecrosis. Patches of bone die, but this may not become visible on radiographs for at least 3 months and may appear only after 5 years following diving. Initially, the patient has no symptoms until the joint begins to collapse. In the usual case, this may occur after about 2 years. Once the femoral or humeral head fractures, the joint cartilage is damaged and severe degenerative joint disease follows.

LUNGS

Some of the bubbles formed in the vasculature of systemic tissues are carried by venous blood to the lungs. Most of these bubbles lodge in small pulmonary vessels, although a fraction may reach the systemic arterial circulation. In most cases of decompression sickness, no pulmonary manifestations appear even though bubbles may be detected in venous circulation. The degree of pulmonary embolization by gas necessary to cause symptoms is unknown; release of vasoactive substances and reflex mechanisms probably contribute to pathogenesis.

The pulmonary syndrome is called "the chokes" by divers and is characterized by substernal chest pain, dyspnea, and cough. Symptoms are aggravated by deep inspiration and by smoking. In animals, clinical signs of the syndrome are accompanied by increased pulmonary arterial pressure and hypoxemia. Pulmonary edema may also occur. The chokes is an extremely serious form of decompression sickness. Without recompression, circulatory collapse and death may follow, whereas recompression results in complete relief within minutes in most cases.

SKIN

"Skin bends" is sometimes seen in scuba divers but more often follows simulated dives in chambers when the skin is in direct contact with the compressed gas. The affected skin, usually on the back or elsewhere on the trunk, itches and burns. If these are the only manifestations, skin bends is frequently left untreated or is treated by breathing oxygen at 1 atm. If discoloration (marbling) appears, chamber treatment is advisable.

Treatment

The standard treatment for decompression sickness is to place the victim in a hyperbaric chamber and increase the air pressure to 2.8 ATA (equivalent to 60 fsw) over 1 or 2

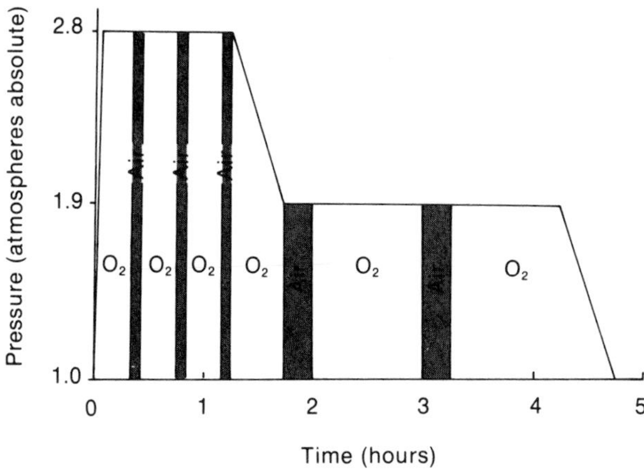

Figure 26–7. For treatment of decompression sickness, chamber pressure is raised and the victim breathes pure oxygen intermittently over several hours. Information based on U.S. Navy treatment table.[13] (*From* Strauss RH (ed): Sports Medicine and Physiology. Philadelphia, WB Saunders, 1979.)

minutes.[13] The patient then breathes pure oxygen intermittently by mask (Fig. 26–7). The increased ambient pressure causes bubbles to diminish in size. Breathing oxygen rather than air increases the gradient for diffusion of inert gas from bubbles and tissue out of the body. Oxygenation of tissues is also increased. However, because increased partial pressures of oxygen can cause oxygen toxicity (ie, convulsions), air is breathed intermittently for periods of 5 minutes or more. Ancillary treatment may include intravenous fluids to increase circulating blood volume.

Treatment can be dramatically effective if it is begun early enough, when symptoms are beginning to develop and tissue damage is mild. As time progresses, however, tissue damage increases and even if all bubbles disappear with hyperbaric treatment, healing requires days or weeks and may not be complete.

Decompression sickness that involves the central nervous system is a medical emergency. The victim should be given oxygen continuously by mask and transported to a recompression chamber by the fastest means possible. If an aircraft is used, cabin pressure should remain as close to 1 atm as possible. The time saved by air transportation is believed to more than compensate for a moderate decrease in ambient pressure. The schedule shown in Figure 26–7 is often used to treat scuba divers. Other schedules are used for deeper dives, but the principles remain the same. Attempts by divers to treat themselves by recompression underwater are usually unsuccessful and dangerous.

The previously mentioned Diver's Alert Network (DAN) is a diving medicine and accident consultation service located at Duke University Medical Center in North Carolina. To use the Network, a diver or physician dials (919) 684–8111 and asks for DAN. (Collect calls are accepted in an actual emergency.) The caller is connected with a diving medicine physician who is available 24 hours a day. The physician may advise the caller directly or refer the caller to a local diving physician. If needed, the physician will work with a DAN regional coordinator to arrange referral and transport to an appropriate treatment facility.

Prevention

During ascent, supersaturation must be controlled so that bubbles do not form and grow sufficiently to cause decompression sickness. After several decades of experience and research, there are now guidelines as to how abrupt a decrease in pressure causes the disease. Thus, divers and others exposed to increased pressure can usually avoid this dan-

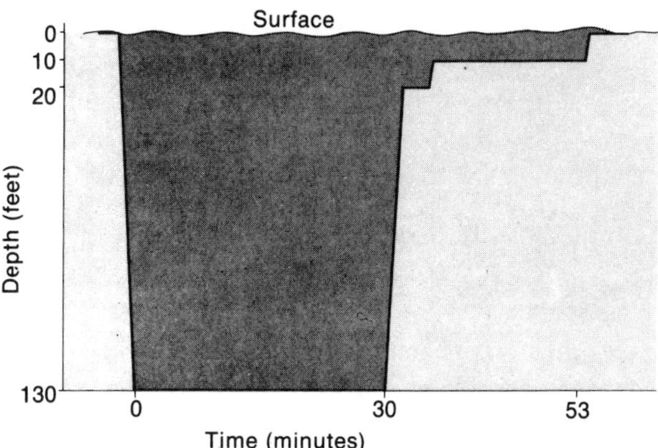

Figure 26–8. Example of decompression: After diving to 130 feet and remaining there for 30 minutes, the diver must stop at several depths during ascent to avoid decompression sickness. Information based on U.S. Navy air decompression table.[13] (*From* Strauss RH (ed): Sports Medicine and Physiology. Philadelphia, WB Saunders, 1979.)

ger by decreasing the pressure gradually (decompressing) (Fig. 26–8). Many divers limit their depth and time underwater so that they can return to the surface without stopping to decompress ("no-decompression limits"). Most careful divers in the United States use the U.S. Navy diving tables as guidelines.[13] Experience has shown that it is a good idea to use these tables conservatively and to avoid approaching no-decompression limits. Even the U.S. Navy is careful to do this, and its master divers usually pad the standard Navy tables with extra decompression. The sport diver should do likewise.

As an alternative, some divers wear decompression "meters" that integrate time and depth information and display decompression guidelines. These electronic meters generally use decompression tables that are more conservative than those of the U.S. Navy, but decompression sickness may still occur. The incidence of decompression sickness among divers using decompression tables and among those using the electronic meters is about the same. A pneumatic analogue meter, which has been on the market for many years, has not been reliable and actually provides less decompression than U.S. Navy tables in dives to depths greater than 80 feet.

Susceptibility to decompression sickness varies among persons and even in the same diver from day to day. Predisposing factors include obesity, exertion, poor physical condition, fatigue, age, cold, dehydration, and injury. Some acclimatization may occur; tunnel workers and commercial divers appear to be less susceptible to decompression sickness when working daily than after an inactive period. Acclimatization, however, has not been observed in sport divers.

Although diving is done in mountain lakes and other bodies of water at altitudes well above sea level, the use of sea level decompression tables becomes less safe as altitude increases. Various decompression methods for altitude diving have been proposed.[14,15] Similarly, flying after diving increases the risk of incurring decompression sickness. Studies by Edel and coworkers[16] led to the conclusion that scuba divers who stay strictly within the depth-time limits recommended by the U.S. Navy tables for dives that do not require decompression will not develop decompression sickness if, after diving, they allow a minimum of 2 hours at the surface before flying in a pressurized aircraft (maximum cabin altitude, 8000 feet). Those who make dives beyond the no-decompression limits should allow a surface interval of 24 hours to avoid the risk of decompression sickness. Commercial pilots are not permitted to fly for 24 hours after scuba diving. It is becoming clear that this is an excellent rule and everyone who expects to fly commercially should probably allow 24 hours after scuba diving before entering an aircraft.

The Undersea and Hyperbaric Medical Society recommends that a woman who is or may be pregnant be discouraged from diving. Fetal risks include not only decompression sickness but also hyperoxia, hypoxia, and hypercapnea.

SOME HAZARDS OF DIVING GASES

The gas mixture that is breathed by a diver must be free of contaminants, such as carbon monoxide and oil vapor. In addition, two gases that are normally breathed—oxygen and nitrogen—become hazardous at increased partial pressures.

Oxygen Toxicity

Breathing oxygen at increased ambient pressures can cause grand mal seizures, which in a scuba diver generally leads to drowning. Therefore, the sport diver should never breathe pure oxygen under water. Occasionally, the U.S. Navy uses a closed-circuit rebreather system to avoid release of tell-tale bubbles into the water. In this system, oxygen is rebreathed after the removal of carbon dioxide. The probability of convulsions increases as ambient pressure and time at pressure increase. The maximal allowable depth using this system is 25 fsw.

Within a hyperbaric chamber, 100% oxygen is breathed at pressures of as much as 2.8 ATA (60 fsw) in the treatment of decompression sickness and air embolism (Fig. 26–7). To avoid inducing convulsions, 5-minute periods of breathing air are interspersed during oxygen breathing. Localized muscular twitching, particularly noticeable in the face, as well as nausea and vertigo, *may* precede convulsions, but often the convulsions occur without warning. If seizures or premonitory signs appear, the oxygen mask is removed and the patient is protected from injury. Seizures are generally brief in duration. After 15 minutes of air breathing, the patient can often return to oxygen treatment without subsequent convulsions. Oxygen-induced seizures appear to be benign, and studies of volunteers who experienced repeated oxygen seizures showed no long-term effects.

The mechanism of central nervous system oxygen toxicity is unclear. Exposure to oxygen at high pressures is associated with several neural changes: the concentration of gamma-aminobutyric acid decreases in the brain; certain enzymes that support oxidative metabolism are altered; and cellular membranes are damaged through oxidation of lipids and sulfhydryl groups. Pulmonary oxygen toxicity is not a problem among scuba divers.

Nitrogen Narcosis

The French call nitrogen narcosis *l'ivresse des grandes profondeurs*—rapture of the deep. It occurs because the nitrogen in air acts progressively as a general anesthetic as its partial pressure increases. Martini's Law, a fanciful rule of thumb, states that each 50-foot increment in depth is equal in effect to one martini on an empty stomach. Manifestations of narcosis occur almost immediately after exceeding about 100 feet and include impairment of judgment, memory, ability to do arithmetic, and fine movements. The mechanism of nitrogen narcosis is unclear. One hypothesis is that nitrogen, which dissolves predominantly in the lipid portion of nerves, causes a small but significant expansion in lipid volume. This, in turn, is believed to alter membrane characteristics in such a way that synaptic transmission is decreased and permeability to ions is increased.

Most other physiologically inert gases, such as neon and xenon, also have narcotic properties at increased pressures. Helium appears to be the single exception. It is substituted for nitrogen as the inert breathing gas in commercial and military dives deeper than 165 to 190 feet. Helium is too expensive for recreational use.

Nitrogen narcosis is one reason to limit sport diving to approximately 130 feet in depth. An intoxicated diver is an unsafe diver. Unfortunately, many divers do not recognize that their judgment is impaired at depths greater than 100 feet.

CARDIOVASCULAR CONSIDERATIONS IN SUDDEN DEATH AMONG DIVERS

Scuba diving is performed by middle-aged as well as young adults and, at times, can place considerable stress on the cardiovascular system. The aquatic environment may stress the body in ways that are not generally associated with equivalent exercise on land, such as cooling. Diving may be particularly hazardous for persons with a propensity for cardiac problems, not only because of increased stress factors but also because the results of incapacitation or unconsciousness underwater are more serious than on land.

After reviewing the records of a large number of diving fatalities across North America, Eldridge[17] concluded that cardiac problems may well be a cause of diving deaths in persons over the age of 40. Her analysis of the physiology involved included the following points. On land, the diver must work hard carrying equipment. In the water, divers sometimes encounter conditions under which they cannot stop swimming even though they may wish to do so. In addition, exposure to cold water leads to increased resistance to blood flow through coronary vessels in persons with coronary atherosclerosis but not in normal persons.[18] Such mechanisms can act to increase the work load of the heart while impairing its blood supply in the presence of atherosclerosis.

A number of factors increase the probability of cardiac arrhythmias among divers. Arrhythmias have been noted among breath-hold divers; even scuba divers sometimes breath-hold, particularly when snorkeling at the surface. This finding may be related to the "diving reflex" that helps to conserve oxygen in mammals such as seals. In these aquatic animals, the act of diving triggers widespread vasoconstriction and profound slowing of the heart rate. As a result, blood is pumped almost exclusively through the lungs, heart, and brain, with lactic acid accumulating in working muscles until the animal surfaces. Bradycardia is found among some human breath-hold divers, but the diving response in humans probably does little to conserve oxygen. Wolf[19] suggested that a variant of the diving reflex in humans may occasionally lead to sudden death, even on land. In susceptible individuals, cardiac arrhythmias also can be triggered by pressure on the carotid sinus, which could be caused by the tight neck of a wet suit or hood. Fatigue also promotes arrhythmias.

Among the fatalities analyzed by Eldridge,[17] a particular behavior pattern appeared repeatedly. The incident often occurred on the surface at the end of a dive when the diver was more likely to be cold and tired. Several victims complained of being tired and were resting or being towed. Many seemed calm just before collapse, in contrast to a panicked individual or one struggling to avoid drowning. Some complained of feeling ill or short of breath, whereas others simply lost consciousness. Frequently, autopsies were not performed or the reports were not available. Among victims with histories such as these, significant coronary occlusion was found sometimes when postmortem examinations were performed.

When death occurs in the water, the cause is often listed as drowning. Important questions are (1) What led to the final event? and (2) How could it have been prevented? An exercise stress test with an electrocardiogram should probably be performed on potential divers over the age of about 35 years. Some workers have suggested adding a cold pressor test as well. Persons with increased cardiac risk factors, such as hypertension, obesity, and smoking, should recognize that diving appears to carry increased risk for them. Persons with known coronary disease or significant dysrhythmias should be discouraged from diving.

OTHER PROBLEMS

Panic, resulting in drowning, is probably the most frequent cause of death among divers. Panic generally is preventable through careful training, knowing one's own limitations, and familiarity with equipment and local conditions, such as waves and currents.

Serious chilling, resulting in a drop in body temperature, is a severe stress encountered by divers in many areas. Hypothermia can impair physical and mental performance. It is prevented through the use of insulating suits and by limiting the length of the dive.

Although divers are rarely attacked by sea creatures, they may accidentally come in contact with stinging jellyfish, sea urchins, or fish with toxic spines. For a more complete discussion of these and other medical problems related to diving, consult the sources suggested under Further Reading.

PHYSICAL EXAMINATION OF THE DIVER

In general, the prospective diver should feel comfortable in the water and be capable of vigorous swimming. It is important for the examining physician to know what kind of diving the applicant intends to do. Entering the water through the surf and swimming in a strong current encumbered by a wet suit is quite different from diving from a boat in calm weather in the warm waters of the Caribbean. However, anyone approved for diving should be capable of sustained hard physical activity in the event of an emergency. Mental, emotional, and physical attributes should be considered. It is particularly important that the gas-containing cavities of the body equalize easily with changing pressure.

Ears and Sinuses

The eardrums should be intact and seen to move when doing the Valsalva maneuver, to ensure patency of the eustachian tubes. The patient should not be suffering from chronic allergies with congested sinuses. With regard to the inner ear, patients with Meniere's disease or other vertiginous conditions should be disqualified from diving.

Eyes

It is important that the patient be able to see well enough to adequately survey the surroundings; to read the tank pressure gauge, watch, and depth gauge; and to find the boat again. Thus, both near and far vision are required. It is perfectly permissible for the patient to wear soft or hard contact lenses or to have corrective lenses fitted into the face plate of the mask. Glaucoma and ocular hypertension need not disqualify the individual if he or she can see adequately. Color vision is unimportant under water. Patients with lens implants following cataract surgery may dive.

Neurologic

It is imperative that the candidate for diving not be epileptic or susceptible to seizures. Epileptic patients on medication who are well controlled and have not had seizures for 5 years or more still should not dive. Changes in oxygen, carbon dioxide, and nitrogen pressures may well predispose to an epileptic seizure in someone with a low threshold. Febrile seizures in infancy that have not recurred are not considered disqualifying. If the patient has a history of stroke, he or she should be disqualified. Faced with a borderline or difficult decision, it is best to consult a neurologist, who can define whether or not the patient would be potentially subject to seizures. Any condition that predisposes the patient to sudden and unexpected loss of consciousness is absolutely disqualifying. Migraine headache may be triggered by decompression. The applicant should be apprised of this.

The patient should not be suffering from any neurologic dysfunction that precludes active swimming. Patients with a history of back injury or a previous history of decompression sickness involving the spinal cord may well be more prone to develop decompression sickness in the spinal cord. Such people should be cautioned to avoid diving near the no-decompression limits and should be cautioned against deep diving.

Psychiatric

The patient's motivation for diving is crucial. The worst situation is where a reluctant spouse has been coerced into learning how to dive in order to join his or her mate on a diving vacation, or when the spouse may have volunteered to do so "to be a good sport." In such cases, the prospective diver may have an underlying fear of the water and may well endanger his or her own life in addition to that of the buddy if panic should occur in an emergency. Be sure to question each prospective diver *in private* about his or her true motivation and feelings about the water. Be suspicious if the person has not previously been active in swimming and/or other in-water activities. The ideal applicant is the true "water rat" who wants to take up scuba diving to further his or her interest. Anyone who enjoys water polo and likes to "horse around" in and under the water is likely to be much safer should an air supply fail or a mask flood.

People with a history of multiple emergency room visits, fractures, motorcycle accidents, and injuries secondary to impetuous behavior are likely to continue being accident-prone while diving. The doctor will be unable to stop these people from diving, but the patient should be apprised of the fact that scuba diving can be brutally unforgiving if the rules are not strictly followed.

Counterphobes are occasionally encountered who have a deep-seated fear of water but want to appear "more normal" and boost their feelings of overall competence by taking up diving. Inquiry into previous aquatic activities may reveal a red flag in this situation.

People with psychotic disorders are unlikely to be candidates for sport scuba diving if they are actively psychotic. However, a history should reveal if the patient has ever taken any kind of psychotropic drug, such as the phenothiazines, lithium, or haloperidol. People taking psychoactive drugs, which can cause somnolence or which could provoke extrapyramidal crises, should not dive. Any drug which makes the diver sleepy also enhances the effects of nitrogen narcosis. Prochlorperazine (Compazine; Smith Kline & French Laboratories, Philadelphia, PA) given to combat seasickness, even in a 5-mg dose, has been shown to cause oculogyric crises in some people. Therefore, Compazine should not be used for seasickness.

Alcohol and Drug Abuse

If the applicant is an addict or chronic heavy user, there should be no problem in deciding to exclude the applicant from diving. One should ask oneself if the applicant who admits to using alcohol or tranquilizers has the common sense to abstain before and during diving. Use of illicit drugs, such as marijuana, angel dust, heroin, and cocaine, are absolute contraindications to diving.

Teeth

The patient should have dentition sufficient to enable him to securely hold a scuba mouthpiece.

Heart

A history of hypertension, per se, is not disqualifying. However, a patient taking a high dosage of beta-blockers or other drugs that preclude maximal exertion should be disqualified.

The diagnosis of myocardial infarction is a contraindication to diving. For a patient over 40 to participate in scuba diving, a stress test would be an ideal prerequisite. The applicant should be capable of achieving at least 14 METS during a stress test. (One MET unit is approximately equal to the individual's oxygen uptake at rest.) Symptoms of angina pectoris or arrhythmias due to coronary artery disease are absolute contraindications to diving.

Patients who have had coronary artery bypass operations have dived successfully when it has been shown that they are capable of high-level exercise and have normal electrocardiograms, and echocardiograms have shown normal heart-wall movement. When closely followed, such patients may not present an increased risk.

Atrioventricular block, such as Mobitz type II block, is disqualifying. Right bundle branch block in the presence of a normal stress test is not disqualifying. Any arrhythmias that could precipitate unconsciousness are disqualifying. Mitral prolapse is not disqualifying but severe aortic stenosis or mitral stenosis should be disqualifying. Mitral regurgitation and aortic insufficiency are not disqualifying if the patient is asymptomatic. It is probably a good idea to disqualify anyone who has intra-atrial or intraventricular septal defect. In such conditions, bubbles may pass from the right side of the heart to the left side during decompression, resulting in gas embolism.

Pacemakers function well under increased pressure, and patients with sequential pacemakers, which allow sinus rate to increase with exercise, can sometimes be approved for sport diving. However, anyone requiring a pacemaker should have a full evaluation by their cardiologist before diving.

Lungs

Any condition of the lungs that may cause air trapping is disqualifying. Active asthma, cold-induced asthma, or exercise-induced asthma are all absolute contraindications to diving. Even though the patient is normally asymptomatic, the breathing of cold dry scuba air while exercising vigorously may provoke an asthmatic attack underwater. It is important to note that the scuba diver can change depth with great rapidity. It is possible to go from 33 feet to the surface in less than 5 seconds. This ascent would require complete exhalation in 5 seconds because the volume is doubled on going from 33 fsw to the surface. For this reason, limiting the potential applicant to "shallow-water diving only" is meaningless in terms of mitigating danger. The most dangerous changes in volume occur within a few feet of the surface. Lung rupture is possible on rising from a depth of 4 feet to the surface.

The patient should be disqualified if there is a history of pneumothorax, because if one were to occur underwater, returning to the surface might prove fatal. If a spontaneous pneumothorax has occurred on one side, there is good likelihood that blebs exist in the opposite lung.

Abdomen and Its Contents

Most bowel, liver, and kidney diseases pose little additional risk underwater as opposed to the surface. However, it is important that paraesophageal or sliding hiatal hernias do not incarcerate, as the portion of the stomach protruding through the hernia could rupture on ascent with catastrophic consequences. Inguinal and umbilical hernias, which may become gas-filled and incarcerate, are also disqualifying.

Gynecologic

There is no contraindication to diving while menstruating, and menstrual blood does *not* attract sharks. All evidence points to the fact that diving while pregnant should be avoided, as there can be very significant risks to the unborn fetus from inert gas uptake and subsequent bubbling.

Endocrinologic

Patients with insulin-dependent brittle diabetes should not dive, as they are at risk for an insulin reaction while underwater. Patients on oral hypoglycemic drugs who are not at risk for insulin reactions may dive. Other metabolic disorders should be considered from the standpoint of whether or not they will interfere with hard physical exertion.

Miscellaneous

There are no absolute criteria for approving applicants at either extreme of age. With regard to the younger diver, he or she should be capable of fully understanding the physics and physiology involved in safely using scuba gear, be able to pass all of the examinations required for certification, and show the maturity and responsibility that one would like to see in a diving buddy. The very young diver should be big enough physically and strong enough to manage his or her scuba gear. Because each applicant will serve as someone else's buddy and perhaps have to effect a rescue, this question should be considered regarding each applicant. Older patients are more likely to have cardiovascular disease and, therefore, may be at risk for diseases associated with hypoperfusion. It is well known that advancing age predisposes to decompression sickness. Older applicants should be cautioned to stay well within no-decompression limits and to avoid deep dives. Older individuals may not be as physically fit as younger applicants. Everyone should be able to exert himself in an emergency to effectively assist in resolving whatever situation may arise.

In summary, the applicant for scuba diving should be able to carry out hard physical work as well as know how to swim. The examiner should pay particular attention to the heart, lungs, ears, and sinuses. The physician should be reasonably assured that the patient will not suffer sudden unconsciousness or incapacitation while in the water.

FURTHER READING

Introductory books intended for the practicing physician include *Diving Medicine*[20] and *Diving and Subaquatic Medicine.*[21] A more complete research-oriented text is *The Physiology and Medicine of Diving and Compressed Air Work.*[22] Diving techniques are described in detail in the *U.S. Navy Diving Manual*[13] and the *NOAA Diving Manual.*[23] Another source is the

Physician's Guide to Diving Medicine.[24] A book popularly used in the training of recreational divers is the *New Science of Skin and Scuba Diving.*[25]

REFERENCES

1. Craig AB Jr: Summary of 58 cases of loss of consciousness during underwater swimming and diving. Med Sci Sports 8:171, 1976.
2. Schaefer KE, McNulty WP Jr, Carey CR, et al: Mechanisms and development of interstitial emphysema and air embolism on decompression from depth. J Appl Physiol 13:15, 1958.
3. Kruse CA: Air embolism and other skin diving problems. Northwest Med 62:525, 1963.
4. Atkinson JR: Experimental air embolism. Northwest Med 62:699–703, 1963.
5. Dutka AJ, Mink R, Hallenbeck JM: Dexamethasone prevents secondary deterioration only when given 3 hours prior to cerebral air embolism [abstract]. Undersea Biomed Res (Suppl) 15:14, 1988.
6. Evans DE, McDermott JJ, Kobrine AI, et al: Effects of intra-venous lidocaine in experimental cerebral air embolism [abstract]. Undersea Biomed Res (Suppl) 15:17, 1988.
7. Leitch DR, Greenbaum LJ, Hallenbeck JM: Cerebral arterial air embolism I, II, III & IV. Undersea Biomed Res 11(3):221–274, 1984.
8. Hart GB: Treatment of decompression illness and air embolism with hyperbaric oxygen. Aerospace Med 45(10):1190–1193, 1974.
9. Kindwall EP: Unpublished data, 1987.
10. Triger M: Influence de l'air comprimé sur la santé. Annales d'Hygiene Publique (Paris) 33:463, 1845.
11. Rivera JC. Decompression sickness among divers: An analysis of 935 cases. Milit Med 129:314, 1964.
12. Gorman D, Edmonds CW, Parsons DW, et al: Neurological sequelae of decompression sickness—a clinical report. *In* Bove AA, Bachrach AJ, Greenbaum LJ (eds): 9th International Symposium on Underwater and Hyperbaric Physiology. Bethesda Undersea & Hyperbaric Medical Society, 1987, pp 993–998.
13. U.S. Navy Diving Manual. Washington DC, US Government Printing Office, 1985.
14. Buhlmann AA, Schibli R, Gehring H: Experimentelle Untersuchungen uber die Dekompression nach Tauchgangen in Bergseen bei vermindertem Luftdruck. Schweiz Med Wochenschr 103:378, 1973.
15. Boni M, Schibli R, Nussberger P, et al: Diving at diminished atmospheric pressure: Air-decompression tables for different altitudes. Undersea Biomed Res 3:189, 1976.
16. Edel PO, Carroll JJ, Honaker RW, et al: Interval at sea level pressure required to prevent decompression sickness in humans who fly in commercial aircraft after diving. Aerospace Med 40:1105, 1969.
17. Eldridge L: Sudden unexplained death syndrome in cold water scuba diving. Undersea Biomed Res (Suppl) 6(1):41, 1979.
18. Mudge GH Jr, Grossman W, Mills RM Jr, et al: Reflex increase in coronary vascular resistance in patients with ischemic heart disease. N Engl J Med 295:1333, 1976.
19. Wolf S: Sudden death and the oxygen-conserving reflex. Am Heart J 71:840, 1966.
20. Bove AA, Davis JC (eds): Diving Medicine. Philadelphia, WB Saunders, 1990.
21. Edmonds C, Lowry C, Pennefather J: Diving and Subaquatic Medicine. Mossman, Australia, Diving Medical Centre, 1981.
22. Bennett PB, Elliott DH: The Physiology and Medicine of Diving and Compressed Air Work, ed 3. San Pedro, CA, Best Publishing, 1982.
23. NOAA Diving Manual. Washington, DC, US Government Printing Office, 1979.
24. Shilling SW, Carlston CB, Mathias RH: Physician's Guide to Diving Medicine. New York, Plenum Press, 1984.
25. National Council for Cooperation in Aquatics, Smith RW (ed): New Science of Skin and Scuba Diving, ed 6. Champaigne, IL, Leisure Press, 1989.

SECTION V

SPECIAL GROUPS OF PARTICIPANTS

27

CHILDREN AND SPORTS

Paul G. Dyment, MD

Children are not just small adults, and this frequently made observation by pediatricians is also valid in the field of sports medicine. Their physiology is different from adults, so their responses to exercise and training are different; their size makes their sports injury patterns different; and their psychological processes cause them to react to sports stresses in different ways. These and other results of the growth and development of children are the subjects of this chapter.

MATURATION AND READINESS TO PLAY

"Doctor, is my 7-year-old son ready to play football?" Before attempting to answer this question, physicians should know that there is very little science to apply to questions concerning whether a child is *neurodevelopmentally ready* to play a sport.

Much easier to respond to is "Will my son be a very good hockey player?," as sport- and task-specific performance tests, which can predict the most proficient players in certain sports, have been evaluated in children.[1] But these tests are only able to predict degrees of success, not sports readiness. They were derived by subjecting players to a variety of performance tests of skills deduced by a task analysis of the sport. Then, the most important tests, as far as ability-prediction was concerned, were statistically separated.

The problem with predicting sports readiness in the child is that at least two other factors can negate neurodevelopmental readiness: the child's social development (Can the child respond to coaching?); and cognitive ability (Can instructions be learned?). A disturbed, defiant, acting-out boy is unlikely to be able to develop the cooperative skills required for team sports, and the slow-learning child may have difficulty mastering the rules of the sport. In both of these cases, the children may be neurodevelopmentally ready, but perhaps they should not be subjected to the stresses of attempting to participate and failing.

Simple levels of motor development are therefore inadequate to predict sports readiness, and instead, the physician must either apply a comprehensive biosocial perspective to answer the question, or take the tack (on more solid scientific grounds) that the question cannot be reliably answered one way or another. The counsel, "If your child wants to, let him or her try," will probably be correct more times than it is incorrect. Arbitrarily deciding that a child is "too young" or "too immature" is more likely to be a product of the physician's personal biases and prejudices.

Children progress through the development of motor, and therefore athletic, skills in a fairly uniform manner. Seefelt[2] evaluated eight fundamental motor skills to decide when children were most likely to be able to perform specific tasks. Their study demonstrated the ages by which 60% of boys and girls could perform each of the following tasks:

throwing, kicking, running, jumping, catching, striking, hopping, and skipping. They reported that although preschool children can perform some of these tasks, most can be performed by early elementary school, and the child is therefore ready to improve these motor skills through repetitive practice. It was apparent that there was an inborn progression of motor skill acquisition as blind children unable to observe other playing children developed the skills in the same order.

MATURATION AND EXERCISE TRAINING

The effects of repeated exercise on the child's maturational process are complicated and difficult to prove. This is in contrast with the reverse, the effect biologic maturation has on the ability to compete in athletics. It is clear that at least the early-maturing boy has a distinct competitive advantage in most sports during early adolescence, whereas the late-maturing girl has an apparent advantage in gymnastics, at least during early adolescence.

"Maturation" needs to be differentiated from "growth." It refers to the progress toward the complete state of development and includes the degree of sexual maturation, whereas "growth" merely refers to the changes in size of the body or its parts. Although both maturation and growth are mostly under genetic control, there are environmental influences, such as nutrition, altitude, and disease, which affect them. Physical exercise does not affect somatic maturity (ie, progress toward adult stature), as young athletes grow at the same rate and achieve the same final heights as do young nonathletes.[3] However, although their heights may be the same, the percent body composition of fat has been found to be lower in athletic children.[4]

Of great concern during the past decade has been the question whether exercise training can affect sexual maturation. This was sparked by the reports that elite young girl athletes frequently had delayed menarche. There was even a relationship derived in equating the number of active training months with the longer time to menarche. This has been seen most consistently in girl swimmers.[5] Although there has been a strong association shown statistically, an association does not always imply a cause-and-effect relationship. For instance, assume two girls both began serious athletic training at age 8 years. One happens to have her menarche at age 11 and the other at age 13, both at times predetermined by their own genetic clocks. Both of these times are within the normal range, but an association can be shown with years of training. That is, the late menarcheal girl had been training for 5 years, whereas the early menarcheal girl had only been training for 3 years.

Another explanation for the association is that delayed maturation may contribute to girls' choices of sports, as there are certain ones, such as gymnastics, dance, and track, in which these girls' structural and performance traits are positively related to success due to the particular characteristics of each of those sports. The physiologic implications of delayed menarche and other menstrual irregularities associated with exercise training are addressed in more detail in Chapter 31.

In some ways, the male of the species has a more clear-cut association between athletics and biologic maturity. The earlier maturing boy is athletically superior at that time, but this is because of his physical advantages of size and strength over his classmates. It is not the athletics which precipitated the early sexual maturation. There is some evidence that males are more sensitive than females to environmental influences on growth and development,[6] and a recent study has demonstrated exercise-induced changes in reproductive function in adult male athletes.[7]

One recent review of the interrelationships between maturation, exercise training, and competitive sports came to the conclusion that:

Training is a significant factor influencing body composition and performance, but not size (stature), physique, and biological maturation. Thus, given the available data, it is difficult to implicate intensive training and the stress of sports competition as critical influences on the biological maturation of children and youth.[8]

THE IMPACT OF PUBERTY

Puberty refers to the physical and biologic changes associated with sexual maturation, whereas *adolescence* refers to the psychosocial process through which a child becomes an adult, a period extending from the onset of puberty to at least the end of the teen years. Prior to puberty, boys and girls grow at the same rate with little real difference in body size between the sexes. Girls enter puberty anytime between 8 and 14 years, and once begun, this physical process is generally complete within 3 years. Boys, on the other hand, start about 2 years later, resulting in a brief period when the average girl of 12 and 13 years of age is heavier and taller than most of the boys in her classroom. Of great importance is the fact that puberty in boys takes about 6 years to complete, so that during the high-school years, similar-age boys are in varying degrees of puberty. A class of 14-year-old boys can vary by as much as 100 lb in weight and 5 years in bone age, yet be within normal limits for both of those parameters. Girls in high school, however, are pretty well all postpubertal.

Tanner,[9] in his monumental work studying the progression of puberty, developed a set of easily identifiable physical characteristics indicating the stages in the normal progression of puberty. He described stages of breast development in girls and genital size in boys, but it is his pubic hair stages which are the most easily employed by a physician, and they can even be fairly reliably assessed by self-evaluation by the athlete. When a "Tanner stage . . ." without further qualifying adjective is recorded, it is the pubic hair scale which is being used (Figs. 27–1 and 27–2).

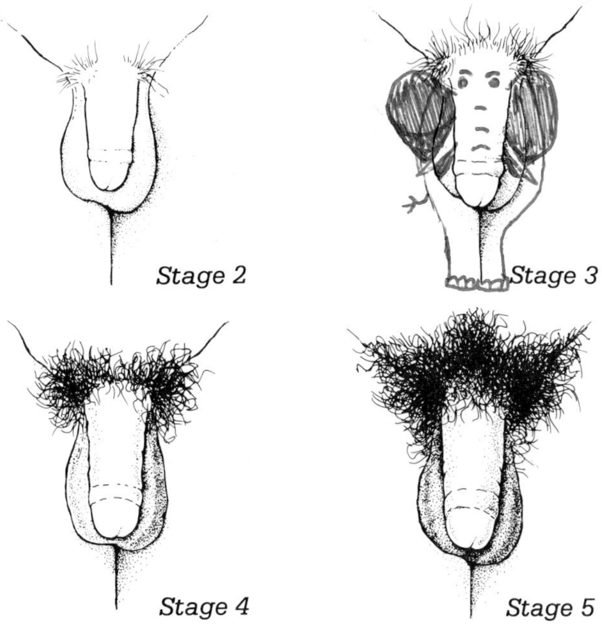

Figure 27–1. Pubertal development of male pubic hair. (Stage 1, prepubertal, not illustrated) Stage 2: Slightly pigmented hair lateral to the base of the penis, usually straight. Stage 3: Hair becomes darker, coarser; begins to curl; and spreads over the pubes. Stage 4: Hair is adult in type, but does not extend onto the thighs. Stage 5: Hair extends onto the thighs and frequently up the linea alba. (*Adapted from* Tanner JM: Growth of Adolescence, ed 2. Oxford, Blackwell Scientific Publications, 1962. Illustration reproduced from Committee on Sports Medicine, American Academy of Pediatrics: Sports Medicine: Health Care for Young Athletes, 2nd ed., in press with permission of the American Academy of Pediatrics, Elk Grove Village, Illinois.)

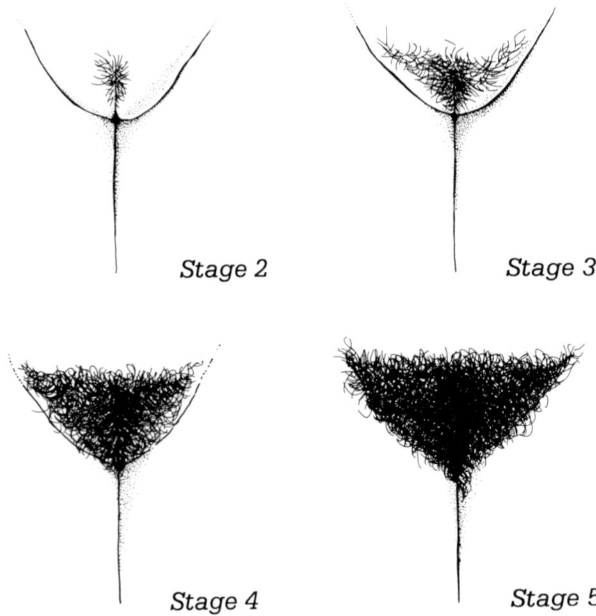

Figure 27–2. Pubertal development of female pubic hair. (Stage 1, prepubertal, not illustrated) Stage 2: Long, slightly pigmented, downy hair along the edges of the labia. Stage 3: Darker, coarser, slightly curled hair spread sparsely over the mons pubis. Stage 4: Adult type of hair, covering a smaller area than an adult, that does not extend onto the thighs. Stage 5: Adult distribution including spread along the medial aspects of the thighs. (*Adapted from* Tanner JM: Growth at Adolescence, ed 2. Oxford, Blackwell Scientific Publications, 1962. Illustration reproduced from Committee on Sports Medicine, American Academy of Pediatrics; Sports Medicine: Health Care for Young Athletes, 2nd ed., in press with permission of the American Academy of Pediatrics, Elk Grove Village, Illinois.)

For males, the growth spurt begins at stage 3, reaches a peak at stage 4, and is practically complete by stage 5, although some young men can continue to add another centimeter or two in height after puberty. The strength spurt does not come until the end of stage 4. Nocturnal emissions begin to occur during stage 3, as can ejaculation with masturbation. Acne, adult body odor, and voice-deepening occur during stage 4. It takes the average boy 2 years to progress from stages 3 to 4, and another two between stages 4 and 5.

For females, the growth spurt begins at the onset of stage 2, reaches a peak at stage 3, and ends at stage 5. Menarche usually occurs during stage 4.

Although girls maintain a fairly constant hematocrit throughout puberty, boys have a steady rise which is directly related to their Tanner stage rather than to their age (Fig. 27–3). This is because it is principally androgenic effect on the bone marrow which results in adult men having higher hemoglobin levels than do adult women. It should be noted that blacks normally have a hemoglobin level about 1 g/dL lower than whites after infancy and throughout life. This relationship of hematocrit and pubertal stage in males can produce a unique clinical situation illustrated by the following case:

CASE 1

Fred and John are two 15-year-old boys of similar height and weight, with similar hemoglobin levels of 13 g/dL. Both are experienced endurance runners, and both are in normal stages of puberty for their age. Fred has only recently entered puberty and is in Tanner stage 2, whereas John has a deep voice, shaves, and is in Tanner stage 5. Are either of these boys anemic?

The answer is that only John has an anemia of some kind, as a hemoglobin of 13 g/dL is abnormally low for a postpubertal male, although it is quite normal for a boy such as Fred still in early puberty.

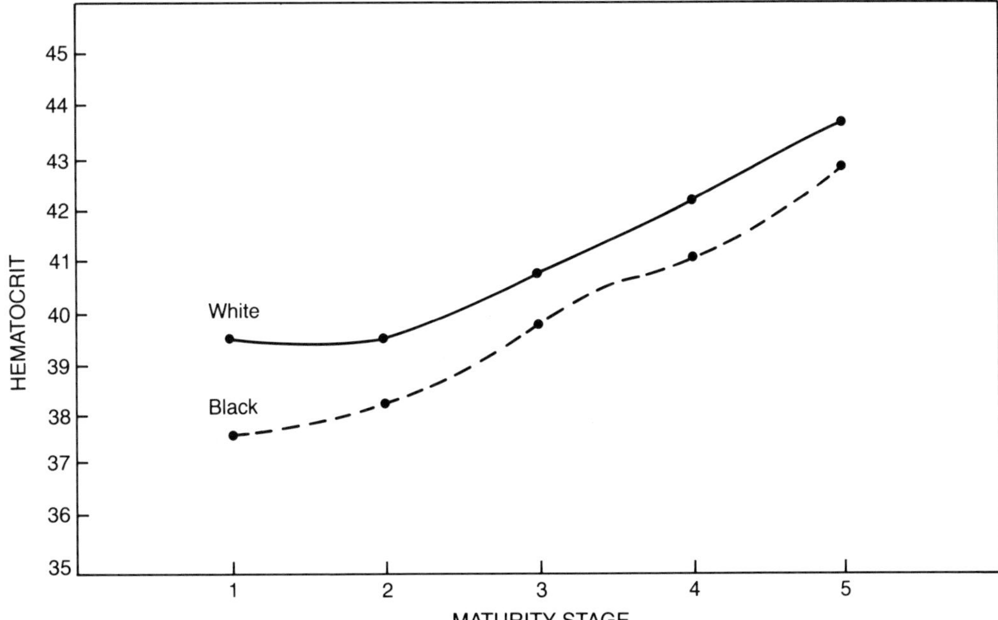

Figure 27–3. Relationship of hematocrit to Tanner stage during adolescence. (*From* Daniel WA: Hematocrit: Maturity relationship in adolescence. Pediatrics 52:388, 1973. Reproduced with permission of Pediatrics.)

The Tanner stages can also be used at the time of a preparticipation examination of a young adolescent athlete if it is being performed in a physician's office where privacy and time allow some anticipatory guidance as part of a complete health maintenance examination. Youth are interested in knowing how they are developing, and this is an opportunity to both instruct and relieve anxieties. After the teenager is dressed, the physician could tell a boy in Tanner stage 2 that he will be growing most rapidly when his pubic hair meets in the midline above the penis, sometime in the next year or two. He should know that he will be most vulnerable to epiphyseal injury during his peak height velocity in stage 3 or 4, that he will really only be adding muscle size and strength after the peak of his height increase, and that he will then be twice as strong as he was before he began the growth spurt. He could also be advised that extensive weight training or weight lifting before that time will do little to give him the muscular body he desires.

Girls beginning puberty can be instructed on the entire progression of events as it occurs in such a brief period of time for them.

STRENGTH TRAINING

It is probably universally accepted that there are no sports in which strength training will not improve performance in at least the postpubertal adolescent or adult. By "strength training," we mean "the use of progressive resistance methods (body weight, free weights, machines) to increase one's ability to exert or resist force."[11] "Weight-lifting" is a competitive sport and is not included in this definition. Until recently, in the absence of data to the contrary, it had been believed by sports medicine professionals that the prepubescent child (ie, Tanner stage 1) did not benefit from strength training. There was thought to be an insufficient amount of circulating androgen necessary for muscle development.

Although some of the data are conflicting, there are enough recent studies to conclude that both muscle strength and endurance can be enhanced in the prepubescent boy as a result of strength training.[11,12] By inference, and not as a result of research, it could also be concluded that the child's lean body mass must also increase in response to strength training as otherwise the increase in muscle strength could not have occurred. By high-school age, not only can increases in muscle strength and endurance be demonstrated, but the number and severity of knee injuries in football players can be significantly reduced as a result of proper strength training and conditioning programs. Proper strength training should therefore be encouraged in all late adolescent and adult athletes. If a boy in an early Tanner stage has the dedication to undergo such a program, he, too, can be encouraged although his gains will be primarily in the cognitive area (ie, how to strength train, something which will be an advantage when he is an older athlete).

There is some increased risk of acute and overuse injury as a result of strength training by people of any age, but this can be reduced to an acceptable level in the child or adolescent by insisting that the program be appropriately designed by an experienced professional (ie, certified athletic trainer, knowledgeable physician), that the athlete undergo a preparticipation examination by a physician (looking particularly for hypertension or a history of blackouts), that proper supervision occur at all times, and that it be part of an overall conditioning program for fitness.

Weight lifting by preadolescents and early adolescents should be discouraged as they are subject to serious injury, not so much from "strains," but from accidentally dropping the weights onto themselves. This is most likely to occur when boys are "competing" in someone's basement without any adult supervision.

PROBLEMS OF THE EARLY-MATURING BOY

In any group of 12-year-old boys, there will be a small number who began their pubertal development when only 10 or 11 years old. These boys are now bigger and stronger than their classmates. Due to the nature of athletic competition, they can become extremely successful in sports. The peer culture present in both junior (and senior) high school can result in this success being transferred to other areas of school life where the athlete can readily become a school leader. This exposure to early success gives these boys a step-up in their emotional security, an advantage which can actually be demonstrated decades later. Studies have shown that men in their 20s and 30s who were early maturers continued to demonstrate an advantage in measures of emotional stability and cognitive ability.

Some of these early-maturing boys, however, are not so lucky, at least if they have developed expectations of continuing their early athletic success through high school and college, and possibly have dreamed of a professional sports career, as time will eventually catch up to them. "The early light burns out first"; and when his classmates finally also physically mature, he will have lost his athletic advantage. His father or coach, not understanding this process, may even berate him: "You aren't as good as you used to be; you are not trying hard enough," etc.

The physician performing a preparticipation examination can recognize this situation if the appropriate questions are asked when a 12- or 13-year-old boy is noticed to be in Tanner stage 4 or 5. Anticipatory guidance should then be delivered to both the boy and his parents about what to expect when his peers "catch up" to him. Until that time, opportunities to compete in teams made up of individuals of similar maturational age should be encouraged, such as allowing mature junior high school students to play with the junior varsity team at the high school.

PROBLEMS OF THE LATE-MATURING BOY

Athletic success in early adolescence is related directly to advanced pubertal stage rather than innate athletic abilities. The Tanner pubic hair stages do correlate with muscle strength and epiphyseal maturity, so the physician can use athletes' Tanner stages when advising about the wisdom of their competing. This is usually only really useful when considering whether a young adolescent boy should compete in a collision sport, such as football or ice hockey, where he may be more likely to be injured by playing against similar age but more physically mature boys who are both bigger and stronger. This is rarely a clinical question when counseling a young adolescent female athlete. My belief is that such a late-maturing young adolescent male should not be denied permission to play by the examining physician, but rather the boy and his parents should at least be advised of the increased theoretical risk of serious injury. If they all are willing to accept that risk, then I would approve his participation. Football and ice hockey are high-risk sports in the first place, and the fact that the boy and his parents have consented to his competing before the examination means they have already accepted a certain degree of risk; the boy's small size is just an additional one.

There are sports in which body size, strength, and endurance are not of overriding importance, and it is to these that the late-maturing young adolescent should be directed—soccer, certain track events, racquet sports, and diving.

Not all late-maturing boys are small. Some are obese and these may be tempted to try out for a position in the center of the defensive line of the football team. The school coach may even be urging the boy to compete, viewing his weight as an advantage in that position. But his lack of muscle mass and epiphyseal strength are two risk factors for a sports injury.

Another subset of late-maturing boys are tall ones, destined for heights well over 6 feet. These boys enter puberty with the long legs so dear to a basketball coach's heart. However, their limited muscle mass and strength makes them susceptible to injury, and their lack of endurance makes them unable to compete effectively for an entire game.

COMPETITION BETWEEN BOYS AND GIRLS

There is little difference in the size and strength of populations of prepubertal boys and girls of similar age. Therefore, it is reasonable to allow boys and girls to compete with each other and participate in coed teams prior to age 11 or 12 years.

However, once circulating androgens start to give boys an advantage in strength, body size, and muscle mass, then competition between males and females is no longer appropriate in most sports, particularly in those contact sports where collisions can produce injuries. This would appear to be self-evident, and most high schools have in the past had rules precluding a girl from competing for a position on a boys' team. These rules were well-meaning in their intent, which was to prevent injuries to girls. However, with the advent of federal legislation mandating equal opportunities for girls to compete, more girls have been competing not only in their "own" sports, but they occasionally have been asking to compete in sports in which there was a boys' team but not one for girls (ie, they want to try out for a "boys' sport," such as football or ice hockey). After repeated court decisions consistently supported these girls against schools enforcing gender-discriminatory rules, school administrators pretty well accept as their legal obligation the allowing of girls to compete for positions on boys' teams in sports in which there are no teams allowing girls in the school. This not only makes legal, but also physiologic, sense. In every school, there will be a small number of girls who are both bigger and stronger than many of the boys; yet there was not a rule preventing small boys from trying out for the team, even though they are as likely to be injured as a girl of similar size.

This even means that schools should allow girls to compete on high-school wrestling teams, although in a mixed-sex contest there are undoubted sexual overtones, which are difficult to ignore. Certainly the boys on a wrestling team who are about to compete against a team with a girl on it could benefit from some anticipatory guidance from the team physician or a sensitive coach: "Listen boys, let's talk about how we're going to feel if we are going to wrestle a girl . . . How will we feel if we lose? . . . Let's be sure that regardless of the sex of the competitor we will compete as hard as ever. . . ."

The reverse situation of boys being allowed to compete for positions on girls' teams in sports in which there are no boys' teams is not so clear-cut. Allowing this on the basis that if girls can compete on boys' teams, then it only seems fair to allow boys to try out for the girls' teams as well, can produce a situation, such as in field hockey, in which the team with the greatest number of boys will most likely win. Another concern is that each boy on that team is denying some girl the opportunity to experience the benefits of the athletic team experience. As boys have historically had more opportunities for sports participation than have girls, about half of the court cases in which such situations have been argued have decided that it is legal to discriminate against boys attempting to cross this gender line.[13] However, half of the cases have had rulings the other way, allowing boys to compete on such girls' teams, so this will continue to be a tough question for a school to decide.

COUNSELING THE "SISSY"

Not all boys are enthusiastic participants in rough-and-tumble play, team sports, and other activities considered "appropriate" for their gender. This can result in such an elementary school–age boy becoming socially isolated from his male classmates, his feelings about his own self-worth diminishing. He may begin showing signs of stress in the form of psychosomatic or chronic anxiety symptoms. Counseling the parents of these boys should include the advice not to "push" the boy forcefully to such activities. The virtues of gentle encouragement should be extolled instead, and above all, a parent should be urged to continue to demonstrate both physical and verbal signs of their love of the child regardless of his interest, or lack of it, in "boys' play." Time usually takes care of this problem. Eventually, either the boy spontaneously develops an interest in such games, or he may reach a high school that is large enough to have a peer group of similarly inclined "nonjocks" with whom he can feel comfortable.

There is a much smaller subset of prepubertal boys who display other signs of effeminate behavior in addition to a dislike and avoidance of boys' games. The physician should inquire about such activities if the parent indicates there is a problem in this area. These boys persistently put on girls' clothes, use lipstick, prefer to play with girls rather than boys, play with dolls, engage in female gestures, and express a desire to have been a girl.

Several prospective studies of such effeminate boys whose behaviors have been serious enough to precipitate a referral to a psychiatrist or psychiatric clinic have shown that most of these boys grew up to be adult homosexuals.[14] These studies have generally concluded that psychological factors could *not* explain this behavior. Instead, their homosexuality is most likely a congenital condition, with its origins either genetic (but not hereditary) or as a result of an incident in fetal life. One should remember, however, that most adult homosexuals are not effeminate. The significance of this group of boys for the primary care physician is that when counseling parents of such boys, a referral to a child psychiatrist may well be in order. However psychiatrists will be more successful in teaching the family how to *cope* with this behavior than they will be in "changing" the boy.

INJURIES

Participation in athletics carries with it a risk of injury. This risk is related to age (really the size of the athlete), the kind of sport, and the athlete's sex. Sports participation is the second most common cause of injury-related emergency room visits and hospital admissions of children.

One large study in Springfield, Illinois,[15] reported that, each year, 6% of school-age children and adolescents sustained a sports injury requiring at least first aid. The injury rate increased with age: 3% for those in elementary school, 7% for those in junior high school, and 11% for those in high school. The study by Goldberg and colleagues[16] of youth football in boys 8 to 15 years of age showed that 5% sustained a "significant" injury, defined as causing greater than 7 days of restriction. They compared this to other reports of similar significant injury rates of 16% for high school football, and 27% for college football.

The reasons for the association of increase in age with increase in injury rate is undoubtedly primarily due to the consequences of the Newtonian concept that the force of a moving object is directly proportional to the product of its mass and its velocity. Thus, when two 50-lb 6-year-old boys running at a speed of 5 mph collide on the football field, the forces stressing their musculoskeletal system are very much less than when two 150-lb high-school boys running at a speed of 10 mph collide. Another reason for the increased injury rate with increase in age is a motivational one—the drive to compete aggressively in order to win seems to increase with age, and this aggressiveness can lead to more injuries.

Most epidemiologic surveys of sports injuries have shown that football are by far the most common cause of them. The detailed study by McClain and Reynolds[17] of 1 year in a large high school revealed an overall injury rate of 22% for the 1283 student athletes taking part in 24 different sports, defining "injury" as trauma serious enough to cause the athlete to either be unable to complete a practice or a game or causing the athlete to miss the subsequent practice or game. Table 27–1 lists the sports with the greatest risks of injury.[17]

Most physicians probably believe that the benefits of the athletic experience outweigh the risks. These benefits include the following maturing experiences: both losing and winning, competing against others while cooperating with teammates, socializing with teammates, gaining a feeling of respect for the physically fit body, gaining the personal disci-

TABLE 27–1. SPORTS WITH GREATEST RISK OF INJURY DURING A 1-YEAR PERIOD IN A HIGH SCHOOL

Sports (Sex)	% of Athletes with Injuries
Football	61
Gymnastics (girls)	46
Gymnastics (boys)	40
Wrestling	40
Basketball (boys)	37
Basketball (girls)	31
Track (girls)	18
Volleyball (girls)	17
Soccer (girls)	17

Adapted from McClain LG, Reynolds S: Sports injuries in a high school. Pediatrics 84:446–450, 1989. Reproduced with permission of Pediatrics.

pline to fulfill a rigorous training schedule, and handling the many diverse stresses of athletic experiences.

REFERENCES

1. Hermiston RT, Gratto J, Teno T: Three hockey skills tests as predictors of hockey-playing ability. Can J Appl Sport Sci 4:95–97, 1979.
2. Seefelt V: The concept of readiness applied to motor skills acquisition. *In* Magill RA, Ash MJ, Smoll FL (eds): Children in Sports, ed 2. Champaign, IL, Human Kinetics, 1982, pp 31–37.
3. Plowman SA: Maturation and exercise training in children. Pediatr Exerc Sci 1:303–312, 1989.
4. Boileau RA, Lohman TG, Slaughter MH: Exercise and body composition of children and youth. Scand J Sports Sci 7:17–27, 1985.
5. Stages JM, Robertshaw D, Miescher E: Delayed menarche in swimmers in relation to age at onset of training and athletic performance. Med Sci Sports Exerc 16:550–555, 1984.
6. Stinson S: Sex differences in environmental sensitivity during growth and development. Yearbook Phys Anthropology 28:123–147, 1985.
7. Cumming DC, Wheeler GD, McColl EM: The effects of exercise on reproductive function in men. Sports Med 7:1–17, 1989.
8. Malina RM: Competitive youth sports and biological maturation. *In* Brown EW, Branta CF (eds): Competitive Sports for Children and Youth, Champaign, IL, Human Kinetics, 1988, p 240.
9. Tanner JM: Growth at Adolescence, ed 2. Oxford, England, Blackwell, 1962, pp 32–33.
10. Daniel WA: Hematocrit: Maturity relationship in adolescence. Pediatrics 52:388–394, 1973.
11. Cahill BR (ed): Proceedings of the Conference on Strength Training and the Prepubescent. Chicago, American Orthopedic Society for Sports Medicine, 1988.
12. Sewall L, Micheli LJ: Strength training for children. J Pediatr Orthop 6:143–146, 1986.
13. Legal opinion on file. Elk Grove Village, IL, American Academy of Pediatrics, 1987.
14. Zuger B: Early effeminate behavior in boys: Outcome and significance for homosexuality. J Nerv Ment Dis 172:90–97, 1984.
15. Zaricznyj B, Shattuck LJ, Mast TA, et al: Sports related injuries in school-aged children. Am J Sports Med 8:318–324, 1980.
16. Goldberg B, Rosenthal PP, Robertson LS, et al: Injuries in youth football. Pediatrics 81:255–261, 1988.
17. McClain LG, Reynolds S: Sports injuries in a high school. Pediatrics 84:446–450, 1989.

28

THE PREPARTICIPATION EXAMINATION OF THE YOUNG ATHLETE

Paul G. Dyment, MD

The preparticipation examination should be part of an overall health care plan for young athletes of school and college age. There is a substantial risk of injury in athletic participation, and the purpose of the "sports physical" is to "prevent life-threatening or disabling injuries by identifying predisposing factors, recommending preparatory and/or rehabilitative measures, and assisting in matching the participant with an appropriate sport and/or position."[1] These goals can be accomplished fairly effectively, but only if the physical examination includes a detailed musculoskeletal evaluation and there is also the time and privacy to offer individual counseling. *If a musculoskeletal assessment is performed, as many as 10% of high school athletes will be found to have an abnormality necessitating advice regarding rehabilitation.*[2] The traditional sports physical in which cursory examinations are performed upon a long line of students in a high-school locker-room are totally inadequate. Under these conditions, there is no time to take a personal medical history, a musculoskeletal evaluation is generally not performed, and there is no individual counseling regarding such topics as the effect of delayed puberty on athletic performance or whether a particular sport is a wise choice for a particular athlete. The effectiveness of the preparticipation examination as it is usually performed has been the subject of several recent commentaries.[3–5]

Studies have shown that over 80% of student athletes perceive the sports physical as their "annual physical examination," and they do not see a physician again for a year, until the time for their next preparticipation examination. Adolescent athletes receiving a locker-room physical examination will not have the opportunity to receive counseling from their personal physician regarding medical subjects (eg, acne) or lifestyle problems (ie, sex, sexuality, drugs, and high-risk behavior), something which they should receive during a *health maintenance examination.* Anticipatory guidance can really be provided only in the privacy of a physician's office. If all preparticipation examinations could be performed as part of an annual health maintenance examination, in a physician's office, with the physician including a musculoskeletal assessment in addition to the usual components of a physical examination, and with anticipatory guidance, then the athlete would receive maximal benefit from the encounter. However, with over 15 million participants of college age or younger in organized sports, it is not realistic to assume all could receive such a personalized examination.

A very effective way to examine a number of athletes is the "stations format," in which a health care team is located at a single site, and each member performs part of the examination. The personnel involved include nurses, physicians (either in primary care or orthopedic surgery), and certified athletic trainers. One comparative study found that far more abnormalities were detected by such teams of providers than by private physicians performing individual examinations.[6] The disadvantages of this technique are that a complete medical history is not obtained, anticipatory guidance cannot be offered, and follow-up care or assessment of the athlete with an abnormality is not provided.

FREQUENCY

How often the physical examination should be performed is a controversial subject. Experts in adolescent medicine generally recommend an annual health maintenance examination. The preparticipation assessment should be a component of that annual examination. However, if the examination is just a preparticipation assessment, which is being done in either a physician's office or in groups (either by the stations or locker-room format), then it really is only necessary *when a person is new to a school* (ie, on entry into high school); but *an interim medical history is necessary before each sports season* to determine whether any injuries or illnesses have occurred since the last complete assessment was done, and then to decide if another physical examination needs to be performed. An athlete at a school that requires only an annual sports physical and who undergoes that examination in the summer could well sprain his ankle during football season, and then participate in basketball that winter without any system in place to assess whether the injury had even occurred much less been rehabilitated adequately.

LABORATORY EVALUATION

Urinalysis

Although the urinalysis for many years was considered an important part of the sports physical examination, there is a general consensus today that this test produces significant findings very infrequently; false-positive findings and minor abnormalities are very common. Therefore, a urinalysis is *not recommended* as part of a sports preparticipation examination.

Hemoglobin

Iron deficiency is not uncommon in postpubertal females, but it has to be quite severe before the body's compensatory mechanisms fail to maintain an appropriate supply of oxygen to the tissues, thereby impairing athletic performance. Screening athletes with a hemoglobin or hematocrit is therefore *not recommended* as part of a sports physical, although it may well be indicated during a complete health maintenance examination at intervals during adolescence. Much more common than iron deficiency anemia is nonanemic iron deficiency, particularly in cross-country runners. Studies indicating whether athletic performance is impaired by decreased iron stores are contradictory, but there is enough supportive evidence to justify the expense of a serum ferritin level on at least national-level competitors, particularly women. Those athletes who are hypoferritinemic are treated with ferrous sulphate after an evaluation of the etiology of the condition.

Sickle Cell Screen

Screening for sickle cell trait in all athletes from populations at risk would seem reasonable. However, whether there is an actual increased risk from an ischemic complication during athletics is controversial, although exercise at a high altitude certainly is a risk.[7] Screening of populations at risk with a sickle hemoglobin solubility test should be considered an ideal and *not an essential* component of a sports physical examination.

MEDICAL HISTORY

Figure 28–1 is an example of a form which can be used by a school system for the interim history preceding a sports season. This should be reviewed by the team or school physician, who then decides which athletes need to undergo a complete preparticipation physical examination. Figure 28–2 is an example of a medical history form which should be completed by the athlete (and the parent if the athlete is a minor) prior to a preparticipation examination. Figure 28–3 is an example of a form which can be used for the actual physical examination and which can be readily used either for an office examination or by those taking part in stations format examinations. In the latter situation, the examiners initial their individual components, and the physician who reviews all of their findings at the end of the process makes the ultimate decision regarding ability to participate.

PHYSICAL EXAMINATION

When performing the sports preparticipation examination, the physician should remember that *most sports injuries are reinjuries,* and that the detection of incompletely rehabilitated previous injuries is one of the principal goals of this examination. This means that a thorough assessment of the musculoskeletal system must be performed in a consistent manner. The examination should be performed at least 4 to 6 weeks before the beginning of the athletic season so that if old injuries are detected, rehabilitative exercises can be recommended to prevent reinjury by strengthening the appropriate ligaments and musculotendinous units.

Stations Format

If the sports participation examination cannot be performed in a private office as part of a health maintenance examination by the athlete's personal primary care physician (who is knowledgeable about the musculoskeletal assessment), then the stations format is the next preferred kind of examination. These are usually organized by the team physician, who arranges for a group of volunteer examiners to be present one evening, and the entire team is assessed at one time.

There should be a waiting room large enough to accommodate all of the athletes simultaneously and where instructions can be given at one time. A series of examining rooms should be adjacent, each one labeled with a large-sized identifying number. Each station should have at least a chair and a clipboard, and the room in which the abdominal examination is performed also needs an examination table.

Thirty or more athletes can be examined within 2 hours if the team includes two physicians and at least four nonphysician medical personnel, such as nurses and certified athletic trainers. The coaches should also be present to direct traffic and to control unruly behavior.

Boys should be dressed in gym shorts and girls in gym outfits. High school–aged athletes must have their medical history signed by a parent prior to the examination; college-aged athletes can complete the form while waiting.

The athletes move from station to station in the order described below. The actual number of stations depends upon the number of examiners available. For instance, if

SPORTS HEALTH RECORD: INTERIM HISTORY

This form may be used prior to participation in any new sport during the interval between preparticipation examinations. Positive responses should prompt a physical examination.

NAME ____________________ AGE ________ DATE ____________

ADDRESS ____________________ PHONE ____________

1. Over the next 12 months I wish to participate in the following sports:

   a. ____________ b. ____________ c. ____________ d. ____________

2. Have you missed more than 3 consecutive days of participation in usual activities because of an injury this past year? Yes ____ No ____

   If yes, please indicate:

   a. Site of injury ____________________

   b. Type of injury ____________________

3. Have you missed more than 5 consecutive days of participation in usual activities because of an illness or have you had a medical illness diagnosed that has not resolved in this past year? Yes ____ No ____

   If yes, please indicate:

   a. Type of illness ____________________

4. Have you had a concussion or been unconscious for any reason in the last year? Yes ____ No ____
5. Have you had surgery or been hospitalized in this past year? Yes ____ No ____

   If yes, please indicate:

   a. Reason for hospitalization ____________________

   b. Type of surgery ____________________

6. List all medications you are presently taking and what condition the medication is for.

   a. ____________________

   b. ____________________

   c. ____________________

7. Are you worried about any problem or condition at this time? Yes ____ No ____

   If yes, please explain: ____________________

____

____

____

I hereby state that to the best of my knowledge my answers to the above questions are correct.

____________________ ____________

Signature of athlete Date

____

Signature of parent

Figure 28–1. Interim history form. (*Adapted from* Sports Medicine: Health Care of the Young Athlete, ed 2. Elk Grove Village, Illinois, American Academy of Pediatrics, 1991, in press; with permission.)

SPORTS PREPARTICIPATION HEALTH RECORD

This examination is to determine sports readiness. It should not replace regular health examinations.

NAME ______________________ AGE ______ GRADE ______ DATE ______________

SPORTS ____

HISTORY: To Be Completed by the Athlete and Parent

	YES	*NO*
1. Have you ever had an illness that:		
a. required you to stay in the hospital?	____	____
b. lasted longer than a week?	____	____
c. caused you to miss 3 days of practice or a competition?	____	____
d. is related to allergies? (ie, hay fever, hives, asthma, insect stings)	____	____
e. required an operation?	____	____
f. is chronic? (ie, asthma, diabetes, etc)	____	____
2. Have you ever had an injury that:		
a. required you to go to an emergency room or to see a doctor?	____	____
b. required you to stay in the hospital?	____	____
c. required x-rays?	____	____
d. caused you to miss 3 days of practice or a competition?	____	____
e. required an operation?	____	____
3. Do you take any medication or pills?	____	____
4. Have any members of your family under age 50 had a heart attack or heart problem or died unexpectedly?	____	____
5. Have you ever fainted, passed out, been unconscious, or had a concussion?	____	____
6. Can you run ½ mile (2 times around the track) without stopping?	____	____
7. Do you:		
a. wear glasses or contacts?	____	____
b. wear dental bridges, plates, or braces?	____	____
8. Have you ever been told you have a heart murmur, high blood pressure, or a heart abnormality?	____	____
9. Do you have any allergies to any medicine?	____	____
10. Do you have both kidneys?	____	____

11. When was your last tetanus booster? ______________________

12. *For Women:*
    a. At what age did you experience your first menstrual period? ______________________
    b. In the last year, what is the longest time you have gone between periods? ______________

EXPLAIN ANY "YES" ANSWERS ____

____

____

Parent Signature ______________________ Athlete Signature ______________________

Figure 28–2. Sports preparticipation history form. (*Adapted from* Sports Medicine: Health Care of the Young Athlete, ed 2. Elk Grove Village, Illinois, American Academy of Pediatrics, 1991, in press; with permission.)

SPORTS PREPARTICIPATION PHYSICAL EXAMINATION FORM

NAME ______________ DATE __________ AGE ______ BIRTHDATE __________

Height ______________ Vision: R ____/____, corrected ______, uncorrected ______

Weight ______________ L ____/____, corrected ______, uncorrected ______

Pulse ______________ Blood Pressure ______________ Percent Body Fat (optional) ________

	Normal	Abnormal	Initials
1. Eyes			
2. Ears, Nose, Throat			
3. Mouth & Teeth			
4. Neck			
5. Cardiovascular			
6. Chest and Lungs			
7. Abdomen			
8. Skin			
9. Genitalia—Hernia (male)			
10. Musculoskeletal-ROM, strength, etc.			
a. Neck			
b. Spine			
c. Shoulders			
d. Arms/hands			
e. Hips			
f. Thighs			
g. Knees			
h. Ankles			
i. Feet			
11. Neuromuscular			
12. Physical Maturity (Tanner Stage)	1 2 3 4 5		

Comments re: Abnormal Findings: ______________

PARTICIPATION RECOMMENDATIONS

1. No participation in: ______________
2. Limited participation in: ______________
3. Requires: ______________
4. Full participation: ______________

Physician Signature ______________

Telephone Number ______________

Address ______________

Figure 28–3. Sports preparticipation physical examination form. (*Adapted from* Sports Medicine: Health Care of the Young Athlete, ed 2. Elk Grove Village, Illinois, American Academy of Pediatrics, 1991, in press; with permission.)

there are three physicians, they can cover stations 4, 5, and 7 (listed below); but if only two physicians attend, then stations 4 and 5 can be combined into a single station.

Station 1. ***Blood Pressure (Nurse).*** Right arm, sitting, measurements greater than the following values require repeat determinations:

6–11 years	>135/80 mm Hg
≥12 years	>145/90 mm Hg

Station 2. ***Visual Acuity (Nurse).*** Uncorrected vision less than 20/40 requires referral for further evaluation. If uncorrected vision is 20/200, the physician should consider the patient as functionally blind in that eye; therefore, contact/collision sports might not be recommended.

Station 3. ***Skin-Mouth-Eyes (Physician, Nurse, or Athletic Trainer).*** At this station, the examiner checks for pustular acne, herpes, dental prosthesis, severe caries, pupil inequality, rashes, and fungal infection.

Station 4. ***Chest (Physician).*** The physician reviews cardiopulmonary-related history and performs lung and heart examination.

Station 5. ***Lymphatics-Abdomen-Genitalia (Physician).*** At this station, the physician performs an examination for cervical adenopathy; abdominal organomegaly; testicular abnormalities and inguinal hernia (in males). Tanner pubic-hair ratings should be determined for males at least, particularly those competing in collision/contact sports (see Chapter 27).

Station 6. ***Musculoskeletal (Physician or Athletic Trainer).*** This examination generally takes only 2 minutes to perform. The examination form included in this chapter (see Fig. 28–3) includes spaces to record this entire component.

Station 7. ***Review (Physician).*** A physician (generally the most knowledgeable about athletic injuries) is at this last station. He or she reviews the examination form and may choose to repeat those tests which revealed abnormalities. The decision is then made about the athlete's degree of sports participation.

SUDDEN DEATH ON THE PLAYING FIELD

This chapter will not review the different components of the physical examination, but a few words should be said about sudden unexpected death during athletics. Most of these are due to cardiac abnormalities, but only a few are of a type that could be detected during a routine physical examination of the heart. In fact, an underlying cardiovascular condition detected or suspected prior to death occurs in only about 25% of such deaths, and even more rarely was the correct diagnosis known. The most common cardiovascular causes of unexpected sudden death in athletes are listed in Table 28–1.

Hypertrophic cardiomyopathy (HCM), previously called idiopathic hypertrophic subaortic stenosis (IHSS), is the most common cause of unexpected death on the playing field.

TABLE 28–1. MOST COMMON CAUSES OF SUDDEN DEATH IN ATHLETES

Hypertrophic cardiomyopathy
Aortic rupture in Marfan's syndrome
Aberrant left coronary artery syndrome
Atherosclerotic coronary artery disease

Adapted from Braden DS, Strong WB: Preparticipation screening for sudden cardiac death in high school and college athletes. Physician Sportsmed 16:128–140, 1988; with permission.

One large series reviewing the circumstances surrounding sudden death in this condition indicated that almost half of these persons were engaged in moderate-to-intense physical activity just before death.[9] Although the echocardiogram is a relatively sensitive test for this condition, there are usually no clues as to its presence, so there is no indication for that test. There are some items in the history and physical that should alert the physician to its presence, however. A family history of sudden unexpected death in a parent or sibling younger than 50 years of age can be found in a quarter of those who die suddenly from hypertrophic cardiomyopathy. A history of syncope (especially after vigorous exercise) and palpitations is also suspicious. There is frequently a high-pitched systolic ejection murmur from subaortic obstruction heard best at the left sternal border, which increases in intensity during late Valsalva maneuver or when the athlete moves to the sitting position from the supine, a maneuver that decreases the left ventricular volume.

By the time the patient with *Marfan's syndrome* is approaching the third decade, many of these stigmata will be present: tallness; heart murmur of aortic or mitral insufficiency; ectopia lentis; arachnodactyly; and upper body (top of symphysis pubis to top of head) to lower body (pubis to floor) ratio decreased from a normal value of 0.92 for whites and 0.85 for blacks. Also, most patients will have a family history of this condition. An athlete presenting with several of these signs should undergo a thorough cardiac evaluation, including an echocardiogram, as sudden death due to aortic rupture is a known complication.

The *aberrant left coronary artery* is a congenital anomaly associated with sudden death in young persons. In this condition, the left coronary artery takes an aberrant course between the aorta and right ventricular infundibulum, and blood flow to its branches is compromised during exercise, resulting in myocardial ischemia. Physical examination of these people is entirely normal. However, most cases have had a history of fainting *during*

TABLE 28–2. CLASSIFICATION OF SPORTS

		Noncontact		
Contact/Collision	**Limited Contact/Collision**	***Strenuous***	***Moderately Strenuous***	***Nonstrenuous***
Boxing	Baseball	Aerobic dancing	Badminton	Archery
Field hockey	Basketball	Crew	Curling	Golf
Football	Bicycling	Fencing	Table tennis	Riflery
Ice hockey	Diving	Field*		
Lacrosse	Equestrian	Running		
Martialarts	Field*	Swimming		
Rodeo	Gymnastics	Tennis		
Soccer	Handball	Track		
Wrestling	Racquetball	Weight lifting		
	Skating			
	Ice			
	Roller			
	Skiing			
	Cross-country			
	Downhill			
	Water			
	Softball			
	Squash			
	Volleyball			

*Field events: Jumping events, such as pole vaulting and high jumping, are limited contact/impact sports; others are noncontact strenuous sports.

Adapted from Sports Medicine: Health Care of the Young Athlete, ed 2. Elk Grove Village, IL, American Academy of Pediatrics, 1990; with permission.

TABLE 28–3. RECOMMENDATIONS FOR PARTICIPATION IN COMPETITIVE SPORTS

			Noncontact		
Condition	**Contact/ Collision**	**Limited Contact/ Impact**	***Strenuous***	***Moderately Strenuous***	***Nonstrenuous***
Atlantoaxial instability	No	No	Yes*	Yes	Yes
Acute illnesses	†	†	†	†	†
Cardiovascular					
Carditis	No	No	No	No	No
Hypertension					
Mild	Yes	Yes	Yes	Yes	Yes
Moderate	†	†	†	†	†
Severe	†	†	†	†	†
Congenital heart disease	‡	‡	‡	‡	‡
Eyes					
Absence or loss of function of one eye	§	§	§	§	§
Detached retina	‖	‖	‖	‖	‖
Inguinal hernia	Yes	Yes	Yes	Yes	Yes
Absence of one kidney	No	Yes	Yes	Yes	Yes
Enlarged liver	No	No	Yes	Yes	Yes
Musculoskeletal disorders	†	†	†	†	†
Neurologic					
History of serious head or spine trauma, repeated concussions, or craniotomy	†	†	Yes	Yes	Yes
Convulsive disorder					
Well controlled	Yes	Yes	Yes	Yes	Yes
Poorly controlled	No	No	Yes¶	Yes	Yes**
Absence of one ovary	Yes	Yes	Yes	Yes	Yes
Respiratory					
Pulmonary insufficiency	††	††	††	††	Yes
Asthma	Yes	Yes	Yes	Yes	Yes
Sickle cell trait	Yes	Yes	Yes	Yes	Yes
Skin					
Boils, herpes, impetigo, scabies	‡‡	‡‡	Yes	Yes	Yes
Enlarged spleen	No	No	No	Yes	Yes
Absent or undescended testicle	Yes§§	Yes§§	Yes	Yes	Yes

*Swimming: no butterfly, breast stroke, or diving starts.

†Needs individual assessment (eg, in the case of an acute illness, one must consider factors such as contagiousness to others and risk of worsening illness).

‡Patients with mild forms of hypertension can be allowed a full range of physical activities; patients with moderate or severe forms, or who are postoperative, should be evaluated by a cardiologist before athletic participation.

§Availability of American Society for Testing and Materials (ASTM)-approved eye guards may allow competitor to participate in most sports, but this must be judged on an individual basis.

‖Consult ophthalmologist.

¶No swimming or weight lifting.

**No archery or riflery

††May be allowed to compete if oxygenation remains satisfactory during a graded stress test.

‡‡No gymnastics with mats, martial arts, wrestling, or contact sports until not contagious.

§§Certain sports may require the use of protective cup.

Adapted from Committee on Sports Medicine, American Academy of Pediatrics; Sports Medicine: Health Care of the Young Athlete, ed 2. Elk Grove Village, IL, American Academy of Pediatrics, 1991, in press; with permission.

exercise (fainting *after* exercise is more likely to be due to hyperventilation); thus, this question should be part of a sports preparticipation history.

Atherosclerotic coronary artery disease is much less common than the first three conditions discussed above, but it can produce sudden death during exercise in previously asymptomatic young athletes. The only clue is a history of anginal pain during activity, but even this is missing in many cases of such deaths. If anginal pain is present, an exercise stress test should be performed before advising athletes about the wisdom of sports participation.

RECOMMENDATIONS FOR PARTICIPATION IN COMPETITIVE SPORTS

In 1988, the American Academy of Pediatrics (AAP) proposed a set of guidelines to assist the physician in deciding whether an athlete should be allowed to compete in a specific sport. They divided athletic events into groups depending upon their degrees of strenuousness and probability for collision (Table 28–2). Various medical and surgical conditions were then considered as to whether they should result in a denial to participate (Table 28–3). Certain sports, such as skiing, are not generally considered contact/collision. However, if the skier hits a tree, then the sport has suddenly become a collision one; so such events were considered as belonging to the "limited contact/impact" group of sports.

These recommendations should only be used as a guideline and are no substitute for a physician's clinical judgement.

REFERENCES

1. Linder CW, DuRant RH, Seklecki RM, et al: Preparticipation health screening of young athletes: Results of 1268 examinations. Am J Sports Med 9:187–193, 1981.
2. Thompson TR, Andrish JT, Bergfeld JA: A prospective study of preparticipation sports examinations of 2670 young athletes: Method and results. Cleve Clin Q 49:225–233, 1982.
3. Rowland TW: Preparticipation sports examination of the child and adolescent athlete: Changing views of an old ritual. Pediatrician 13:3–9, 1986.
4. Samples P: Preparticipation exams: Are they worth the time and trouble? Physician Sportsmed 14:180–187, 1986.
5. Risser WL, Hoffman HM, Bellah GG, et al: A cost-benefit analysis of preparticipation sports examinations of adolescent athletes. J Sch Health 55:270–273, 1985.
6. DuRant RH, Seymore C, Linder CW, et al: The preparticipation examination of athletes: Comparison of single and multiple examiners. Am J Dis Child 139:657–661, 1985.
7. Eichner ER: Sickle cell trait, exercise, and altitude. Physician Sportsmed 14:144–151, 1986.
8. Braden DS, Strong WB: Preparticipation screening for sudden cardiac death in high school and college athletes. Physician Sportsmed 16:128–140, 1988.
9. Maron BJ, Roberts NC, Epstein SE: Sudden death in hypertrophic cardiomyopathy: A profile of 78 patients. Circulation 65:1388–1394, 1982.

29

ORTHOPEDIC PREPARTICIPATION SCREENING EXAMINATION OF THE YOUNG ATHLETE

James G. Garrick, MD

Preparticipation medical examinations are required in many athletic activities. A portion of such an examination is orthopedic screening (Figs. 29–1 through 29–13), which in most instances is performed not by an orthopedist but rather by a primary care physician. Unfortunately, that is often the portion of the examination that is most uncomfortable for the primary care physician, who may have recently been bombarded with literature and lectures describing sophisticated tests for determining joint instability and muscular deficiencies and imbalances.

It is important to bear in mind that any preparticipation screening examination cannot be all things to all people. Just as the cardiovascular portion of such an examination cannot represent a complete cardiac workup, neither can musculoskeletal screening be a thorough orthopedic evaluation. The examination represents, rather, a minimum standard, the performance of which is well within the capabilities of any physician and even most nurse practitioners, athletic trainers, and physical therapists. It is not a substitute for the scheduled, periodic examinations recommended for children and adolescents.

The examination is designed to identify congenital and acquired musculoskeletal problems that may either be adversely affected by sports participation or compromise attempts at athletic endeavors. From a pragmatic standpoint, it is aimed at identifying the residuals of previous musculoskeletal injuries.

Abnormalities found by the examination merit a directed orthopedic examination. Although many of the conditions identified will ultimately not result in disqualification, they may prompt specific efforts at conditioning or rehabilitation. In some instances, a condition may prompt a reassessment of athletic choices or goals. For example, a 12-year-old female gymnast with a history of an elbow dislocation and a 10-deg loss of elbow extension might be first placed on a range of motion and strengthening program. If that fails to result in normal motion, the athlete might be counseled to consider competitive diving, as her future as a successful elite-level gymnast is significantly compromised. The same condition in a football lineman would be of little consequence.

Thus, final decisions and advice should be left to those with an intimate knowledge of the orthopedic aspects of sports participation as well as the musculoskeletal demands of the sports activities.

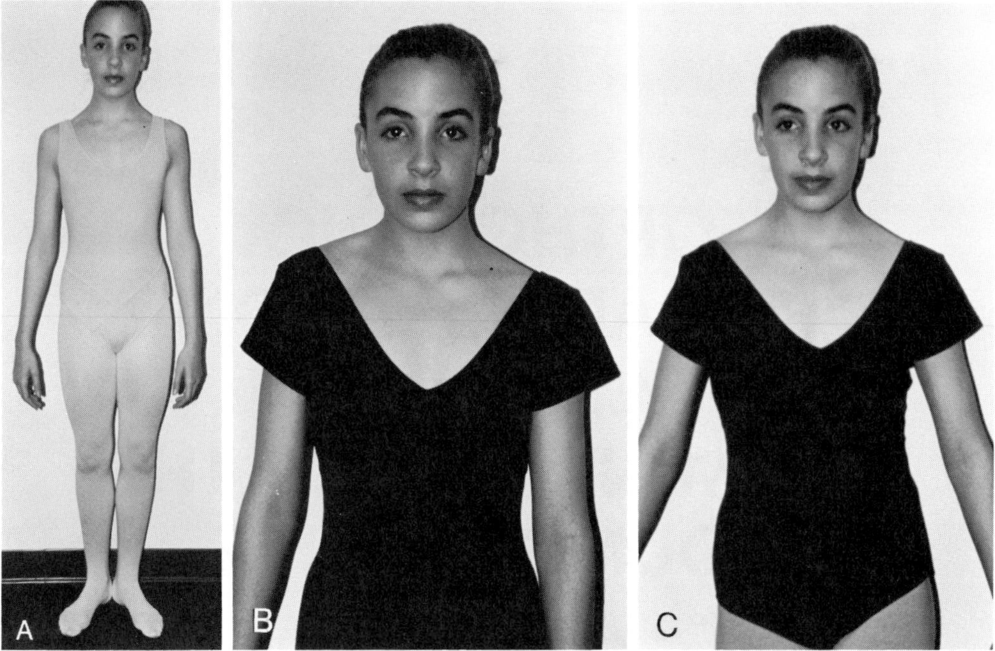

Figure 29–1. A: Athlete stands facing examiner, arms at the sides. Head tilted or rotated to the side may indicate trapezius or paracervical muscle spasm. **B**: Shoulders at different heights identifies trapezius spasm or shoulder weakness. Enlarged acromioclavicular or sternoclavicular joint identifies residual of previous sprain. **C**: Asymmetric indentation at waist may indicate scoliosis or leg-length discrepancy.

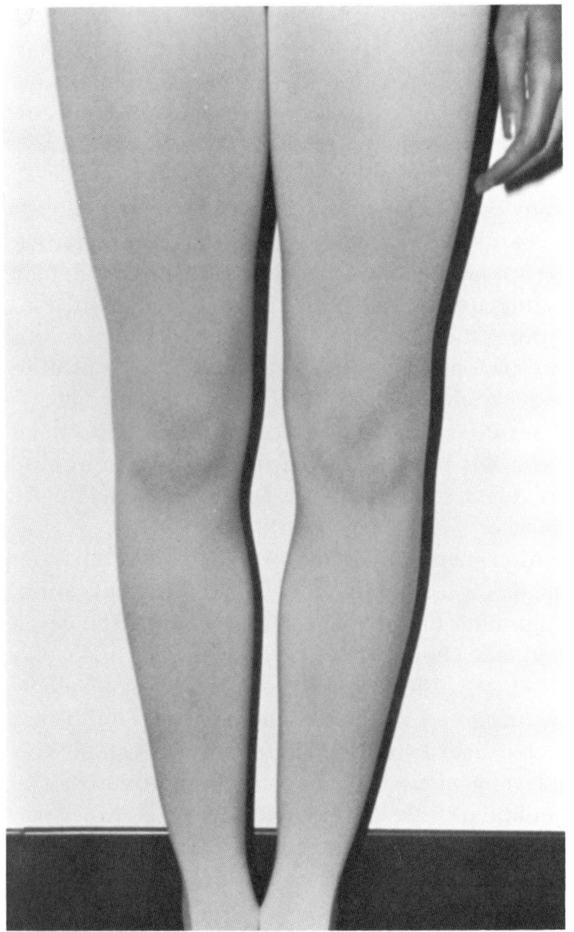

Figure 29–2. Asymmetric knee contours or obvious swelling identifies effusion or Osgood-Schlatter disease. Asymmetric ankle contours indicate effusion. Athlete contracts (tightens) quadriceps. Asymmetric quadriceps muscles (especially vastus medialis) identify residual atrophy or weakness from knee injury.

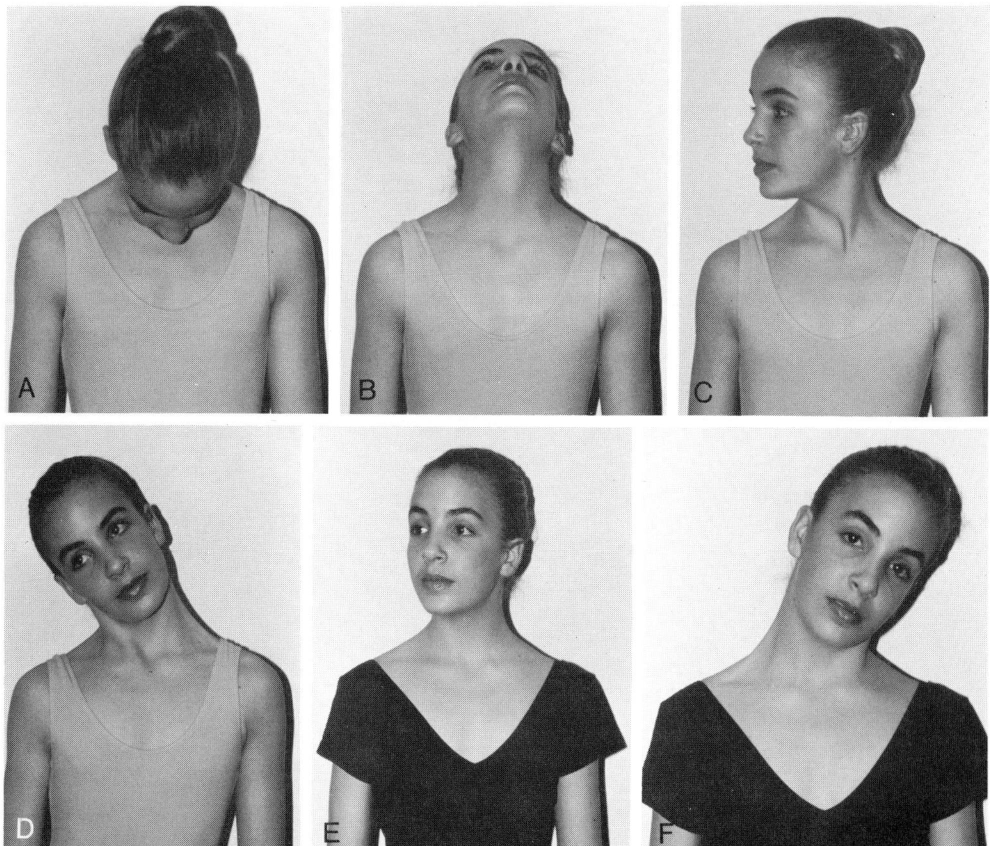

Figure 29–3. Demonstrate neck range of motion. **A**: Flex; look at floor. **B**: Extend; look at ceiling. **C**: Rotate; look over left shoulder, then right shoulder. **D, E,** and **F**: Lateral bending; place left ear on left shoulder, then right ear on right shoulder. Asymmetric or restricted motion may indicate muscle spasm or weakness.

The preparticipation examination does not attempt to evaluate such matters as joint laxity, whether congenital or acquired. The reasons are twofold: There is no universally agreed upon means of determining the degree of inherited laxity that might predict an increased likelihood of injury; and postinjury laxity is not only difficult to evaluate, but once documented, its relationship to reinjury often remains to be determined.

Thus, the goal of the screening examination is to identify those who might have problems with sports participation and to bring them to the attention of the appropriate specialist. The examination should be held at least 2 weeks in advance of the first practice to allow time for consultations and tests if necessary.

HISTORY

Perhaps the most important portion of the examination is the elucidation of an accurate history of prior musculoskeletal injuries. Indeed, the actual physical examination might be viewed as being nothing more than an adjunct and quality control of the history.

The history consists of a series of redundant questions dealing with previous musculoskeletal injuries and problems. The redundancy is intentional because of the unreliability of many youthful historians. The following is a suggested list of questions:

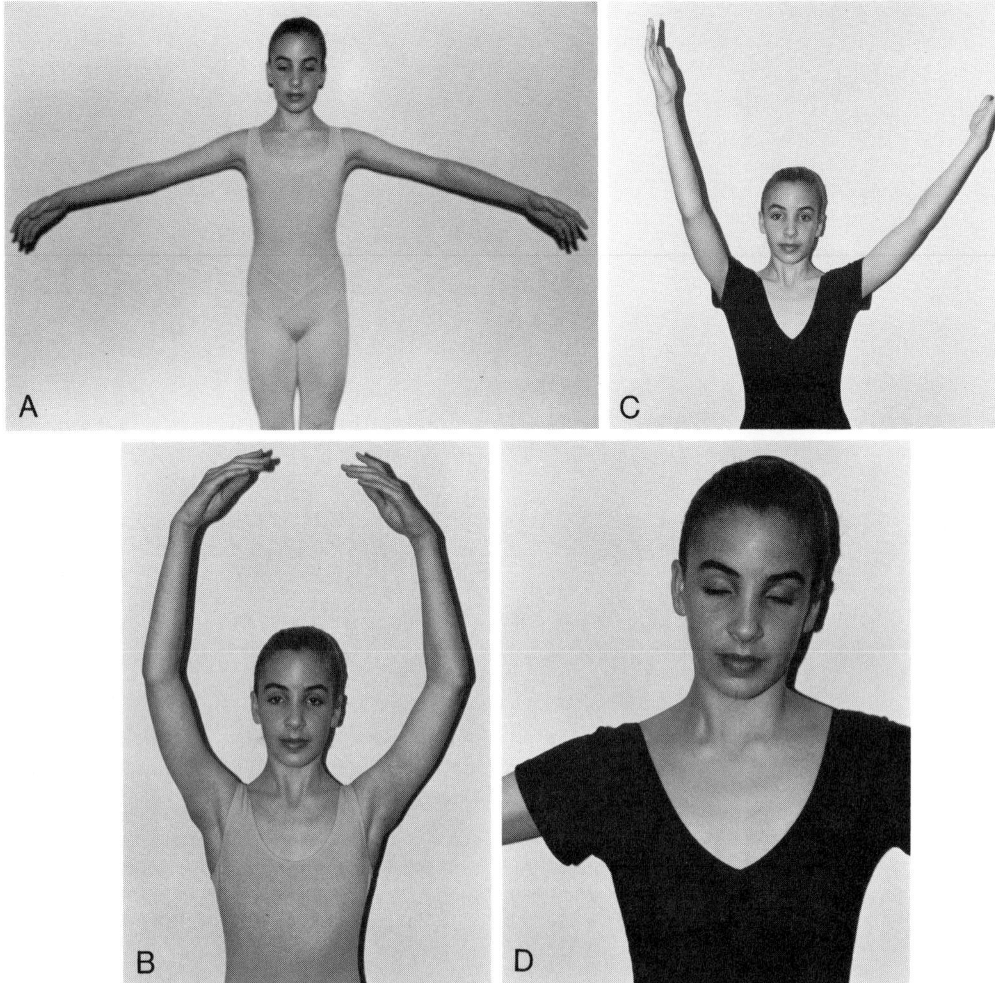

Figure 29–4. **A** and **B**: With elbows extended, athlete raises arms and touches hands over head. **C** and **D**: Asymmetric elevation of shoulders or premature shoulder elevation indicates limited or painful motion.

Have you ever—
- been a patient overnight in a hospital?
- been a patient in an emergency room?
- had an injury that required x-rays?
- had an operation?
- had an injury that caused you to miss a game or practice?
- had an injury that required a doctor's care?

Are you now under the care of a physician?

Do you have any medical problems or injuries at the present time?

Have you ever had—
- a broken bone?
- a torn ligament?
- a muscle pull?
- a "pinched nerve"?
- a head or neck injury?
- a back injury or "back problems"?

PHYSICAL EXAMINATION

Boys should wear trunks or a swim suit, girls a leotard or two-piece swim suit. Although it is tempting to line up four or five athletes and perform a mass screening, it is less time-consuming to examine one person at a time.

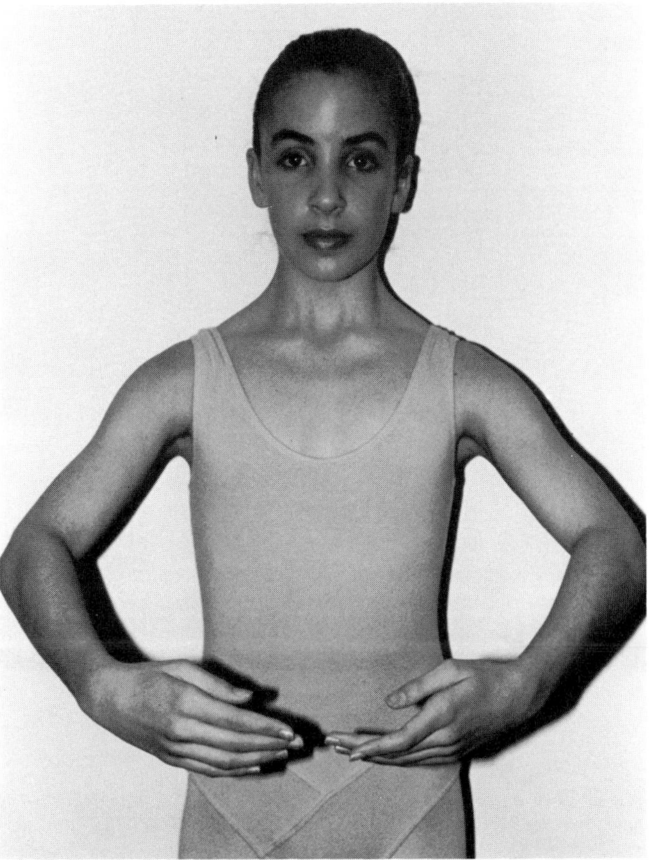

Figure 29–5. Athlete holds arms horizontally in front of body. Atrophy or fasciculation of anterior deltoid identifies weakness or shoulder impingement.

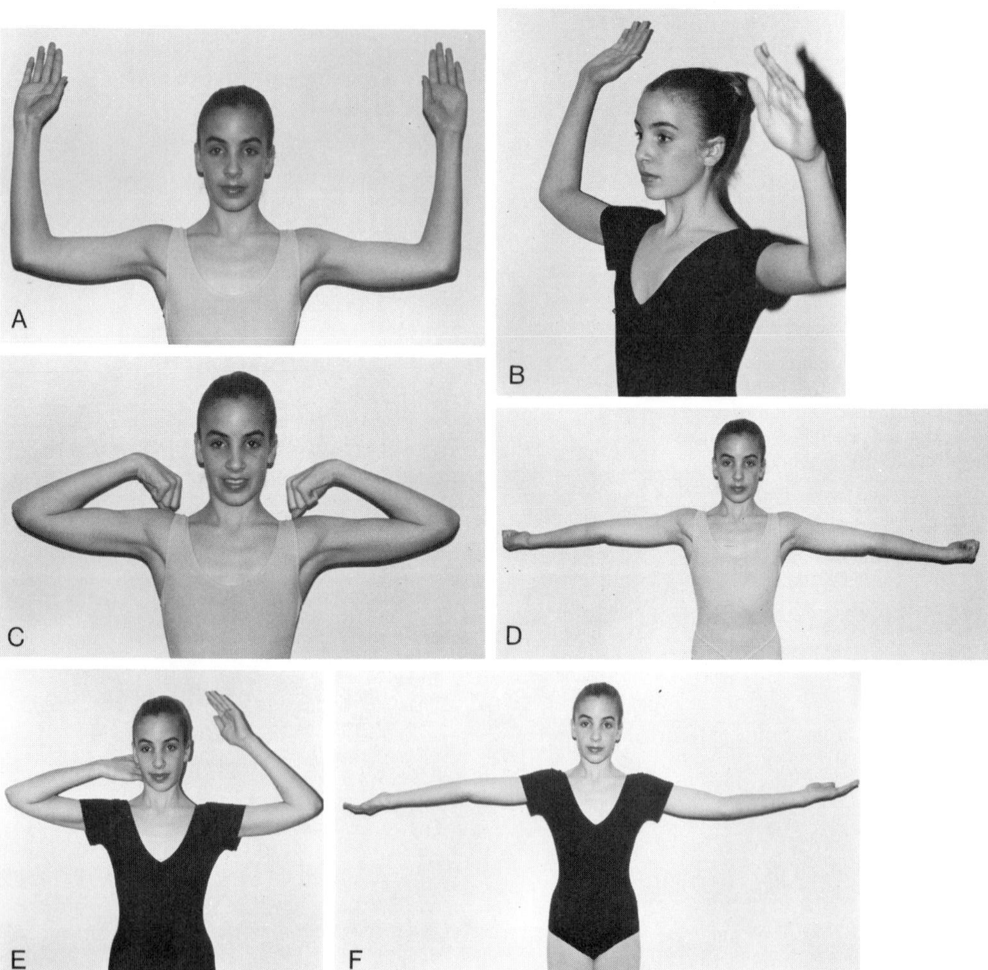

Figure 29–6. A: Athlete holds arms horizontally from the sides with hands up and elbows flexed 90 degrees. **B**: Reluctance to rotate forearm externally to vertical indicates shoulder subluxation or dislocation. **C** and **D**: In this position, athlete fully flexes and extends elbow. **E** and **F**: Lack of full flexion or extension (unilateral) identifies previous elbow trauma, osteochondritis dissecans, or "Little League elbow."

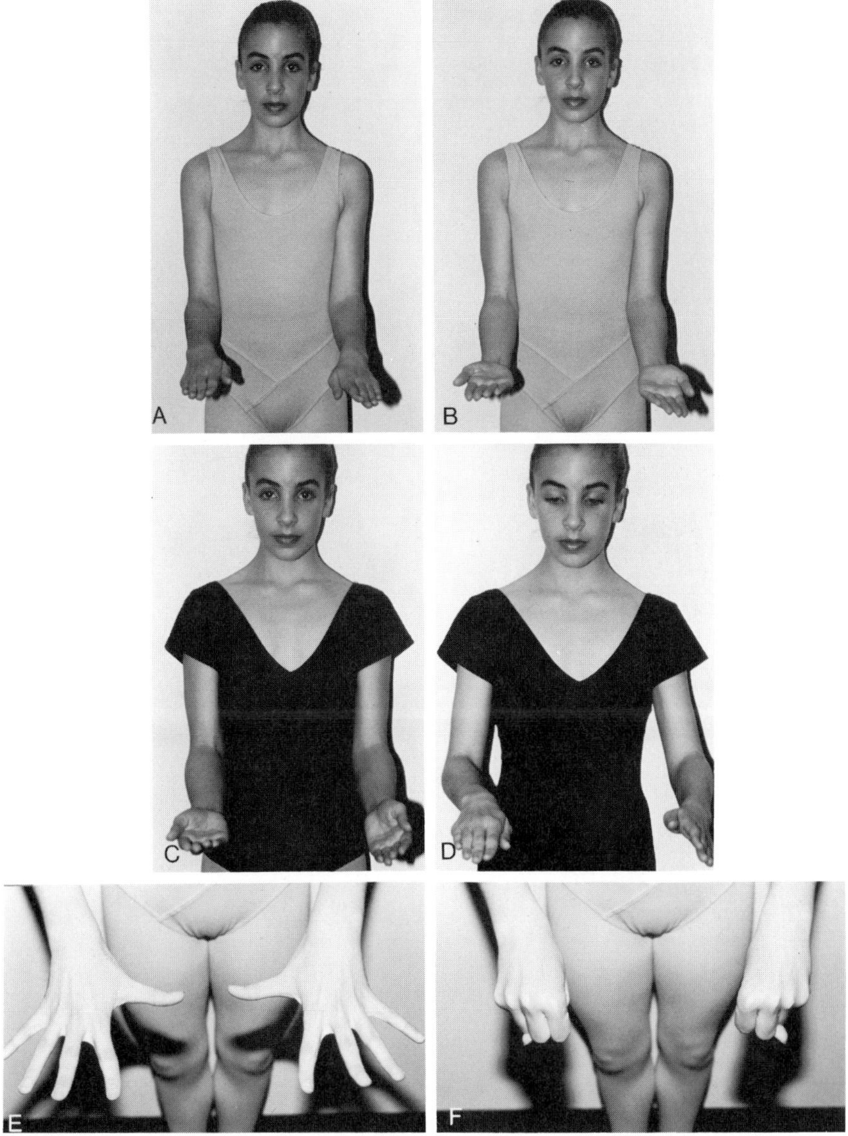

Figure 29–7. Arms at side, elbows flexed 90 degrees, **(A)** pronate (palms facing floor), and **(B)** supinate (palms facing ceiling). **C** and **D**: Asymmetry of extremes of motion indicates previous elbow or wrist injury, osteochondritis dissecans of elbow, or "Little League elbow." **E**: Spread fingers. **F**: Make a fist. Asymmetry of metacarpal-phalangeal or interphalangeal joints of flexion and extension indicate residuals of sprains or fractures.

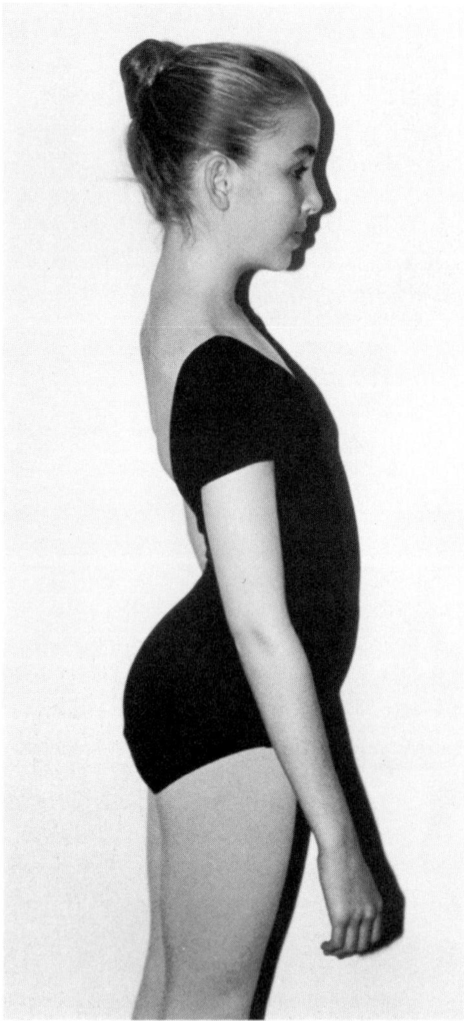

Figure 29–8. Lordosis ("swayback") may indicate spondylolysis. Unilateral lack of full knee extension identifies effusion or postinjury hamstring spasm.

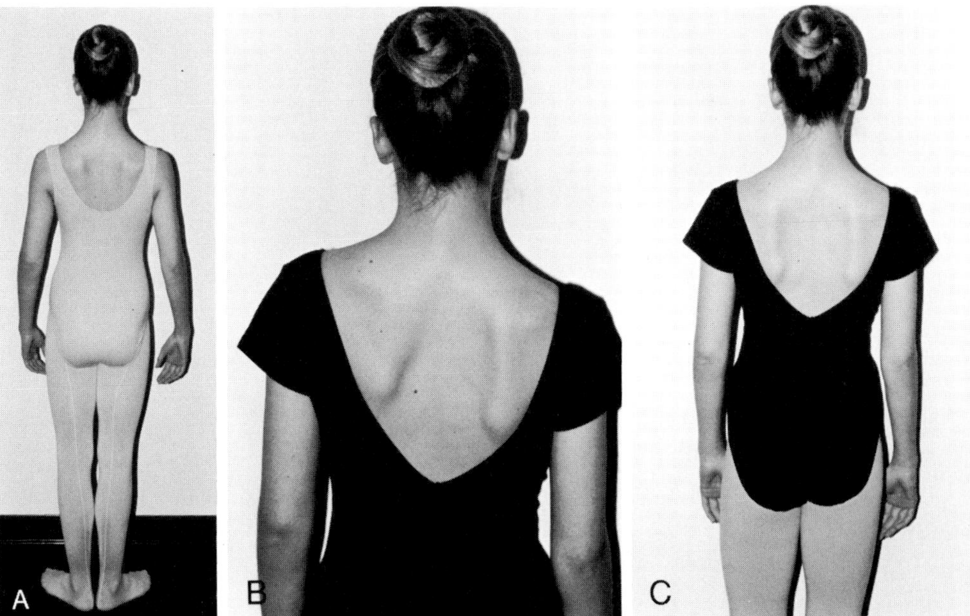

Figure 29–9. A: Athlete stands facing away from examiner. **B** and **C**: Examiner observes shoulder heights, waist indentation, and posterior chest prominence for indications of scoliosis, shoulder weakness, or spasm.

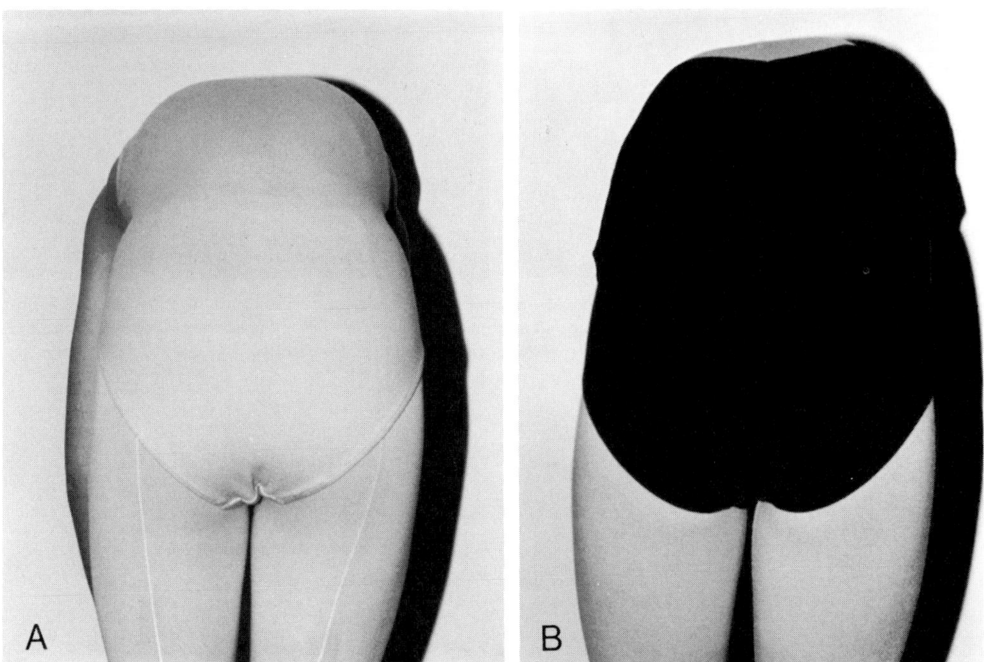

Figure 29–10. A: Athlete bends at waist (touches toes). **B**: Asymmetry of posterior rib cage indicates scoliosis. Limited flexion, inability to obliterate lumbar lordosis, or discomfort indicates tight hamstrings or spondylolysis. Spine rotation with attempted flexion indicates paraspinous muscle spasm.

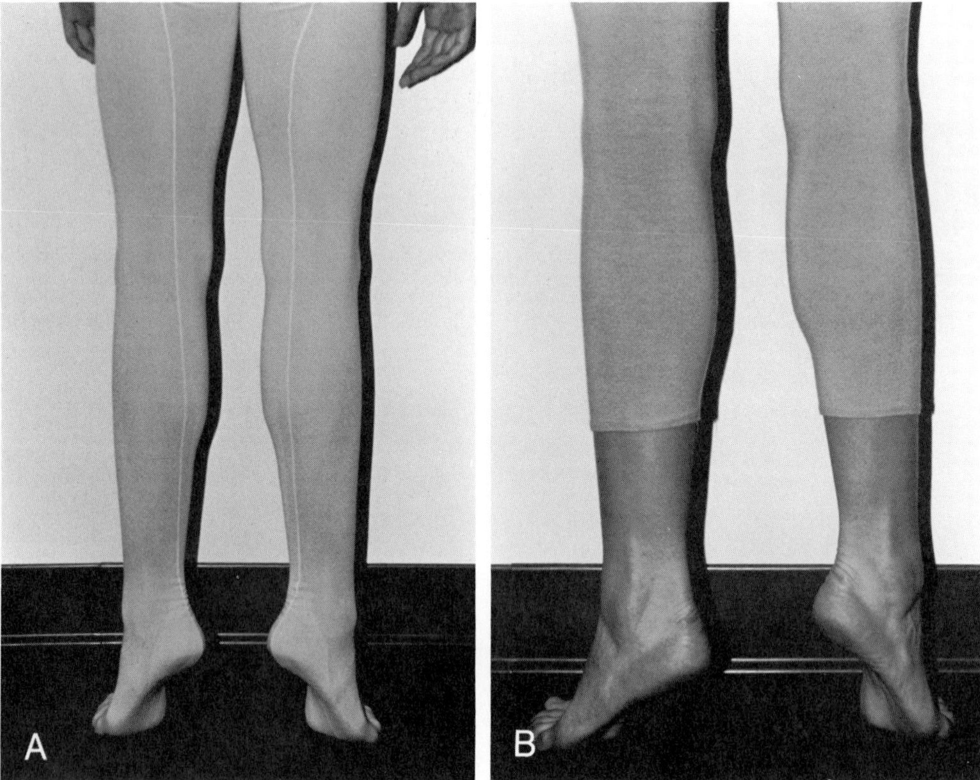

Figure 29–11. A: Athlete stands on toes. **B**: Asymmetry of heel elevation indicates postinjury loss of ankle motion or weak calf muscles. Asymmetry of gastrocnemius (upper calf bulge) identifies postinjury weakness (ankle sprain residual). Asymmetry of Achilles tendon width indicates tendonitis.

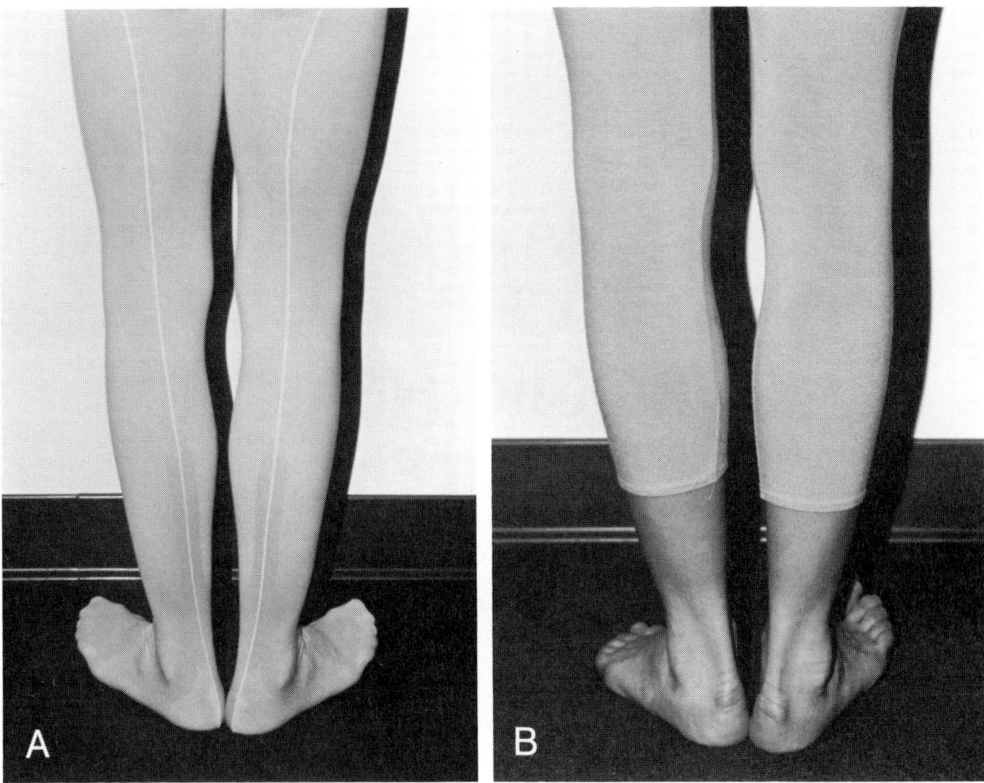

Figure 29–12. **A**: Athlete stands on heels. **B**: Asymmetric forefoot elevation may indicate tight or weak calf musculature or postinjury loss of ankle motion.

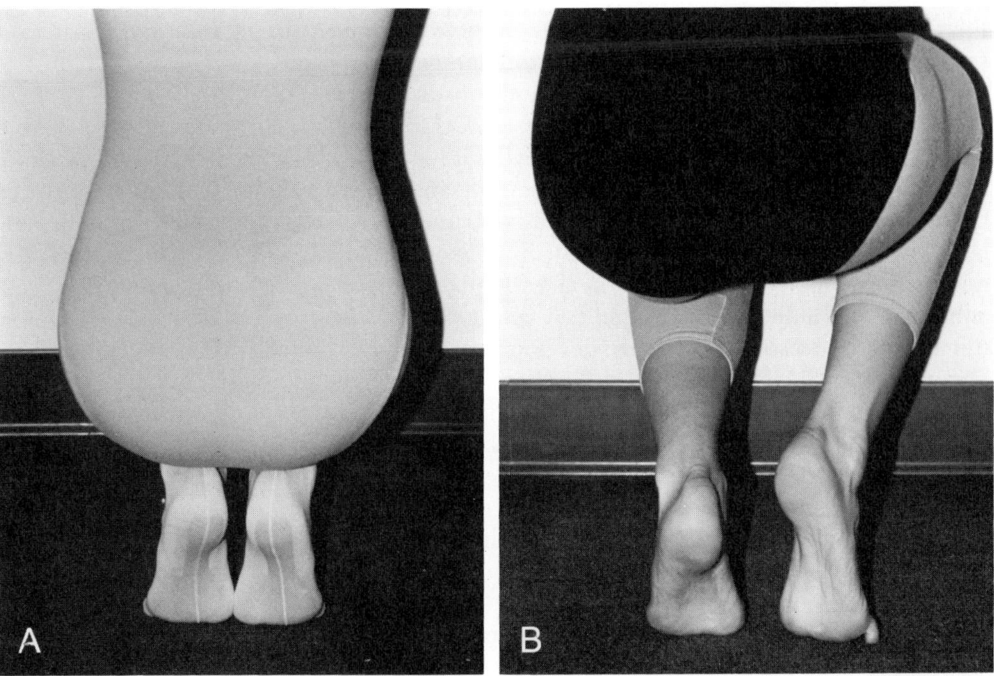

Figure 29–13. **A**: Athlete assumes a squatting position. **B**: Asymmetry of thigh-to-heel distance or heel-to-floor elevation indicates loss of ankle motion (postsprain or fracture); lack of knee flexion from quadriceps spasm or weakness or knee effusion; or chondromalacia of patella. As athlete rises from squatting position, examiner notes asymmetry of knee motion, which indicates chondromalacia patella, quadriceps weakness, or internal derangement.

30

SPORTS PARTICIPATION FOR THE CHILD WITH A CHRONIC HEALTH PROBLEM

John H. Kennell, MD
Wayne Rusin, MD

To keep the body in good health is a duty . . . otherwise we shall not be able to keep our mind strong and clear. Buddha

Argue for your limitations and sure enough, they're yours.
Richard Bach

Physical activities play an important role in the development of all children. During the second year of life, for example, the toddler has a tremendous desire to climb and explore. This activity increases strength and coordination and therefore confidence. Even in the first year, infants have a great urge to kick, roll, crawl, and move about. There is new evidence that there is a definite rhythmic pattern to the movements of newborn infants, which we have previously considered random. This same rhythmic pattern has been shown in fetal movements.[1] Infants gain knowledge first about their own bodies and later knowledge of persons and objects in their expanding world. As a child grows, kinesthetic and tactile sensations form the foundation upon which the beginnings of self-awareness and individuality are built. A young child's play provides external evidence of the internal processes of cognitive development. Much of the play of young children has importance for their physical growth, muscle development, and conditioning as they participate in activities such as swinging on swings, climbing trees, and chasing each other around the playground. This play activity is also valuable for their intellectual development because it permits them to explore their environment, to learn about objects, and to solve problems. Play activity also advances their social development. Their activities with other children help them to develop self-control and to learn to play by the rules of the social game. Peers are a source of information about these rules and about how well the child is playing the game. Peers provide a different perspective than the family. Just as parents do, peers influence the development of a child through reinforcement and modeling. In addition, they may serve as a standard against which children can evaluate

This work was supported in part by the William T. Grant Foundation, Bureau of Maternal and Child Health, and the National Institute of Child Health and Human Development, RO1-HD16915.

themselves, using others as a "yardstick." This process of social comparison is one basis for the development of the child's self-image and self-esteem. Failure to gain mastery and competence may clearly have a negative influence on the child's development of body image and self concept.

During the middle years of childhood, from grades 1 to 7, or from ages 6 to 12 years, the child's weight doubles and boys and girls acquire many major and minor motor skills. There is a great drive and pleasure in physical skill mastery. To ride a two-wheel bicycle may be more important to a child's self-esteem than learning to read and write. This is also the period when a child learns to roller skate and ice skate; to play baseball and football; to swim and dive; and to hang by the knees, spin tops, jump ropes, snap fingers, and whistle. In the process, boys and girls gain an increased sense of self and an increased integration of who they are and their place in society. Boys and girls become distinct individuals during this period, and they become more empathic and less egocentric. Children at this age need to feel that they are growing more capable and that they are mastering skills.

During these years, children have a special separate subculture with traditions, games, values, loyalties, and rules of its own. This is frequently overlooked as parents often impose highly organized, tightly scheduled activities, such as music lessons, dance lessons, horseback riding lessons, Little League baseball and Pop Warner football league, and visits to the orthodontist, in addition to school homework. Continuing into the adolescent years, teenagers begin to loosen ties to their home and parents and begin to seek the approval of their peer group. A wish to do well in sporting activities is often an expression of the adolescent's need for approval by peers and by adults.

We can begin to get a small inkling of the problems of a child with a chronic health problem if we consider the needs of the typical child of 6 to 12 years and compound them with the special needs of children with a chronic condition. Failure of a child with a chronic disease to achieve a satisfying level of physical competence and mastery may be derived from three sources:

1. *Medical effects:* Children with a chronic disease may fail to maintain the medical regimen or may have inadequate medical supervision.
2. *Parental response:* Parents may respond to the child with a chronic disease with distortions that include overprotection, overcompensation, or rejection.
3. *Personal distress of the child:* This can include denial, withdrawal, decreased motivation, and a general sense of incompetence and helplessness.

For example, children with epilepsy or diabetes have the additional concerns of controlling their bodies, losing consciousness, and requiring long-term medication. Many children with musculoskeletal disorders may find it difficult carrying out some of the traditional activities of childhood or may be restricted from sports activities. Chronic disease does not only apply to physical handicaps. Young people with attentional difficulties, such as attention deficit hyperactive disorder (ADHD), and young people with mental retardation (MR) may experience great frustration in organized sports. In the past, children with mental retardation were excluded from traditional activities and from sports. We need to ask ourselves how many children who have chronic health problems or attentional problems or who are mentally retarded have also developed secondary problems (eg, obesity or inappropriate social behavior) because they have been excluded from the subculture and physical activities of the school-aged child. Three basic principles should be adhered to in all of children's sports. First, all children want to play, not sit on the sidelines and watch. Second, all children need sports to be scaled down to their level to insure fun and mastery. Third, children need less emphasis on winning and more emphasis on skill acquisition and enjoyment. While it is the theme of this chapter to encourage sports participation in children with health problems, it is necessary to distinguish between participation in athletic activities and participation in competitive sports. Competition is often highly motivating and is one means for promoting self-satisfaction and developing muscles and coordination, but this is true only if the child has a chance of achieving success. If children who are healthy or who have a chronic health problem are condemned to constant failure because of limitations in strength, endurance, range of motion, or coordination, participation in competitive activities can be destructive to their self-image. The healthy child with limited ability or a child with a chronic health problem should be guided to an appropriate level of activities with no competition or with a goal of competition against previous performance. The child with a serious handicap usually recognizes that she or he has little opportunity to succeed in sports competition with healthy children of the same age. However, the child with a mild handicap may not have this perception and may experience considerable frustration and discouragement when she or he continues to make these comparisons.

It is in situations like these that the roles of the parent and physician become extremely important. When we consider the significant developmental accomplishments that usually take place between 6 and 12 years, we can appreciate the crucial significance of the decisions made by parents and physicians about whether an individual child should take part in physical activities. If we are aware of the important molding, reinforcing, standard-setting role of the peer group, we will further appreciate the importance of arranging for the child with a chronic health problem to have the opportunity to participate in a sports activity successfully. This will make the youngster's childhood as normal as possible

A child with a chronic health problem who is not weighed down by restrictions from parents and physicians may be able to participate in almost all normal activities with a peer group. It is thus possible for this child to then have a normal healthy passage through the school years with a strong self-image and self-esteem.

Children should be allowed to participate in formal and informal athletic activities with children of their own age according to abilities and interests. Any action that keeps a child from full participation with peers should be considered carefully. If restrictions are necessary, the reasons should be explained as clearly and reassuringly as possible. The duration of the restriction should be spelled out whenever possible. Substitute activities should be proposed to keep the child involved with peers in group activities that offer some competition, excitement, or potential for muscle building or development of coordination. Some parents of children with chronic disorders have a tendency to introduce restrictions or continue them contrary to the advice or intention of a physician.[2]

Studies have also shown that patients and their parents may misunderstand the physician's reasons for recommending restrictions and may have unwarranted concerns about the patient's health.

Other parents push their healthy child or a child with a chronic health problem into activities because of their own, rather than the child's, desire. A discussion with the parents and child should be arranged to find out who wants the youngster to participate in what activity and why. Shaffer[3] has proposed a classification of sports or athletic activities that would be helpful when making plans for a child with a chronic health problem. A modification of this is shown in Table 30–1. With this information, a discussion with a physical education director, and a careful clinical evaluation of the child, the physician can counsel the parents and the child about the problems associated with the physical activity of a person with a particular handicap. Although all children with chronic health problems face these adjustment problems, particular health problems present specific concerns and require individual attention. Some of the more common chronic disorders will be discussed in this chapter.

TABLE 30–1. CLASSIFICATION OF SPORTS

Strenuous Contact Sports	Strenuous Limited Contact Sports
Football	Basketball
Ice hockey	Field hockey
Lacrosse	Racquetball/squash
Martial arts (karate, judo)	Soccer
Rugby	Volleyball
Wrestling	**Moderately Strenuous Sports**
Strenuous Noncontact Sports	Badminton
	Baseball (limited contact)
Aerobic dancing	Curling
Crew	Equestrian*
Cross-country	Golf
Cycling*	Skateboarding
Diving*	Table tennis
Fencing	**Nonstrenuous Sports**
Gymnastics*	Archery
Skiing*	Auto racing*
Swimming*	Bowling
Tennis	Motorcycling*
Track and field	Riflery
Water polo*	
Water skiing*	
Weight lifting*	
Windsurfing*	

*Increased risk if loss of consciousness occurs as with hypoglycemia, seizure, syncope.

Adapted from Shaffer TE: The health examination for participation in sports. Pediatr Ann 7:670, 1978; with permission.

DIABETES

Early efforts with the patient, parents, and other family members are often pivotal in the management of a child with a chronic health problem such as diabetes. The diagnosis results in shock and a series of turbulent emotional reactions. All members of the family need abundant opportunity to express their fears, concerns, and feelings of guilt before they are able to understand explanations about the physiology of the disease and the philosophy and plan of management. Many of the psychological problems occurring during the later periods of care can be traced to inadequate introduction to diabetes during the first episode of illness. The family and the patient who have a thorough understanding of the disturbed physiology, the natural history of the disease, and the aims and goals of the physician are in the best position to handle this chronic disease process effectively.

Right from the start it is desirable to stress that the child with diabetes should be allowed to lead as normal a life as any other child with the exception of the need for some attention to diet, insulin, blood and urine testing, and illnesses. Part of this discussion should emphasize the value of peer activities and make it clear that the diabetic child can take part in all normal, traditional activities, including participation in sports activities appropriate for the child's age. Because this may be difficult for the parents to accept at first, it is important to meet with the parents to listen and to provide them with an opportunity to express their guilt, anger, sadness, and anxieties. This interested and concerned listening may be very beneficial in the long run.

Benefits of Exercise

Children whose diabetes is properly controlled have normal growth and development. Regular exercise can improve exercise tolerance. As a result of exercising by diabetic patients, the extra energy expenditure helps consume stored calories and improves sensitivity to insulin. In general, the same beneficial effects afforded to nondiabetic children and adolescents who exercise are realized by exercising diabetic persons. Specialists who manage diabetic children agree that exercise remains an important part of treatment. Participation in traditional peer activities and in sports and athletic activities does much to enhance the child's self-image.

Precautions

Exercise should preferably take place after a meal and should be relatively regular. Because the child is taking insulin, it is necessary to match up the caloric intake and the insulin. The current use of blood glucose meters adds an important safety factor. By checking blood glucose levels before and after exercise, the physician working with the family can decide whether to decrease insulin or to increase snacks. Special instruction is needed for dietary management during participation in competitive sports or strenuous exercise to avoid hypoglycemic episodes. A distinction should be made between isolated periods of exercise and the effect of a regular exercise program. Because there seems to be an increased sensitivity to insulin with ongoing exercise, one may anticipate a reduction in insulin requirements.

Eating patterns are important in exercising individuals, as food may be necessary before, during, and after exercise to avoid hypoglycemia. Special care needs to be taken when exercise is done before bedtime to avoid hypoglycemia during sleep. Insulin sensitivity remains for up to 12 hours, so a bedtime snack is indicated. Specific recommendations for changes in insulin and diet in relation to exercise need to be established by trial and error. However, in general, a reduction in insulin or increase in calories should be considered on days of strenuous exercise. The timing of the exercise will determine whether to decrease regular or long-acting insulin. Excess release of insulin from injection sites, particularly in the legs, has been shown to occur during exercise contrary to the normal physiologic reduction of plasma insulin during exercise.[4] Injection of insulin in the abdomen preferably, but next best in the arms, may be helpful in reducing these effects.[5] Availability of a handy carbohydrate source (eg, juice packs, glucose tablets, sugar cubes) may save embarrassment. Candy is traditionally used for this purpose but may present an unnecessary conflict of willpower, particularly for smaller children. Parents should talk to coaches about diabetes and what to do if the child becomes disoriented or shows other symptoms of hypoglycemia. They must insist on the child's absolute right to stop and get sugar.

Children and adolescents with diabetes can participate in virtually all athletic activities. The only exceptions are those that present an immediate personal hazard if hypoglycemia occurs. Therefore, no deep-sea diving, no piloting of airplanes, and no sky diving are allowed.

Diabetes in itself should not limit the type of excercise or sports event.[6] Patients with severe complications should discuss their individual plans for exercise and sports activities with their physician. Diabetic patients who are in poor control are not good candidates for strenuous exercise. Exercise during hyperglycemia with ketosis may actually increase blood glucose and ketone levels. It should be stressed, however, that once a reasonable degree of control is attained, control is generally improved by regular exercise. When diabetic neuropathy is present, awareness of peripheral injuries may be diminished. It is desirable to teach all diabetic children to take care of their extremities, particularly if they are in sports activities. They must be taught to give prompt attention to lacerations and abrasions, burning or freezing of the feet; to trim toenails evenly with the end of the toes; and to avoid tight shoes or socks which interfere with the circulation or cause calluses.

PROBLEMS OF DEPENDENCY

In working with a child with a chronic illness, such as diabetes, a major concern is the dependency on the part of both parents and child. It is not unusual for mothers and fathers to focus many of their frustrations, anxieties, and problems on the chronic illness and the chronically ill child. This often manifests itself as excessive concern over certain aspects of care. A mother may find it difficult to allow the child out of her sight.

There are rich opportunities for such children to establish a dependent relationship with a family when they have a chronic illness, such as diabetes mellitus, because of the complicated interrelations between nutrition, medication, and physical activity. It is necessary for the physician managing children and adolescents with diabetes to keep in mind the normal developmental sequences through which a healthy child passes in the establishment of independence. For example, what may be considered normal dependency for a 3-year-old child may be clearly abnormal for one who is 12 years of age.

Problems of dependency are reduced when the family, school personnel, and friends understand from the beginning that the diabetic child should be able to participate in all athletic activities. Of course, the physician needs to explain that he or she will help the family with adjustments in insulin dosage and in diet. It is desirable for children with diabetes to participate with other children in all activities; however, in the first summer or two of the illness, many children benefit from attending a summer camp for diabetic children in which normal camp activities are stressed and in which the diabetic aspect is minimal. After that, the child should be able to attend a regular summer camp that accepts diabetic children who are able to care for themselves. In the adolescent years, a session or two at a camp that stresses self-care and education may help prepare the adolescent for independent living.

With adolescence, the child is usually self-motivated toward greater independence. This period of life, which is regularly one of stress for the healthy child, is even more stressful for the chronically ill child. The conflict between dependency and independence is heightened because of the diabetic child's greater needs. Early in adolescence is the appropriate time for children to be responsible for more and more of their care, to give their own insulin injections, to test their own blood and urine, and to keep their own records. At this time, it is advisable for the physician to work almost entirely with the child rather than through the mother as in the preadolescent period. The tendency of adolescents to overlook the fact that they have an illness, to eat with abandon, and to skip some doses of insulin has to be anticipated.

EPILEPSY

Epilepsy may result from a large number of underlying medical problems. The largest proportion of children have seizures of unknown etiology. The range of seizure types is broad. Some are brief with little or only partial visible alteration in the child's behavior or consciousness, so that the patient or bystanders may not be aware of them. While these brief seizures might occur several times a day, the child may be at little or no disadvantage in her or his activities. In contrast, many children have major motor (grand mal, tonic-clonic) seizures associated with unconsciousness. This type of seizure presents a medical problem with regard to athletic activity because of the small but realistic possibility that a head injury or other injury may occur at the onset of a seizure.

During the past three decades, there has been progressive improvement in the drug control of epileptic seizures. An improved ability to define the type of seizure and the development of more effective antiepileptic medication have contributed to a better prognosis for epileptic patients. The majority of children and adolescents are now seizure-free for extended periods. The quality of seizure control is a major factor in deciding on the type of sports participation for the child or adolescent with epilepsy. The child with frequent major motor seizures despite careful medical management may not be a candidate for competitive athletics but should not be restricted from lighter physical activity, such as physical education. Between the two extremes of absence seizures (petit mal and grand mal), there is a spectrum of seizure states, the nature and severity of which require that each child receive individual consideration of daily activities.

Early in the course of the disease, it is necessary for the child with epilepsy and the family to recognize that certain adjustments in the daily routine may be necessary. There should be a frank discussion with every child with epilepsy about the hazards of overfatigue, skipped meals, excessive alcohol intake, and "street drugs." In making these alterations, the aim is to strike a balance between the needs of the child to participate with peers in daily activities and the limitations that any restriction may impose. If it is possible to achieve optimal control of seizures, the child with epilepsy, as with other chronic illnesses, should be able to develop the self-confidence necessary to live independently in the community as an adult.

There is general agreement among physicians and educators that most children with epilepsy belong in regular school classes. When seizures are under adequate control and there are no associated intellectual or emotional deficits, there is no need for special facilities, arrangements, or restrictions.

Fortunately for children with epilepsy, physical and mental activities appear to be seizure deterrents. Many epileptic patients have fewer seizures when they are active than when they are sleeping or resting. Although this is a characteristic that may vary with individual children, it leads to a general recommendation that most epileptic children should participate in all physical activities that do not impose a significant risk of injury to themselves or others (see Table 30–1).

A great majority of children and adolescents with epilepsy participate in physical activities with no difficulty.[7] A concern about hyperventilation should not be a deterrent to exercise. By producing the need for greater gas exchange, physical activities do not alter body chemistries in the same way as voluntary or forced hyperventilation, which may precipitate petit mal spells. It is fortunate that many school systems make little distinction between epileptic and nonepileptic children in athletic programs.

Every effort should be made to minimize restrictions. There is an increased risk with participation in sports, but it is minimal. Most children and adolescents and their families have accepted this risk and have determined that it is worth taking compared with the greater physical and mental risk of inactivity and alienation. A truthful discussion with all concerned and mutual trust are better than arbitrary rules. The following are guidelines to use in such discussions:

1. *Contact sports:* There is generally no reason to restrict the epileptic child from contact sports. Boxing, with its potential for head trauma, should be avoided in all children including those with epilepsy.

2. *Gymnastics:* There is general agreement that a child with epilepsy should not perform athletic activities in which a fall, due to a seizure, could result in serious injury. These would include such activities as rope climbing and gymnastics, particularly the parallel bars. Individualization is crucial in these sports.

3. *Swimming:* The child with epilepsy should be allowed to participate in swimming activities with the understanding that he or she, like all other children, should always be under supervision.

4. *Skiing and bicycle riding:* Most children and adolescents can participate in these popular activities with suitable precautions, such as bicycle riding off the street, or skiing on the lower slopes.

Each child with epilepsy should be receiving health supervision by a physician experienced with managing this disorder. Contact with the school health service, principal, and teacher is essential so that unnecessary concerns or restrictions will not be placed on the child thereby preventing him or her from appearing "different." In this way, home and school environments will remain consistent and present fewer adjustment problems for the child. The school authorities should be informed about what to do in case of a seizure so they will not be alarmed and will carry out the necessary emergency measures. Community resources, such as the Epilepsy Foundation, may also be of value in providing information about the characteristics of seizures and their management.

The risks involved in athletic participation should be considered by the parents, the physician, and the child with the risks weighed against the harmful psychological effects of unnecessary restriction. Parents should participate in the making of all decisions by joint conferences with the school and with the child's physician. But the child's own wishes must also be considered to the degree appropriate for his or her age and judgment. These children must realize that there is a calculated risk of injury and, in some instances, they should be prepared to impose voluntary restrictions on themselves, depending on the nature and frequency of the seizures. Recommendations should be individualized based upon a given child's seizure history. At all times, the therapeutic benefits of allowing the child to participate in normal physical education activities versus the harmful effects of forbidding them to participate should be kept in mind. Often, a trial period can provide a sound basis for long-term planning when the decision about participation is not clear. The occurrence of a seizure during the trial period rarely has significant consequences beyond the episode itself.

Adolescent young men and young women with no chronic health problems are intensely concerned about their bodies and about achieving control of them. They also want to be reassured that they are normal like other young men and women. When adolescents have epilepsy, there is a special reason for attending to their needs. They need to be encouraged to accept more and more responsibility for their care, and the parents usually need to be helped to release their control of the adolescent. It is necessary to make a special effort to establish good communication with the young man or young woman so that there can be frank discussions every 6 to 12 months about why medications are being given, the dangers of stopping abruptly, and why it is necessary to continue this medication. In spite of this, the rebellious nature of an adolescent may result in skipped doses and temporary discontinuation of the medication as if to prove there really is no problem. When a seizure does result, it is usually a powerful reminder that a problem is present and medication is often taken reliably after that, in part to avoid the embarrassment of a seizure. If no seizures result, it is appropriate to consider with the adolescent whether there can be a trial with gradual reduction of medication.

MUSCULOSKELETAL DISORDERS

A physician's recommendation concerning athletic activities for normal, healthy children must take into account a wide range of individual differences in size, age, coordination, stage of maturation, and level of physical and mental development. However, when the child has a musculoskeletal abnormality, the physician must also consider the broad spectrum of variations of the disorder itself. For example, a child with rheumatoid arthritis may be in acute pain with systemic symptoms, such as persistent fever; have no evidence of activity; have mild monarticular arthritis that terminates after 2 or 3 years; or have every joint involved without letup for 10 years.

Several years ago, the members of the Committee on Sports Medicine of the American Academy of Orthopaedic Surgeons agreed to the following recommendations about types of athletic competition for children with common skeletal abnormalities:

1. Mild athletic competition (walking, bicycle riding, jogging).
2. Moderate athletic competition (tennis, roller skating, ice skating, baseball, volleyball, swimming).
3. Vigorous competition (football, skiing, soccer, gymnastics).

Kingsbury Heiple, John Makley, Thomas McLaughlin, and C. L. Nash of the Department of Orthopaedics of Case Western Reserve University have reviewed and slightly modified these recommendations. The Academy surgeons emphasize that no decisions are "cut and dried," radiographs or history alone is usually not sufficient, the clinical findings should be correlated with radiographs, and recommendations should be individualized. The recommended activities for some conditions follow.

Osgood-Schlatter Disease (Osteochondrosis)

Children should be allowed to participate in vigorous athletic competition up to their pain tolerance. If the condition is acute, this generally means mild or no competition; if the condition is chronic, mild or moderate activity is advised.

Spondylolisthesis

If the condition is asymptomatic, moderate or vigorous athletic competition usually can be permitted when the student has achieved a proper level of conditioning. However, patients with spondylolisthesis should not participate in gymnastics. If children with spondylolisthesis are symptomatic, they should be treated, usually with a back support and corrective exercises. If treatment renders the child asymptomatic, he or she may be allowed to try to return to basketball or football while wearing a back support. Basketball can be as stressful as football for a patient with spondylolisthesis, and the twisting motion of baseball may incapacitate the child. Regardless of the status of the student's symptoms, he or she must be under the ongoing care of an orthopedist.

Spinal Problems

Patients with mild scoliosis (30 degrees Cobb measurement or less) who are asymptomatic can participate in moderate conditioning types of weight lifting (even if they are in brace treatment, assuming the activity is done during the prescribed "out-of-brace" time). Other sports activities, such as swimming, during the out-of-brace time will help the young person keep in good condition (and sometimes excel) at the same time during which treatment is proceeding. For skeletally immature children who have spinal problems, weight lifting should be only repetitive with weights of 10 to 15 lb or less. Any exercise (or machine exercise) that applies a vertical (axial) or rotary loading to the spine should be limited to weights of no more than 10% to 15% of the child's body weight. Bench pressing can be allowed up to 50% of the body weight. Once the child reaches skeletal maturity, lifting can become more vigorous within the limits of the individual's capacity. Excessive weight lifting has been thought by some to cause or exacerbate spinal deformity (spondylitis with hyperkyphosis) and hypertension.

Congenital Subluxation of the Hip, Legg-Perthes Disease, Slipped Capital Femoral Epiphysis

In general, the recommendations for children who have these conditions are the same. With mild deformity of the femoral head, there can be moderate-to-vigorous athletic competition; with moderate deformity, mild-to-moderate competition; and with severe deformity, mild or no competition. However, the compensation by the acetabulum and the amount of motion in the hip are other important considerations. Clinically, if there is mild limitation of motion in the hip, if the joint space is good, and if muscle function about the hip is strong, the child should be able to compete through the high school level without difficulty. However, if there is moderate limitation of motion in the hip, the child is not a candidate for collision sports, such as football and wrestling, and is probably not a candidate for basketall. If the child is too active, recurring hip pain will develop and restriction of activity to a level where there is no hip pain and no spasms will be required. Swimming and non–weight-bearing activities, such as bicycling, will be tolerated by all children with these conditions.

Rheumatoid Arthritis

When the disease is quiescent with complete functional recovery, moderate-to-vigorous activity is allowed. If the disease is quiescent with minimal or moderate crippling, mild-to-moderate activity (especially ice skating or swimming) is allowed. If there is complete functional recovery but the patient is still on therapy with nonsteroidal anti-inflammatory agents, mild-to-moderate activity is recommended. If the patient is asymptomatic with mild effusion, experiences synovial changes in the weight-bearing joints, and is on nonsteroidal anti-inflammatory medication, mild activity with participation at her or his own level of tolerance is permitted. As with the hip diseases, evaluation of symptoms should be the main criterion.

It is a good general rule to avoid simply examining a child at the beginning of the season and deciding what he or she can or cannot do. The physician should arrange to observe these patients during the activity and see how they respond to this increased physical exertion. If the physician attempts to predict how the child will do without this observation, the activities of some children will be limited unnecessarily and other children will get into trouble because they were allowed to participate in an activity that caused increased symptoms. The physician must follow the child and change recommendations on the basis of the child's response to the activity.

It is wise for physicians to be alert to energetic and enthusiastic physical education teachers who demand excellence of all their children, some of whom do not have the coordination abilities, strength, and muscle power to excel in sports. These children, whether they are healthy or have a musculoskeletal problem, may be pushed to the point where they are not successful and may experience considerable emotional stress as a result of this.

RESPIRATORY DISEASE

Asthma and Exercise-induced Bronchospasm

The goal of asthma therapy during childhood is to achieve a degree of control of symptoms which will permit as normal a life-style as possible. Normality includes the capacity to engage in exercise and even athletic competition. Asthma is not a contraindication to participation in sports. A minority of children with asthma, less than 10%, will have difficulties with control that precludes strenuous exercise.[8]

Exercise-induced bronchospasm (EIB) occurs in 70% to 90% of asthmatics and 35% to 40% percent of atopic (nonasthmatic) children. The U.S. Olympic Team for the XXIII Olympiad had 67 of 597 (11%) of the athletes who demonstrated EIB.[9] Obviously, disqualification from sports simply because of a history of asthma or EIB is not justified.

EIB classically follows 3 to 8 minutes of significant exercise challenge and continues after termination of the exercise. The symptoms and signs of EIB include coughing, chest tightness, wheezing, and difficulty breathing.

There are several nonpharmacologic techniques that may lessen the frequency and intensity of EIB. Physical training has been shown to increase resting airway function. The impact of EIB is greatest in the poorly conditioned athlete. A vigorous warm-up is used by some athletes to precipitate EIB during warm-up. Following warm-up, athletes will be refractory to EIB for 2 to 3 hours. Athletes in endurance events have been known to run through their EIB. Intake of food less than 2 hours prior to an athletic event has been shown to increase the likelihood of EIB. Warm, humid air causes far less bronchoconstriction than cold, dry air.[10] Face masks can be used for rebreathing warm air.

Complicating factors for young people with EIB and asthma may include upper respiratory tract infections (URIs); sinusitis; allergens, such as dust, ragweed, and mites; and pollutants, such as smoke, chlorine, ozone, and sulfur dioxide. The use of propranolol (a beta-blocker), which is being used more for juvenile migraine, may potentiate bronchospasm to a dangerous level.

The therapy of children with asthma matches drug selection with the severity of the disease. Adrenergics, theophylline anticholinergics, cromolyn, and corticosteroids can be used in various combinations in the day-to-day treatment program. Individuals with asthma and EIB as well as individuals with only EIB may achieve excellent control with preexercise medication[11] (Table 30–2). Asthma medications are now available in convenient, safe metered-dose inhalers and can be taken 10 to 15 minutes before exercise.

In summary, advances in pathophysiology, pharmacology, and delivery of medications for asthma and EIB has resulted in an improved outlook for a young person's participation in athletics. It is a rare young person whose disease prohibits their participation.

Cystic Fibrosis

Young people with cystic fibrosis and advanced lung disease may experience dyspnea with exercise. Exercise performance is often limited and is in direct relation to the severity of their disease. Children with cystic fibrosis often develop airway obstruction, hyperactive airways, and pulmonary-induced heart disease. The use of exercise in the therapy of children with cystic fibrosis has demonstrated a number of benefits (Figs. 30–1 and 30–2) including improved clearance of mucus, increased endurance of respiratory muscles, reduced airway resistance, and improved exercise performance.[12,13] Many studies have also reported a marked subjective improvement with a greater sense of well-being and self-confidence. Young people with cystic fibrosis will benefit from an exercise assessment prior to starting an exercise program. The need for an individualized approach is critical

TABLE 30–2. PREEXERCISE TREATMENT OF EXERCISE-INDUCED BRONCHOSPASM

- $Beta_2$-agonist aerosol (use any one of the following)
  - Albuterol MDI
    - 2–3 puffs 10–15 minutes before exercise
  - Metaproterenol MDI
    - 2–3 puffs 10–15 minutes before exercise
  - Terbutaline MDI
    - 2 puffs 10–15 minutes before exercise
- $Beta_2$-agonist tablets or syrup (if aerosols are unavailable or too difficult)
  - Albuterol (Proventil, Ventolin)
    - Syrup: 5.0–7.5 mL 1 hour before exercise
    - Tablets: 4 mg 1–2 hours before exercise
  - Metaproterenol (Alupent, Metaprel)
    - Syrup: 10–20 mL 1 hour before exercise
    - Tablets: 4 mg 1–2 hours before exercise
  - Terbutaline (Brethine, Bricanyl)
    - Tablets: 2.5–5.0 mg 2 hours before exercise

Abbreviation: MDI = metered-dose inhaler.

because of the wide variation in pulmonary function in young people with cystic fibrosis. The hope, yet unproven, is that exercise will slow down the progression of the disease.

The favorable effects of exercise in patients with cystic fibrosis show once again that parents and physicians should be cautious about restricting activities, and excluding children and adolescents from sports and athletic activities, unless there is clear evidence that the activity would be harmful. Even with conditions, such as cystic fibrosis, that result in breathlessness with mild exertion, the evidence that there is increased function and an improved state of well-being should challenge us to find activities and to develop programs of physical training that will be appropriate and beneficial for these young women and young men. Indeed, two cystic fibrosis patients in our program run cross-country and another bicycles 50 miles at a time.

As with other individuals who are "out of shape," it is wise to start exercise and athletic activity at an appropriately low level and then make gradual increases. Children, adolescents, and young adults with cystic fibrosis have greater sweat electrolyte losses; thus,

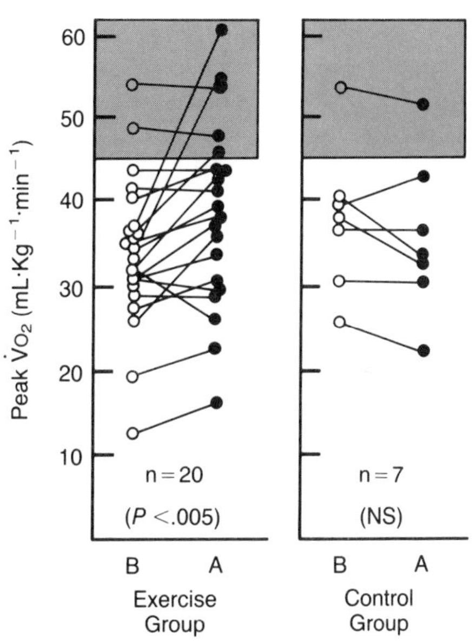

Figure 30–1. Peak oxygen consumption of exercise group *(left)* and control group *(right)* before (B) and after (A) a 3-month conditioning program. Shaded area indicates normal range. (*From* Orenstein DM, Franklin BA, Doershuk CF, et al: Exercise conditioning and cardiopulmonary fitness in cystic fibrosis. Chest 80:394, 1981; with permission.)

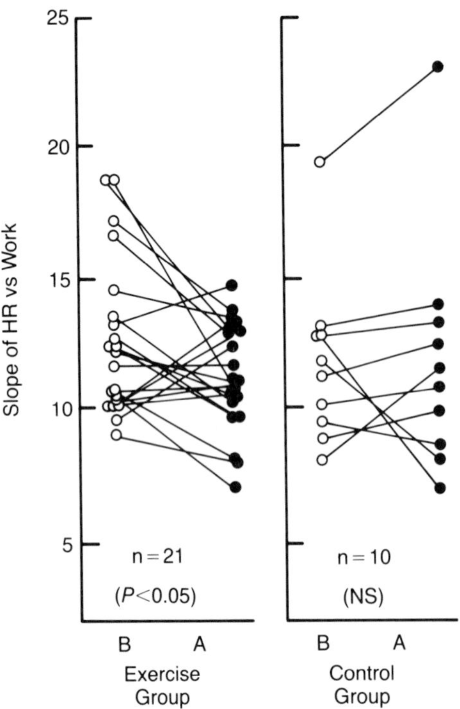

Figure 30–2. Slope of heart rate versus work curve (beats per minute (bpm)· kilopond-meter per minute $(kpm)^{-1}\cdot min^{-1}$) for exercise *(left)* and control group *(right)* before (B) and after (A) a 3-month conditioning program. (*From* Orenstein DM, Franklin BA, Doershuk CF, et al: Exercise conditioning and cardiopulmonary fitness in cystic fibrosis. Chest 80:395, 1981; with permission.)

they and their athletic supervisors (eg, gym teachers) should be advised about the need for free access to salt or salty foods (not salt tablets). In contrast to most other individuals who are exercising, individuals with cystic fibrosis should avoid a large consumption of free water if it is not accompanied by increased salt intake.

HEART DISEASE

The increased emphasis on sports, exercise, and physical fitness nationwide in the last two decades is a remarkable development with potential benefits for children with chronic health problems, including cardiac disease. The proliferation of sports camps, fitness and health spas, and joggers everywhere reflects a change in understanding and attitude about the value of sports and exercise. The average parent's appreciation of the importance of regular aerobic exercise for adults with coronary heart disease makes it easier now than 10 or 20 years ago for the physician to encourage physical exercise for a child with heart disease. However, just as in the past, when the physician gives any indication that a child has a cardiac problem, the concerns of the parents will often lead to pressures on the child to avoid all-out exertion or, in some cases, to refrain from specific activities associated with a cardiac death of a family member or friend. The parents' concerns may lead directly or indirectly to restrictions on the child's activities that are more appropriate for an adult with angina or other ischemic heart disease (eg, "Don't shovel the snow," "Don't run too fast," "Don't get overheated"). When a child with a heart murmur or a past history of either definite or suspected heart disease has a routine evaluation, the wise physician will inquire about physical exercise and competitive athletics.

Shaffer and Rose[14] have reported that roughly 85% of young athletes have ejection-type murmurs, on the basis of their own experience. This presents the physician with the challenge of identifying a small number of hemodynamic abnormalities from this high incidence of murmurs.

Cardiovascular Evaluation

The following is one systematic approach to this challenge. The primary physician who has been consulted about participation in athletic activities will start the cardiovascular evaluation by obtaining the history of the child or adolescent's normal physical activities and his or her response to the usual exertion of daily activities. This should include information about the presence of any cardiac symptoms in the past or a family history of cardiac problems.

A thorough cardiac examination will include the evaluation of vital signs and the inspection, palpation, and auscultation of the cardiovascular system:

Vital signs: These will include height and height percentile, weight and weight percentile, resting heart rate, respiratory rate, and blood pressure.

Inspection: This will provide evidence about the general state of health, features of posture, facial appearance, and minor or major abnormalities characteristic of syndromes associated with cardiac defects, such as Marfan's, William's, or Noonan's syndrome. A careful inspection of the precordium may identify abnormal impulses or configuration of the heart.

Palpation: The simultaneous palpation of the femoral and brachial artery pulses will usually rule out or provide clues to the presence of coarctation of the aorta. A thrill may be found when the carotid arteries and suprasternal notch are palpated. Palpation of the precordium for the area and intensity of the left ventricular impulse, the right ventricular impulse, and the outflow area of the right ventricle may provide more valuable information than is gained from auscultation.

Auscultation: The next step is usually the examination of the heart rate and rhythm followed by evaluation of the normal S_1, S_2, and S_3 heart sounds and extra sounds, such as ejection and nonejection clicks. As a rule, a murmur is not holosystolic if the first sound can be auscultated easily. The intensity and splitting of the second heart sound (S_2) are extremely important aspects of the cardiac evaluation.[15]

By using these simple screening techniques, the primary care physician can eliminate most of the pathologic causes in evaluating young athletes with a systolic heart murmur. The intensity of the murmur and of cardiac activity can be increased by any factor that increases cardiac output. Recent physical exertion, anxiety about the examination, or fever will change the normal cardiovascular examination. After the young man or woman has had time to rest or relax, the cardiac findings may be changed on reexamination.

An electrocardiogram (ECG) and chest radiograph are indicated when there is a suspected abnormality of the cardiovascular system. When these are normal, this is usually reassurance that there is no cardiovascular problem that will limit physical activity. In mild acyanotic congenital heart defects, the electrocardiogram and roentgenogram may be normal. A history of syncope during exercise or immediately thereafter, or a family history of premature atherosclerosis or hypertrophic cardiomyopathy, requires further assessment by a lipoprotein profile or echocardiogram, respectively.

Most of the young men and women with suspected heart disease will be evaluated and counseled by the primary care physician. When should there be an evaluation by a cardiologist prior to participation in sports? When definite heart disease is present or when the issue of normality versus abnormality cannot be settled, referral to a pediatric cardiologist is wise. Activity guidelines for many of the congenital cardiac defects found in children and adolescents were published by the Inter-Society Commission for Heart Disease Resources. The authors of this report stated:

> Poor adjustment and anxiety are related more to parental anxiety than to the actual degree of incapacity. This emphasizes the importance of the physician's explanation to the family of this condition, what is expected of them and their child and how they may foster the child's functioning with self-limitation of activities.
>
> A child with congenital heart disease rarely requires restrictions of physical activity other than those imposed by himself. This is particularly characteristic of preschool children and the cyanotic child at any age. On the other hand, older children and the adolescent patient may need guidance. Possible exceptions to this generalization are children with aortic stenosis and those with complete heart block.[16]

The authors stress that repeated exercise testing to determine changes in exercise tolerance that result from medical or surgical intervention may provide helpful guidelines for long-term follow-up. It is an important principle to avoid undue restriction of activity without jeopardizing the patient's safety. The child with severe valvular heart disease, whether congenital or acquired, will require restricted physical exertion. Aortic stenosis is a particular concern as are coarctation of the aorta with hypertension, advanced mitral stenosis, and congenital defects that might cause an atrioventricular conduction disorder or that are complicated by severe pulmonary vascular disease.[17]

To repeat, referral to a cardiologist is appropriate for any young man or woman who has a previously recognized cardiac defect. Referral is also appropriate when the primary physician has doubts about the presence of a cardiovascular abnormality or the significance of possible abnormal findings. It is much better to obtain a definite opinion from a pediatric cardiologist than to leave any doubts in the minds of the athlete, the family, or the primary care physician. Full, active interscholastic competition is possible and often desirable for young men and women with rheumatic heart defects and congenital heart defects that do not cause hemodynamic impairment.

Arrhythmias

Most of the cardiac arrhythmias in children or adolescents arise from ectopic beats and have an atrial, ventricular, or junctional origin. Sinus arrhythmia, wandering pacemaker, and intermittent junctional rhythms are usually normal and due to increased vagal activity caused by factors ranging from athletic conditioning to asthma to abdominal distention. Less frequently, arrhythmias may be due to paroxysmal supraventricular tachycardia and atrioventricular block.

In general, ectopic beats that are ventricular or supraventricular in origin are benign. They present no reason for concern if they are unifocal and if they disappear with exercise. When normal children are exercised to a heart rate greater than 140 beats/min, all ectopic beats disappear or decrease in number. However, this does not always hold for premature ventricular contractions. With low-grade exercise in some individuals, the premature ventricular contractions may increase, whereas in others they may decrease. The diagnosis of myocarditis should be considered carefully whenever an ectopic rhythm appears in a child who has previously been well, but the diagnosis should be based on more evidence than just an arrhythmia.

A child with paroxysmal supraventricular tachycardia should be allowed to have full participation in sports if the arrhythmia can be controlled. It is wise to obtain an exercise ECG to evaluate the response of the cardiac rhythm to intense exercise. A child with congenital complete heart block can usually participate in normal activities. The ability of the heart to supply the oxygen requirements of the body during intense activity will define whether the young person can take part in competitive athletics. Consultation with a cardiologist is often wise when the rhythm disorders are complex. As a general rule, the primary physician and the cardiologist should allow the child or adolescent to participate in athletic activities rather than impose restrictions that might lead to long-term psychological harm, which usually has much more serious long-term consequences than would come from the risk of permitting participation.[17]

Surgically Corrected Cardiac Defects

With the advances that have occurred in cardiac surgery, many children who have had surgical correction of a cardiac defect may be able to participate fully in athletic activities. For example, Goldberg and associates,[18] reporting on a variety of cardiac defects, indicated that most patients demonstrated considerably increased maximal endurance postoperatively, but their mean postoperative score on the maximal endurance test was lower than that of normal children. Shah and Kidd,[19] and Mocellin and coworkers[20] both found considerable improvement in exercise performance; thus, children with surgically corrected cardiac defects should be able to take part in school sports. However, their performance was below the level for healthy controls. The maximal oxygen uptake of the patients was 85% of that of healthy controls matched for age and height.

Blood Pressure

The measurement of the blood pressure is part of almost every medical examination to determine whether a child should participate in sports and athletic activities. Many factors make the evaluation of the blood pressure difficult. Because the biceps and triceps of some athletes are unusually large and some athletes have long upper arms, it is necessary to use the appropriate blood pressure cuff. A systolic and/or diastolic blood pressure that exceeds the 95th percentile for age and is confirmed by three consecutive measurements is defined as significant hypertension. A systolic and/or diastolic blood pressure that exceeds the 99th percentile for age and is confirmed by three consecutive measurements is considered severe hypertension. Curves defining the age-specific distribution of systolic and diastolic blood pressure for boys and girls are described in the "Report of the Second Task Force on Blood Pressure Control in Children—1987."[21]

Blood pressure levels in normal children increase continuously from birth to adolescence, and information is being accumulated about the blood pressure levels in different population groups. The 99th percentiles as defined by the Second Task Force are as follows: ages 6 to 9 years, 130/86 mm Hg; ages 10 to 12 years, 134/90 mm Hg; ages 13 to 15 years, 144/92 mm Hg; and ages 16 to 18 years, 150/98 mm Hg. Individuals with mild elevations of blood pressure should have their blood pressure measured weekly to establish the range of their blood pressure values. However, limitation of sports participation is not warranted in these individuals. Actually, there is some evidence suggesting the opposite: sports participation may have beneficial effects.

Studies in adolescents have demonstrated that both aerobic training and strength training (not power lifting, ie, single repetition, maximum effort) may provide beneficial effects on elevated blood pressure. This is especially true if the youngster is initially obese and the training is associated with a loss of weight.[22–24] There are few to no data to suggest that intense aerobic activity is detrimental to blood pressure status. However, there have been reports of morbidity and mortality associated with hypertensives participating in weight-lifting training or competition.

The recommendations are not as clear-cut when there is moderate-to-severe hypertension above 170/100 mm Hg, or secondary hypertension. Although there are almost no data to suggest an increased risk from athletic participation, it would be wise to follow a cautious approach, particularly if the hypertension is secondary to renal disease and the examination is preparatory for participation in a contact or strenuous sport. The young athlete with moderate hypertension requires more extensive evaluation and carefully supervised stress testing. With severe hypertension, competitive athletics are usually contraindicated because of concern about the effect of the severe blood pressure elevation on the kidney, heart, and brain.

For all young women and men with a blood pressure above the normal upper limits, a history that includes the family history is important. The physical examination including palpation of the femoral pulses may provide a diagnostic clue. Laboratory studies should include, as a minimum, blood counts, urinalysis, and serum potassium, blood urea nitrogen, and creatinine levels. In addition, an echocardiogram should be obtained to measure left ventricular wall (LVW) thickness. If LVW thickness exceeds normal limits, it is an indicator of end-organ effect, and some would recommend pharmacologic treatment of this subset of youngsters with elevated blood pressure. At this time, it is not clear what the blood pressure levels should be to result in a definite recommendation not to participate in strenuous scholastic competition. However, for individuals with moderate hypertension or secondary hypertension, it would seem wise to rule out participation in activities that are primarily isometric (eg, wrestling, gymnastics, line blocking in football, and weight lifting).

Restrictions in Heart Disease

As we approach the twenty-first century, the greatest concern of parents and physicians should be focused on the fear produced by the diagnosis of heart disease and the avoidance of unnecessary limitations. For many years, a large number of young men and women have been unnecessarily prohibited from participating in sports and, as a consequence, they have suffered from detrimental effects on their self-esteem and physical health. The preceding paragraphs presented some specific contraindications for sports participation, but these represent a small percentage of the children who come to a physician for examination. In most of these situations, before imposing a restriction that may have a very drastic effect on the future life of that young man or young woman, the physician should obtain consultation with a pediatric cardiologist.

The incidence and severity of rheumatic fever and acute rheumatic carditis have decreased in the United States over the last 30 to 40 years. During this same period, there has been increasing evidence of the benefits and safety of encouraging children to be active physically after the acute inflammatory process has subsided. The advantages of this approach compared to the earlier philosophy of restricting physical exertion still serves as a guide for the management of children with rheumatic fever as the number of cases has risen in recent years. Mitral valve prolapse is of particular concern because of a prevalence rate of about 5% in the general population. Based on the overall available clinical evidence, which indicates a favorable outcome and lack of severe problems with strenuous exercise, mitral valve prolapse is considered a benign cardiac condition in most instances. Except under rare conditions,[17] patients with mitral valve prolapse should be encouraged to participate in all competitive sports.

In the last 15 years, the care of children who have had Kawasaki disease has again raised the issue of limiting sports and physical activity because of concern about cardiac involvement. Fifteen to twenty percent of patients who have had Kawasaki disease develop coronary aneurysms. It is generally accepted that children who show no evidence of aneurysms by echocardiogram during the subacute phase of the illness should be encouraged to resume full activity after recovery. However, if coronary artery aneurysms are detected, the wise physician will seek the guidance of a pediatric cardiologist about the appropriate level of physical activity for these patients and for children with myocarditis. The challenge of restraining an energetic young child plus the harmful long-term psychological consequences demonstrated with restricted rheumatic heart disease patients make it likely that fewer of these children will be restrained from full athletic activity as experience accumulates.

An excellent source of information concerning athletics and cardiovascular problems entitled, "Cardiovascular Abnormalities in the Athlete: Recommendations Regarding Eligibility for Competition," is available from the American College of Cardiology.[17]

ATTENTION DEFICIT HYPERACTIVE DISORDER

The number of children with attentional problems in the United States has been estimated at 5% to 10%. Children with attentional difficulties are defined not only by their academic difficulties but also by information-processing weaknesses and poor behavioral and social adjustment.[25]

Although attentional difficulties are not usually defined as a chronic disease, attention deficit hyperactive disorder (ADHD) is a chronic dysfunction of control systems that regulate learning and adaptation.

Children with attentional difficulties often have problems with the integration of activity and attention, distractibility, impulsivity, poor memory strategies, and underresponsiveness to social feedback cues, all of which may predispose to a low self-esteem and poor self-image. The negative self-concepts often create a reluctance to participate in sports because of concerns about failure.[26] Sports which are team-oriented, requiring position play, or sports with complex rules, such as basketball or football, often present overwhelming problems for children with attentional disorders. At our Behavioral Pediatric Clinic, we are impressed with the number of children with attentional problems who are no longer participants in sports because of negative past experiences.

Attentional difficulties for most children are not "grown out of" but persist into adolescence. Two adolescents at our clinic demonstrate the problems a young athlete with attentional difficulties may encounter. One 17-year-old boy with good physical skills failed to make the football team because he could not remember the plays. The second, a talented swimmer, was dismissed from the swimming team because of his inability to show up for practice on time due to his lack of good organizational skills. When there exists in our culture a deeply rooted connectedness between athletic participation and personal growth and development, lack of success in sports may contribute to poor self-esteem and withdrawal from sports participation.

Children with attentional difficulties need to be individually evaluated to determine specific strengths and deficiencies. Sports that are more individual, such as karate, archery, swimming, or long-distance running, may be mastered more easily than team sports. The use of coaching strategies that emphasize cooperation, having fun, and adapting the sport to make the requirements more appropriate for the young person, will avoid creating neurodevelopmental cripples.

MENTAL RETARDATION

Recreation and athletic activity are important for all children, regardless of their mental capacity. A physician's recommendation about athletic activities for mentally retarded children, as with all children, must take into account the differences in size, coordination, degree of physical fitness, and physical health. The stage of maturation, level of mental development, and the emotional stability of the child are all important considerations when organizing activities for children who are mentally retarded. Children with average mental development usually have multiple opportunities for athletic activities and recreation without special planning. Mentally retarded children and adolescents have had fewer opportunities. Recent efforts to "mainstream" activities has resulted in some improvement. How many of the problems of emotional and social immaturity reflect in part a lack of experience with other children? How much of the poor coordination, lack of physical fitness, and obesity seen in children who are mentally retarded is due to this exclusion? These conditions become progressively more severe as the retarded child grows older, partly as a result of limited opportunity for athletic activity. The majority of mentally retarded children can and should participate safely and productively in athletic activities when appropriate supervision is provided.

Parents of children who are mentally retarded are often confused and uncertain about what to expect from their child. Some tend to restrict their youngsters from physical activities, and others may push their children at too rapid a pace. However, most parents are anxious for guidance to help determine what is best for their child. The pediatrician is in a unique position to advise these parents because he or she is likely to know the family and to understand the emotional and personal needs of the child and his or her physical capabilities. Federal legislation mandating early intervention for infants with disabilities and their families will provide a special opportunity and responsibility for physicians.

When developing a program for retarded children, it is important to distinguish between individual and team sports in competitive and noncompetitive athletic activities. Mentally retarded children usually find a greater degree of success participating in individual and dual sports rather than team sports. Activities that require gross rather than fine motor coordination can be stressed. Competition is often highly motivating and may be a means of promoting self-satisfaction, self-confidence, and self-esteem and of developing gross motor coordination. The Special Olympics has shown with great success how retarded children can compete against each other. Regardless of intellectual capacity, there is a wide range of athletic ability; some children are remarkably coordinated and others are extremely clumsy. Competition with children who are not retarded may be appropriate for some mildly or moderately retarded children, but it will mean repeated failure for most unless all competitors are well-matched. If children continually fail, their self-image, which should be supported by participation in athletic activity, may be damaged. Nevertheless, there are mutual benefits when retarded children engage in noncompetitive sports with more normal children. When planning joint activities, it should be remembered that there is some correlation between developmental levels and persistence, attention span, emotional control, and understanding the rules of the game. Children who are mentally retarded usually perform best and enjoy themselves most with children of the same developmental level, not of the same chronologic age.

A special concern in children with Down syndrome is atlantoaxial instability. Atlantoaxial instability has been found in 15% of individuals with Down syndrome. Lateral cervical spine radiographs in neutral, flexion, and extension positions identify most of the affected children starting at 4 to 6 years of age. If instability is identified, activities that may involve head and neck trauma should be avoided. These include contact sports, gymnastics, and the breast stroke, butterfly, and diving starts in swimming.

Every retarded child needs a continuing program of physical maintenance with regular exercise and supervised athletic activities. If they are not able to participate in basketball, football, or baseball, they may be able to compete in track and field events or in basic skills development, such as shooting baskets, kicking, or playing catch. Swimming, hiking, camping, archery, soccer, tennis, bicycling, folk dancing, and boating are examples of athletic activities that can give a retarded youngster the satisfaction, sense of participation, social contacts, and physical exercise that can be most profitable.

Games elicit more interest than simple exercises. Simplification of the rules facilitates understanding and encourages increased participation. Games may be modified so that most of the children are interacting most of the time, which is often necessary with retarded children who may have a shorter attention span. In addition, participation of other children who are mentally retarded may enhance a youngster's self-esteem and develop group identity. Cratty[27] points out that keeping records of personal improvement, counting, and similar intellectual activity on the part of retarded children may provide ancillary intellectual benefits from participation in vigorous physical efforts. He has valuable, practical suggestions about facilities, equipment, playground markings, fitness activities, and selected exercises. The Department of Education is also a rich source of information about physical education and recreation programs for the mentally retarded. The Kennedy Foundation provides information about specific model programs, such as the Special Olympics Program.

Many programs for the mentally retarded are best planned at the community level. Communities that take on this responsibility have the added opportunity of providing activities for retarded and nonretarded children to participate together and thus, decrease the isolation that has often ensued for the mentally retarded. The general population lacks knowledge about the mentally retarded, and children of normal intelligence generally do not have the experience that must be provided to encourage understanding and the development of favorable human attitudes. Children who are retarded are often rejected because of a lack of personal and social skills, which partly results from their relative isolation from other children. Interactions with other children would help to develop these needed skills.

The reaction of people over the centuries to the retarded, and to others who are different, has been one of rejection. For too long, children who were mentally retarded have been segregated from those who were not. With efforts being made to ameliorate other prejudices, it is important to expedite the integration of these children into the general population to continue the momentum started by Public Law 94-142, which was designed to equalize educational opportunity by mainstreaming. Every effort should be made to include the mentally retarded child in all appropriate recreational activities. If this were the case, many of the problems of the mentally retarded (eg, poor physical fitness, boredom, restlessness, social immaturity, hyperactivity) would be lessened. All could share in a sense of accomplishment.

STRESS REDUCTION

A relatively new challenge in children's sport is stress control or the child's ability to cope with the competitive situation.[28] The need to help children cope with the stress of competiton, errors, wins and losses, and unfulfilled expectations would be absurd in many cultures but is a necessity in ours. A recent survey of youth sport leaders revealed that understanding and helping young athletes cope with competitive stress are two of the most important issues in today's youth sports.[29] Stress control programs can be of great benefit to young athletes but are required as a result of society's inability to allow children to live and grow playfully as children. The inability to manage stress and competition in a healthy way can result in some serious problems at any age.

Stress in athletics can arise from any of four areas. These areas include situational factors, cognitive factors, physiologic factors, and behavioral factors. Stress reduction strategies need to focus on all four of these areas. Individual stress reduction strategies should include education (what is stress), voluntary muscle relaxation skills, cognitive therapy (self-talk strategies), and skill rehearsal. Additionally, modification of the sport[30] to increase chances of success and dealing with unrealistic coaches and parents' demands and expectations may be critical. The Coaches' Effectiveness Training (CET)[31] and the American Coaching Effectiveness Program[32] illustrate this approach. The four-part philosophy includes the following principles:

1. Winning isn't everything, nor is it the only thing.
2. Failure is not the same thing as losing.
3. Success is not synonymous with winning.
4. Success is found in striving for victory and is related to effort.

These issues of stress may become even more apparent when compounded in the issues related to a chronic disease. In view of the negative consequences of stress for self-esteem, strategies that help to minimize stress and promote more effective coping skills may be the critical determinant in a young person's athletic success.

CONCLUSION

In summary, the overriding goal of the physician caring for a child with a chronic health problem should be to make it possible for the young man or woman to lead a normal life and to participate in as many recreational or athletic activities as possible. In making plans for athletic participation for a child with a chronic health problem, a thorough clinical evaluation should be completed. Then, it is desirable for the pediatrician or primary care physician to discuss the sports plan with the parents, the child, and the physical education director at school. When consulted by a family, the wise physician will attempt to find out the family's reasons for allowing their child to participate in a particular sports activity. The physician should encourage each child to take part in typical childhood activities as well as other athletic pursuits with peers. The individual's limitations should be known so that the physician can find an acceptable sports or athletic activity for children and young adults with a chronic health problem.

ACKNOWLEDGMENTS

The authors express their appreciation to Elaine Corbin, for her secretarial assistance; and thanks to Drs. Robert Bilenker, Gordon Borkat, William Dahms, Kingsbury Heiple, Samuel J. Horwitz, Carolyn Kercsmar, Douglas Kerr, John Makley, Thomas McLaughlin, and C. L. Nash, for their critical comments and suggestions about portions of this chapter. Particular thanks to Dr. William Strong for his contribution of information about sports for children and adolescents with heart disease.

REFERENCES

1. Robertson SS, Dierker LJ, Sorokin Y, et al: Human fetal movement: Spontaneous oscillations near one cycle per minute. Science 218:1327, 1982.
2. Kennell JH, Soroker E, Thomas P, et al: What patients of rheumatic fever don't understand about the disease and its prophylactic management. Pediatrics 43:160, 1969.
3. Shaffer TE: The health examination for participation in sports. Pediatr Ann 7:670, 1978.
4. Vranic M, Berger M: Exercise and diabetes mellitus. Diabetes 28:147, 1979.
5. Koivisto V, Felig P: Effects of leg exercise on insulin absorption in diabetic patients. N Engl J Med 298:79, 1978.
6. Stein R, Goldberg N, Kalman F, et al: Exercise and the patient with type I diabetes mellitus. Pediatr Clin North Am 31:665–673, 1984.

7. Bar-or O: Pediatric Sports Medicine for the Practitioner: From Physiologic Principles to Clinical Applications. New York, Springer-Verlag, 1983, pp 227–246.
8. Ellis EF: Asthma: Current therapeutic approach. Pediatr Clin North Am 35(5):1041–1052, 1988.
9. Pierson WE, Voy RO: Exercise-induced bronchospasm in the XXIII summer Olympic games. New Engl Reg Allergy Proc 9(3):209–213, 1988.
10. Strauss RH, McFadden RG, Ingram RH, et al: Enhancement of exercise-induced asthma by cold air. N Engl J Med 297:743, 1978.
11. Pierson WE: Exercise-induced bronchospasm in children and adolescents. Pediatr Clin North Am 35(5):1031–1040, 1988.
12. Keens TG, Krastins IRB, Wannamaker EM: Ventilatory muscle endurance training in normal subjects and patients with cystic fibrosis. Am Rev Respir Dis 116:853–860, 1977.
13. Orenstein DM, Franklin BA, Doershuk CF, et al: Exercise conditioning and cardiopulmonary fitness in cystic fibrosis. Chest 80:395, 1981.
14. Shaffer TE, Rose KD: Cardiac evaluation for participation in school sports. JAMA 228:398, 1974.
15. Strong WB, Steed D: Cardiovascular evaluation of the young athlete. Pediatr Clin North Am 31:665–673, 1984.
16. Engle MA, Adams FH, Betson C, et al: Resources for optimal long-term care of congenital heart disease. Circulation 44:A205, 1971.
17. Cardiovascular abnormalities in the athlete: Recommendations regarding eligibility for competition. J Am Coll Cardiol 6:1186–1232, 1985.
18. Goldberg SJ, Adams FH, Hurwitz RA: Effect of cardiac surgery on exercise performance. J Pediatr 71:192, 1967.
19. Shah P, Kidd L: Hemodynamic responses to exercise and to isoproterenol following total correction of Fallot's tetralogy. J Thorac Cardiovasc Surg 52:138, 1966.
20. Mocellin R, Bastanier C, Hofacker W, et al: Exercise performance in children and adolescents after surgical repair of tetralogy of Fallot. Eur J Cardiol 4:367, 1976.
21. Report of the Second Task Force on Blood Pressure Control in Children—1987. Task Force on Blood Pressure Control in Children. Pediatrics 79:1–25, 1987.
22. Hagberg UJM, Ehsani AA, Goldring D, et al: Effect of weight training on blood pressure and hemodynamics in hypertensive adolescents. J Pediatr 104:147–151, 1984.
23. Hofman A, Walter HJ, Connelly PA, et al: Blood pressure and physical fitness in children. Hypertension 9:188–191, 1987.
24. Rocchini AP, Katch V, Anderson J, et al: Blood pressure in obese adolescents: Effects of weight loss. Pediatrics 82:16–23, 1988.
25. Levine MD: Developmental Variation and Learning Disorders. Cambridge, MA, Educators Publishing Service, 1987.
26. Ross DM, Ross SA: Hyperactivity: Current Issues Research and Theory. New York, Wiley Interscience, 1982.
27. Cratty, BI: Improving the physical fitness of retardates. *In* Pearson PH, Williams CE (eds): Physical Therapy Services in the Developmental Disabilities. Springfield, IL, Charles C Thomas, 1972, p 338.
28. Scanlon TK: Competitive stress and the child athlete. *In* Silva JM, Weinberg RS (eds): Psychological Foundations of Sport. Champaign, IL, Human Kinetics, 1984, pp 118–129.
29. Sport for children and youths. *In* Weiss M, Gould D (eds): The 1984 Olympic Scientific Congress Proceedings, vol 10. Champaign, IL, Human Kinetics, 1986.
30. Garfield C: Peak Performance: Mental Training Techniques of the World's Greatest Athletes. Boston, MA, Houghton Mifflin, 1984.
31. Smith NJ, Smith RE, Smoll FL: Athletic stress: Developing coping skills through sports. *In* Kidsport: A survival guide for parents. Reading, MA, Addison-Wesley, 1983, pp 132–148.
32. Marten R: American coaching effectiveness program. Sportsline, July–Aug 1981, pp 2–3.

SOURCES OF INFORMATION

1. Special Olympics International
   1350 New York Avenue, NW, Suite 500
   Washington, DC 20005
   (202) 628–3630
2. National Handicapped Sports and Recreation Association
   Farragut Station, P.O. Box 33141
   Washington, DC 20036
   (301) 652–7505

3. American Diabetes Association
   Diabetes Information Service Center
   1660 Duke Street
   Alexandria, VA 22314
   (800) ADA-DISC
4. American Heart Association
   7320 Greenville Avenue
   Dallas, TX 75231
5. Epilepsy Foundation of America
   4351 Garden City Drive
   Landover, MD 20785
6. American Lung Association
   (Check regional associations)
7. New Games Foundation
   P.O. Box 7901
   San Francisco, CA 94120
8. American Academy of Pediatrics
   Committee on Sports Medicine
   Sports Medicine: Health Care for Young Athletes
   Evanston, IL, American Academy of Pediatrics, 1983
9. American Alliance for Health, Physical
   Education, Recreation and Dance, 1990
   Association Drive
   Reston, VA 22091
   (703) 476–3400
10. U.S. Olympic Committee Drug Control Hotline
    (800) 233–0393
    (Information regarding approved and restricted drugs)

31

FACTORS IMPORTANT TO WOMEN ENGAGED IN VIGOROUS PHYSICAL ACTIVITY

Ralph W. Hale, MD

Involvement of large numbers of women in programs that stress some form of vigorous exercise is a relatively recent phenomenon. During the last two decades, high schools and colleges have started to develop extensive athletic programs for women, beginning with physical education classes and extending to competitive sports. Within the last decade, we have also seen a marked increase in the number of women participating in recreational exercise programs after completing school. At the Olympic and international level, many of the teams have begun to include increasing numbers of female athletes.[1] The International Olympic Committee has recently stated that their goal for 1996 and beyond is to increase the number of sports for women.

One of the first widespread recognitions of the ability of women to perform tasks requiring strength and endurance occurred during World War II. With the large number of men in the armed forces, women had to be trained to fill the jobs. As they did so successfully, most industrial companies realized that women could perform many of the tasks that had previously been reserved for only men. It was a small adaptation for these same women to use their new skills in the world of sports and exercise.

In 1896, during the first of the modern Olympics, there were no female participants. By 1932, the amount had risen to only 4%. During this time, there were few women recognized as outstanding athletes, such as Babe Didrikson Zaharias, and they were considered exceptions. By 1968, the number of female participants in the Olympics had risen to almost 14% and there were large numbers of outstanding athletes, especially in swimming, gymnastics, track and field, and figure skating. However, there are still concerns among international-sport supervising bodies regulating women and sports participation. This is evidenced by the current lack of a marathon (until 1984) and the exclusion of other events, such as women's water polo and the decathlon.

As a result of the increasing ability of women to compete in organized sports, there has been a slow but gradual increase in the number of athletic programs available at the national, collegiate, and high school levels. We have also witnessed a number of modifications in training techniques, and these changes have improved performance. As an example, there was little or no emphasis upon weight training for women swimmers from the United States prior to the 1964 Olympics. After the unexpected East German domination, our swimming coaches rapidly adopted weight training as an integral part of the female competitive swimmer program. In the future, we will see more of these advances as women seek to become better athletes.

Another major impetus to women's programs has been enactment and enforcement of Title IX of the Educational Assistance Act of 1972. This act requires all institutions receiving federal money to offer equal opportunities to women for their programs, including athletics. As a result, new programs have been developed and funded in many schools. This has increased the ease with which female students of all ages can be exposed to a variety of exercise and competitive programs and learn about the benefits of sports. It has also given these students the opportunity to continue their sport at the collegiate level rather than stop at the end of high school. Other legislation on nondiscrimination and equal employment has further advanced women by opening up job opportunities in organizations in which physical fitness is a requirement.

This change of attitudes and laws has not been an easy task. Women have encountered tremendous resistance in attempting to break these barriers. Unfortunately, most of this resistance comes as a result of emotional or social factors and not as the result of physiologic or anatomic differences. Some of the resistance forced women to engage in precedent-setting lawsuits. In 1971, for example, the Little League of New Jersey was taken to court because it prevented a young woman from competing on a Little League boys' team. There was never any argument about the girl's ability, only an attempt to prove that she was not capable of competing with the young men and that her participation could result in injury. Much evidence was introduced by the Little League attorney to support their case. Many allegations could not be proved, and one major contention—that female bone was weaker—was based upon studies of Japanese cadaver bone. In another important and similar case, an Ohio court in 1977 ruled that girls could participate on high-school football teams.

As more women become participants in all levels and types of sports, there has been a diminishing of these psychosocial barriers as well as the legal and legislative ones. The classic view of an athletic young girl as being a "tomboy," with its negative implications, is changing. Numerous studies now indicate that peer acceptance and family understanding have helped to place the female athlete on a par with her classmates. In some areas, she even reaches the level of popularity traditionally reserved for the male athlete. Continued parental and school acceptance of the female athlete will go even further to help destroy these barriers. Parents should be actively encouraged to accept this new role for their daughters. However, there are still gains to be made. An Australian study presented during the 1979 meeting of the American College of Sports Medicine reported that women still view athletics as a social outlet compared with men, who compete to win. This attitude is changing as the desire to win or to strive for achievement goals becomes more socially acceptable for women.

Unfortunately, many of the "scientific" decisions regarding participation of women in sports and exercise programs have been made on the basis of scant, limited, or absent physiologic information. Research about women and exercise was very limited until the last few years, and even now it is in its infancy. As a result, there are still many myths and outdated concepts that persist about women and exercise. This chapter reviews the current available research data and attempts to correlate its application to exercise programs. It is hoped that in the future, a greater understanding about women and their participation in strenuous exercise programs will evolve. It seems superfluous but necessary to remind the reader that what is known about men cannot always be extrapolated to women and that programs of exercise designed for men are not always appropriate for women.

ANATOMIC AND PHYSIOLOGIC CONCERNS

Skeletal System

The skeletal system of the female is distinctly different from that of the male in a number of areas (Table 31–1). Although some of these differences are related to the gynecoid shape of the female pelvis, which is necessary for easy delivery of a child, the others are not and reflect key differences between the sexes.

Female bone is less dense than male bone. When weighed on an equal-volume basis, male bone is 1.25 to 1.50 times heavier than female bone. As a result, a woman weighs less than a man of the same size because she has a lighter body frame. Because women are also shorter, they have a lower center of gravity, which is helpful in exercise that requires strength and balance, such as in gymnastics. The female has shorter limbs relative to body length. She has an increased "carrying angle," which can also influence the use of the arms as a lever (Fig. 31–1). As a result of an increased shoulder slope, her lower arms do not hang vertically, and she has different upper arm mechanics when throwing. These changes may cause her to have more of a sidearm or "whip" throw and make it difficult for her to replicate the male overhand throw.

Because of its gynecoid shape, the female pelvis is wider than the male's and has a greater slanting of the femur toward the knee with less bowing of the leg. This can result in different running mechanics. When a female who has an accentuation of this slant is running, she will appear to swing her lower leg in a slight circle. These anatomic configurations have been reported, but not proved, to increase the potential danger of injury to the knee. The gynecoid shape of the pelvis results in less support and less of a fulcrum effect when using lower body strength. The acetabulum is also smaller and more delicate, so that the potential for hip injury may be increased, although this potential has not been documented.

A female usually shows maturation of the long bones earlier than a male of comparable age. When she reaches pubescence and begins estrogen production, the epiphyses begin to close. As a result, she seldom grows more than 2 inches beyond her height at the time of menarche. At one time, this knowledge was used as the basis for prescribing estrogens for tall girls in an attempt to shorten their height. We know that this is rarely effective unless given before the growth spurt occurs and totally ineffective if given after menses. Therefore, in almost all instances, this type of therapy should be discouraged.

The joints and ligaments of the female are responsive to the cyclic effects of the circulating hormones. These have only minimal effect in the nonpregnant female but can be a major factor in pregnancy, which will be discussed later in this chapter.

TABLE 31–1. SKELETAL CHARACTERISTICS IN WOMEN COMPARED WITH MEN*

Item	Result
Size: usually smaller, shorter	Lower center of gravity Lighter body frame
Pelvis: wider	Different running mechanics
Thighs: slant inward toward knees	Injury may be more likely because of knee instability
Lower leg bones: less "bowed"	
Limbs (relative to body length): shorter	Shorter lever arm for movement—important for use of implements
Shoulder: narrower, greater sloping	Different mechanics of upper limb motion
Upper arms: do not hang vertically	
Elbows: marked "carrying angle"	Important in throwing pattern

*Information courtesy of C. Wells, Arizona State University.

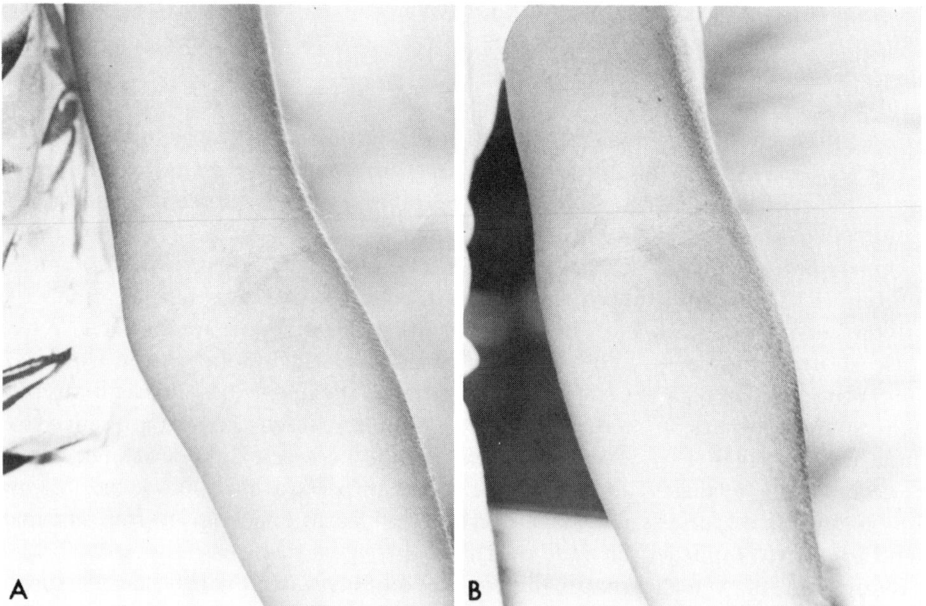

Figure 31–1. Carrying angle (elbow) for female **(A)** and male **(B)**.

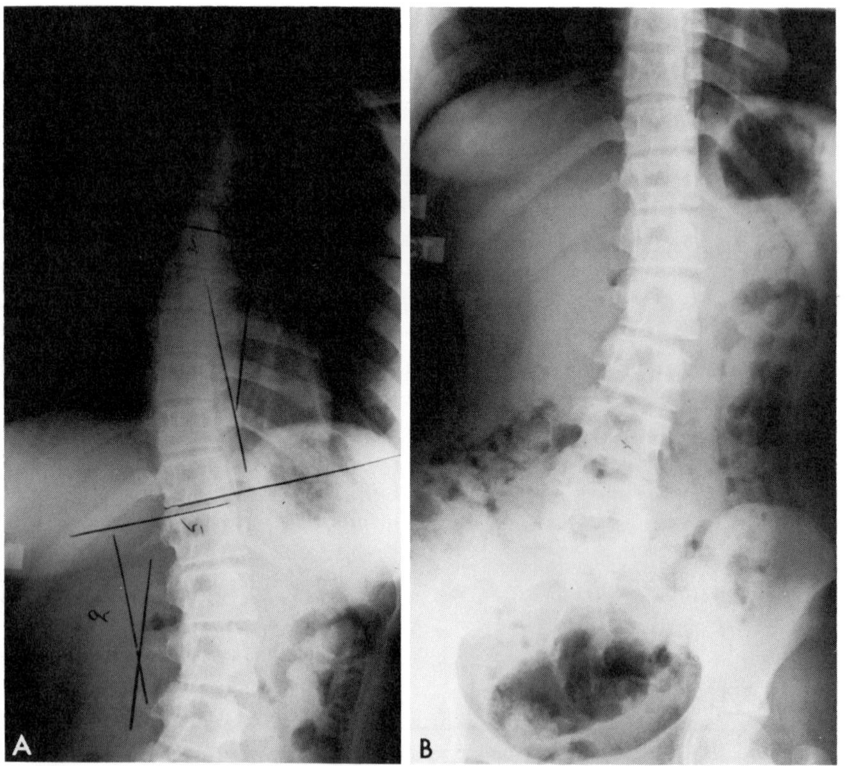

Figure 31–2. A, B: Two examples of scoliosis.

A skeletal deformity that may also affect the female's ability to participate in vigorous exercise is scoliosis (Fig. 31–2). This lateral curvature of the spine occurs more frequently in women than in men. In its mildest form, a woman may note few problems with exercise, but when it causes greater than 1 to 2 inches of curvature, there will be added strain to the back muscles, altered stability, shortened stature, and a change in normal biomechanics. This topic is discussed more thoroughly in textbooks of orthopedics. It is important, however, to be aware that it can occur. Onset is usually in the early teens when women are most active.

Muscular System

Because most exercise programs require strength and endurance, one of the key concerns for women is muscle mass and the ability to train their muscles. The typical woman has had little opportunity to become involved in a program of weight training. What strength she has developed reflects more her lifestyle and activities than any specific program. Even in highly competitive athletics, the introduction of a weight training program for women is a relatively recent innovation. As a result, the average woman has less muscle mass and less strength than the average man. Wilmore[1] found that the average woman's upper-body strength is only 30% to 50% of the values obtained in men; lower-body strength averaged only 70% of that in men of identical size. Therefore, the composite strength pattern of a woman is 30% to 40% weaker than the comparable man.

The discrepancy between the upper-body strength and the lower-body strength has been explained as a result of the lack of use of the upper body by most women, whereas the lower body is constantly used. Others speculate that hormones play a significant role in this difference because women have less lean body mass.

SPECIAL NUTRITIONAL CONCERNS

Women in a vigorous exercise program have the same nutritional requirements as men. Whenever a woman begins an exercise program, diet should be reviewed. Depending upon her daily diet, she may need supplemental items. Many young women are on very poor diets, eat at irregular intervals, or fast repeatedly "to lose weight." It is important to explain to these women the rationale of a regular eating pattern. They should also be aware that exercise as a weight-loss mechanism is a slow process. When they first start, they will replace fat with muscle, which weighs 1.3 to 1.5 times more per unit volume. Therefore, they may be losing fat but may perceive themselves as failing to lose weight and become discouraged. We have found that the use of a skinfold caliper is very helpful in this situation.

For the highly competitive athlete, a dietary history is also important. The top-level athletes tend to be susceptible to food fads. As a result, they may experiment with bizarre diets in an attempt to improve their performance. The general nutritional requirements of an athlete are explained in chapter 16. There are, however, several special concerns.

It has been shown that estrogen alters the metabolism of vitamin C. As a result, women have a higher requirement than men. Vitamin C is also needed in greater quantities in the presence of stress, such as vigorous exercise. These levels have never been adequately defined, but we recommend an additional 60 mg per day of ascorbic acid.

Iron is another special nutritional need for women who exercise. In most textbooks, the normal hemoglobin level for women is listed as a minimum of 10.5 or 11.0 g/dL. Anemia is usually diagnosed at a level of 10 g/dL. Neither of these minimums is sufficient for the exercising woman. She needs a minimum level of 13 g/dL of hemoglobin, or she should be started on supplemental iron. Over a period of 5 years at the University of Hawaii, we have found that our athletes feel better and perform better when they maintain hemoglobin level of 13 g/dL or higher.

Exercise itself does not affect the total serum iron. Studies have shown that pre- and post-training levels of total serum iron are unchanged. Exercise can, however, give an artificial alteration. When a patient is actively exercising, she may become dehydrated. As a result, the hematocrit and hemoglobin concentration increase and she gives the appearance of polycythemia. After the 1979 Honolulu marathon, we obtained samples from runners immediately after the finish of the race. Some women had hematocrit results of 50% to 60%. As hydration is accomplished, the opposite effect may occur.[2] Prior to dispersal of fluid into the extravascular spaces, the dilutional effect may give low levels of hemoglobin. It is preferable that all women have a hemoglobin and hematocrit evaluation obtained prior to starting any vigorous exercise program. It is equally important that this be obtained on a day when the patient has not exercised and is in a state of normal hydration. We routinely perform a urine specific gravity test at the same time as the blood test to determine the state of hydration.

Once an exercise program is initiated, women should be periodically rechecked especially if symptoms occur. During menstruation, the average female loses 35 to 60 mL of blood per cycle. If this causes even a 1- to 2-g/dL drop in hemoglobin levels, it will significantly alter oxygen-carrying capacity and affect performance.

Another nutritional concern is increased caloric intake. As the woman exercises, she will usually ingest a commensurate increase in calories. When she stops or reduces exercise, she must also reduce the calories; otherwise, she will rapidly increase her weight.[3]

It would be incomplete to discuss nutritional concerns without mentioning the eating disorders.[4] Anorexia nervosa and bulimia are conditions which can affect athletes. Until a few years ago, most physicians either were unaware of or ignored these conditions. However, we now know that they can occur in athletes just as in nonathletes. Most of these cases are reported in young women.

Loss of weight and "thinness" are usually associated with strenuous exercise in a healthy individual. It has become socially acceptable to be thin and to restrict dietary intake while engaging in exercise. Anorexic and bulimic patients have recognized these phenomena and are more and more often hiding their basic eating disorder by "exercising." As a result, the physician has a difficult time in differentiating the actual etiology of the weight loss. The following case presentations illustrate this problem (Cases 1 and 2).

CASE 1

LC is a 19-year-old college student. When she came home for her Christmas break, her mother was concerned about the excessive weight her daughter had lost. She was told it was because she was engaging in a strenuous exercise program as part of an intercollegiate varsity program. The mother refused to accept this rationale and sought professional help. The daughter was actively exercising but not to a degree that would justify a loss of over 30% of her body weight. A detailed investigation including a referral to an eating disorder clinic eventually led to the diagnosis of anorexia.

CASE 2

BS is a 17-year-old swimmer. Her coach weighs each swimmer once a week and ridicules her if any weight gain occurs. As a result, BS began to use induced vomiting after every meal as a means of weight control. She was recently brought to the hospital emergency room with symptoms of hypoglycemia and hypokalemia. Her hemoglobin was 8.4 g/dL. When confronted with these findings, her teammates reported that they had been aware of her activities for several years but did not want to report the situation.

These are just two cases that reflect the problems associated with eating disorders. Although they are not caused by vigorous exercise, it is easy to conceal them in an exercise program. The dilemma facing the physician is how to differentiate. Unfortunately, there is no easy way. First, an actual exercise diary is necessary. Excessive weight loss with a moderate exercise program is often the first indication. A food diary is also helpful, but the physician should realize it will probably be falsified. Evaluation of performance times can also assist. In the final analysis, however, the only factor we can rely upon is awareness and a high index of suspicion.

REPRODUCTIVE SYSTEM

Women who begin an exercise or competitive athletic program may have all of the same problems with the reproductive system as those women who are sedentary. The physician should always be aware of this and not overlook a serious problem by attributing it to exercise. We treated a 50-year-old active woman who was menopausal and started bleeding after running. She was found to have an adenocarcinoma, but she had attributed it to her exercise and did not come in until her routine semiannual visit.

It is also obvious that any difficulty with the reproductive system may have a special significance to an athlete. In a competitive event, where hundredths of a second determine the winner, a seemingly minuscule problem may have major ramifications. For this reason, it has been my experience that women who exercise and compete are far more aware and concerned about changes in body function than the average sedentary female, whether these changes are real or only imagined. The higher the caliber of the athlete, the more aware she is of her body and body functions.

Menarche

In the United States, the average age of menarche is 12.2 to 12.6 years. As more and more young girls become involved in strenuous exercise programs, concern has been voiced as to the effect of these programs upon the age of menarche.

Data obtained at the 1976 Olympics and U.S. National Championships indicate that these athletes had a later onset of menses than the nonathletes in the United States or in their home country.[5] It has also been found that athletes in certain sports tend to start menstruation later. For example, volleyball players had an average age at menarche of 14.18 years. Further investigations have also shown a later onset of menses, although a much smaller difference, for some college athletes and for some other sports. Runners, for example, had a later onset than gymnasts, and both had a later onset than did swimmers.

The question that arises is whether the exercise caused the delayed menses or whether girls with later menses were better athletes. Tall girls make better volleyball players, so that perhaps the delayed menses was only coincidental. On the other hand, a late-maturing girl will have increased long bone growth and a slightly different physique than the average early-maturing girl. This physique may also be a factor in good athletic performance.

Some observers[6] have also shown that even in a specific sport, for example, running, the age of onset of menses varies with the type of runner. It is important to remember, however, that regardless of a delay in menses, the other secondary sexual characteristics are not delayed.[7] A young woman with an absence of secondary sexual characteristics does not usually have an exercise-induced delayed menarche, and she should be evaluated for other causes.

What, then, is the cause of a delayed menses? A number of factors may be involved. The young girl may not have adequate body fat to convert her androgens to estrogens. Several authors have investigated this phenomenon, and although the data are not consistent, it does appear that body fat plays a role. Another factor may be an "energy drain."[8] Just how it would occur and what its mechanism would be are still speculative.

Fortunately, even though strenuous exercise undertaken before menarche may delay its onset, there is no evidence that this is a significant health factor. No adverse occurrences have been described. When the young girl reduces her physical activity, menses will usually occur within 3 to 6 months. If menses does not occur and secondary sexual characteristics have been present for 12 to 18 months, an investigation is indicated.

Menstruation

Menses is a concern of most women who participate in any exercise program. Because the average duration of flow is 5 to 7 days, women cannot avoid exercise and still maintain a consistent training schedule. As a result, most women continue to exercise throughout menses. Data are accumulating that show that world and national records have been set at all phases of the cycle, including menses. Most observers have recorded no difference in performance during menses and no contraindication to practice or competition. We do not recommend any change in training or competition schedules because of menses.

There is some evidence to suggest that vigorous exercise may have a beneficial effect on menses. In a review at the U.S. Military Academy, women reported that their strenuous exercise program had caused many favorable changes in their menses.[9] These included less flow, which will be discussed later, and a generally better feeling.

At the time of menses, many women undergo a variety of changes, including depression, malaise, bloating, and irritability. These have been lumped under the general term *premenstrual tension* (PMT). The etiology is thought to be the effect of antidiuretic hormone (ADH) on sodium excretion; as sodium is retained it also retains fluid. When this fluid is extravascular, it causes swelling of tissues. Women with severe degrees of PMT may retain 2 to 5 lb of excess fluid. One of the effects of exercise appears to be a reduction in the levels of ADH and, consequently, reduction in fluid retention. In a preliminary study that we performed, women with significant PMT had lower ADH levels after exercise and a subjective feeling of an easier menses. This work needs to be expanded and repeated; however, there is no evidence that PMT worsens with exercise. Diuretics have historically been used for this problem. In the woman who is exercising, diuretics can cause dehydration and electrolyte imbalance, which may have a much more adverse impact upon performance than the retained fluid. For nonathletes, I personally encourage all women with PMT to start an exercise program.

Frequently, a woman may request that the physician delay a menses because of a major athletic event. It has been my experience over the years that this is difficult to accomplish. Inevitably, breakthrough bleeding occurs with the medication, or the excess progesterone will cause an increased water retention with its added weight. As a result, I find that starting the menses early by use of progesterone withdrawal with medroxyprogesterone acetate, 10 mg twice daily for 3 to 5 days, is much more effective. Whenever possible, I prefer to start a month early but even when that is not possible, beginning withdrawal in the same month can be successful.

Dysmenorrhea (painful menstruation) is one of the greatest concerns of the female athlete. In a study by Malina and associates,[5] it was found that Olympic level athletes reported twice as much dysmenorrhea as high school athletes or sedentary controls. In our review of records of athletes at the University of Hawaii, athletes report more dysmenorrhea than the nonathletic students. The relevance of these data is difficult to assess, however. The trained athlete is much more aware of her body and the potential negative effect that dysmenorrhea may play. As a result, some authors believe that for most women, dysmenorrhea is more of a perceived problem with performance than an actual problem. The higher the level of competition, the greater the perception.

The etiology of dysmenorrhea in athletes and nonathletes is prostaglandins (Fig. 31–3). The release of prostaglandins begins just prior to the onset of flow and lasts for 2 to 3 days in a gradually reduced amount. The uterus, in most cases, reacts to these prostaglandins with muscle contraction, which, in turn, causes ischemia and pain. However, it is at least theoretically possible that the athlete can release prostaglandins from other sources, which can accentuate the problem by supplementing the level of uterine prostaglandins. We have seen several athletes who had varying degrees of dysmenorrhea, depending upon their training cycle, regardless of competition. When the training was intense, they had severe dysmenorrhea; when training was normal, they had mild dysmenorrhea.

In the woman who has severe dysmenorrhea associated with her menses, treatment should be instituted. A number of years ago, several athletes at the University of Hawaii reported a reduction in pain while undergoing treatment for injuries with the antiprostaglandins. As a result, we began the routine use of antiprostaglandins for dysmenorrhea about 6 to 8 years ago with good results. In addition to specific therapy, we also asked these patients to keep a careful calendar to document their cycle. If menses is to occur at an inappropriate time, we begin withdrawal therapy. Although they can be used, oral contraceptive pills are rarely indicated except for contraception.

During menses, most women who exercise rely upon tampons for fluid absorption. Exercise is difficult with a pad, even with the newer minipads. It is important to reassure these women that tampons are safe. Adverse publicity about toxic shock syndrome has

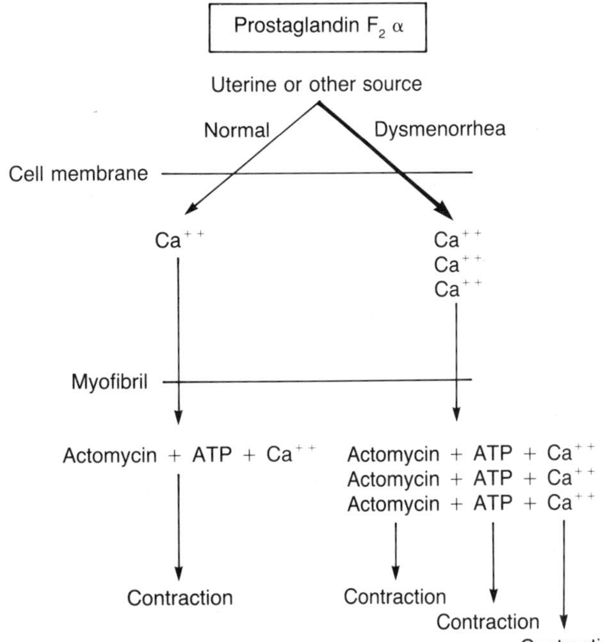

Figure 31–3. Effect of prostaglandins in the female with dysmenorrhea.

created a dilemma for many athletes. I personally recommend that the athlete who has never delivered a child use one of the tampons that becomes longer with swelling rather than thicker. Long periods of usage should be avoided by changing tampons a minimum of three times a day, including before and after each exercise or competition session. The superabsorbent fibers should also be avoided.

Oligomenorrhea

One of the major problems associated with women who participate in a vigorous exercise program is its effect upon cycle length.[10] This problem has been primarily reported in long-distance runners, but it can also occur in other sports. During the initial evaluation, it is important for the physician to remember that women who exercise can also have the same problems as women who do not exercise. It should also be noted that other abnormalities of bleeding have not been reported with exercise. Heavy bleeding, clotting, and spotting are usually symptoms of other conditions.

The definitions of oligomenorrhea are not universally accepted. For consistency in this chapter, secondary amenorrhea will mean that the patient has fewer than two menses in a consecutive 12-month period. Oligomenorrhea will mean fewer than six menses in a consecutive 12-month period. There will obviously be patients who do not fit either category or others who have different problems. These are the exceptions and must be dealt with on an individual basis.

Oligomenorrhea associated with athletics was first described in 1962 in European athletes. This was followed shortly thereafter by other articles from a variety of countries. The incidence is unknown, although it is probably more common than most physicians realize. Its occurrence appears to be related to the intensity of the exercise, diet, and stress. It may also occur when an athlete is given an injectable corticosteroid for an injury. We have seen numerous patients who have had oligomenorrhea following a cortisone injection.

Most studies of this problem have been done with runners. A major determinant appears to be the number of miles run per week. When the runner exceeds 30 to 60 miles per week, she has a 25% to 45% chance of developing amenorrhea. Once it develops, continued exercise at this level will keep the patient amenorrheic.

Body fat and weight are also apparent factors. We know that peripheral fat is an important site for the conversion of circulating androgens to estrogens. When the body fat decreases, the estrogens also decrease and the androgens increase. This sets up an endocrinologic profile that results in cessation of menses. The necessary amount of fat loss is still a subject of investigation. It has been reported that an actual weight loss of 25 lb is sufficient. Others believe that the percentage of fat loss is more important and suggest that a 30% decrease of fat levels to below 20% of total body weight are associated with these changes. Whatever the level, it appears that a loss of body fat does result in menstrual abnormalities. The exact levels and percentages probably vary from one patient to another.

Body fat and weight, on the other hand, are not the only factors. Many runners have elevated levels of prolactin, and this hormone can also stop menstruation. A reduced protein intake may interfere with the normal cycle. Other researchers have proposed that a vigorous exercise program creates an energy drain, which, in a nonspecific way, can interfere with normal menses. Finally, there has been a suggestion that the elevated core temperature associated with vigorous exercise may play a part by altering ovarian steroidogenesis. In our own experience, we have seen rectal temperatures of 105 to 107°F following a marathon. It is obvious that there is still much work needed in this area to determine the exact role of all of these observations as well as to elucidate any other factors.

TABLE 31–2. MENSTRUAL ABNORMALITIES ASSOCIATED WITH EXERCISE

Month	1976	1977
July	86% Normal	82% Normal
September	73% Amenorrhea	75% Amenorrhea
December	41% Amenorrhea	45% Amenorrhea
August	7% Amenorrhea	8% Amenorrhea

Adapted from Anderson FL: Women's sports and fitness programs at the U.S. Military Academy. Physician Sportsmed 7:72, 1979; with permission.

As a special note, the role of psychological stress must always be considered when evaluating the patient with oligomenorrhea. Studies at the U.S. Military Academy[9] have shown a high incidence of amenorrhea even a year after entrance into the Academy and after initiating a vigorous exercise program (Table 31–2). These same women are reported to have no significant change in body fat percentage. This area of investigation needs much more research.

Once a patient approaches the physician with a complaint of oligomenorrhea, the physician must do a careful evaluation before diagnosing the cause as vigorous exercise. First, other systemic disease must be eliminated. Pregnancy, hypothyroidism, reproductive system anomalies, diabetes, and other endocrinopathies are just a few of the many systemic conditions that may also cause a cessation of menses. If there is no evidence of these or any other problems, and bleeding resumes while the patient is still exercising or within 2 to 3 months after she reduces her exercise, no further evaluation is needed at this time. She should be seen in 6 months for reevaluation. If bleeding persists, we would do nothing further (Fig. 31–4).

For the patient who has amenorrhea even after she reduces exercise, an evaluation is indicated (Fig. 31–5). This would initially include a serum prolactin measurement to rule out a tumor. If the prolactin level is normal, progesterone withdrawal is indicated. No further evaluation is necessary at this time if a menses occurs. We would, however, reevaluate the patient in 6 months, including a repeat prolactin test even with a normal bleeding pattern. Should bleeding fail to resume with progesterone withdrawal, the next

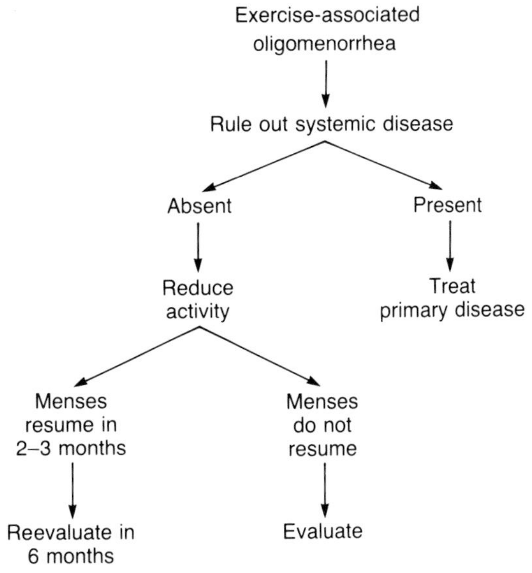

Figure 31–4. Evaluation of exercise-associated oligomenorrhea.

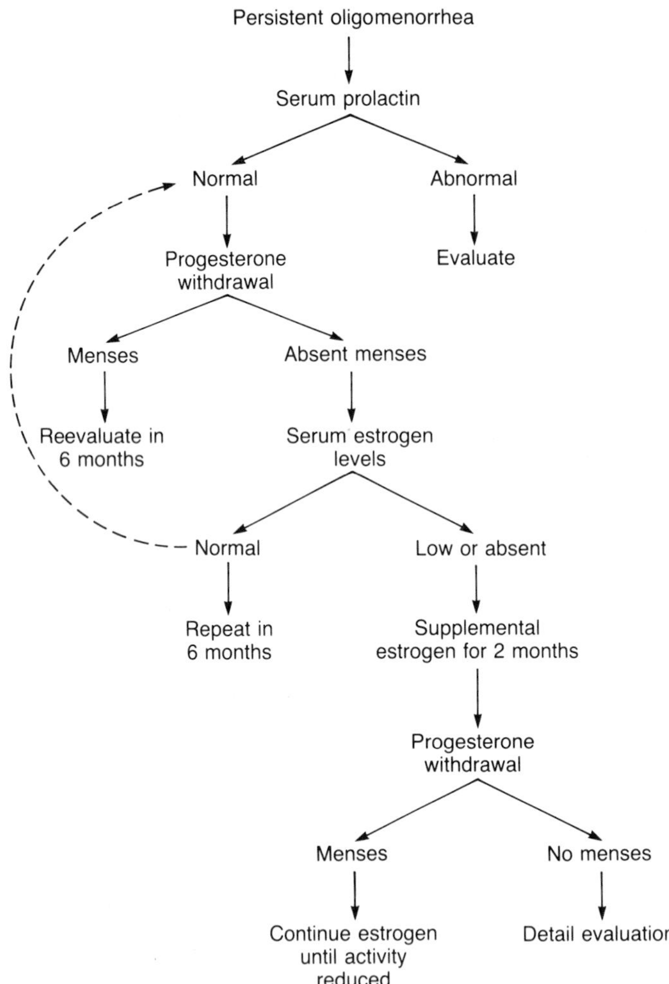

Figure 31–5. Evaluation of persistent exercise-associated oligomenorrhea.

step would be a determination of serum estrogen (E_2) levels. If estrogen levels are normal, the patient should be observed for 6 months and the evaluation repeated. If the levels of estrogen are low or absent, the patient should be given supplemental estrogens. There is no evidence that these women will suffer any of the effects of premature menopause. However, it does not appear physiologically correct to allow young women to persist in a hypoestrogenic state. Two months after starting supplemental estrogens, the withdrawal should be repeated. If bleeding ensues, no further therapy other than estrogens is indicated at this time, although a complete reevaluation is needed in 6 months, including repeat withdrawal. If the patient reduces exercise significantly, she should be reevaluated at that time and further therapy will be dependent upon her future plans.

Pelvic Infections

Women who engage in vigorous exercise programs appear to have a slightly greater frequency of vaginal infections. The majority of these are a vulvovaginitis as a result of a fungal infection, commonly referred to as *Monilia.* The reason for this is unstudied, but it is probably due to an accentuation of the same factors that predispose all women to infections of this area. These factors include prolonged exposure to wet shorts and underpants, increased heat and sweat in the area, and the potential for irritation. Women should be aware of this problem and avoid prolonged use of wet clothing; likewise, they should wear absorbent underpants. In aquatic sports, women should change to dry suits whenever possible. If an infection occurs, treatment is the same as for the nonathlete. In addition, the use of topical corticosteroids is always indicated. This will reduce the external irritation and allow continued exercise participation. There is no effect on competition other than this irritation.

Women who exercise can also acquire other pelvic infections. The etiology is usually the same as in nonathletic women, and there is no increase in the incidence because of exercise. This includes the venereal diseases. One manifestation of the most common of these, gonorrhea, is of concern to physicians who care for women athletes. Gonorrhea can occasionally result in a migrating polyarthritis. If a careful history is not obtained, the joint involvement may be misdiagnosed as an injury. The differential diagnosis is helped by a history of multiple joint involvement. As an example, one of my patients, a tennis player with a swollen elbow joint, was initially misdiagnosed as having "tennis elbow." Gonorrhea was later diagnosed and treated when the injury cleared spontaneously but reappeared in the knee.

The only reported pelvic infection that is specifically related to exercise is "waterskiing salpingitis." The cause is water being forced into the vagina and uterus when the skier is pulled through the water while the vagina is still submerged. This is a rare occurrence, and the diagnosis should be made only if all other causes of salpingitis can be eliminated.

SEXUAL ACTIVITY AND CONTRACEPTION

Several studies indicate that as many as 60% to 70% of women are sexually active by the age of 18. Sexual activity expends an amount of energy estimated to be approximately equivalent to a 50- to 100-yard dash. As such, this energy drain is small and should have little or no effect upon an exercise program. It is the accompanying emotional drain that may be a factor, depending upon the relationship. Athletes, both male and female, are reported to have more sexual activity than nonathletes and to enjoy it more. This is assumed to be a result of their greater body awareness.

Women who exercise use the same types of contraceptive methods as those who do not. Some of these methods can have implications for the exercising female, but the available information is very sparse. The barrier and chemical methods of contraception should have no effect on an exercise program, and they should not be affected by exercise. Occasionally, a woman may develop a vulvar irritation secondary to contraceptive cream and jelly, but this should clear rapidly when no longer in use.

Intrauterine contraceptive devices (IUDs), on the other hand, can have a profound effect on the exercising woman and have been associated with a high degree of pelvic pain and abnormal bleeding. The pain may persist for some time, and when it occurs, performance will be hindered. These devices are also associated with pelvic infections. However, the most significant impact of the IUD is the potential for heavy, prolonged, and/or frequent bleeding. In some studies, as many as 75% of users report abnormality of flow, and in a third of these, it is clinically significant. For women in an exercise program, this blood loss can lower hemoglobin levels and thereby alter oxygen-carrying capacity. Any alteration that reduces the oxygen available to tissues will affect training and performance. In one case, a young woman who was training for a marathon was seen because of exhaustion and inability to run. Her hemoglobin level 4 months prior to this visit had been 13.6 g/dL; the current hemoglobin level was 9.4 g/dL. She had had an IUD inserted 3 weeks after the first determination and experienced heavy periods every 2 weeks following insertion.

Oral contraceptive pills cause many physiologic changes. These are well documented in the medical literature. However, few studies have been performed that attempt to correlate the use of the pill with exercise or to discover any effects of exercise on the pill. All that is known is that changes take place.[11] Among those changes that may potentially exert an influence on exercise are an increased blood volume and an increased cardiac output. There are only minimal changes in respiratory measurements.

What role these observations play is unknown. It is possible that oral contraceptive pills may actually be advantageous. Based on current knowledge, there is no reason to use or to prohibit the use of the pill in women who are exercising.[11] The determination should be made on the basis of contraceptive need and appropriateness, not the exercise.

Although they are seldom used for contraception in the United States, long-acting progesterone injections are used in other parts of the world. At present, there is no information about their effect. It is known that they frequently cause irregular bleeding and can cause fluid retention. Neither of these is desirable in a female athlete engaged in a strenuous exercise program.

SPORTS INJURY

Breast

Although potential injury to the breast is of great concern to most women in vigorous exercise programs, there were no reports of any significant injury in a review of women's sports at the University of Hawaii for a 6-year period. In a questionnaire to more than a thousand women competing in a marathon, none of them reported any problems. The only sport in which the breast might be significantly injured is archery, and that is not due to the sport but to the equipment.

Anatomically, the breast is composed mostly of fatty tissue. As a result, a woman who has reduction in her total body fat will notice a change in breast size after she begins an exercise program.

There are two minor problems that runners or women in running sports may encounter. The first of these is nipple abrasion. As the breasts move with running, the nipple can be rubbed until it loses its epithelial lining. Some women counter this by placing tape or Band-Aids over the nipple area before exercising. Other women with large breasts occasionally use nursing pads in their bras. Another minor problem is shoulder pain. This is seen in women with large pendulous breasts and is a result of the breast's weight pulling downward. This effect as well as the nipple abrasion can be reduced or prevented by the use of a well-fitted bra. Fortunately, a number of manufacturers now produce excellent bras for women who exercise.

X-ray Effects

Caution should be used when dealing with women who injure themselves during exercise. X-rays can have an effect on the ovaries. This danger should be minimized by the use of lead shields for the lower abdomen any time a woman is having a radiograph taken of any other part of her body.

MENOPAUSE

Women in the United States reach menopause at an average age of 51 to 52 years. For 6 to 8 years prior to this, many women will go through a series of changes referred to as the climacteric. The symptoms of this syndrome include insomnia, irritability, depression, menstrual irregularity, and hot flushes. For the majority of women, this period of transition from a reproductive female to a menopausal female is a central point in their life. With proper evaluation and support, it does not have to be traumatic.

One very helpful aspect of this transition can be an active exercise program. Women who are exercising at least three times per week appear to have less symptoms, or at least are less affected by these symptoms, than sedentary women. The exact etiology for this difference is unknown. Speculation has implicated a "healthier frame of reference," alteration in the neuroendocrine system, as well as other less scientific reasons. Because there is no actual data to support any of these reasons, we are left with anecdotal reports as a basis for our conclusion.

What is known however, is that menopause is not a contraindication to continuation or initiation of an exercise program. For those who have had an active program before menopause, there is little need to make any changes. For the woman who is just starting, a complete physical examination emphasizing the orthopedic and cardiovascular systems with standard lab studies, including an electrocardiogram, is indicated. Exercise is stressful and before undertaking a program, a woman needs to be in a state of moderate good health.

Evidence has shown that postmenopausal women who are not on replacement estrogen therapy have a much more significant loss of calcium with subsequent development of osteoporosis. By maintaining an active exercise program, this loss of calcium can be slowed.[12] Several studies now report good results in maintaining bone density by engaging in a vigorous exercise program.

A frequent question asked by patients is, "How long should I continue to exercise?" There is no easy answer to this question. In general, I advise my postmenopausal patients to continue to exercise until they either can no longer do exercise for health reasons, or a vigorous exercise program is incompatible with their life-style. On the other hand, for this latter group, I counsel them on less vigorous forms of exercise and discourage them from quitting altogether.

During an average woman's life, she will spend 40 years in a potentially reproductive capacity (age 12 to 52). She will also spend 26 years (age 52 to 78) as a menopausal female. This is a significant part of her life and it should be a period of continuity of exercise.

REFERENCES

1. Wilmore JH: The application of science to sport: Physiological profiles of male and female athletes. Can J Appl Sport Sci 4:103, 1979.
2. Dressendorfer RH, Wade CE, Amsterdam EA: Development of pseudoanemia in marathon runners during a 20-day road race. JAMA 246:1215, 1981.
3. Brown CH, Wilmore JH: The effects of maximal resistance training on the strength and body composition of women athletes. Med Sci Sports 6:174, 1974.
4. Lyons HA, Cromey R: Compulsive jogging: Exercise dependence and associated disorder of eating. Ulster Med J 58:100, 1989.
5. Malina RM, Spirduso WW, Tate C, et al: Age at menarche and selected menstrual characteristics in athletes at different competitive levels and in different sports. Med Sci Sports 10:218, 1978.
6. Dale E, Gerlach DH, Wilhite AL: Menstrual dysfunction in distance runners. Obstet Gynecol 54:47, 1979.
7. Frisch RE, Gotz-Welbergen AV, McArthur JW, et al: Delayed menarche and amenorrhea of college athletes in relation to age of onset of training. JAMA 246:1559, 1981.
8. Warren MP: The affects of exercise on pubertal progression and reproductive function in girls. J Clin Endocrinol Metab 51:1150, 1980.
9. Anderson JL: Women's sports and fitness programs at the U.S. Military Academy. Physician Sportsmed 7:72, 1979.
10. Hale R: Exercise, sports and menstrual dysfunction. Clin Obstet Gynecol 26(3):728–735, 1983.

11. Lehtovirta R, Kuikka J, Pyorala T: Hemodynamic effects of oral contraceptives during exercise. Int J Gynecol Obstet 15:35, 1977.
12. Sinaki M: Exercise and osteoporosis. Arch Phys Med Rehabil 70:220, 1989.
13. Garlick MA, Bernauer EM: Exercise during the menstrual cycles: Variations in physiological baselines. Res Q 39:533, 1968.
14. Littler WA, Bojorges-Bueno R, Banks J: Cardiovascular dynamics in women during the menstrual cycle and oral contraceptive therapy. Thorax 29:567, 1974.

32

EXERCISE DURING PREGNANCY

Raul Artal, MD

Women's life-styles have changed significantly in the past years and pregnant women are increasingly attempting to maintain an active life-style. Consequently, pregnant women are frequently turning to their physician for advice. Most activities can be continued during pregnancy; nevertheless, there are certain anatomic and physiologic changes that occur in pregnancy that could interfere with or reduce the ability to engage in some physical activities.

In this chapter we will review the pertinent anatomic and physiologic changes that may affect pregnant women and provide a scientific rationale for exercise prescription in that pregnancy.

Exercise prescription requires proper knowledge of work capacity and recognition of potential associated risks. We will review maternal and fetal responses to exercise and the potential benefits, risks, and contraindications for exercise during pregnancy.

ANATOMIC AND PHYSIOLOGIC CHANGES OF PREGNANCY

Pregnancy is associated with significant anatomic changes. Most significant and pertinent to exercise prescription is the progressive shift in the point of gravity that results in an exaggerated lordosis, which frequently precipitates low back pain. The following changes lead to this complication: From a strictly pelvic organ at 12 weeks' gestation, the uterus becomes an abdominal organ, displacing the intestines and distending the abdomen. Progressively, the point of gravity shifts anteriorly and cephalad. In addition to lordosis, the pelvic bones progressively rotate on the femur to prevent forward falling. Pregnancy is associated with increases in progesterone and elastin that affect to various degrees the composition of the connective tissue, resulting in progressively looser joints and ligaments.[1] Thus, how strong and large the individual muscles are becomes critical for the prevention of instability of the joints with its potential for injury. In evaluating the biomechanical factors related to exercise in pregnancy, it is important to remember that other factors can influence exercise in pregnancy, among them the progressive increase in weight and the accumulation of interstitial fluid in the lower extremities. These changes produce greater internal forces and joint torques during the acceleration of the body mass, thus requiring greater muscular effort. One mechanism for avoiding injuries related to these anatomic changes is the ability to balance the involvement of additional muscles in each activity against lower loading conditions.

FUEL METABOLISM IN PREGNANCY AND ENDOCRINE RESPONSES TO EXERCISE

Fuel metabolism in pregnancy is balanced between the needs of the mother and fetus. The progressive fetal needs are modulated by hormones that have been recognized as diabetogenic. These hormones increase fat storage, delay glucose clearance, and decrease energy expenditure; cortisol has the most gluconeogenic effect. The other hormones include estrogen, progesterone, prolactin, and somatotropin. All these changes accompany the facilitated diffusion of glucose across the placenta. In contrast, amino acids are actively transported across the placenta. Either hypoglycemia or hyperglycemia may affect fetal growth and produce structural and/or functional abnormalities. Infants of diabetic mothers may have a malformation rate of 9.0% compared with a rate of only 2.1% in the normal population.

The energy cost of pregnancy is estimated at about 80,000 kcal, or 300 kcal/day.[3] Women exercising during pregnancy need proportionately more calories (Fig. 32–1). Adequate weight gain is the most practical indicator of caloric intake. A healthy primigravida gains an average of 15.3 kg by the end of her pregnancy.[4] Maternal weight appears to be an important factor in determining fetal birth weight in nonobese women (<135% of ideal body weight). It is thus recommended that at least 11 kg of weight be gained in pregnancy. Conversely, low maternal prepregnancy weight (<90% of ideal body weight) is associated with lower fetal birth weight.[4] Excessive maternal weight gain with fat accretion does not appear to correlate with birth weight.[5]

Assessing fuel utilization during exercise in pregnancy is essential because of the possible effects of exercise-induced maternal hypoglycemia on the fetus.

Higher respiratory exchange ratios (R) observed during exercise in pregnancy suggest preferential utilization of carbohydrates.[6,8] R is a respiratory variable that reflects the ratio between carbon dioxide output and oxygen uptake ($\dot{V}O_2$), and provides information on the proportion of substrate derived from various foodstuffs. If carbohydrates are completely oxidized to CO_2 and H_2O, one volume of CO_2 is produced for each volume of O_2 consumed. An R value of 1.0 would indicate that only carbohydrates are being used (Fig. 32–2). Comparative measurements by indirect calorimetry in pregnancy indicate preferential use of carbohydrates during cycle ergometry (non–weight-bearing) exercise.[9] Dur-

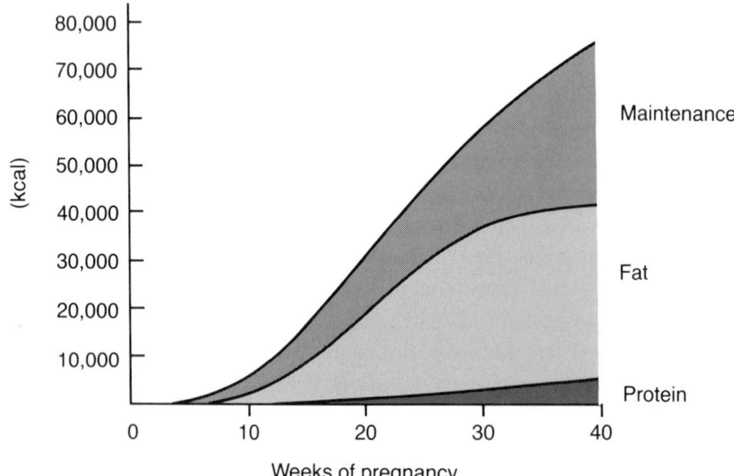

Figure 32–1. The cumulative energy cost of pregnancy and its components. (*From* Hytten FE: Nutrition. *In* Hytten FE, Chamberlain G (eds): Clinical Physiology in Obstetrics. Oxford, Blackwell, 1980, p 166; with permission.)

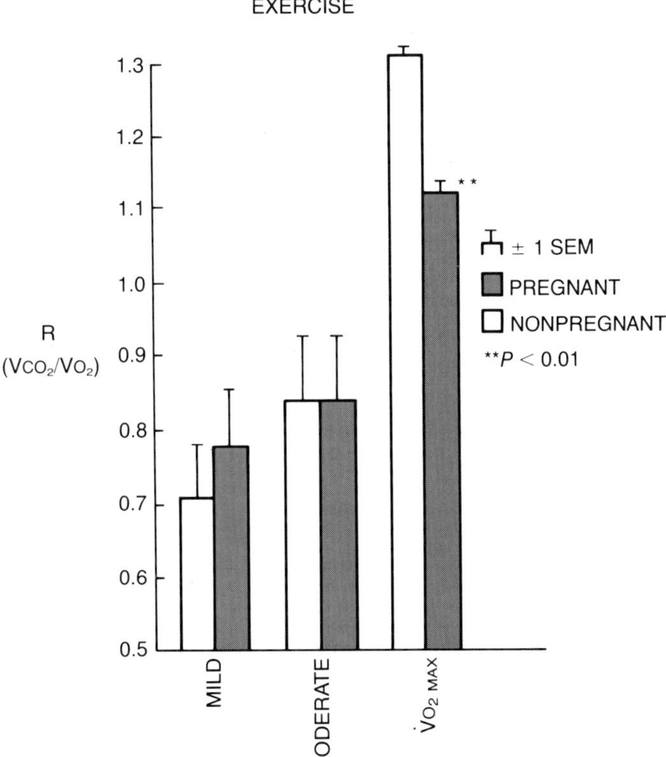

Figure 32–2. Comparison of respiratory exchange ratios (R) during mild, moderate, and $\dot{V}O_{2max}$ exercise. (*From* Artal R, Wiswell R, Romem Y, et al: Pulmonary responses to exercise in pregnancy. Am J Obstet Gynecol 154:378–383, 1986; with permission.)

ing light-to-moderate exercise in pregnancy, plasma glucose levels remain constant; during prolonged or strenuous exercise, glucose concentrations fall significantly (Fig. 32–3). Recognizing patterns for glucose utilization in pregnancy can be applied directly to improve glycemic control in pregnant women with type II diabetes.[10]

Catecholamines promote both glycogenolysis and lipolysis. Epinephrine modulates the release of glucagon and free fatty acids (FFAs). During prolonged exercise, FFAs provide an important energy substrate and, indeed, during prolonged exercise in pregnancy, their levels increase significantly.[11]

The heavier the work load, the greater is the sympathoadrenal activity. Significant increases in norepinephrine (but not epinephrine) parallel the increase in work load.[12] The potential increase in circulating norepinephrine has clinical relevance because norepinephrine can precipitate uterine activity. Thus, women at risk for premature labor are advised not to exercise in pregnancy. Levels of plasma norepinephrine are a crude index of the sympathetic nervous activity that consistently relates to heart rate and to the percent of $\dot{V}O_{2max}$; at the same time, it has an inverse relationship with the splanchnic blood flow.[13] Pregnant women respond to exercise with significantly higher concentrations of plasma norepinephrine.[12] It is conceivable that such higher concentrations have significantly greater restrictive effects on the splanchnic, renal, and uterine blood flow.

PULMONARY FUNCTION IN PREGNANCY AND EXERCISE

The second half of pregnancy is characterized by significant changes that result in the expansion of the chest circumference. These changes lead to an increase in inspiratory

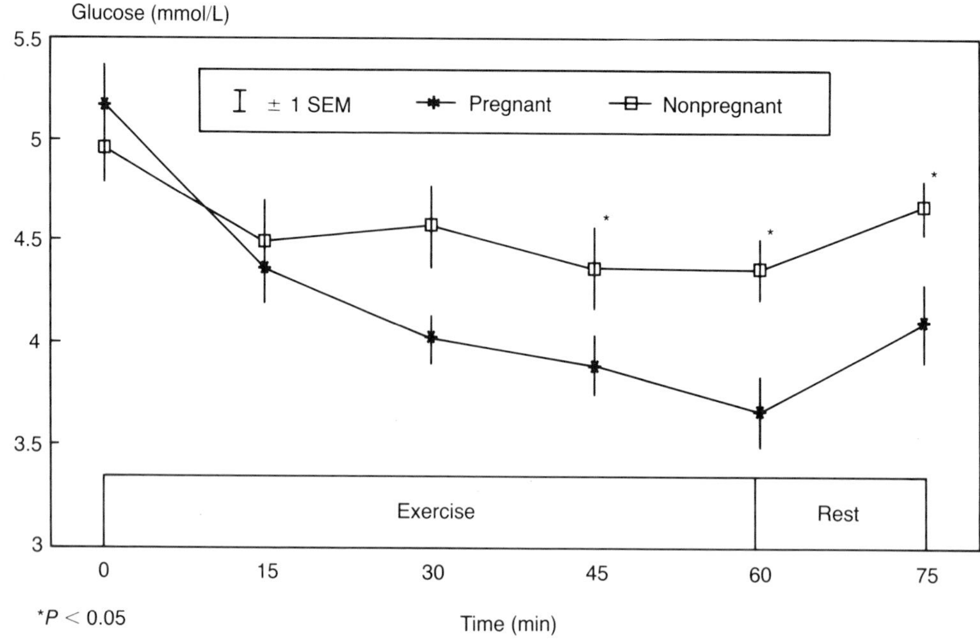

Figure 32–3. Glucose concentrations during prolonged exercise: pregnant versus nonpregnant. (*From* Soultanakis HN: Glucose homeostasis during pregnancy in response to prolonged exercise. Postdoctoral thesis, University of Southern California, 1989; with permission.)

capacity of 300 mL (tidal volume plus inspiratory volume) and a reduction in functional residual capacity. Oxygen consumption increases in pregnancy by 10% to 20%. The combination of the above changes results in a lower oxygen reserve. Such reserve can be further reduced or compromised during strenuous exercise.

The primary physiologic purpose of the state of hyperventilation in pregnancy is to reduce arterial P_{CO_2}. The arterial pH is maintained at approximately 7.44. The mild maternal alkalosis facilitates placental gas exchange. Any increase in alkalosis can lead to fetal hypoxia.

When conducting exercise studies during pregnancy, it is important to distinguish between weight-bearing and non–weight-bearing activities. Similar to nonpregnant women, pregnant subjects experience increases in respiratory frequency, minute ventilation, and tidal volume with exercise. A similar decrease in respiratory frequency has been observed only during $\dot{V}O_{2max}$ exercise.[6] Oxygen consumption (Fig. 32–4) and tidal volume (Fig. 32–5) responses to mild and moderate exercise do not differ between pregnant and nonpregnant controls; however, these responses are significantly decreased in pregnant subjects during strenuous $\dot{V}O_{2max}$ exercise when indexed for weight. $\dot{V}O_{2max}$ values (L/kg) are lower during exercise in pregnancy.[6] The disproportionate increase in minute ventilation as compared with oxygen consumption is reflected in a relatively high ventilatory equivalent for oxygen.[6]

MATERNAL HEMODYNAMICS AND EXERCISE

One major concern related to exercise during pregnancy is the hemodynamic response to exercise, which includes redistribution of blood flow to the exerting muscles and away from the visceral organs and the uterus. Orthostatic hypotension may occur more frequently in pregnancy, particularly after standing or after exercising in the supine position.

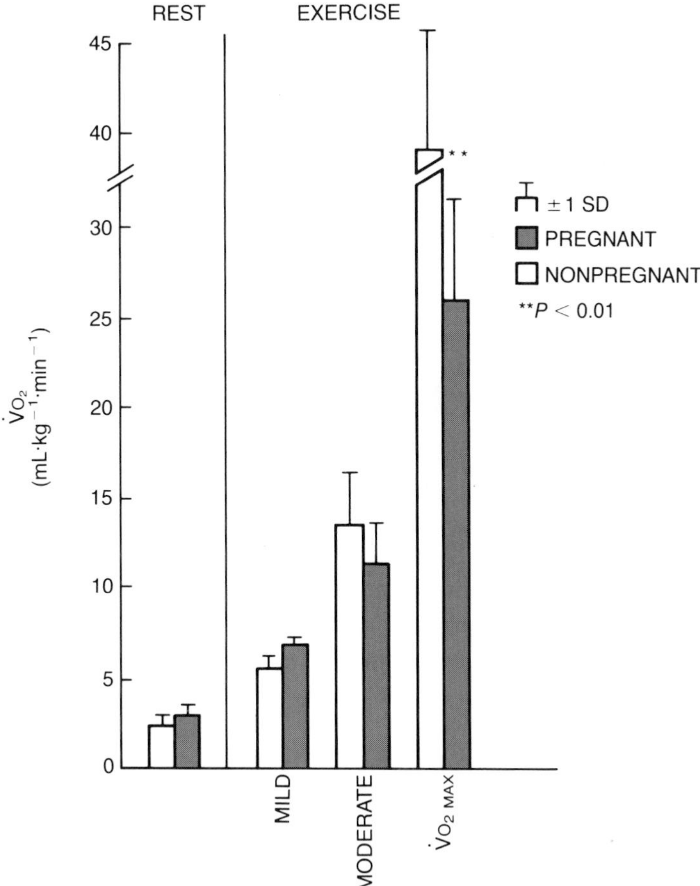

Figure 32–4. Oxygen consumption during mild, moderate, and $\dot{V}O_{2max}$ exercise. (*From* Artal R, Wiswell R, Romem Y, et al: Pulmonary responses to exercise in pregnancy. Am J Obstet Gynecol 154:378–383, 1986; with permission.)

In the second half of pregnancy, lying in the supine position can result in the aortocaval syndrome as a result of impingement of the uterus on the aorta and vena cava; this causes diminished blood return to the heart, potential hypotension, and reduced blood perfusion of the visceral organs. Thus, exercises in the supine position should be avoided in pregnancy.

Pregnancy is characterized by major hemodynamic changes. Early in pregnancy, the cardiac output increases in excess of the increment in uterine blood flow. Cardiac output reaches maximum values by midpregnancy and becomes highly variable in the third trimester. The supine position causes symptomatic reductions in cardiac output in about 5% of the pregnant women.[14] It is logical to assume that exercise in this position could significantly increase the incidence of hypotension.

Using the CO_2 rebreathing technique, we found that during cycle ergometry exercise in pregnancy, there are different kinetic adjustments augmented by increased maternal weight.[15,16] The relative increases in cardiac output and stroke volume are similar in pregnant and nonpregnant subjects. However, during strenuous exercise, the cardiac output response appears to be blunted in pregnancy. It was demonstrated in these studies that, at low exercise intensities, cardiac outputs in pregnancy are compensated by higher heart rates, whereas at higher exercise intensities, the contribution is primarily the increased stroke volume. Similarly, Sady and co-workers[17] have demonstrated higher cardiac outputs

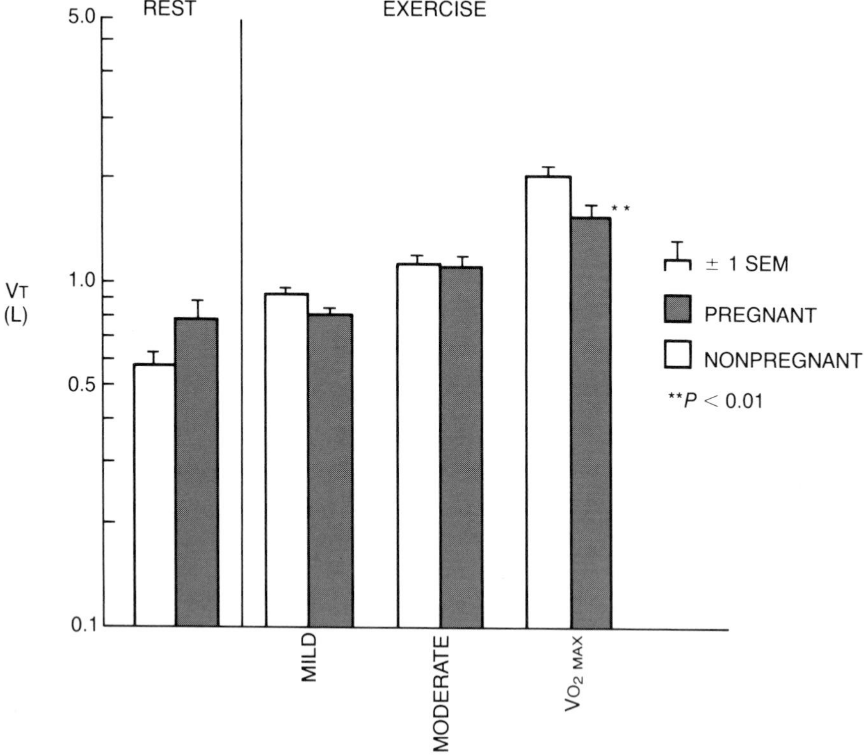

Figure 32–5. Comparison of tidal volumes during mild, moderate, and $\dot{V}O_{2max}$ exercise. (*From* Artal R, Wiswell R, Romem Y, et al: Pulmonary responses to exercise in pregnancy. Am J Obstet Gynecol 154:378–383, 1986; with permission.)

during pregnancy by 2.2 to 2.8 L/min at rest, and proportionately higher at increasing work loads. At lower intensity exercise, the contributions to increased cardiac output were a reflection of increments in heart rates and stroke volumes; during higher intensity exercise, the elevated cardiac outputs were the result of higher stroke volumes.

In human pregnancy, the heart rate is elevated by approximately 20 beats/min in all three trimesters and declines to prepregnancy levels in the postpartum period. Along with the increase in the heart rates, there is an increase in myocardial oxygen requirement. This increased demand is probably insignificant in normal women, but it may be consequential in the presence of cardiovascular pathology. These physiologic adaptations were taken into account by the panel that drafted the American College for Obstetricians and Gynecologists (ACOG) guidelines for home exercises. They recommend that during unsupervised exercise in pregnancy, heart rate should not exceed 140 beats/min (approximately 60% to 70% of $\dot{V}O_{2max}$ for the pregnant population).[18]

One other important aspect of hemodynamics during exercise in pregnancy is the cardiac output distribution to different organs. Limited human[19] or animal[20–22] data are available to demonstrate that, indeed, there is a significant impact on uterine blood flow during exercise in pregnancy. It is important, then, to point out that uterine blood flow increases significantly in the human and at term reaches 500 to 600 mL/min. Approximately 90% of this flow reaches the placenta while the remaining 10% perfuses the myometrium. In the presence of such abundant blood flow, it is very unlikely that changes which occur during mild-to-moderate exercise have any impact on the healthy fetus. A study published by Morris and associates[19] suggested a 25% reduction in the perfusion of the human pregnant uterus during brief mild bicycle exercise in a semireclining position.

Some of this blood flow reduction could certainly be attributed to the aortocaval syndrome that impacts on cardiac output while the subject is in the supine position. Nevertheless, these data are consistent with those obtained by Rowell[13] in nonpregnant subjects. Clapp[20] observed no change in uterine blood flow during mild exercise in sheep but did record a 28% flow decrease during strenuous and prolonged exercise. Hohimer and colleagues[21] reported a 32% decrease in blood flow during exercise in pygmy goats in which maternal heart rate increased from 129 to 195 beats/min.

In another animal study, Lotgering and associates[22] demonstrated that the uterine blood flow depends on the intensity and duration of the exercise and inversely correlates with the heart rate. Mean uterine blood flow decreased significantly by 13% during a 10-minute exercise period at 70% $\dot{V}O_{2max}$; 17% during 10 minutes at 100% $\dot{V}O_{2max}$; and 24% near the end of a 40-minute period at 70% $\dot{V}O_{2max}$.

Studies conducted in experimental pregnant animals should be carefully interpreted when applied to humans, especially because most of these animals are restrained and catheterized during the experiments; consequently, they are already stressed. Responses to the additional stress of exercise may be limited or inconsequential.

FETAL RESPONSES TO MATERNAL EXERCISE

To maintain its metabolism during hypoxia, the fetus depends on anaerobic metabolism to maintain its energy requirements. Prolonged anaerobic metabolism may lead to exhaustion of carbohydrate stores and to metabolic acidosis. Thus, the main concern related to maternal exercise is that any of the potential benefits could be offset by potential fetal risks (Table 32–1).

The crux of the theoretical risks is related to the selective redistribution of blood flow during exercise to the exercising muscles and away from the visceral organs. Stuaies conducted in nonpregnant[13] and pregnant[19] individuals confirm that blood flow selectively redistributes during exercise. These are the unanswered questions: To what extent, if at all, does the blood flow redistribution affect oxygen transfer across the placenta; and, if it does, could it adversely affect the fetus? The indirect evidence is that healthy fetuses of healthy mothers in the absence of either obstetric or medical complications can tolerate brief periods of hypoxia with no evidence of lasting effects.

In the experimental animal, a reduction in uterine blood flow by 50% or more can lead to fetal respiratory acidosis.[23] Theoretically, such conditions could be created in the human pregnancy during either strenuous or prolonged exercise. Alterations in uterine blood flow could result in acute fetal changes (fetal distress, fetal heart rate changes) and chronic fetal changes (intrauterine growth retardation). Fetal demise may theoretically occur as a result of either of the above instances, but is more likely to occur in the latter chronic condition. Most of the studies addressing fetal responses examined fetal heart rate (FHR) changes during or after exercise.[24] The consistent FHR response to maternal exercise is an increase of approximately 10 to 30 beats/min. Such increases in FHR may persist for as long as 30 minutes.

Typical FHR changes are believed to occur in the presence of fetal distress or, con-

TABLE 32–1. THEORETICAL FETAL RISKS OF EXERCISE IN PREGNANCY

Fetal distress
Prematurity
Intrauterine growth retardation
Congenital malformations

versely, to reflect fetal well-being. Fetal well-being is generally ascertained by a reactive FHR pattern that includes, in a 10-minute window, two accelerations that last at least 15 seconds with the peak of the acceleration at least 15 beats/min above a baseline of approximately 140 beats/min. Conversely, fetal distress is suspected in the presence of any late FHR deceleration (a decrease in FHR after a uterine contraction). Significant decelerations are defined as heart rate decreases of at least 30 beats/min below the baseline that have a duration of at least 15 seconds. During prolonged decelerations, the FHR falls at least 40 beats/min below baseline and this lasts for more than 1 minute. During more severe conditions, prolonged decelerations occur during which the heart rate must fall at least 40 beats/min below the baseline and last in excess of 1 minute, or the FHR falls to a rate of less than 90 beats/min for more than 1 minute.

Fetal bradycardia is defined as a heart rate below 120 beats/min for 2 minutes or longer. This is to distinguish it from a deceleration, which refers to a decrease in FHR below 120 beats/min for less than 2 minutes.

To date, published data on FHR responses to maternal exercise include 22 studies.[25] Fetal bradycardia has been reported with an incidence of 8.9%. There are several reports of FHR monitoring obtained during maternal exercise. It is not yet clear whether episodes of fetal bradycardia are a common occurrence during maternal exercise, and the mechanism by which they are triggered can only be speculated upon.

Transient hypoxia, caused by cord compression, fetal head compression, or vagal stimulation, is only one of the possible mechanisms suggested that might trigger these changes in FHR. These reports have naturally generated significant concerns, primarily owing to the inaccessibility of the fetus to evaluate the real impact of these events. More recently, umbilical artery Doppler velocimetry was undertaken to evaluate fetal umbilical artery blood flow resistance immediately prior to and after maternal exercise.[26–28] Owing to technical difficulties, these studies are inconclusive. In the future, this research tool may become a valuable screening tool to determine brief or long-lasting effects on the fetal circulation.

Physical fatigue and psychological stress have been recognized for a long time as potential etiologic factors in precipitating premature labor.[29] It is not clear at this time if engaging in recreational physical activities increases the risk for premature labor and delivery. Nevertheless, it is important to recognize that the incidence of preterm labor is between 5% and 10%, and that it accounts for 75% of perinatal deaths.[30] Bed rest has been used clinically with various degrees of success to prevent preterm labor, particularly in patients with twin gestation. The benefit of reduced activity in preventing preterm labor remains to be addressed prospectively. Nevertheless, in the absence of definitive data, it behooves us to recommend against any physical activity in individuals at risk for premature labor. We must also recognize that higher levels of circulating norepinephrine as generated by exercise can precipitate premature labor. Increasing levels of circulating plasma norepinephrine are known to cause increased uterine activity.[31]

One other concern is the effect of heat stress generated by exercise on the developing fetus. It has been well established in the experimental animal that hyperthermia has a teratogenic effect[32]; however, owing to obvious ethical considerations, this effect has never been adequately studied in the human. All the human data implicating hyperthermia in excess of 39°C as teratogenic have come from case reports,[32] which may suggest an association, but cannot prove causality. These reports suggest a strong association between hyperthermia and defects of the central nervous system (anencephaly, encephalocele, and spina bifida). These malformations are the result of a failure of closure of the neural tube in the phase of embryogenesis. Closure of the anterior neuropore occurs at 25 days after conception, and closure of the posterior neuropore occurs at 27 days. It appears, therefore, that hyperthermia should be avoided early in gestation although other theoretical risks of hyperthermia have been recognized to threaten the fetus throughout gestation.

Hyperthermia in the experimental animal leads to an increase in fetal umbilical circulation to facilitate dissipation of fetal heat.[33] This increased circulatory demand often leads to fetal tachycardia, a symptom of fetal distress. At the same time, umbilical arteriovenous temperature and oxygen content gradients decrease. In the experimental animal, this chain of events can lead to fetal circulatory collapse.

While most of the interaction between maternal exercise and the fetus may be transient, questions remain as to the long-lasting effects on the fetus. One manifestation of long-lasting effects is intrauterine growth retardation (IUGR). Clapp[28] reported that women who continued strenuous exercise throughout pregnancy gained less weight and delivered earlier (by 8 days), and their infants had a consistently reduced birth weight (by approximately 500 g).

A review[25] of all published studies evaluating outcome of pregnancies of mothers who exercise throughout pregnancy confirms the above and consistently reveals certain trends:

1. Women who exercise prior to pregnancy and continue to do so while pregnant weigh less, gain less, and deliver smaller babies than the control group.
2. All women decrease their physical activity as pregnancy progresses.
3. No information is available to assess or suggest that active women have better pregnancy outcomes than sedentary women.
4. Physically active women appear to tolerate labor pain better.

To answer critical questions related to maternal exercise, future studies will have to include a large enough sample size with a proper population mix; record incidence of complications; and quantify exercise history, type, intensity, and duration and its relation to $\dot{V}O_{2max}$.

EXERCISE PRESCRIPTION IN PREGNANCY

The absence of proven benefits of exercise during pregnancy and absence of definitive data on fetal risks resulted in prudent recommendations by the ACOG[18] that are very much in line with recommendations for the nonpregnant general population. As demonstrated by Blair and co-workers,[34] the health benefits of exercise can be obtained also at exercise intensities considerably lower than those recommended[35] for increasing aerobic power. The ACOG guidelines are intended for the general population. The original educational bulletin "Exercise During Pregnancy" was published in May 1985 following deliberations of an educational task force of eight experts. The bulletin describes the anatomic and physiologic changes that occur during pregnancy and their relation to exercise. It suggests how to develop an exercise prescription for pregnant women to maintain aerobic ability, and it also describes the potential maternal and fetal risks that are described in this chapter.

The following section describes the essentials of these recommendations, which can serve as a basis for any exercise prescription in pregnancy. The ideal exercise program should offer a variety of options: walking, swimming, stationary cycling, and modified forms of dancing or calisthenics. No single exercise or exercise program will be able to meet the needs of all women. It is incumbent upon the physician taking care of the pregnant woman to assess each individual's ability to engage in physical activities and to advise a program that maintains the highest level of fitness consistent with maximum safety.

The essential points of the ACOG bulletin are summarized below:

1. Any exercise program offered to pregnant women must be safe and fun to do. In the absence of clear benefits for pregnancy outcome, safety is the main concern. It cer-

tainly can be assumed that the same exercise-related health benefits derived by nonpregnant individuals could be derived by pregnant women as well.

2. One important ethical principle emphasized in the guidelines is that when uncertain, always err on the safety side.

3. Exercise programs for pregnant women can benefit them by promoting strength and coordination, both of which decrease in pregnancy. By strengthening the abdominal and back muscles, pregnant women can prevent the low back pain that is common in pregnancy.

4. Regular exercise is preferable. Nevertheless, sedentary women are not discouraged from engaging in physical activities, although moderation is advised. Pregnancy is a particularly suitable time to introduce behavior modification.

5. Pregnant women are advised not to exceed a heart rate of 140 beats/min while exercising in an unsupervised environment. This limit approximates 60% to 70% of the maximum aerobic capacity in the general population. Several considerations formed the basis for this recommendation. Primarily, it is precautionary advice to avoid cardiovascular complications in the unsupervised pregnant woman. It is recognized that cardiovascular complications are more likely to occur with strenuous exercise. The need for intensive and strenuous training is limited to very few individuals and for them, recommendations should be individualized. Furthermore, the correlations between $\dot{V}O_2$ and heart rates appear to differ in pregnancy and, at times, are poor.[36]

6. To prevent musculoskeletal injuries, warm-up and cool-down are recommended. The progressive laxity of joints and ligaments predisposes pregnant women to injuries. The rationale is the same for recommending against excessive stretching in pregnancy.

7. Pregnant women should be advised that the strenuous portion of their exercise routine should not exceed 15 minutes. This is precautionary advice to prevent hyperthermia and musculoskeletal injuries. Exercise can be resumed after brief periods of rest.

8. Emphasis should be placed on proper caloric and fluid intake. When engaging in any physical activity, pregnant women have to compensate for the additional caloric cost. Proper hydration is essential for preventing hyperthermia and maintaining normal homeostasis.

9. Any exercise program should warn of constraints. In the absence of complications, pregnant women may continue to engage in the same type of physical activities as prior to pregnancy. Pregnancy may impose certain limitations. To avoid potential risks, pregnant women should avoid the following:

Exercise in the supine position
Exercises that involve the Valsalva maneuver
Hyperthermia—not to exceed body core temperatures of 38°C
Ballistic movements

Contraindications to exercise during pregnancy are listed in Table 32–2. Additional contraindications should be determined by the physician on an individual basis.

A recent review by the same group of experts that drafted the original ACOG guidelines indicates that new scientific knowledge has not shown any need to change the recommendations for the general public and that the guidelines are still pertinent.

The medical need for intensive and strenuous training is limited in pregnancy, especially since it has been demonstrated in nonpregnant subjects that health benefits can be derived from moderate exercise. The goal of exercise in pregnancy is to balance the highest level of fitness against maximum safety.

The information gathered as of today supports the position that pregnancy should not be a state of confinement. Nevertheless, there are limitations and constraints that may vary from one individual to another and interfere with the ability to engage in all forms of exercise.

TABLE 32–2. CONTRAINDICATIONS TO EXERCISE IN PREGNANCY

Absolute Contraindications
Active myocardial disease
Congestive heart failure
Rheumatic heart disease (class II and above)
Thrombophlebitis
Recent pulmonary embolism
Acute infectious disease
At risk for premature labor, incompetent cervix, multiple gestations
Uterine bleeding, ruptured membranes
Intrauterine growth retardation or macrosomia
Severe isoimmunization
Severe hypertensive disease
No prenatal care
Suspected fetal distress
Relative Contraindications*
Essential hypertension
Anemia or other blood disorders
Thyroid disease
Diabetes mellitus
Breech presentations in the last trimester
Excessive obesity or extreme underweight
History of sedentary life-style

*Patients may be engaged in medically supervised exercise programs.

REFERENCES

1. Caloaneri M, Bird HA, Wright V: Changes in joint occuring during pregnancy. Ann Rheum Dis 41:126–128, 1982.
2. Mills JL, Knopp RH, Simpson JL, et al: Lack of relation of increased malformation rates in infants of diabetic mothers to glycemic control during organogenesis. N Engl J Med 318:671–676, 1988.
3. Hytten FE: Nutrition. *In* Hytten FE, Chamberlain G (eds): Clinical Physiology in Obstetrics. Oxford, Blackwell, 1980, p 165.
4. Abrams BF, Laros RK: Prepregnancy weight, weight gain and birth weight. Am J Obstet Gynecol 154:503–509, 1986.
5. Langhoff-Ross J, Lindmark G, Gebre-Medhin M: Maternal fat stores and fat accretion during pregnancy in relation to infant birthweight. Br J Obstet Gynaecol 94:1170–1177, 1987.
6. Artal R, Wiswell R, Romem Y, et al: Pulmonary responses to exercise in pregnancy. Am J Obstet Gynecol 154:378–383, 1986.
7. Sady M, Haydon D, Sady S, et al: Maximal exercise during pregnancy and postpartum [abstract]. Med Sci Sports Exerc 20:511, 1988.
8. Clapp JF III, Wesley M, Sleamaker RH: Thermoregulatory and metabolic responses prior to and during pregnancy. Med Sci Sports Exerc 19:124, 1987.
9. Artal R, Masaki DI, Khodignian N, et al: Exercise prescription in pregnancy: Weight-bearing versus non–weight-bearing exercise. Am J Obstet Gynecol 161:1464–1469, 1989.
10. Artal R, Masaki DI: Exercise in gestational diabetes, a new therapeutic approach. Practical Diabetology 8(2):7–14, 1989.
11. Soultanakis HN: Glucose homeostasis during pregnancy in response to prolonged exercise [postdoctoral thesis]. University of Southern California, 1989.
12. Artal R, Wiswell RA (eds): Exercise in Pregnancy, ed 1. Baltimore, Williams & Wilkins, 1986, pp 143–144.
13. Rowell LB: Human Circulation Regulation During Physical Stress. New York, Oxford University Press, 1986, p 232.
14. Kerr MG: The mechanical effects of the gravid uterus in late pregnancy. J Obstet Gynaecol Br Commw 72:513–529, 1965.
15. Artal R, Khodignian N, Kaumurlo R, et al: Cardiopulmonary adaptations to graded exercise in pregnancy. Society for Gynecologic Investigation Proceedings 66, 1986.
16. Artal R, Khodignian N, Rutherford S, et al: Cardiopulmonary and metabolic responses to bicycle ergometry in pregnancy. Society for Gynecologic Investigation Proceedings 48, 1987.

17. Sady SP, Carpenter MW, Thompson PD, et al: Cardiovascular response to cycle exercise during and after pregnancy. J Appl Physiol 66:336–341, 1989.
18. American College for Obstetricians and Gynecologists: Home Exercise Programs, 1985.
19. Morris N, Osborne SB, Wright HP, et al: Effective uterine bloodflow during exercise in normal and pre-eclamptic pregnancies. Lancet 2:481–484, 1956.
20. Clapp JF III: Acute exercise stress in the pregnant ewe. Am J Obstet Gynecol 136:489–494, 1980.
21. Hohimer AR, Bissonnette JM, Metcalf J, et al: Effect of exercise on uterine blood flow in the pregnant pygmy goat. Am J Physiol 246:H207–H212, 1984.
22. Lotgering FK, Gilbert RD, Longo LD: Exercise responses in pregnant sheep: Oxygen consumption, uterine blood flow and blood volume. J Appl Physiol 55:834–841, 1983.
23. Wilkering RB, Meschia G: Fetal oxygen uptake, oxygenation and acid-base balance as a function of uterine blood flow. Am J Physiol 244:H749, 1983.
24. Artal R, Romem Y, Wiswell R: Fetal heart responses to maternal exercise. Am J Obstet Gynecol 155(4):729–733, 1986.
25. Artal R, Wiswell AR, Drinkwater B (eds): Exercise in Pregnancy, ed 2. Baltimore, Williams & Wilkins, 1990, pp 213–225.
26. Moore DH, Jarrett JC, Bendick PJ: Exercise-induced changes in uterine artery blood flow, as measured by Doppler ultrasound in pregnant subjects. Am J Perinatol 5:94, 1989.
27. Veille JC, Becevice AE, Wilson B, et al: Umbilical artery waveform during cycle exercise in normal pregnancy. Obstet Gynecol 73:957, 1989.
28. Clapp JF, Dickstein S: Endurance, exercise, and pregnancy outcome. Med Sci Sports Exerc 16:556–562, 1984.
29. Papiernik E: Proposals for a programmed prevention policy of preterm birth. Clin Obstet Gynecol 27:614, 1984.
30. Fuchs F: Prevention of prematurity. Am J Obstet Gynecol 126:809, 1976.
31. Zuspan FP, Cibils LA, Pose SY: Myometrial and cardiovascular responses to alterations in plasma epinephrine and norepinephrine. Am J Obstet Gynecol 84:841–846, 1962.
32. Edwards MJ: Hyperthermia as a teratogen. Teratogenesis Carcinog Mutagen 6:563–582, 1986.
33. Cefalo RC, Hellegers AE: The effects of maternal hyperthermia on uterine and placental blood flow. *In* Moawad AM, Lindheimer MD (eds): Uterine and Placental Blood Flow. New York, Masson Pub, 1982, pp 185–191.
34. Blair SN, Chandler JY, Ellisor DB, et al: Improving physical fitness by exercise training programs. South Med J 73:1594–1596, 1980.
35. American College of Sports Medicine: Guidelines for exercise testing and prescription, ed 3. Philadelphia, Lea & Febiger, 1986.
36. Wiswell RA, Artal R, Romem Y, et al: Hormonal and metabolic response to exercise in pregnancy. Med Sci Sports Exerc 17(2):206, 1985.

33

THE MALE GENITOURINARY SYSTEM

Jeffrey P. York, MD

The kidneys are seemingly well protected from direct injury. Laterally, the rib cage surrounds the upper third of the right kidney and the upper half of the left kidney. Posteriorly, the kidneys are protected by the quadratus lumborum, sacrospinalis, and latissimus dorsi muscles. Anteriorly, they are protected by the abdominal viscera as well as the internal and external obliquus and transversus abdominis muscles. Despite this protection, renal injury is found in 1 of every 3000 hospital admissions,[1] with 60% to 70% of these injuries due to blunt trauma.[2] The urinary bladder is protected from external injury during sports by its low abdominal and pelvic position and the fact that the bladder is usually empty during sports events.

Nevertheless, kidney and bladder injuries are fairly common in male athletes of all ages. Children are particularly prone to renal damage owing to the relatively large size of their kidneys and the incomplete ossification and strength of the rib cage. Approximately 30% of pediatric renal injuries are caused by sports activity.[3,4] In contrast, the risk of significant bladder abnormalities is higher in men than in boys and increases with age and increasing degree of hematuria.

This chapter discusses common male urologic injuries and abnormalities that may be seen by primary care physicians. Some of these problems are the direct result of athletic activity; others are as common in athletes as they are in the general population.

KIDNEYS

Types of Injuries

Examples of renal injuries (Fig. 33–1) include contusions, lacerations, shattered kidneys, and pedicle injuries. Physical findings suggestive of renal damage include tenderness in the flank or upper abdomen or a palpable abdominal mass. Flank contusion or ecchymosis (Grey Turner's sign) may indicate a retroperitoneal collection of blood. Radiographic evidence of a fractured rib or lumbar spine transverse process, loss of the psoas shadow, or a "ground glass" appearance in the region of the renal bed also suggests damage. Contusions and minor lacerations account for over 90% of all renal trauma cases. Treatment is conservative: enforced bed rest, hydration, and analgesics for a few days. It is imperative that the athlete refrain from strenuous activities for 2 to 3 weeks. Classically, rebleeding from the injury occurs 15 to 21 days after injury, concomitant with clot resolution. An athlete who participates strenuously before tissue is completely healed risks rebleeding and subsequent rehospitalization, with even more lost playing time. Rest and recuperation usually lead to complete recovery.

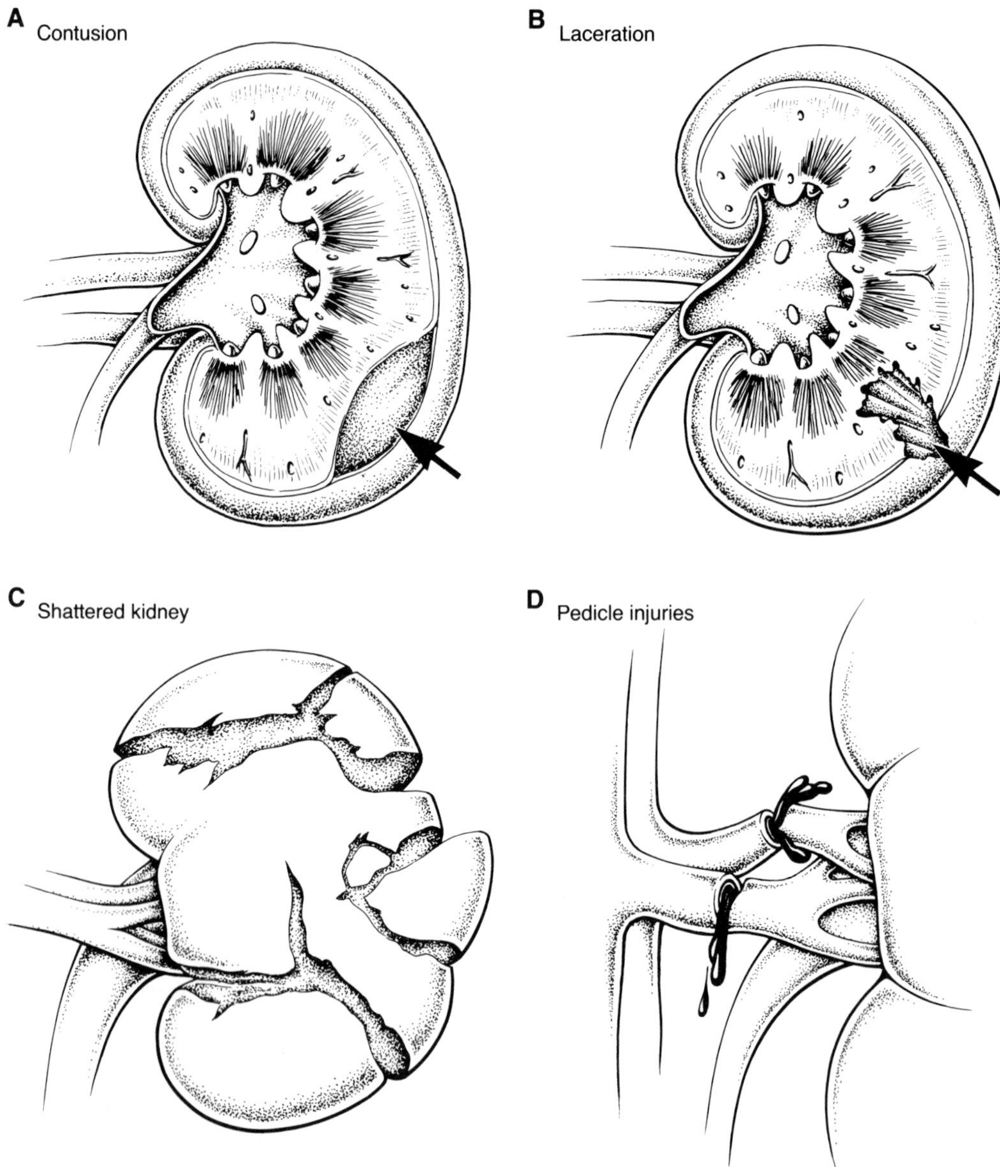

Figure 33–1. Coronal section of left kidney showing examples of renal trauma. **A**: Contusion; **B**: laceration; **C**: shattered kidney; and **D**: pedicle injuries.

Conservative management may be sufficient for major lacerations, although the possibility of delayed bleeding (15.0%) and postinjury hypertension (0.7% to 33.0%) are arguments in support of early surgical intervention.[5] Surgical exploration for pedicle injuries and shattered kidneys is well accepted.

Trauma-Induced Hematuria

Although hematuria is considered the hallmark of renal trauma, the degree of hematuria may not indicate the extent of injury. Microscopic evaluation has not been proved superior to dipstick evaluation, with the latter having a greater than 97.5% sensitivity and specificity for detection.[6] Controversy exists as to the need for radiographic evaluation for microscopic hematuria following trauma. More than 90% of these patients have a renal contusion at most and may be spared the possible morbidity of contrast studies. Further studies are warranted if there is gross hematuria or if microscopic hematuria is associated with signs or symptoms of shock, a dropping hematocrit, or a retroperitoneal mass that is increasing in size.[7] A high-dose bolus urogram with nephrotomography has been the standard for staging renal trauma[8]; however, computed tomographic (CT) scanning has largely replaced this technique owing to its ability to partially evaluate the renal pedicle and to assess the rest of the abdomen and retroperitoneum.[9]

Recently, a 14-year-old soccer player presented with gross hematuria, nausea, and flank pain following a minor flank trauma. An excretory urogram (Fig. 33–2) showed no contrast uptake by the left kidney. A CT scan (Fig. 33–3) showed a large left renal pelvis and perirenal extravasation of urine and probably blood. This was found to be secondary to a ureteropelvic junction (UPJ) obstruction (Fig. 33–4) that subsequently was surgically repaired.

Although significant renal trauma is unusual in most sports, boxing appears to be an exception. In studies of more than 900 professional boxers, Amelar and Solomon[10] and Kleiman[11] found that over 70% of the athletes had microscopic hematuria following a bout. The finding of significant hematuria (>6 red blood cells [RBCs] per highpower field [HPF]) depended on the length of the fight: Seventeen percent occurred in fights that lasted fewer than four rounds, 40% in 6 to 8 rounds, and 44% in 10 or more rounds. In addition, albuminuria was found in 68% of the boxers. Excretory urography on 100 of

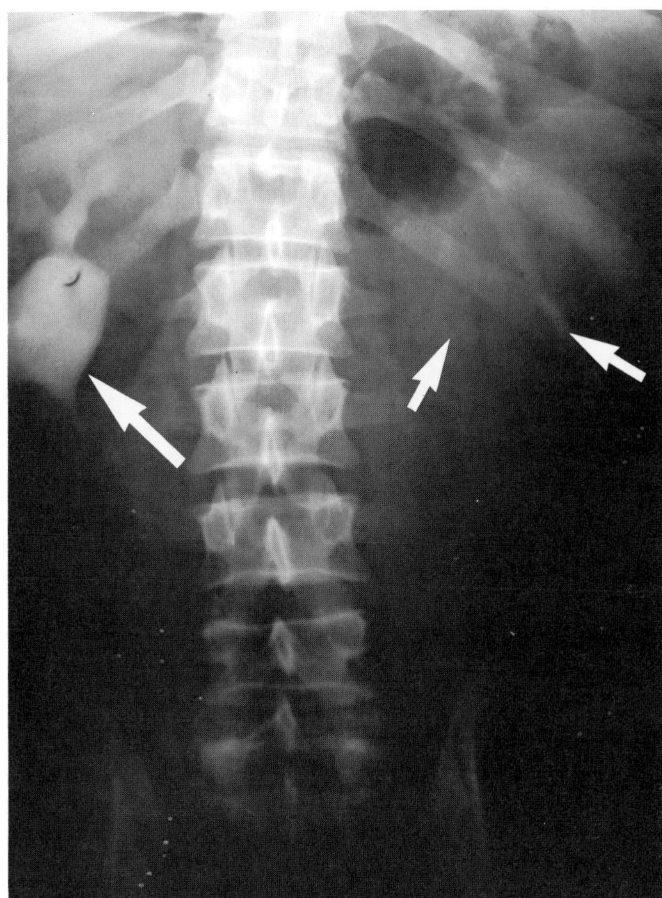

Figure 33–2. Excretory urogram of a 14-year-old soccer player with minimal flank trauma shows normal right kidney *(large arrow)* but no contrast uptake by the left kidney *(small arrows)*.

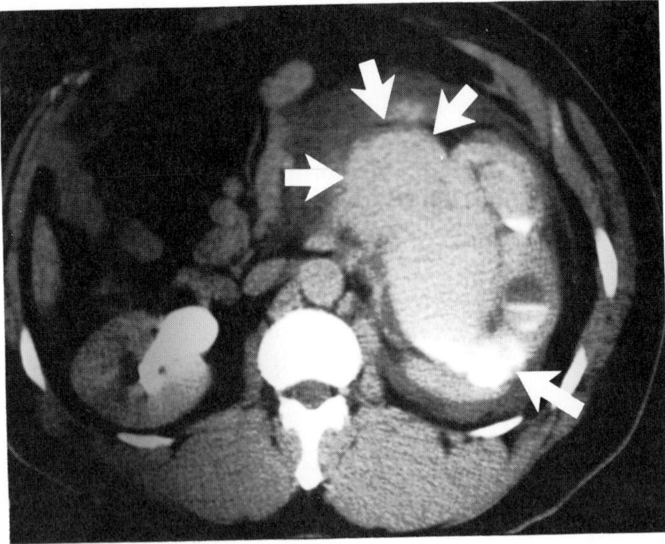

Figure 33–3. CT scan of patient in Figure 33–2. A large left renal pelvis *(small arrowheads)* is seen with extravasation of contrast medium from the collecting system *(large arrow)*.

the boxers revealed renal hypermobility in 33% and hydronephrosis and signs of renal contusion in 26%. None of the injuries required surgical intervention.

Underlying Renal Abnormalities

When the injury is not in proportion to the force of the trauma, an underlying renal abnormality should be suspected. In a review of 240 children, 28% of the renal injuries

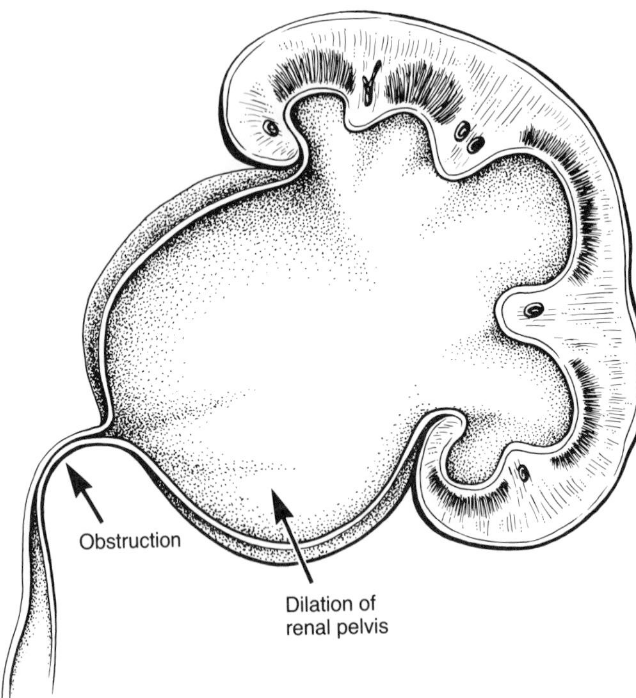

Figure 33–4. Ureteropelvic junction obstruction causing dilation of renal pelvis.

were due to sports.[3] Of the nine patients who had surgery, five of the patients had underlying renal abnormalities, including horseshoe kidneys, megaureter, renal malignancy, and UPJ obstruction.

UPJ obstruction is usually caused by an intrinsic narrowing at the junction of the renal pelvis and the ureter, leading to impaired urine drainage from the kidney. Although 25% of cases are found in the neonatal period,[12] this disorder is not uncommonly found in young adults, who often have symptoms of intermittent flank pain that is sometimes associated with the diuresis induced by excessive drinking. A patient with these symptoms should be restricted from strenuous physical activity, especially contact sports, until the symptoms resolve or the patient is cleared by urologic evaluation.

Renal Infections

Pyelonephritis is not common in the young athlete, but if found it demands a complete urologic evaluation of both upper and lower tracts. An excretory urogram or renal ultrasound is usually sufficient to rule out upper-tract stones, tumors, or congenital renal abnormalities. A good history will elicit symptoms such as incontinence, urgency, decreased urinary stream, or feelings of incomplete voiding that may indicate a neurogenic bladder. Most renal infections originate from bladder colonization, which is not uncommon in young sexually active females.

Stone Disease

Patients with stone disease most often develop the disorder after the fourth decade of life. Calcium stones are found 80% of the time, with the rest primarily of uric acid components. Although stone disease is uncommon in athletes, stones do form when the urine becomes supersaturated with the solute. I have seen renal colic in a number of athletes who have a high-protein diet and tend to become dehydrated. Uric acid stones were found in most of these cases. Presumably, the high-protein diet leads to hyperuricuria, and fluid restriction (practiced by bodybuilders, wrestlers, and boxers) exacerbates it.

Tretment in these cases should be directed toward increased urine output (2 L daily) and, perhaps, alkalinization of the urine with sodium bicarbonate because uric acid crystallizes in an acid environment. If calcium stones are found, the physician should order a 24-hour urine collection to evaluate calcium, oxalates, uric acid, and citrate content.

A common mistake made by physicians is to empirically recommend dietary restriction of calcium. If the stones are calcium oxalate in nature, dietary restriction of calcium may lead to hyperoxaluria with a paradoxic worsening of the stone disease. This is due to increased dietary absorption of oxalates that would otherwise be bound in the gut to calcium as an insoluble salt.

BLADDER

Exercise-Induced Hematuria

Gross hematuria seen after strenuous jogging or marathons is called "runner's bladder." Blacklock[13,14] reported on 18 patients presenting with gross hematuria following 10,000-meter runs. Cystoscopically, he found "kissing lesions" consisting of a rim of contused tissue encircling a central area of normal urothelium on the posterior bladder wall, bladder neck, and trigone. He postulated that repeated trauma of the posterior bladder wall on the prostatic base causes this contusion. Apparently, these lesions resolve within 1 week and become cystoscopically normal.

Patients prone to this abnormality have been cautioned not to run with an empty bladder, which may worsen the situation. Patients presenting with gross hematuria, however, should be carefully evaluated with urography and cystoscopy to rule out potentially more serious causes. In addition, urinary sediment should be screened for casts and protein, which may indicate primary parenchymal disease coexisting with the suspected trauma.

Sometimes a patient presents with smoke- or tea-colored urine after minor athletic endeavors. Gardner[15] described this finding in 1956 and called it "athletic pseudonephritis." It has not been reproduced in animal models, but it may be due to a combination of hematuria, hemoglobinuria, and myoglobinuria. These findings appear to be common in walking-running events[16] and have been attributed to continuous minor renal trauma, increases in renal vein pressure, dehydration, or even transient renal ischemia.[17] These exercise-related benign causes of hematuria usually resolve without sequelae within 24 hours and require no further evaluation.

Urinalysis

It is well known that normal individuals excrete erythrocytes in their urine. Larcom and Carter[18] determined that a normal excretion of erythocytes would correspond to 2 RBCs/HPF of a spun urine sediment. Large studies from insurance companies indicate that normal excretion for men would be 1 to 2 RBCs/HPF, and for women, 4 to 5 RBCs/HPF. Therefore, any values exceeding these would warrant evaluation.

In athletes under age 35, an intensive evaluation for microscopic hematuria is not cost-effective. Nevertheless, repeated urinalyses that are positive for hematuria after a sports activity (within the guidelines above) or episodes of hematuria that are not associated with a lower urinary tract infection warrant evaluation. A good history should be obtained to elicit medication use (analgesics, anticoagulants), previous oropharyngeal infections (poststreptococcal glomerulonephritis), family history of blood dyscrasias, history of trauma, and history of urinary infections or abnormal voiding patterns. A serum creatinine level (or, if proteinuria exists, a creatinine clearance) should be obtained. If a history of possible streptococcal infections exists, an antistreptolysin-O titer, complement levels, and possibly erythrocyte sedimentation rate should be obtained. If the patient is black or of South European or Mediterranean ancestry, a test for sickle cell anemia should be performed. Urine should be sent for cytologic evaluation for possible malignancy. The upper tracts should be evaluated with an excretory urogram. If the excretory urogram shows no abnormalities, cystoscopic examination should be done. If no cause is found, it is important to follow these patients. Carson and colleagues[19] found that 16% of patients with initially negative workups for microscopic hematuria had significant lesions within 2 years.

MALE GENITALIA

The male genitalia, although not anatomically protected as are the kidneys and bladder, are seldom injured during athletic activity. Nevertheless, athletes are susceptible to all urologic problems.

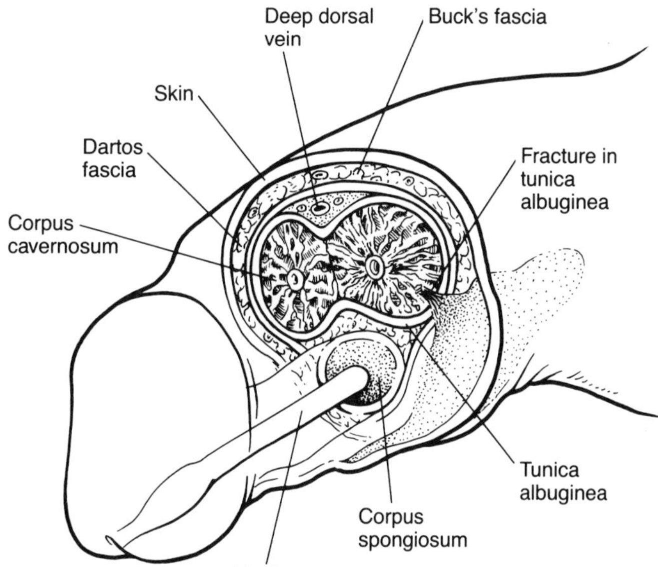

Figure 33–5. Cross section of penis. Fracture of the tunica albuginea occurs when the erect penis is subjected to trauma.

Penis

The nonerect penis is a highly mobile organ and is rarely injured except in farm machinery accidents. When erect, however, the penis is susceptible to acute trauma with resultant fracture of the tunica albuginea (Fig. 33–5). The area of the fracture is acutely swollen and ecchymotic, and the penis is usually bent to that side. This is a true urologic emergency necessitating evacuation of the clot and repair of the tunical tear.

Historical data from the patient is notoriously inaccurate in these injuries. The patient usually neglects to mention the sexual activity that caused the fracture and ascribes the injury to a work- or sports-related trauma.

Direct blows to the flaccid penis or perineum may lead to vascular injuries and potency abnormalities. St. Louis and co-workers[20] described a case in which direct injury to the ventral base of the penis in a 19-year-old man during a basketball game led to total occlusion of the dorsal and deep penile arteries bilaterally. These vascular injuries are more likely to be caused by straddle-type injuries or direct blows to the pubis, such as spearing with football helmets. These same mechanisms may lead to total disruption of the male urethra, although this has not been described during sports activities. The injury is classically within Buck's fascia, and patients have a butterfly-type ecchymosis on the perineum.

When such an injury is encountered, the primary diagnostic tool is a retrograde urethrogram performed with a mixture of radiopaque contrast medium and sterile water-soluble jelly. Depending on the extent of the injury, primary repair may be an option; however, recent reports[21] indicate that insertion of a transcutaneous suprapubic catheter leads to resolution of the urethral tear in approximately 20% of cases. A secondary repair after resolution of the pelvic hematoma may result in increased rates of potency.

I have seen a number of long-distance cyclists who describe a paresthesia and numbness in the perineum and phallus following prolonged cycling. Bicycler's penis resolves spontaneously with no apparent sequelae other than a mild loss of enthusiasm before the next race. Altering the angle of the bicycle seat to decrease perineal pressure may decrease the severity of this malady. O'Brien[22] reported on a number of young men who demonstrated transient urinary retention or decreased force of voiding after vigorous cycling. The problem resolved after a short hiatus from the activity. Salcedo[23] thought that hematuria in a 13-year-old boy was related to continued trauma due to "dirt-bike" racing and added this as a possible cause of hematuria in the adolescent.

Testicles

The organs protected most by the male athlete may be the testicles. These paired structures develop in the retroperitoneum adjacent to the fetal kidney and usually descend into the scrotum during the eighth fetal month. The embryologic site of development explains the referred pain of ureterolithiasis into the testicles, and the groin and flank discomfort seen with testicular trauma. Owing to crossover of the mesenteric ganglia and the vagal nerve, testicular trauma may also lead to nausea and vomiting.

Most male athletes use an athletic supporter to elevate the testicles and decrease discomfort in the freely hanging organs. Plastic cups are also usually worn by baseball catchers, hockey and lacrosse goaltenders, and other athletes who require added scrotal protection. As Vermooten[24] pointed out, individuals who previously had a contusion of the testes usually use this added protection.

A direct blow to the scrotum may lead to significant injury—usually testicular contusion with ecchymosis and swelling that responds to elevation of the scrotum and bed rest. Direct application of a towel-wrapped ice pack to the scrotum for 24 hours after injury markedly decreases the pain. If there appears to be an expanding mass that cannot be transilluminated, if the epididymis cannot be separated from the testicle, or if the pain seems out of proportion to the injury, a diagnosis of fracture of the testicle or epididymis should be considered.

Scrotal ultrasound may show disruption of the tunica albuginea or epididymis, but may be falsely negative. Radionuclide testicular scanning is usually not helpful except in a delayed evaluation when viability of a testicle is in question. When ultrasound or clinical findings warrant exploration, this should be accomplished rapidly with a generous scrotal incision and deliverance of the testicle and spermatic cord into the surgical field. Usually an orchiectomy is performed; however, if minimal testicular tissue is lost, or in the case of a solitary testicle,[25] defunctionalized seminiferous tubules can be removed and a primary repair performed.

In the last 2 years, I have treated five patients who had testicular trauma associated with sports: two during softball/baseball games, two during karate activities, and one from "dirt-bike" racing. Injuries ranged from an epididymal laceration to a complete rupture with subsequent necrosis of the testicle (direct blow from a baseball-pitching machine). Three orchiectomies and two primary repairs were performed. Figure 33–6 shows a fracture of the superior pole of a testicle struck by a softball. Devitalized tissue was removed, and the tunica albuginea was surgically closed. A postoperative testicular radionuclide scan 2 months later revealed good function of the remaining testicular tissue.

Preexisting scrotal abnormalities may predispose the testicle to an increased risk for injury; thus, preparticipation physical examinations should not neglect the genitalia. Undescended testicles may lie within the inguinal canal or adjacent to the pubic tubercle and be in a direct line between the skin and pubic bone. Braumrucker[26] found cryptorchidism in 0.8% of U.S. Army recruits.

When a testicle is not found within the scrotum, three explanations exist: anorchia, retractile testes, or undescended testes. Unilateral anorchia is found in 5% of boys presenting for surgical exploration. The contralateral testicle is usually slightly larger. Anorchia is most often due to torsion of the testicle and infarction prior to birth; no hormonal or fertility abnormalities will occur. Surgical exploration reveals a vas deferens and sper-

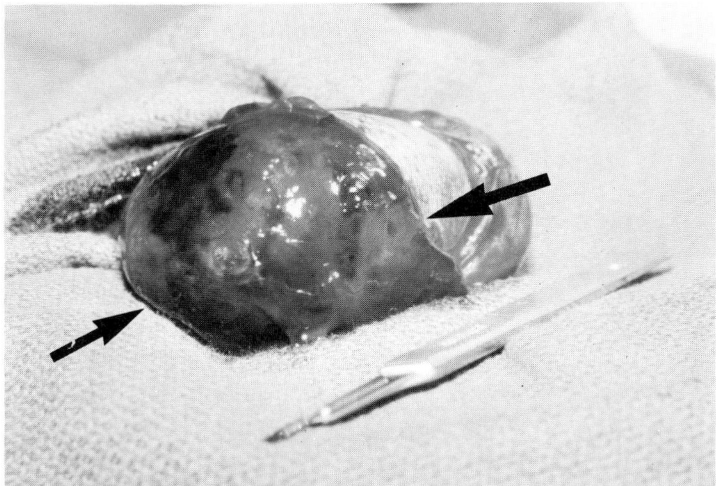

Figure 33–6. A ruptured upper pole of the testis due to a softball injury. Seminiferous tubules *(between arrows)* are extruding from the lower pole of the partially fractured testis.

matic vessels attached to a bud of scar tissue. Rarely, agenesis of the testicles occurs. Contrary to popular belief, testicular agenesis is not related to renal agenesis, despite the close embryogenesis of the testicles and kidney. If a kidney does not develop, however, in 10% to 15% of cases, the testicle on that side will not have an intact vas deferens or epididymis (structures that develop from the embryonic mesonephric ridge).

Often, a nonpalpable testicle is retractile and within the inguinal canal; it can be gently pulled into the scrotum, but it promptly returns to its inguinal position. These testicles remain in the groin owing to excessive cremasteric activity and usually spontaneously descend into the scrotum during puberty. They rarely require surgery.

Most commonly, the undescended testicle resides permanently within the inguinal canal or just inside the internal inguinal ring and, in contrast to retractile testes, cannot be gently pulled into the scrotum. These testicles usually require surgical repair. Patients with undescended testicles are at increased risk for the development of testicular cancer as well as decreased fertility. Surgical repair may not reverse this risk, but it may allow easier access for frequent palpation.

Scrotal Masses

Referral for evaluation of a scrotal mass is not uncommon in the male athlete. Testicular cancer is the most common solid malignancy in 16- to 35-year-old males, and the fear associated with this disorder should engender early urologic consultation. The presence of a mass in the testicle, separate from the cord and epididymis (Fig. 33–7), is probably due to a malignancy and demands prompt inguinal exploration.

A mass separate from the testicle should be evaluated by transillumination with a bright light. Masses that cannot be transilluminated should be evaluated with ultrasound examination and possibly with surgical exploration.

Varicoceles (Fig. 33–8) may be present in 9% to 19% of all men. These lesions are varicosities of the internal spermatic veins and may be described as a "bag of worms" adjacent to the testicle and cord. There is significant debate as to the pathologic consequences of a varicocele. Seventy percent are on the left side, 20% are bilateral, and 10% are on the right side. Current teaching indicates surgical correction or transcutaneous

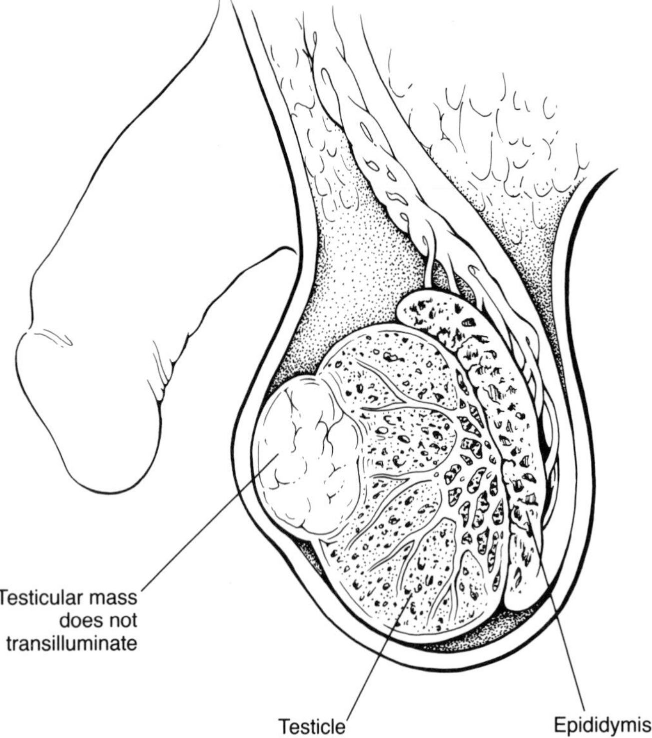

Figure 33–7. A testicular mass separate from the cord and epididymis demands prompt exploration.

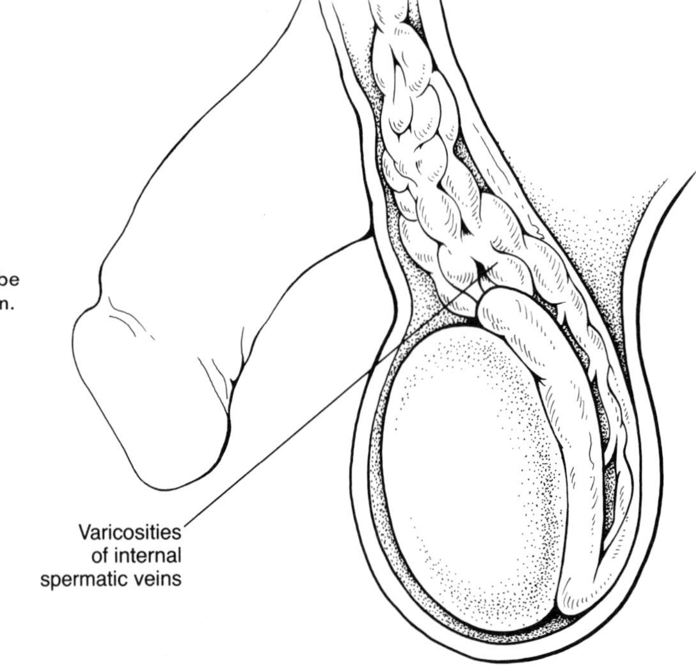

Figure 33–8. Varicoceles may be present in 9% to 19% of all men.

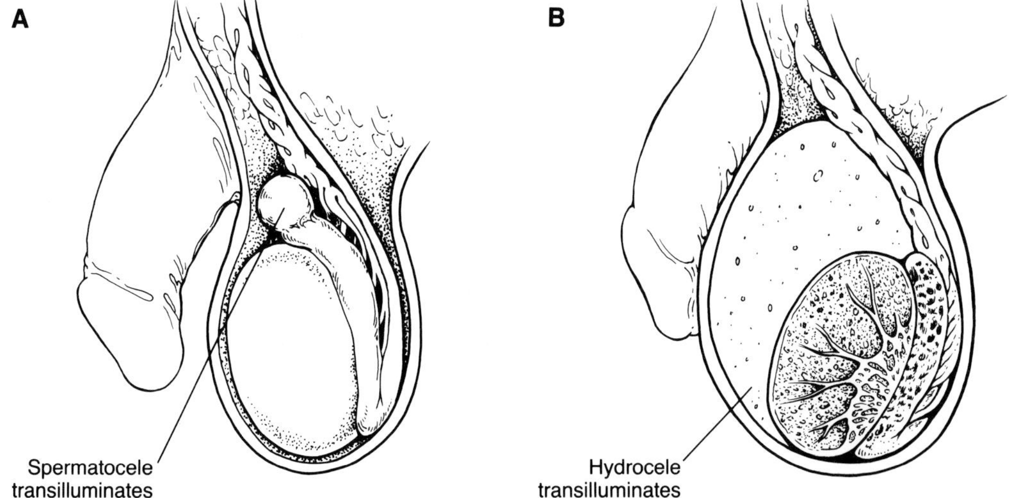

Figure 33–9. **A**: Spermatocele. **B**: Hydrocele.

embolization of these lesions for pain, diminished ipsilateral testicular size or growth, or subfertility. In the absence of these problems, varicoceles do not require treatment.

Cystic masses within the epididymis or adjacent to the testicle are probably spermatoceles (Fig. 33–9A) caused by extravasation of sperm from the epididymis following trauma or infection. They require no treatment unless they are extremely large or painful. A solid noncystic mass within the epididymis is usually a benign sperm granuloma and requires no further treatment.

A cystic mass encompassing the testicle and epididymis is usually a hydrocele (Fig. 33–9B) caused by decreased absorption of the normal tunica vaginalis secretions due to trauma, infections, or tumors. An acute hydrocele without evidence of underlying epididymitis may harbor an underlying malignancy and should be investigated with ultrasound and, possibly, surgical exploration. Rarely, traumatic or infectious hydroceles may become large enough or cause sufficient discomfort to warrant treatment. Although aspiration with or without sclerosing agents may be tried, more often surgical correction is necessary.

Epididymitis

Testicular pain is another common urologic complaint of the male athlete. The practitioner must distinguish epididymitis from testicular cord torsion. Early in epididymitis, a tender, indurated epididymis may be felt; later, it may become hard and fixed to the skin. The spermatic cord is often swollen and indurated. The patient may be clinically ill and is usually febrile with an elevated leukocyte count. Urinalysis is usually positive for leukocyte esterase, and frank pyuria may exist.

Treatment for acute epididymitis is bed rest with sitz bath of the scrotum and antibiotic therapy. Support of the scrotum on towels or a "Bellevue bridge" hastens recovery.

The etiologic agent in men under age 35 is usually *Chlamydia* and in men over age 35, *Escherichia coli.* Cultures should also be analyzed for gonococci. If gonococcal or gram-negative organisms are not implicated, treatment with doxycycline (100 mg twice a day) or tetracycline (500 mg four times a day) may be instituted for 10 days to 2 weeks.[27] If the diagnosis of epididymitis is in question and the urine is acellular an analysis, the diagnosis of testicular cord torsion must be more strongly considered.

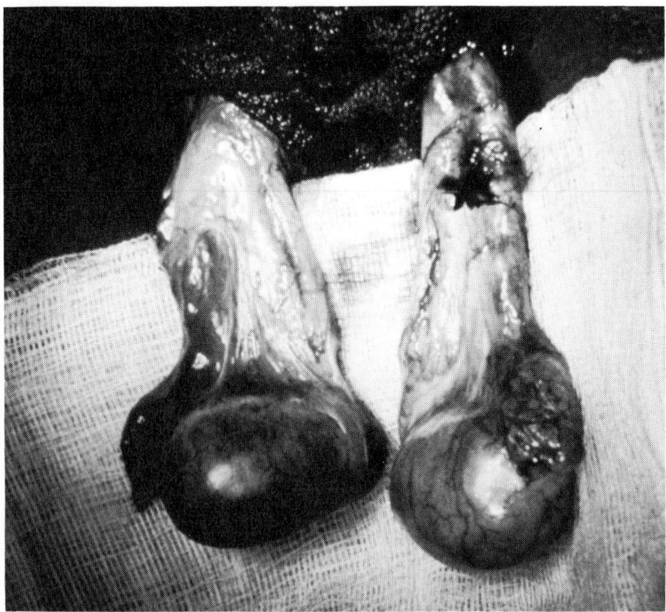

Figure 33–10. Torsive testicle *(left)* and nontorsive testicle.

Testicular Cord Torsion

The patient with acute testicular pain, a high-riding testicle, possible obliteration of the space between the epididymis and the cord, an abnormal position of the epididymis, or induration of the overlying scrotal skin is likely to have testicular cord torsion. Though many patients relate a history of testicular cord torsion to some vigorous activity,[28] it is unlikely that activity is responsible. Testicular cord torsion is a true emergency and warrants prompt urologic evaluation. If presentation is within 4 to 6 hours, cooling of the scrotal skin, lidocaine cord block (Xylocaine; Astra Pharmaceutical Products, Westboro, MA), and manual detorsion may be accomplished, but should not delay surgical exploration and repair.

Radionuclide scanning may help distinguish torsion from epididymitis; however, clinical suspicion should override a negative scan. In no instance should surgical exploration be delayed to obtain the scans. Although, in the past, these torsive testicles have been surgically detorsioned and sutured in place, recent data indicate that if left in place, an ischemic testicle may lead to infertility secondary to a contralateral testicular defect.[29] Figure 33–10 contrasts a normal testicle with a torsed testicle. The torsive testicle was surgically detorsioned but then removed because normal blood flow did not return.

SEXUALLY TRANSMITTED DISEASES

Urethritis

Sexually transmitted diseases are the most common urologic problem of the athlete. Nongonococcal urethritis (NGU) is the most common offender. Patients usually present with dysuria and urethral discharge. In addition to serologic testing for syphilis and culturing for gonococcus with a blood-agar medium, a noncotton urethral swab should be used to obtain a mixed culture of *Chlamydia* and *Ureaplasma.* Chlamydial infections usually respond to a 7-day course of tetracycline (500 mg orally four times a day) or doxycycline (100 mg orally twice a day). A sexual history should be taken because these infections may be reportable depending on state laws. Prudence dictates concomitant treatment of the sexual partner. Patients should be cautioned to either abstain from sexual activity or use condoms during treatment, until a follow-up culture is negative.

Gonococcal urethritis treatment has undergone significant change owing to the prevalence of penicillinase-producing gonococci and tetracycline-resistant strains. Concomitant chlamydial infection is found in up to 45% of cases. Culture-documented gonococcal infections should be treated with a single 250-mg intramuscular dose of ceftriaxone (Rocephin; Roche Laboratories, Nutley, NJ) followed by doxycycline, 100 mg orally daily for 7 days. In addition, all infected patients should have serologic testing (fluorescent treponemal antibody absorption or Venereal Disease Research Laboratories) for syphilis. Human immunodeficiency virus (HIV) testing should also be offered to the patient.

Venereal Warts

In our clinical practice, condyloma acuminatum is the most commonly seen sexually transmitted disease. The increased finding of abnormal cervical Pap smears due to this papilloma virus has sent many unsuspecting male partners to us for evaluation. Clinically apparent warts are seen as papillary growths on the shaft of the penis, perineum, scrotum, and anal verge. If no lesions are visible, the genitalia are wrapped with 2% acetic acid–soaked gauze for 10 minutes and examined under magnification. Areas of papilloma virus will appear bright white. Treatment includes freezing, electrical hyfercation, laser ablation, or local application of podophyllin. If podophyllin (10% to 25%) in benzoin is used, the patient should be cautioned not to apply the medicine to normal skin and to wash thoroughly 1 hour after application. Recurrence rate is up to 80%, regardless of the type of treatment, perhaps because subclinical lesions may not be completely treated. I favor treatment with ablation using the CO_2 laser at 1 to 2 W. This seems to lead to fewer recurrences with minimal ulceration and scar formation. I also recommend condom use for 3 months with frequent examination during that time. Intraurethral lesions can be treated with urethroscopy and neodymium:yttrium-aluminum-garnet (Nd:YAG) laser ablation or daily intraurethral instillation of 5-fluorouracil (5%) for 1 month.

Herpes Simplex

Herpes progenitalis is a chronic disease with no known cure and presents as an edematous wheal with small vesicles that resolve in 7 to 10 days. These lesions are usually painful and may become secondarily infected. Topical application of acyclovir ointment or cream may be used to decrease the pain and works best when applied at the first prodrome or within 2 days of symptom onset. Oral acyclovir (200 mg five times daily for 7 to 10 days) may decrease pain or shorten the active period, but it will not abolish the virus, which resides in the nerve ganglia. Patients who exhibit more than six recurrences per year have been treated with daily suppression with acyclovir (200 mg two to five times daily), with nearly 75% showing significant reduction in recurrence rates.[30] Current guidelines from the Centers for Disease Control recommend this treatment for no more than 1 year. Acyclovir-resistant strains have appeared with suppression, but only in immunocompromised patients. Because these lesions are extremely contagious, patients should abstain from sexual activity during the infectious period.

REFERENCES

1. Mertz JH, Wishard WN Jr, Nourse MH, et al: Injury of the kidney in children. JAMA 183:730–733, 1963.
2. Mendez R: Renal trauma. J Urol 118(5):698–703, 1977.
3. Kuzmarov IW, Morehouse DD, Gibson S: Blunt renal trauma in the pediatric population: A retrospective study. J Urol 126(5):648–649, 1981.
4. Mandour WA, Lai MK, Linke CA, et al: Blunt renal trauma in the pediatric patient. J Pediatr Surg 16:669–676, 1989.
5. Peterson NE: Complications of renal trauma. Urol Clin North Am 16(2):221–236, 1989.
6. Mee SL, McAninch JW: Indications for radiographic assessment in suspected renal trauma. Urol Clin North Am 16(2):187–192, 1989.
7. Glenn JF, Harvard BM: The injured kidney. JAMA 173(7):1189–1195, 1960.
8. Mahoney SA, Persky L: Intravenous drip nephrotomography as an adjunct in the evaluation of renal injury. J Urol 99(5):513–516, 1968.
9. Bretan PN Jr, McAninch JW, Federle MP, et al: Computerized tomographic staging of renal trauma: 85 consecutive cases. J Urol 136(3):561–565, 1986.
10. Amelar RD, Soloman C: Acute renal trauma in boxers. J Urol 72:145–148, 1954.
11. Kleiman A: Hematuria in boxers. JAMA 168(12):1633–1640, 1958.
12. Williams DI, Karlaftis CM: Hydronephrosis due to pelvi-ureteric obstruction in the newborn. Br J Urol 38(2):138–144, 1966.
13. Blacklock NJ: Bladder trauma in the long-distance runner: "10,000 metres haematuria." Br J Urol 49(2):129–132, 1977.
14. Blacklock NJ: Bladder trauma from jogging. Am Heart J 99(6):813–814, 1980.
15. Gardner KD Jr: Athletic pseudonephritis: Alterations of sediment by athletic competition. JAMA 161(8):1613–1617, 1956.
16. Bruce PT: Stress haematuria. Br J Urol 44(6):724–725, 1972.
17. Javitt NB, Miller AT: Mechanism of exercise proteinuria. J Appl Physiol 4:834–839, 1952.
18. Larcom RC, Carter GH: Erythrocytes in urinary sediment: Identification and normal limits with a note on the nature of granular casts. J Lab Clin Med 33:875–879, 1948.
19. Carson CC III, Segura JW, Greene LF: Clinical importance of microhematuria. JAMA 241(2):149–151, 1979.
20. St. Louis EL, Jewett MA, Gray RR, et al: Basketball-related impotence. N Engl J Med 308(10):595–596, 1983.
21. Morehouse DD: Delayed management of external urethral injuries. *In* Cass A (ed): Genitourethral Trauma. Oxford, Blackwell Scientific Publications, 1988, pp 209–222.
22. O'Brien KP: Sports urology: The vicious cycle [letter]. N Engl J Med 304(22):1367–1368, 1981.
23. Salcedo JR: Huffy-bike hematuria [letter]. N Engl J Med 315(12):768, 1986.
24. Vermooten V: Sports injuries to the genitourinary tract. Am J Surg 98:457–462, 1959.
25. Goldman MS: Repair of shattered solitary testicle. Urology 24(3):229–231, 1984.
26. Braumrucker GO: Incidence of testicular pathology. Bull US Army Med Dept 5:312, 1946.
27. Berger RE, Alexander ER, Monda GD, et al: *Chlamydia trachomatis* as a cause of acute "idiopathic" epididymitis. N Engl J Med 298(6):301–304, 1978.
28. Skoglund RW, McRoberts JW, Ragde H: Torsion of the spermatic cord: A review of the literature and an analysis of 70 new cases. J Urol 104(4):604–607, 1970.
29. York JP, Drago JR: Torsion and the contralateral testicle. J Urol 133(2):294–297, 1985.
30. Medical Letter 30(757):10, 1988.

34

EXERCISE AND AGING

Arthur J. Siegel, MD

> *[O]ne of the most useful reforms which could be introduced into the present constitution of society would be that the advice of the physician should be sought and paid for while in health, to keep the patient well, and not, as now, while in sickness, to cure disease, which might in most cases have been avoided or prevented.* Lemuel Shattuck, 1850

The last decade is witnessing a virtual discovery of important information on the relationship between exercise, physical fitness, and the aging process. The consensus based on available information 10 years ago was that exercise might improve the quality of life, but there were few data to prove that exercise had any direct impact on either morbidity or mortality with regard to specific diseases or from a statistical overview. Common sense has long dictated that physicians should recommend various life-style changes to enhance health, such as following prudent diet guidelines and refraining from smoking; however, physicians have waffled on the exercise recommendation. Many physicians have been uncertain about the impact of exercise on the aging process and have regarded physical fitness as an endeavor that should be reserved for youth. Exercise skeptics have viewed regular sports participation in older individuals—whether it be running, swimming, skiing, or even dancing—as frivolous or even dangerous. The good news is coming in fast. Exercise is safe and beneficial. It may even serve as an antidote to the aging process.

CAN EXERCISE ALTER THE AGING PROCESS?

Until recently, this notion seemed more in the realm of clinical speculation rather than scientific hypothesis. There is, however, growing awareness that many conditions that have been traditionally considered as biomarkers of the aging process may indeed be influenced by behavioral as well as environmental factors. Social changes, economic policies affecting the consumer movement emphasizing personal responsibility for health, and the accumulating evidence for the efficacy of certain specific preventive health measures have led to a renewed emphasis on the positive impact of beneficial health maintenance activities. Physicians are increasingly drawn back to the important task of providing advice and procedures for patients to maximize the health of each individual. The importance of routine annual checkups for early diagnosis was the popular prevailing concept in the 1970s. Pertinent screening, detection, diagnosis, and treatment of various illnesses at an early stage were deemed responsible for improvements in general health and increased life expectancy.[1]

Studies in many fields indicate that a substantial part of the age-related decline in physiologic function is due to misuse or disuse rather than to chronologically determined decrements in exercise capacity. The purpose of this chapter is to review relevant information suggesting that physical fitness can function as an antidote to the aging process.

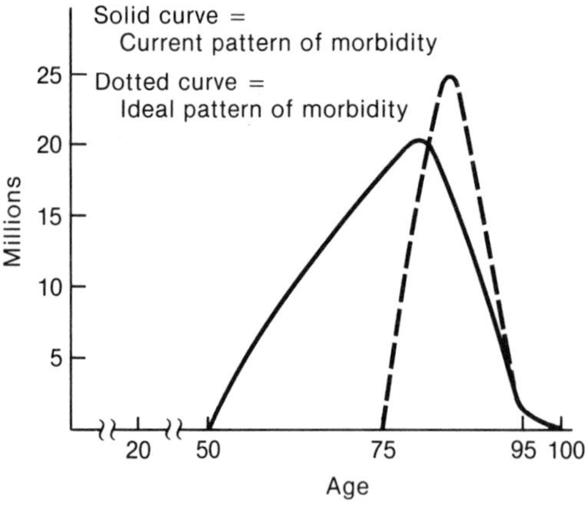

Figure 34–1. As morbidity and disability are delayed through health promotion, the period of morbidity *(solid curve)* is compressed to the latest years in life *(dotted curve)*. (Reprinted with permission from the Geriatrics Society, The changing scope of prevention in late life, by Robinson BE [Clinical Report on Aging, 2:1–21, 1988].)

This includes "squaring off" the so-called mortality curve, leading to modest increases in life expectancy (Fig. 34–1). More importantly, physical fitness can lead to improved organ function and enhancement of the elder "health span," with a delay in the onset of morbidity from various illnesses from midlife to later life. Exercise therefore contributes not only to a longer life but also to a higher quality life.

The Aging Population: Does Exercise Have Anything to Offer?

Senior citizens are a growing and ever more active segment of the general population. Men and women older than age 65 now make up 12% of the nation's population, and forecasters predict that this figure will increase to 20% by the year 2030.[2] The absolute numbers of older people have increased dramatically from 18 million in 1965 to nearly 30 million in 1990. The nation's median age has increased from 16 years in 1820 when such data were first collected to 32 years in 1986, with an expected rise to 40 years by the second decade of the next century. Population specialists are forecasting the arrival of the "elder boomers" sometime after the turn of the century. Around the year 2010, the first wave of the nation's largest generation ever—the 76 million individuals born between 1946 and 1965—will be reaching their mid-60s. The "exercise-aging connection" may be as important in the 1990s as the diet–heart disease connection has been in the last decade. The evidence that exercise and physical fitness can reduce morbidity from various specific diseases and have a positive impact on all-cause mortality will be reviewed in this chapter.

The old view of aging is shown in Figure 34–2, with the obligate declines in organ function with age. This represents loss of functional capacity in various organ systems on an age-dependent basis. Table 34–1 documents organic system decompensation with aging as if engraved in stone. The case for exercise summarized in the following sections challenges these old assumptions.

New evidence indicates that positive life-style interventions, such as exercise, can achieve the primary goal of disease prevention, which postpones illness and disability. The modest increase in life span is multifactorial and due to reduction in heart disease mortality from cholesterol reduction, diet intervention, smoking cessation, and treatment of high blood pressure. The specific and real impact of physical fitness, however, is to preserve the quality of life by postponing illnesses of disuse and by decreasing morbidity from various illnesses. Figure 34–3 summarizes the prototypic lingering chronic illness pattern associated with disuse during aging. The underlying drawing shows the effect of post-

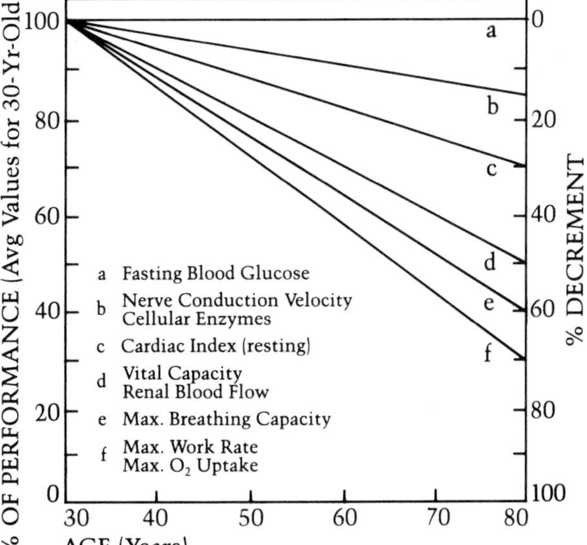

Figure 34–2. Decrements in physiologic functions in normal men aged 30 to 80 years, expressed in percent of average values for 30-year-olds. (*From* Shock NW: Physiological and chronological age. *In* Dietz AA (ed): Aging—Its Chemistry. Washington, D.C., American Association for Clinical Chemistry, 1980; with permission.)

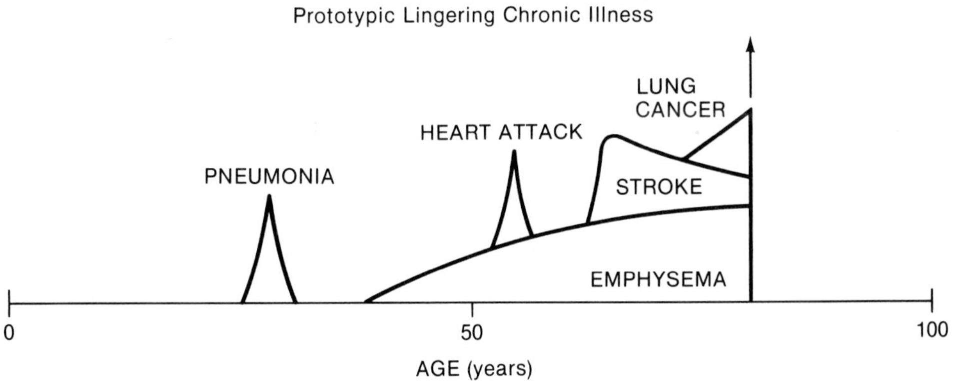

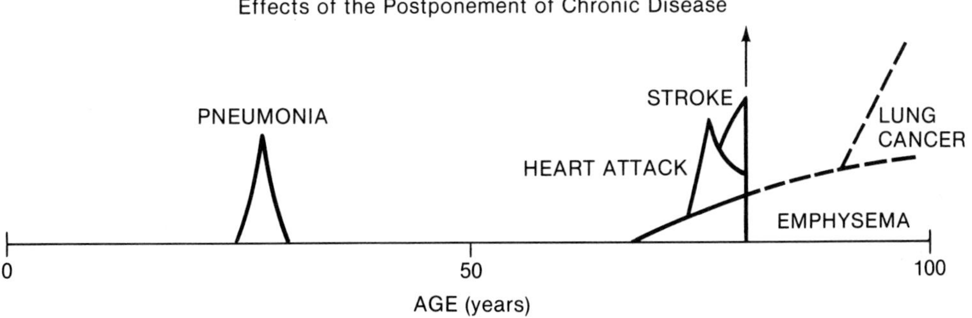

Figure 34–3. Summary of the prototypic lingering chronic illness pattern associated with disuse during aging and the effects of the postponement of chronic disease. (*From* Fries JF: Aging Well. Reading, MA, Addison-Wesley, 1989, ©1990. Reprinted by permission of Addison-Wesley Publishing Co., Inc., Reading, MA.)

TABLE 34–1. SOME CHANGING PARAMETERS NOTED WITH AGING IN VARIOUS ORGAN SYSTEMS

Brain
- Weight decrease of 10% to 12% during a normal long life
- Gray/white matter ratio
  - Age 20, 1.28:1
  - Age 50, 1.13:1
  - Age 100, 1.55:1
- Decline in cerebral blood flow
  - Age 17–18, 79.3 mL/min per 100 g brain tissue
  - Age 57–99, 47.7 mL/min per 100 g brain tissue
- Neurofibrillary tangles and senile plaques
  - Up to age 50, uncommon
  - Age 90, found in 90%

Heart
- Left ventricular wall: up to 25% thicker at age 80 than at age 30
- Cardiac output: decreases 40% between 3rd and 8th decades, or a little less than 1%/year
- Maximum heart rate
  - Young adult, 195 beats/min
  - Average 65 year old, max 170 beats/min
- Blood pressure
  - Mean, age 20–24: females 116/70, males 122/76
  - Mean, age 60–64: females 142/85, males 140/85

Lungs
- Residual volume: increases 100% between 3rd and 9th decades
- Vital capacity: decreases by 17 to 22 mL/yr
- Forced expired air volume in 1 sec (FEV_1): falls progressively: males, 32 mL/yr; females, 25 mL/yr
- Maximal breathing capacity: reduced by 40% between 20 yr and 80 yr
- Maximum amount of O_2 utilized under stress: reduced 50% by age 80

Kidneys
- Weight: age 60, 250 g; age 70, 230 g; age 80, 190 g
- Number of glomeruli per kidney: birth:age 40, 500,000–1,000,000; by 7th decade ⅓ to ½ less
- Renal blood flow: 2nd decade, 670 mL/min; 8th decade, 350 mL/min
- Glomerular filtration rate: decreases 46% from age 20 to age 90
- Maximum specific gravity of urine: youth, 1.032; age 80, 1.024

Ovaries
- Weight
  - In reproductive years, 10 g
  - In old age, 4 grains
- Oocytes
  - At birth, about 500,000
  - Age 50, $<$10,000
- Urinary estrogen excretion

	Estradiol	Estrone	Estriol
Age 20–29	9.6 ± 1.6	6.1 ± 1.2	16.6 ± 2.8
Age 50–59	3.7 ± 0.8	2.2 ± 0.5	4.9 ± 1.1
Age 80+	1.9 ± 0.3	1.6 ± 0.3	3.3 ± 0.5

Muscles
- Cells making up voluntary muscle: decrease by 50% at age 80
- Weight of skeletal muscle: age 21–30, 45% of body wt; age 70+, 27%

Bones
- Rate of bone loss/decade: men, 3%; women, 8%
- Average height loss: age 65–74, 1.5″; age 85–94, 3″

Adapted from Sleepscope, Sleep and Aging, no 1. Used with permission of Roche Laboratories, Nutley, NJ 07110.

ponement of chronic illness and associated disability, which compresses morbidity into the latest phases of life. The evidence continues to mount that the old adage, "Use it or lose it," is true for exercise and aging in general. The strong message is that physical fitness enables us to live better as well as longer.

Physical Fitness and Normal Aging: The Positive Exercise-Aging Hypothesis

Physical activity has been associated with the prevention and control of several medical conditions that are the major causes of death and disability in the United States. Table 34–2 lists the major diseases that are traditionally associated with the aging process and are responsible for significant morbidity and mortality over age 65. Regular exercise leading to physical fitness may be associated with an amelioration or postponement of such conditions as coronary heart disease (CHD), hypertension, non–insulin-dependent diabetes mellitus, osteoporosis, obesity, and mental health problems.[3] In the past, uncertainty has existed with regard to the role of physical fitness in improvements in disease-specific and all-cause mortality. Several large prospective studies have employed statistical analysis to adjust for the independent impact of age, smoking habits, cholesterol levels, systolic blood pressure, fasting blood glucose levels, parental history of coronary heart disease, and exercise on mortality rates.[4] Because CHD is the leading cause of mortality in the United States today, the supportive role of physical activity in reducing CHD is of particular importance as a public health intervention.

Estimates of attributable risk for disease-specific and all-cause mortality indicate that low physical fitness is an important risk factor for early mortality in both men and women. Higher levels of physical activity appear to promote longevity, especially due to the lowered rates of cardiovascular disease. In addition, exercise can contribute to a decrease in morbidity and disability, as shown in Figure 34–3, which has a positive impact on functional life span associated with higher physical fitness profiles.[5]

An extensive study of leisure-time physical activity has shown that even moderate exercise can be protective in this regard.[6] Recent data indicate a 30% to 40% greater risk of death from CHD or all other causes in sedentary men than in those who expend more than 1000 kcal per week during leisure-time physical activity. This translates into walking 10 miles per week, or roughly 40 minutes of walking three or four times per week. Light leisure-time activity on a consistent basis seems to confer the maximal benefit, with a definite de-emphasis on strenuous physical exertion, which can lead to cardiovascular and other complications. A high level of athleticism is beyond the scope required to maintain the benefits of cardiovascular health.[7]

TABLE 34–2. SOME DISEASES ASSOCIATED WITH THE AGING PROCESS

Atherosclerosis	Parkinson's disease
Hypertension	Alzheimer's disease
Nephrosclerosis	Osteoporosis
Maturity-onset diabetes	Osteoarthritis
Emphysema	Cataracts, presbyopia
Neoplasia	

NORMAL AGING

The human life span, experts suggest, is either fixed or increasing at a very slow rate, perhaps a month each century. In an ideal world free of disease and accidental death, the human life span is still limited by a decline in functional reserve of multiple organ systems to levels insufficient to maintain the internal physiologic milieu. The functional reserve in young adult life of organ systems such as the heart, lungs, and kidneys is four to ten times that required to maintain normal homeostasis.

Parameters associated with aging in various organ systems are outlined in Table 34–2. Physiologic measurements of decrements in performance or function which accompany these organic changes are shown in Figure 34–2. There is an almost linear decline in functional reserve in all parameters beginning after the age of 30. The decrements in function in normal men expressed relative to 100% of function at age 30 are shown by decades. These losses in functional reserve are interactive and define an upper limit of attainable age.

Research on normative aging begins with this observation of declining function. The next question is to ask whether factors in life-style, such as regular exercise, can maintain higher levels of function or performance, which vary among healthy persons of similar age. Selection of special individuals, such as master athletes (older than age 50), may reflect an influence of exercise specific to these individuals and may not apply to a cohort of nonathletes of similar age. World records for high-performance athletes by age are an example of this selection effect in the extreme. World marathon records for men by age show a linear decline in maximum performance from ages 30 to 70 (Fig. 34–4), perhaps reflecting age-related declines in maximal attainable heart rate and maximal oxygen consumption. Figure 34–5 shows the relative decline in world records for the 100- and 10,000-meter races with advancing age from age 35 to age 85 or greater in both men and women. World record performances fall off by 50% for the shorter distance events but by a greater figure for more prolonged events, such as the 10,000-meter race. Running records for males in 5-mile, 10,000-meter, and 10-mile events are shown in Figure 34–5. At any level and for any sport involving a wide variety of capacities, similar declines in peak performance with age have been seen. Performance of special individuals, such as aging world-class athletes, may reflect innate physical capacities for training, displaying a genetic endowment as well as environmental factors.

Whether regular exercise, such as running, can indeed stave off or overtake the aging process has been examined in selected athletes in various sports.[7] Physiologic studies conducted in expert older athletes, such as runners, tennis players, and master swimmers,

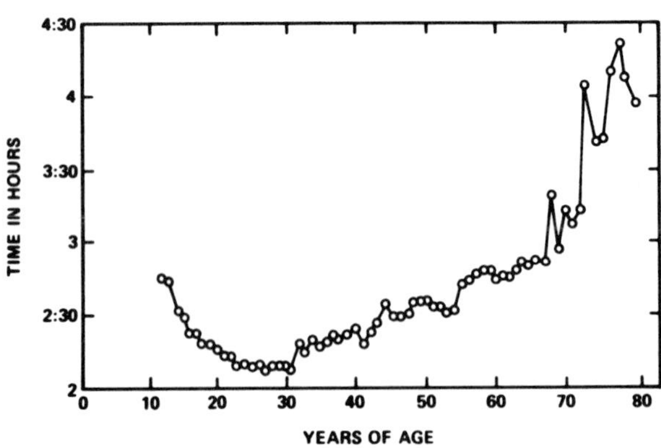

Figure 34–4. World marathon records for men. Note the slow but linear decline in maximum performance between the ages of 30 and 70. (*Adapted from* Fries JF: Aging, natural death and the compression of morbidity. N Engl J Med 303:134, 1980. Reprinted, by permission of the New England Journal of Medicine.)

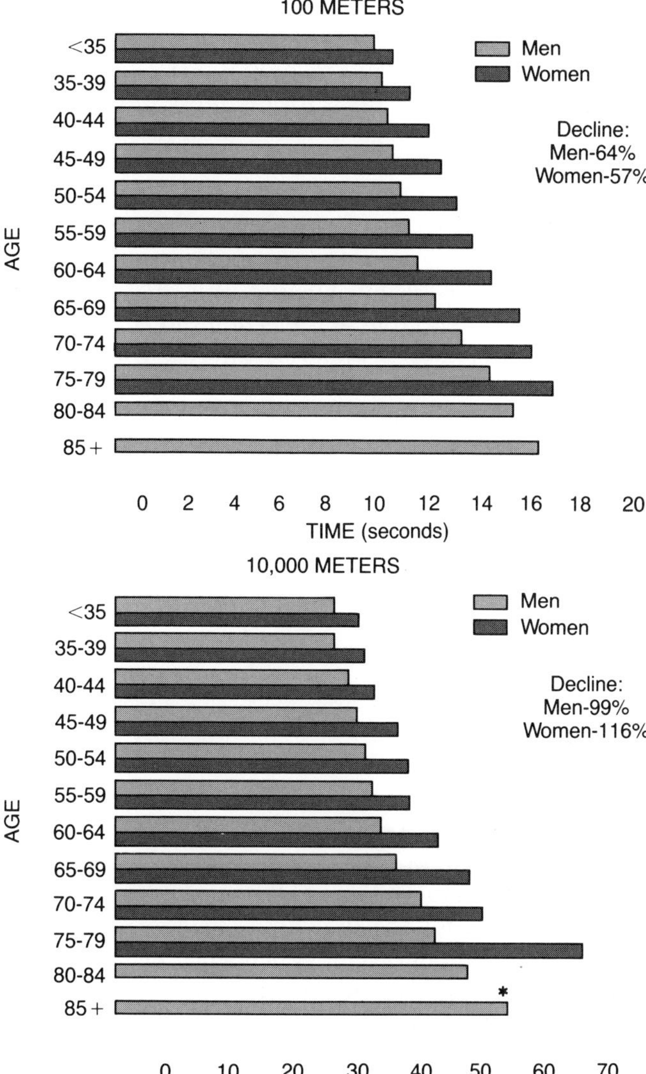

Figure 34–5. Decline in the world records for the 100- and 10,000-meter races with advancing age. (*From* Morley JE, Reese SS: Clinical implications of the aging heart. Am J Med 66:77–86, 1986; with permission.)

show superior fitness for advancing age groups.[8] Decline in maximal attainable heart rate is the major limiting factor on maximum oxygen uptake in such individuals. All show a lesser decline in fitness than observed for sedentary age-related controls. Studies among unselected healthy but inactive subjects show an average loss of 8% in cardiovascular fitness capacity per decade; highly active individuals show a lesser decline in the range of 4%.

One interpretation is that regular exercise retards or postpones the decrement in physiologic capacity seen with normative aging by 50%; another explanation is that active individuals are selected by their life-style for greater-than-average aerobic capacity. Individuals who choose to take part in strenuous exercise on a regular basis may have more efficient cardiovascular systems to begin with than their less active counterparts. Extrapolation of the benefits to less physically active people may lead only to injury or illness.

THE CARDIOVASCULAR SYSTEM

As implied earlier, new information is being gathered on the positive benefits of physical activity in healthy individuals for the prevention of the initial development of several diseases, especially with regard to the cardiovascular system. The report from the U.S. Preventive Services Task Force reviews all literature pertaining to exercise and primary prevention of CHD.[3] The protective effect of physical activity is demonstrated by studies of both occupational and leisure-time activity.[6–10] The most well-designed studies are cohort studies conducted in a prospective fashion and analyzed to assess attributable risk.[7] This type of data addresses the potential criticism that the association between physical activity and CHD may stem from self-selection rather than from a true protective effect of exercise. This selection bias would be the case if persons who chose to be physically active were already inherently more healthy and thus at lower risk of CHD than those who did not choose to be physically active because of such preexisting risk. While it is impossible to fully eliminate this potential source of bias from studies of cohort design, weight of the statistical analysis to minimize such bias favors an independent protective exercise effect. Findings from the Harvard College Alumni Study (HCAS) originally suggested that the protective exercise threshold was at moderate-to-intense exercise.[11] This has been moderated by recent studies showing that expenditure of roughly 100 kcal/day in leisure activity suffices to confer a benefit. Although a cause-effect relationship between physical activity and prevention of CHD has not been proved in a prospective randomized clinical trial, the evidence is strong and positive. These findings warrant advising all asymptomatic adult individuals to adopt a physically active life-style with guidelines for consistency and moderation.[6]

The Exercise Dose-Response Curve for Cardiovascular Health in the Elderly

Prescribing an appropriate exercise program for an elderly patient requires a detailed clinical assessment of cardiovascular function as well as degrees of physical limitation due to other illness. One recent approach adapts the New York Heart Association's functional classifications for CHD (designed in 1962) to assess functional exercise capacity for elderly patients in general.[12]

For anyone above the age of 65 who has been sedentary and wants to be in an exercise program, the process properly begins with an exercise treadmill test. This accomplishes an accurate assessment of the patient's true maximal heart rate and also screens for the possibility of severe CHD in the high-risk population. Patients can be stratified to take into account concurrent medical illness, such as diabetes, arthritis, or renal disease, or other limiting factors. A system of classification can then be stratified as follows.

Class 1. Patients in this group have no known illness or disease that results in limitation in physical activity. The initial exercise should consist of 10 to 15 minutes of flexibility training plus 20 to 30 minutes of low-impact, low-intensity aerobics three to four times per week. Swimming or stationary cycling to achieve a heart rate at 50% of maximum attained heart rate is a safe intensity for initiation of this program. Class 1 patients can increase exercise intensity after 3-month intervals, working up to 60% to 70% of maximum heart rate, and can even supplement stretching and aerobic activity with some coordination or strength training exercises. Strength training should also be of low intensity with patients using weights small enough to allow 20 to 30 repetitions before fatiguing.

Class 2. These patients show a functional impairment at some specific exertion or level. Such patients require more structured exercise and should not exceed a specific heart rate of roughly 10 beats/min below the level at which symptoms arise. Such patients can acquire the skill of monitoring a level of perceived exertion during exercise to be cross-checked with specific heart rate measurements. Reduced intensity and 1 or 2 days of rest between each exercise workout are safe precautions.

Class 3. These patients are ambulatory but experience functional impairment with activities of daily living. The primary goal here is to keep patients active, ambulatory, and flexible to maintain the highest possible level of independence. Appropriate stretching and very-low-intensity aerobics define a safe limit for this group. Strength training to improve function, such as getting up and down stairs or transferring to and from bed, may also be appropriate.

Class 4. Such patients are functionally impaired by illness at rest or with minimal activity. The risks of exercise are likely to outweigh the benefits in this group although stretching and antigravity range of motion exercises will still be beneficial for the musculoskeletal system. Recent cardiovascular research adds another benefit for regular exercise: It produces an increase of plasminogen activator (tPA) in an individual's tissue, offering enhanced protection against thromboses and myocardial infarctions. Findings from a recent study at the University of Washington in healthy subjects show a mean 44% increase in tPA levels with regular exercise in both young and elderly subjects. An increase in tPA activity may be one mechanism by which chronic exercise reduces cardiovascular morbidity.[13]

THE PULMONARY SYSTEM

Changes in lung function attributable to aging alone as distinct from those caused by smoking or specific pulmonary diseases have been reviewed.[14] In healthy individuals, total lung capacity remains virtually constant through life. Vital capacity, however, decreases by 17 to 22 mL per year (Table 34–1, Fig. 34–2); flow measurements, such as forced vital capacity and forced expiratory volume over 1 second, decrease progressively after the mid-30s by roughly 32 mL per year in men and by 25 mL per year in women. Maximum breathing capacity is reduced by 40% between the ages of 20 and 80. There is a corresponding increase in residual volume and in the functional residual capacity, showing a slow loss in elastic recoil, especially at high lung volumes. Age-related loss of lung recoil causes earlier closure of small or terminal airways at higher lung volumes, resulting in imbalance of ventilation and perfusion with the aging process. Arterial oxygen tension may also decline with age but falls into the range of mild hypoxemia only in the presence of underlying disease.[14]

As with other organ systems, during youth there is considerable reserve in lung function, which then becomes progressively compromised with advancing decades. Studies on exercise training and testing in patients with chronic obstructive lung disease confirm that regular exercise can maintain or improve exercise capacity even in the face of static function as measured on formal pulmonary testing. Improvement in exercise tolerance is due to specific muscular training and increased efficiency rather than to objective change in lung mechanics. All types of exercise training are task-specific, so that rehabilitative activities should focus on useful tasks in daily life, such as progress in walking. As with healthy elderly individuals, walking may be sufficient to promote and maintain a training effect that allows increased exercise capacity without objective evidence of disease reversal. Exercise training in patients with chronic lung disease, however, does indicate a benefit with improved exercise capacity even in the absence of demonstrable improvement in pulmonary function parameters.[15]

Recent clinical evidence shows that patients with chronic obstructive pulmonary disease benefit significantly from exercise rehabilitation programs. One such innovative program is called REACH—Respiratory Exercise and Education Activities Create Healthiness.[16] An emphasis on life-style change, including education and regular low-intensity physical activity, resulted in improvement in functional performance, with enhanced quality of life and self-improved image due to increased physical activity levels. This type of improvement indeed reflects the positive outcome of exercising interventions in specific conditions.

DIABETES MELLITUS: EXERCISE IMPLICATIONS

More than 11 million people in the United States (6.6% of the adult population) suffer from diabetes mellitus. The pathophysiology of diabetes mellitus is directly tied into glucose metabolism, which is also affected by exercise. The goal of effective treatment is to provide glucose homeostasis with dietary exercise interventions supplemented by appropriate pharmacologic agents (insulin, sulfonylureas) where appropriate. Non–insulin-dependent diabetes mellitus (NIDDM) is associated with obesity, hyperinsulinemia, and relative insulin resistance. Patients with this condition can benefit from regular exercise to promote an increase in insulin sensitivity, a relative increase in lean body mass, and normalization of glucose tolerance. Appropriate diet with regular exercise is the treatment of choice, which may reduce or obviate the need for pharmacologic treatment.[17]

Exercise recommendations for the NIDDM patient must begin with realistic goals. Previously sedentary individuals as discussed in the cardiovascular section should undergo a general medical examination with an exercise tolerance test prior to launching a physical exercise program. In this manner, previously sedentary patients with a potential for severe or silent myocardial ischemia can be appropriately identified. A modest walking program with incremental exercise up to 20 to 30 minutes three to four times per week as per guidelines from the American College of Sports Medicine is ideal. Elderly and previously sedentary patients with or without underlying diabetes mellitus should take several months to build up this training base.

There are no contraindications to exercise for patients with NIDDM even when complicated by angina pectoris or peripheral vascular disease. Prophylactic treatment with nitrates before exercise and testing of the threshold to claudication will help maintain fitness and increase function with preservation of overall health. The hazards of overexertion and dehydration should be avoided at all times.

Patients with insulin-dependent diabetes mellitus (IDDM) can also undertake aerobic exercise when coupled with proper nutrition and adjustment of insulin dosage. Insulin-dependent or type 1 diabetics should reduce their insulin dosage prior to any prolonged exercise even at modest intensities. For activities lasting more than 60 to 90 minutes, insulin doses should be reduced by one third. In this way, the insulin-dependent diabetic can benefit from fitness without running the risk of hypoglycemic reactions.[17]

Exercise Benefits in Non–Insulin-Dependent Diabetes Mellitus

The predominant form of diabetes in the elderly is the non–insulin-dependent type, which is principally treated through the modalities of diet and exercise. Both the Consensus Development Conference for the National Institutes of Health and the U.S. Preventive Services Task Force recognize and endorse exercise as a key intervention in this condition.[18]

The acute effects of physical activity on glucose metabolism have been well studied. Physical activity leads to an increase in insulin sensitivity with an improved glucose clearance from the circulation. Several studies have looked at the role of physical activity in delaying or preventing the onset of NIDDM, which may be an independent risk factor for death from cardiovascular and cerebral vascular disease. Results from the U.S. Preventive Services Task Force Study suggest that physical activity may have a positive effect on improvements in glucose tolerance and subsequent long-term complications. The evidence is, however, less convincing than that for CHD.[4,18]

OBESITY AND WEIGHT CONTROL

Obesity is a risk associated with advancing age that is connected to but independent from the risk for development of diabetes mellitus.[3] Obesity also carries an increased risk for development of hypertension and cardiac conditions in the elderly, including congestive heart failure. Recent estimates indicate that 34 million Americans are obese, meaning that they are 20% or more over their ideal range of body weight for age and sex.

Recent research suggests that obesity hinges as much on a decrease in basal energy expenditure as it does on an increase in caloric intake.[19] Accordingly, exercise or an increase in regular physical activity should be a key therapeutic component for gradual weight reduction in addition to sound nutritional counseling. A companion study from the National Institutes of Health points out that low energy expenditure is a major contributor to obesity in middle-aged and older adults.[17] Individuals with low activity profiles downregulate their metabolic rates, with reduced caloric expenditure and increased storage of nutrients in fat depots. The low metabolic rate, in turn, predisposes to decreased physical activity and conspires to the development of progressive weight increase. An increase in physical activity can serve to raise the lowered metabolic rate, with an increased caloric expenditure and relative enhancement of lean body mass. In this manner, regular exercise coupled with balanced nutrition can promote normalized weight, provide a safe and effective treatment for obesity, and materially reduce the risk for developing diabetes mellitus. This, in turn, reduces risk for cardiorespiratory and circulatory conditions.

Cholesterol was the central medical focus for intervention in cardiovascular risk in the 1980s. Epidemiologic data indicate that up to 24 million Americans aged 60 years and older are candidates for treatment of high blood cholesterol by current standards.[20] Exercise has a direct and substantial impact on improvement in the lipoprotein profile with elevations of high-density cholesterol and improvement in the risk factor ratio. The National Cholesterol Education Program (NCEP) has stressed the importance of lowering serum cholesterol as an intervention in treatment for all segments of the population, including the elderly.[21]

THE MUSCULOSKELETAL SYSTEM

Traditional knowledge on aging states that muscles atrophy and weaken with age, perhaps by a 10% functional decline per decade after age 65. Recent research on exercise and aging shows, however, that the musculoskeletal system still responds to physical conditioning if disease does not limit exercise participation.[19] The decline in total muscle mass is accompanied by replacement of muscle with adipose tissue, which leads to a change in metabolic parameters. The change in muscle mass may be a key to several of the other so-called age-related changes from bone density, to obesity, and to changes in glucose tolerance. A loss in muscle mass reduces the basal metabolic rate, which affects daily caloric requirements. The ability to do aerobic activity is directly related to and affected by muscle mass, and perhaps equally the health of an individual's cardiovascular system. Even with a sound cardiovascular system, the elderly individual must maintain muscle mass through

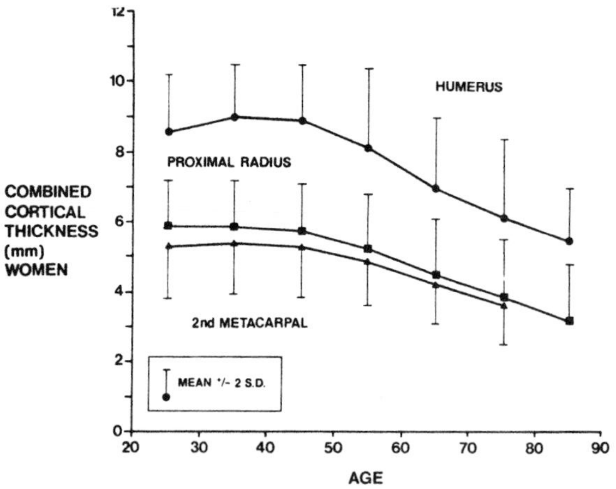

Figure 34–6. Changes with age in combined cortical thickness in three long bones in women.

regular aerobic exercise to support and balance caloric intake. Progressive loss of muscle tissue may be less age-related than behavioral or environmental in origin. Current evidence indicates that regular aerobic activity and even strength training can maintain lean body mass, which is a marker for continued physical activity and a higher metabolic rate. For these reasons, regular physical activity plays as important a role in combatting obesity as does dietary restriction.[4,19]

The impact on bone mass is equally important and impressive. Bone mass declines progressively after age 40, with accelerated losses after age 65, especially losses related to inactivity. This loss can be slowed by exercise and estrogen replacement in postmenopausal women, but it cannot be entirely reversed. Age-induced losses in bone density predispose to fracture from minor trauma, which further impairs exercise capacity and produces the downhill spiral leading to inactivity and increased morbidity from various causes (Fig. 34–6).

Bones, Joints, and Muscles

The influence of aging and the potential benefits of exercise conditioning are perhaps most dramatically demonstrated in the musculoskeletal system, particularly with skeletal muscle. Rather than being consigned to a progressive atrophy with advancing years, skeletal muscle tissue responds to training with functional and biochemical responses to maintain strength and performance.[22]

The training effect on skeletal muscle, including improvements in aerobic capacity as well as isotonic and strength functions with isometric stresses, continues into later years. Athletic performance can also be maintained with training as demonstrated by the evidence on age-specific track performances, which shows modest and moderate declines with advancing age (see Figs. 34–4 and 34–5). Fitness depends on consistency of a training stimulus over time but also on rest and recovery. Evidence both in animal models and in human subjects suggests greater risk for overuse injuries from overtraining with advancing years as a manifestation of an increased requirement for rest as part of the recovery process.[22] While aging reduces skeletal muscle performance and changes selected biochemical measures, exercise conditioning can partially offset these declines. Soft tissue sports-induced injuries result from overtraining, the risk of which may indeed increase with age. Long-term high-intensity exercise, such as high-mileage distance running, can lead to chronicity of overuse injuries with development of functional impairment. Once structural injury to a joint such as the hip has occurred, chronic changes of osteoarthritis may develop superimposed on such injury by a chronic overuse stress.[23] One recent study confirms that osteoarthritis of large weight-bearing joints occurs with some frequency in sports-active runners with advancing age.[24] Evidence continues to indicate, however, that such changes are due to consequences of specific injuries rather than to an overloading effect alone. The protective effects of regular exercise on bone density and its role in prevention of osteoporosis continue to argue strongly for the beneficial effects of regular low-intensity exercise.

Osteoporosis

Osteoporosis is a major health problem which cannot be cured but can be prevented. It is the medical problem par excellence to exemplify the impact of aging and inactivity, with an estimated 1.2 million fractures per year occurring in the United States among the elderly as a consequence of osteoporosis.[25] This serious cause of medical morbidity, especially in older women, can be reduced—if not averted—by adequate estrogen, calcium intake, and appropriate exercise during pre-, peri-, and post-menopausal years. These factors may attenuate the progressive bone loss shown in Figure 34–6.

An exercise program can provide the mechanical stress necessary to stimulate bone remodeling and to maintain bone density. Similar to considerations with regard to cardiovascular risks and benefits, the type and amount of exercise may need to be tailored to an individual's capacity for overall sports participation. Light-to-moderate exercise improves bone density in older women. The consensus report from the National Institutes of Health endorses exercise but stresses the concomitant need for estrogen replacement in the absence of contraindications.[26] Regular low-intensity exercise is the prescription of choice for the elderly to assist in maintaining flexibility, strength, and strong bones. Osteoporosis is a devastating condition for which there is no cure, but active prevention is possible through balanced nutrition, regular exercise, and hormonal therapy (when appropriate).

IMMUNITY AND INFECTION

The effects of aging on the immune system have been a subject of intensive recent research. Most cell-mediated and humoral immune responses decline progressively with advancing age.[27] This includes the T-cell compartment, notably the CD4 subset, which includes helper cells guided by T-cell genetic controls. Advancing age brings with it a decline in immune competence, which can perhaps be mitigated by nonspecific immune stimulation from regular physical activity. The neurochemical and neurohumoral signals activated by exercise may serve to maintain immune competence along a higher profile of readiness. Factors which may account for such benefits are discussed in further detail elsewhere in this volume.

MENTAL HEALTH

Once again, the U.S. Preventive Services Task Force has provided a recent update on studies relating exercise levels, fitness, and mental health parameters.[3] In general, a positive association exists between physical activity and improved affect (mood, depression scale, and anxiety). Exercise participation translates into a more positive self-image as reflected in measures of self-esteem. Exercise certainly plays a major role in stress reduction, which leads to self-reported lower levels of anxiety and more productive or creative thinking. A positive impact of exercise on cognition, however, remains to be established. Physical activity does promote a more positive sense of self, improved coping skills, and reduced anxiety levels.

Additional research will address the relationship between endogenous opioid peptides (EOPs) and psychological parameters. Exercise increases the endorphin response, which has been related to exercise-induced euphoria and the "runner's high." It is as yet unclear whether acute or chronic changes in peripheral levels of EOPs are associated with positive psychological responses.

SPORTS, SEXUALITY, AND AGING

Much research is currently devoted to exploring the relationship between exercise and sexuality, and even fertility.[28] The acute effects of strenuous exercise include elevated levels of testosterone in both men and women although levels may be suppressed with chronic exercise, especially with overtraining states.[29] Participants in various sports, such as running and cycling, continue to report a positive impact on sexual interest and performance from their sports participation.[30] Respondents to surveys in a running magazine showed that roughly 70% felt more sexually attractive and capable because of their sports participation. A recent similar survey (September 1989) reported a crossover between sports participation and a sense of sexual vitality.[31] Relationships between sports participation and sexual performance are unexplored, but they may be related on some level to the release of endorphins as discussed earlier. Athletes report no adverse effects of sexual activity prior to athletic competition.[32]

Surveys of sexual dysfunction in older men show a predominance of neuropathic and vascular causes.[33] As both circulatory and endocrine-metabolic function may be positively affected by exercise, there may be a benefit of delaying or reducing sexual dysfunction through exercise. The positive psychological connection would presumably neutralize the component of reversible impotence due to psychogenic causes.[34] The active life-style promotes a feeling of being more sexual and may be the key to "sex after sixty."[35]

CONCLUSION

The evidence is mounting that exercise has a measurable positive impact on life expectancy with a decrease in cardiovascular disease–specific and all-cause mortality. Perhaps of greater significance is increasing evidence that physical fitness through regular low-intensity exercise can reduce or postpone morbidity from several major medical conditions, such as coronary heart disease, hypertension, non–insulin-dependent diabetes mellitus, osteoporosis, obesity, and mental health problems. Based on this evidence, specific recommendations for regular low-intensity physical exercise should be a foundation and cornerstone of health care in the elderly. Exercise adds to both the quality and the quantity of life. Guidelines for "aging well" are available and should be recommended.[36]

REFERENCES

1. Robinson BE: The changing scope of prevention in late life. Clin Rep Aging 2:1–21, 1988.
2. Roessing W: Anything but retiring. USAIR 11:66–71, 1989.
3. Harris S, Caspersen C, DeFriesce G, et al: Physical activity counseling for healthy adults as a primary preventive intervention in the clinical setting. JAMA 261:3590–3598, 1989.
4. Blair S, Kohl H, Paffenbarger R, et al: Physical fitness and all-cause mortality. JAMA 262:2395–2401, 1989.

5. Fries JF: Aging, natural death, and the compression of morbidity. N Engl J Med 303:130–134, 1980.
6. Slattery ML, Jacobs DR, Nichaman MZ: Leisure time physical activity and coronary heart disease death: The US railroad study. Circulation 79:304–311, 1989.
7. Paffenbarger R, Hyde R, Wing A, et al: Natural history of athleticism and cardiovascular health. JAMA 252:491–495, 1984.
8. Ryan AJ: Senior athletes. Senior Patient July/August:56–61, 1989.
9. Paffenbarger R, Hale W: Work activity in coronary heart mortality. N Engl J Med 292:547–552, 1975.
10. Morris JN, Chave SPW, Adam C, et al: Vigorous exercise in leisure time and the incidence of coronary heart disease. Lancet 1:333–337, 1973.
11. Paffenbarger R, Hyde R, Wing A, et al: Physical activity, all-cause mortality, and longevity of college alumni. N Engl J Med 314:605–613, 1986.
12. Tanji JL: CHD classification helps assess capacity for exercise in the elderly. Intern Med News November 1–14:36–37, 1989.
13. Stratton JR: Exercise pumps up tPA. Med Tribune December 14:6, 1989.
14. Knudson RJ: How aging affects the normal adult lung. J Respir Dis 2:74–78, 1981.
15. Braun SR, Fregosi R, Reddan WG: Exercise training in patients with COPD. Postgrad Med 71:163–167, 1982.
16. Stratton BF: Pulmonary rehabilitation: For the breath of your life. J Cardiopulmonary Rehabil 9:80–86, 1989.
17. Siegel AJ: Exercise and diabetes mellitus: Benefits and risks. Your Patient & Fitness 2:6–11, 1988.
18. National Institutes of Health: Consensus Development Conference on Diet and Exercise in Non–Insulin-Dependent Diabetes Mellitus. Diabetes Care 10:639–644, 1987.
19. Siegel AJ: New insights about obesity and exercise. Your Patient & Fitness 2:6–11, 1988.
20. Sempos C, Fulwood R, Haines C, et al: The prevalence of high blood cholesterol levels among adults in the United States. JAMA 262:45–52, 1989.
21. Palumbo PJ: Cholesterol lowering for all: A closer look. JAMA 262:91–92, 1989.
22. Butler DL, Siegel AJ: Alterations in tissue response: Conditioning effects at different ages. NIH monograph, in press.
23. Eichner ER, Pascale M, Grana W: Does running cause osteoarthritis? An epidemiologic perspective: An orthopedic perspective. Physician Sportsmed 17:147–166, 1989.
24. Marti B: Distance running and osteoarthritis. Br Med J 299:91–93, 1989.
25. Notelovitz M: Exercise and osteoporosis. Your Patient & Fitness 1:10–16, 1987.
26. National Institutes of Health Consensus Conference: Osteoporosis. JAMA 252:799–802, 1984.
27. Weigle W: Effects of aging on the immune system. Hosp Pract 24:112–119, 1989.
28. Schinfeld JS: Effects of athletics on male reproduction and sexuality. Med Aspects Hum Sexuality February:119–126, 1989.
29. Wheeler GD, Wall SR, Belcastro AN, et al: Reduced serum testosterone and prolactin levels in male distance runners. JAMA 252:514–516, 1984.
30. Special survey: Running and sex. Runner 4:26, 1982.
31. Survey. Bicycling September:26–32, 1989.
32. Sztajzel J: Having sex before athletics doesn't appear to hurt performance. Intern Med News December 1–14:1–16, 1989.
33. Mulligan T, Katz G: Why aged men become impotent. Arch Intern Med 149:1365–1366, 1989.
34. Thienhaus OJ: Practical overview of sexual function and advancing age. Geriatrics 43:63–67, 1988.
35. Curtis LR: Sex after sixty. Senior Patient Jan/Feb:38–43, 1989.
36. Fries JF: Aging Well. Reading, MA, Addison-Wesley, 1989.

35

SPORTS AND RECREATION FOR THE PHYSICALLY DISABLED

Roy J. Shephard, MD, PhD, DPE, FACSM, FFIMS
Glen M. Davis, PhD, FACSM

HISTORICAL DEVELOPMENT OF SPORTS FOR THE DISABLED

Sports for the disabled were initially conceived in the context of mental disability, and as far back as 1908, the Playground Association of America had set "play in institutions" as one of its major objectives.[1] The idea that sports might be played from wheelchairs was first promoted by Stafford[2] in the context of corrective physical education, but such programs became increasingly popular during World War II as a means of providing both exercise and encouragement to injured service personnel. Independent initiatives were begun at Veterans Administration hospitals in the United States, at British Army hospitals in Egypt, and at the Stoke Mandeville Hospital near Aylesbury, in England. A World Games for the Deaf was also organized in 1924. More recently, sports for the disabled have spread to encompass amputees, the blind, those affected by cerebral palsy, and "les autres" (includes individuals with a broad range of locomotor disabilities, such as muscular dystrophy, multiple sclerosis, Friedreich's ataxia, arthrogryposis, and osteogenesis imperfecta).

Rehabilitation specialists continue to view adapted sports as a form of therapy, avoiding the complications of a very inactive lifestyle, encouraging a return to gainful occupations, and challenging the disabled not to regard physical obstacles as inevitable limitations.[3–5] However, others (including many of the disabled) have seen the potential of adapted sports as ranging from healthy recreation to the pursuit of excellence, culminating in international competition.[6–8]

Much of both public attention and research study has to date focused upon the wheelchair competitor, although there is now increasing recognition of the need to extend such interest to those with other forms of disability. Sir Ludwig Guttmann of Stoke Mandeville Hospital was a dominant figure in the early development of sports for the spinally injured. He organized the first wheelchair games at Stoke Mandeville in 1948, with 14 male and 2 female participants.[9] Four years later, the International Stoke Mandeville Games Federation (ISMGF) was founded. More than 50 national organizations were soon affiliated, and the growth in participation was such that by 1960 it became necessary to use the Olympic facilities in Rome. Four years later, the Olympic site in Tokyo was again the venue for the paraolympiads, but in 1968, the potential problems of high altitude and lack of support from the Mexican government caused a displacement of the wheelchair games to Tel Aviv. Subsequent international competitions for the disabled have been held on a quadrennial basis with meets in Heidelberg (1972), Toronto (1976), and Arnhem (1980). Blind and amputee athletes were allowed to participate in the Toronto games, which attracted competitors from 38 countries and more than 100,000 paying spectators.[6] Those with cerebral palsy were also admitted to the Arnhem games. In 1984, the ISMGF met at Stoke Mandeville, with about 1000 competitors, while about 3000 adherents to other groups, such as the International Sports Organization for the Disabled (ISOD) met in New York. The various factions of the adapted sports community were reunited in Seoul (1988) at the International Games for the Disabled (IGD). In recent years, the quadrennial international competitions have been supplemented by national contests for the various categories of disability. Regional competitions, such as the Pan-American Paraplegic Games, the Commonwealth Paraplegic Games, the European Games, and the Far East and South Pacific Games, have also attracted ever-growing numbers of enthusiastic participants.

The events comprising typical summer games for the disabled have now become extremely varied. Track events include wheelchair races over distances of 40 to 1500 m. In the Toronto paraolympiad of 1976, six athletes with spinal lesions covered the 1500-m distance in less than 4 minutes, and in the U.S. national wheelchair marathon, the current time of under 2 hours for the 42.2-km distance is substantially better than that achieved by able-bodied runners. Throwing activities for the wheelchair competitor include discus, shot put, and javelin. Athletes with amputations, blindness, or cerebral palsy also compete in jumping events (high, long, and triple jumps). Swimming contests are extremely popular with all categories of the disabled, and other individual sports include archery, bowling, fencing, rifle shooting, snooker (a form of billiards), table tennis, and weight lifting. Team events include wheelchair basketball, wheelchair and standing volleyball (for amputees), wheelchair soccer (for the cerebral palsied), and many adapted team games, such as "goalball" for the blind.

Winter games for the deaf were inaugurated in Austria in 1949. Germany and Austria also showed an early interest in skiing competitions for amputees, commonly using a single regular ski and two small outrigger skis for downhill events. The spread of competition to the United States was hastened by the need to rehabilitate those with casualties sustained in the Vietnam War.[10] By 1984–85, some 1000 racers were attempting to qualify for national competitions. Downhill skiing events are also enjoyed by blind athletes (using a guide), and paraplegics (sitting in a sled or "pulk"). Ice hockey is also played by paraplegics, using small sleds.

Many active recreational pursuits have been adapted to accommodate the special needs of the disabled. Cycling, hill walking, horseback riding, rowing, and waterskiing have all been organized for the blind, while the lower-limb disabled have enjoyed gliding, sailing, and recreational swimming. Adventure sports, such as rock climbing, parachute jumping (over water), and wilderness canoeing, have appealed to special segments of the disabled population,[11,12] whereas others with more modest ambitions have been happy to enjoy five-pin bowling or table tennis as their sources of active recreation.

MEDICAL PROBLEMS ASSOCIATED WITH SPORTS FOR THE DISABLED

In general, the medical problems associated with competitions for the disabled are no greater than those encountered during competitions for the able-bodied, in either summer[13] or winter events.[14] There is a low overall injury rate owing to the absence of contact sports, and the main efforts of medical staff are directed to the treatment of such general conditions as sunburn, dehydration, gastroenteritis, and sprains rather than specific lesions related to the disability.[6,15] Fractures are occasionally sustained in paralyzed lower limbs, but given the absence of innervation, the inconvenience is often less than for an able-bodied athlete. Instability of the atlanto-occipital joint is a specific concern in individuals with Down's syndrome, the blind must be protected from collisions, and some with neurologic disorders must be guarded from both seizures and the side effects of corrective medication. In wheelchair competitors, abrasions and lacerations may arise from hand contact with the brake, armrest, or push rim, and from trapping of the hand between two competing wheelchairs; overuse of hand movements during distance events may give rise to a carpal tunnel syndrome; and, in hot weather, pressure sores may develop on the buttocks and back. Amputees may also develop pressure sores in limb stumps. Finally, lack of active muscle and, in some cases, defects of autonomic regulation increase the vulnerability of the disabled to both heat and cold stress.

CLASSIFICATION OF DISABILITY

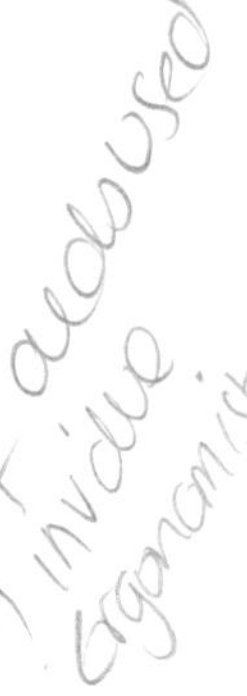

Conferences on adapted sports have spent much time attempting to devise methods that would assure fair competition between individuals variable in the extent of their disability.[15–17] The original approach was to allow competitors individual handicaps, but more recently, emphasis has turned to methods of classifying disability, both for individuals and for teams whose individual players have various amounts of disability. Total fairness remains an elusive goal, given the wide variety of clinical problems, and any exhaustive attempt at categorization is quickly defeated by the resultant lack of an adequate number of entrants in a given category.

Current schemes for the various types of physical disability are discussed in more detail by Shephard.[15] There are three classes of blind athletes: class I ranges from zero light perception to an inability to recognize objects or contours; class II ranges from object recognition to a visual acuity of 2/60, or a visual field having an arc of less than 5 deg; and class III covers a visual acuity of 2/60 to 6/60, or a visual arc of 5 to 60 deg.

Amputee sports recognizes various combinations of upper and lower limb loss; the most modern schema has nine categories of limb disablement for individual summer competitors, and three or four categories for team members. In winter sports, contestants are classified according to the number of skis and outriggers that are used.

Neurologic disorders may be classified on an anatomic, functional, or dynamic basis:

1. An *anatomic classification* is based upon the location and nature of the spinal cord lesion, as determined by observations on trunk balance and muscle strength. This method has serious limitations when comparing individuals with lesions of differing etiology. For example, it fails to consider the differing extent of sensory impairment when muscle paralysis is due to congenital lesions, trauma, or diseases, such as anterior poliomyelitis.[17] Such a schema also makes minimal allowance for incomplete lesions, and for individuals who have regained partial control of posture and other functions by learning to use accessory muscles.

2. A *functional classification* is currently the most popular. It considers the quality and quantity of active muscle mass, supplemented where necessary by strength measurements and the testing of sport-specific tasks (Fig. 35–1). A certified examiner watches trunk control skills, such as picking up a ball from the floor, muscle strength is rated on a six-point scale, and the extent of sensory loss is noted. Discussion of this schema has centered on the optimum qualifications for those making the classification of disability, and the occasional attempts of athletes to simulate problems in order to be assigned to an advantageous disability category.

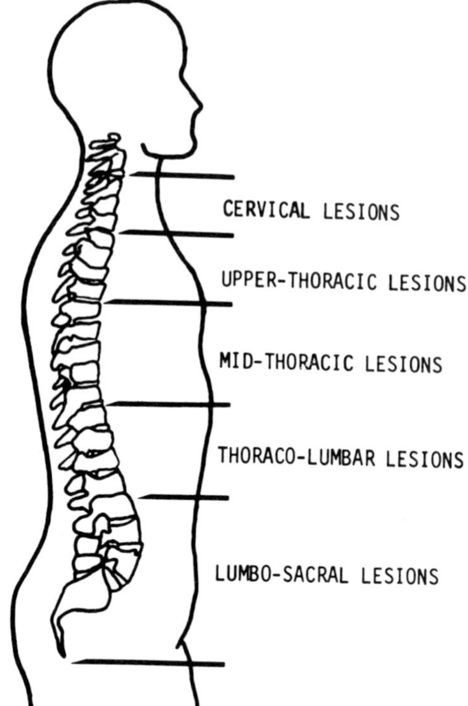

Figure 35–1. Functional classification for wheelchair sport. (*Adapted from* Northeast Wheelchair Athletic Association: Program of the Wheelchair Games, 1980; with permission.)

3. A *dynamic classification* is based on the extent of habitual activity reported by the individual. It has the attraction that it reflects the total consequences of disability, including pyschosocial sequelae; note can be taken of voluntary sports involvement, employment, and daily activity patterns.

Cerebral palsy is perhaps the most difficult of lesions to classify. Eight tests examine the function of the arms and torso, and four additional tests evaluate leg function and stability. Note is taken of response time, speed, coordination, accuracy of movement, and range of motion. Eight basic categories of disability are recognized, the first four of these requiring a wheelchair for both sports and daily activities.

PSYCHOSOCIAL BENEFITS OF SPORTS FOR THE DISABLED

Although few investigators would deny the merits of moderate physical exercise for most categories of the disabled, debate continues on the merits of exposing such individuals to international competition.[15] Some still maintain that given the psychological trauma of the disability itself, it is unfair to expose such groups to the standard type of athletic competition, with the possibility of a further defeat. Rather, any participant should compete only against personal performance, as assessed by a stopwatch or a tape measure. Others argue that the disabled have the normal human desire to move faster or to throw further than their peers, and that this desire is best satisfied by a normal type of competition, albeit appropriately handicapped.

Public competition offers an opportunity for closer integration with society, allowing the spectators fresh insights into both the problems and the potential of the disabled.

Achievements, such as the completion of a marathon competition in under 2 hours, should convince "normal" society that "sickness and disability are not synonymous."[6]

There remains some danger that the usual type of adapted contest can in itself become a kind of ghetto for participants, officials, and spectators; for this reason, there are advocates of full integration of the disabled in all spheres of life, including athletic competition. Sports should serve to promote social integration, offering an opportunity for the disabled person to reenter the mainstream of society. Thus, it is important that all areas of sports and recreational facilities (including the "athletes' village" of major competitive sites) be fully accessible to the disabled.

Studies of psychosocial influences must consider the direct impact of disability upon the individual and (unless the lesion is of congenital origin) the interaction of this major life event with premorbid personality, attitudes, and beliefs.[18–20] There is much stigmatization and stereotyping of the disabled by society, educators, and even those with other categories of disability.[15,21] A poor self-image may encourage the disabled to engage in various adverse forms of life-style, such as the abuse of alcohol and drugs, and relative to the able-bodied, any involvement in sports may rely more upon the provision of external rewards, such as praise from a coach or teacher.[15] Processes of socialization into and by sports also differ between the disabled and able-bodied populations.[15,22] The usual reason for sports involvement of the disabled is the encouragement of a teacher rather than parental involvement; likewise, educational and athletic aspirations account for much of the socializing effects of participation.

Several studies of disabled populations have documented an association between neuromuscular handicap and an abnormal psychological state.[23–28] There are commonly a low ego strength, a poor body image and a reactive depression, with perception of being controlled by circumstances (an "external locus of control").[15] Davis and colleagues[29] observed significant relationships between the level of spinal transection and (1) 5 of 16 variables on Cattell's 16 PF test of personality characteristics, (2) 5 of 7 elements on Kenyon's attitudes towards physical activity questionnaire, and (3) the score for "locus of control." Paraplegics as a whole differ significantly from the general population, but given that such lesions usually have an acute onset, it remains unclear whether such differences antedated the paraplegia and/or contributed to the spinal injury. Spinally disabled athletes are more venturesome and tough-minded than their inactive peers, while the gap between the actual and the desired body image is also smaller for athletes than for inactive individuals.[30] The profile of mood states shows high levels of anger in many wheelchair competitors, while the state of anxiety is also high in some categories of blind athletes at the time of competition.[31] One measure of overall adaptation to disability is employment status. Some recent surveys have suggested that unemployment rates are as high as 50% among disabled populations. The working ability is known only for those who find employment. Nakamura[32] observed that, at one Japanese industrial center, spinally traumatized sports participants had a 2% lower rate of job absenteeism and a 22% greater monthly wage than sedentary disabled workers, suggesting the possibility that sports participation contributed to a successful work history.

The ability to undertake a physical training program also seems to be enhanced by a favorable initial psychological profile.[23] It is logical to anticipate, in turn, that training-induced improvements in physical working capacity would have a beneficial influence upon a number of the psychological disturbances noted above, particularly a poor body image.[33] Relative to able-bodied controls, Ankebrand[34] demonstrated improvements of self-concept and self-acceptance when a group of disabled individuals participated in an 8-week recreational bowling program. Dalton[35] and Goldberg and Shephard[30] offered further suggestive evidence of psychological benefit from training, but conclusive proof is as yet lacking. Moreover, even if we can soon demonstrate benefit, there is still a need to weigh carefully the relative effectiveness of programs that focus upon sports participation, fitness development, and recreation. Likewise, there is need to examine the value of integrated programs relative to those that are specially adapted to a particular type of disability.

PHYSIOLOGIC BENEFITS OF EXERCISE

Methods of Fitness Assessment

In the disabled, as in the able-bodied, an enormous variety of field[36] and laboratory methods[15] have been proposed to measure cardiovascular and muscular fitness. However, the proponents of such methodologies have not always acknowledged the problem of substantial intra-individual variation in test scores, owing to both limitations of the procedures and variations in the individual's condition from day to day. The magnitude of intra-individual variation is such that testing can provide only a very crude indication of a person's physiologic status. On the other hand, grouped results can be helpful in comparing the effectiveness of various training plans, and in assessing such issues as the relationship between physical fitness and a successful return to gainful employment (Noreau and Shephard, 1990).

Cardiorespiratory Performance

During field testing, the hearing impaired and the blind can undertake a 12-minute run of the Cooper type.[37] The assumption is made that everyone runs with comparable mechanical efficiency, although in practice both the deaf and the blind may run less efficiently than the able-bodied. An analogous 12-minute wheelchair run has been described[38] for paraplegics, but the results any given individual achieves for this test are plainly influenced to a great extent by ground conditions, wheelchair design, and experience in making an all-out effort for a 12-minute period. Lesion level may also affect the mechanical efficiency of propulsion and thus the energy cost of covering unit distance. Predictions of maximal oxygen intake can be made from heart rate readings and power output during operation of a portable forearm cranking device, using the Astrand nomogram.[39] Again, mechanical efficiency may vary with the characteristics of the disability; but, in general, the error of predictions relative to direct measurements of peak oxygen intake seems much as in the general population. The portable ergometer has been used to develop norms of oxygen transport for a large sample of wheelchair users in the Toronto area (Table 35–1).[40]

Under laboratory conditions, groups such as the blind and the deaf can follow standard protocols for the measurement of maximal oxygen intake,[37,41–44] although more attention needs to be paid to the preliminary explanation of the test (particularly with blind subjects). Motivation to all-out effort may be difficult to ensure in disabled persons who are not accustomed to vigorous effort, and there are some unique issues of test safety to consider. During submaximal exercise, abnormalities of running gait tend to increase the oxygen cost of running for both the blind[45] and individuals with cerebral palsy[15]; there are corresponding increases in heart rate and respiratory minute volume relative to the figures observed in the able-bodied.

Laboratory tools for the measurement of maximal oxygen intake in the wheelchair population have included forearm cranking devices,[46–49] the mounting of a wheelchair on a modified inclined treadmill[50–53] or low-friction rollers,[54–56] and the coupling of a wheelchair to a cycle ergometer[57–59] or purpose-built ergometer system.[60] The main advantage claimed for the wheelchair devices is that they mimic normal wheelchair use fairly closely.

TABLE 35–1. CLASSIFICATION OF PEAK OXYGEN INTAKE FOR SPINALLY INJURED SUBJECTS

	Peak Oxygen Intake (mL·kg^{-1}·min^{-1})		
Fitness Level	***Females***	***Elite Male Athletes***	***General Male Sample***
Poor (−3.0 to −1.8 sd)	<5.4	<17.2	<10.5
Below average (−1.8 to −0.6 sd)	5.4–16.2	17.2–31.5	10.5–21.9
Average (−0.6 to +0.6 sd)	16.3–27.1	31.6–45.9	22.0–33.4
Above average (+0.6 to +1.8 sd)	27.2–38.0	46.0–60.3	33.5–44.9
Excellent (+1.8 to +3.0 sd)	>38.0	>60.3	>44.9

Abbreviation: sd = standard deviation.

Adapted from Kofsky PR, Shephard RJ, Davis GM, et al: Fitness classification tables for lower-limb disabled individuals. *In* Sherrill C (ed): Sport and Disabled Athletes. Champaign, IL, Human Kinetics Publishers, 1986, p 147; with permission.

Empiric data show a low mechanical efficiency during operation of a wheelchair. The precise value depends upon the type of wheelchair that is used, and the individual's prior experience with vigorous wheelchair propulsion[57,58,61,62]; commonly, efficiency increases in curvilinear fashion with power output, from 6.5% at 5 watts (W) to 10.5% at 25 W.[58] It has been speculated that the wheelchair user might realize a much greater mechanical efficiency and, thus, a higher peak power output through a system of levers or gears, the asynchronous application of force to the two wheel rims, or an alteration in the mechanics of "stroking" the rims.[63–68] But to date, wheelchair research has concentrated mainly on the development of lightweight models with a low air resistance, high maneuverability, a low center of gravity, and interchangeable drive wheels.[69–70]

In the context of cardiorespiratory testing, certain models of the forearm cycle ergometer[71–75] have advantages of portability and a moderate unit cost, although applicability of the peak power outputs thus determined to the task of wheelchair propulsion (either in sports or in daily life) is less certain. The mechanical efficiency for a given power output is generally higher for the forearm crank than for the wheelchair, because (1) inherent neural pathways favor asynchronous limb movements,[64] (2) both flexor and extensor muscles can be used for force generation,[76] (3) torque is transmitted by a handle rather than by pressure on the wheel rim,[65] (4) gear ratios are advantageous,[65,77] and (5) less energy is expended in stabilizing the trunk.[78] Partly because of higher mechanical efficiency, the heart rate, stroke volume, systolic blood pressure, respiratory minute volume, respiratory gas exchange ratio, oxygen consumption, ventilatory equivalent, and blood lactate levels are all lower for arm cranking than for a comparable intensity of submaximal wheelchair ergometry.[48,58–60,76,79,80] On the other hand, either form of stress testing is appropriate for eliciting a maximal cardiorespiratory response. Systematic differences of peak oxygen intake between the two test modes amount to less than 5% for male paraplegics, and less than 10% for male tetraplegics and female paraplegics.[48,81,82]

During submaximal ergometry, the "on-transient" (start-up phase) tends to be longer in the wheelchair-confined than in the able-bodied. A longer testing time may thus be required in order to reach a "steady state." One factor contributing to circulatory "hypokinesis" is venous pooling in the lower extremities due to impairment of the "muscle pump" and a disruption of the sympathetic nerve outflow below the level of the lesion.[75,83,84] If a cord transection has been sustained above the level of the second thoracic vertebra, there is a total loss of sympathetic nerve innervation; increases of cardiac output during exercise then depend largely upon a withdrawal of vagal tone and a slow increase of venous return. Normally, rising blood levels of catecholamines make a major contribution to both the increase of heart rate and the increase of myocardial contractility during vigorous exercise. It is thus important to note that in traumatic paraplegics, the loss of impulses from supraspinal centers leads to greatly reduced plasma epinephrine and norepinephrine levels during vigorous exercise.[85–87]

Muscular Performance

A variety of field tests of muscular performance have been proposed for the physically disabled. But as in the able-bodied, the results are very vulnerable to details of test conditions, opportunities for the learning of technique, and influences of body size; unfortunately, many forms of physical disability are associated with abnormalities of both height and body mass.[15]

In principle, laboratory measurements of anaerobic power and capacity of the wheelchair-disabled could be obtained in a manner analogous to that described by Bar-Or and Inbar[88] for leg effort, using an arm ergometer with a suitable scaling of the flywheel loading. Coutts and Stogryn[89] have recently measured anaerobic power and capacity in a small sample of spinally injured subjects; such data would be particularly important in the evaluation of wheelchair basketball players, of whom rapid accelerations are required. Lakomy and colleagues[90] have suggested that the lactate threshold (the percentage of peak oxygen intake developed at a blood lactate level of 4 mmol/L) is a useful test of an individual's ability to operate a wheelchair over a distance event, such as a 5-km race.

A lack of muscular strength and endurance often limit both the performance of strength events and the daily life of the disabled, whether the cause of disability be cerebral palsy, anterior poliomyelitis, a cerebrovascular catastrophe, or traumatic tetraplegia. Individual muscles have traditionally been evaluated using such methods as the lifting of free weights,[91] dynamometric determinations of handgrip force,[35,64] mechanical cable tensiometry,[81,92,93] and electrical strain gauge measurements of isometric force.[94–96] More recently, isokinetic dynamometers have measured the peak torque, average torque, and endurance of movements at the shoulder, elbow, and wrist joints,[97,98] although there is still discussion of such issues as appropriate gravitational correction of data.[99] The main disadvantages of isokinetic measurements are cost and lack of portability of the measuring equipment. Davis and associates[98] found that in wheelchair users, a single measurement of dominant handgrip force was moderately correlated with the overall upper-body isokinetic strength ($r = 0.79$); correlations between the field and the laboratory measurements were only marginally improved[36] by adding to the grip strength score information on isometric shoulder extension force and isometric elbow extension force ($r = 0.82$).

TYPICAL FITNESS STATUS OF THE DISABLED

Most disabled populations show some reduction of fitness relative to the general population. With groups such as the visually impaired and the mentally retarded, the usual cause of a poor fitness score is overprotection by parents rather than any inherent cardiovascular or muscular deficit.[37,43,100–104]

Cardiorespiratory Fitness

Blind students may demonstrate quite a high level of cardiorespiratory fitness while they are attending a special school with an active program of endurance sports. However, a marked regression of their physical condition occurs during the summer months, when there is no one to supervise and to encourage their physical activity. Cumming and associates[102] suggested that in the young deaf, a lack of sensory input encouraged an increase of habitual activity and, thus, a high level of cardiorespiratory fitness; but a reexamination of their data suggests that the hypothesis was based on a low level of fitness in the comparison group, rather than any outstanding performance on the part of deaf students.[44]

Wheelchair users vary widely in their levels of cardiorespiratory fitness. In theory, their peak oxygen transport is limited by a low maximal heart rate,[105,106] a low stroke volume,[75,84,107,108] a small volume of active muscle, and a poor peripheral circulation.[15] In practice, some wheelchair users with high-level lesions are seriously incapacitated with respect to both employment and the activities of daily living (Noreau and Shephard, 1990); others are able to develop a peak oxygen intake that compares favorably with the scores for moderately trained able-bodied athletes (Fig. 35–2, Table 35–1).[47,52,55,108–110] Lundberg[56] noted that the peak oxygen intake of some disabled Swedish basketball players approached 47 $mL \cdot kg^{-1} \cdot min^{-1}$ and that peak serum lactate concentrations averaged 15.5 mmol/L; in contrast, able-bodied subjects who used the same wheelchair ergometer were only able to develop values of 44 $mL \cdot kg^{-1} \cdot min^{-1}$ and 9.7 mmol/L, respectively.

When wheelchair athletes are compared with their inactive peers, one immediate issue is the extent to which the advantage of the active group is attributable to selection rather than training. As will appear below, peak oxygen transport values are much larger for those who compete in track and swimming events than for those who are involved in "strength" competitions. Nevertheless, a relatively short period of training is enough to carry the inactive individual more than halfway toward the values observed in endurance athletes (Davis, Plyley, and Shephard, in press). Another issue is the impact of lesion level upon aerobic performance. In general, quadriplegics have poorer function than paraplegics. One study of Olympic-caliber athletes showed a progressive gradation of peak oxygen transport from quadriplegia to minimal paraplegia, in the men from 14.1 $mL \cdot kg^{-1} \cdot min^{-1}$ to 37.8 $mL \cdot kg^{-1} \cdot min^{-1}$ and in the women from 11.7 $mL \cdot kg^{-1} \cdot min^{-1}$ to 32.7 $mL \cdot kg^{-1} \cdot min^{-1}$.[81] Others, also, have reported a substantial effect of ISMGF category upon cardiorespiratory function.[6,32–35] On the other hand, in a more representative sample of the disabled population, Kofsky and co-workers observed little impact of lesion level over the range of ISMGF classes II to V. Possibly, the effect of lesion level becomes manifest only *after* function has been maximized by rigorous training.

The cardiorespiratory fitness of amputees depends on age, the reason for surgery (eg, trauma versus peripheral vascular disease), and the extent of other clinical problems.

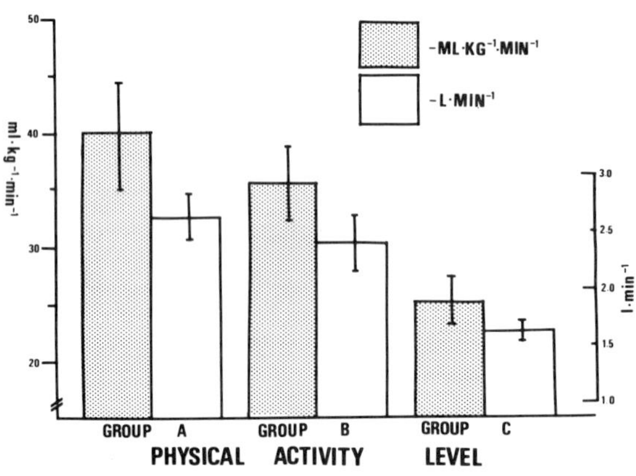

Figure 35–2. Cardiorespiratory fitness of male wheelchair users. Group A: National-caliber athletes (n = 9); Group B: recreational sportsmen (n = 15); Group C: inactive subjects (n = 18).

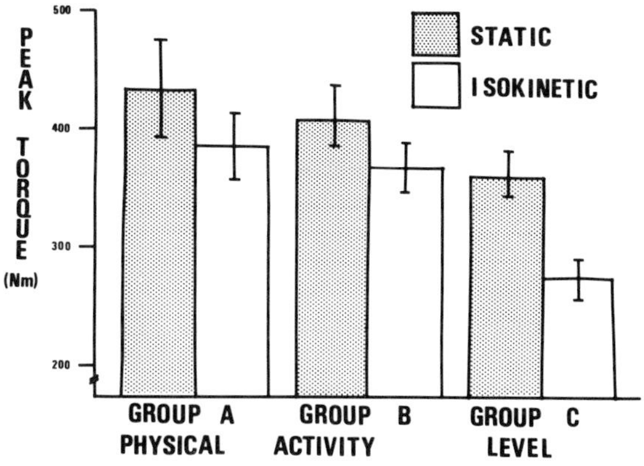

Figure 35–3. Static and isokinetic strength in 42 lower limb–disabled men with varying levels of physical activity. Group A: National-caliber athletes (n = 9); Group B: recreational sportsmen (n = 15); Group C: inactive subjects (n = 18).

Many elderly amputees lack the aerobic power necessary to master the use of a prosthesis.[15,71]

The peak aerobic power is often low in a person with cerebral palsy. Contributing factors here appear to be an increase in cell water and a decrease in lean tissue mass.[113]

Muscle Strength

Muscular strength and endurance differ widely between top athletes and inactive wheelchair-disabled individuals (Fig. 35–3). Cross-sectional studies show a close relationship between strength and activity patterns, without proving which is cause and which is effect. Davis and colleagues[110] demonstrated that the habitual activity of nearly 90% of disabled subjects could be classified correctly on the basis of seven measures of isokinetic strength and endurance (Fig. 35–4). Grimby[109] observed a positive relationship between shoulder abduction torque and deltoid fiber diameter in wheelchair users; the static and dynamic arm strength of participants in wheelchair sports was sometimes 23% to 30% greater than in controls. In confirmation of these observations, Taylor and associates[114,115] reported that the average cross-sectional fiber dimensions of the shoulder muscles in active wheelchair users were two to three times greater than in able-bodied individuals; the hypertrophy apparently affected both type I and type II muscle fibers (perhaps reflecting participation in both strength and endurance events).

Simple field tests of performance suggest that relative to those with normal auditory systems, deaf children have poor static and dynamic equilibrium, motor coordination,

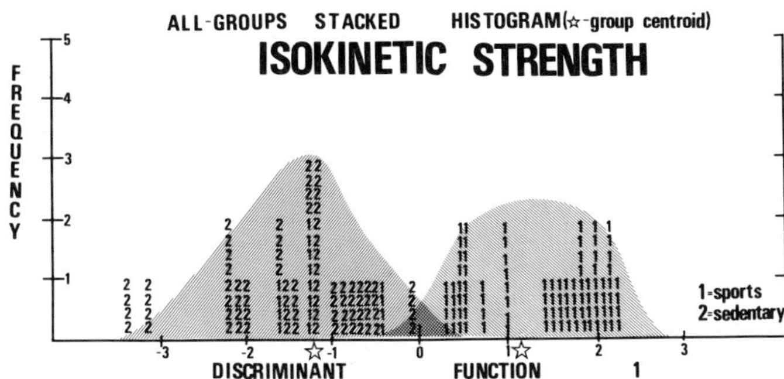

Figure 35–4. Discrimination of habitual activity grouping, based upon seven measures of isokinetic strength. Subjects were 49 male and female wheelchair users, aged 19 to 59 years.

speed, and power.[116,117] Strength is unimpaired, but (perhaps because of vestibular involvement) the muscular endurance may be less than anticipated.[118]

Muscle spasms, athetoid movements, lack of coordination, lack of strength, and impaired fine motor skills may all limit the performance of the person with cerebral palsy.[15] Likewise, muscular dystrophies progressively rob a growing child of strength and endurance.[119] Multiple sclerosis also gives rise to a progressive weakness and a poor tolerance of progressive workouts.

RESPONSE TO TRAINING PROGRAMS

It is now widely accepted that unnecessary restriction of physical activity due to personal or parental fears, segregation, or periods of hospitalization and rehabilitation can all contribute to the low levels of cardiorespiratory fitness, muscle wasting, and accumulations of body fat that are seen in many disabled individuals.[15,50,120–122] Training for appropriately adapted forms of sport thus makes an important contribution to maintenance and even improvement of health in the disabled.

When first seen, many disabled individuals are in poor physical condition, and a substantial training response might be anticipated (Tables 35–1 and 35–2). However, in practice, there are often obstacles to adoption of an effective training program. There may be fear of exercise in general or of specific types of activity, such as pool exercises; technical difficulties, such as poor balance, lack of vision or hearing, and poor comprehension of instructions; activation of a small muscle mass with a corresponding limitation of the cardiovascular stimulus; pooling of blood in regions that are paralyzed or lack sympathetic innervation; and associated disorders, such as ischemic vascular disease, diabetes, or blindness. All of these problems, psychological and physiologic, are compounded by practical barriers, such as lack of transportation, or a limited income for the purchase of clothing and equipment.

The choice of physical activity for a disabled person lies between remedial exercises in a hospital setting, individual supervised training with weights and/or ergometers, and participation in some form of sports or recreation. Considerable self-discipline is needed

TABLE 35–2. UPPER-BODY STRENGTH OF SPINALLY INJURED SUBJECTS*

	Upper-body Strength (N/kg)		
Fitness Level	***Females***	***Elite Male Athletes***	***General Male Sample***
Poor (−3.0 to −1.8 sd)	<1.9	<10.4	<7.1
Below average (−1.8 to −0.6 sd)	1.9–7.5	10.4–16.3	7.1–12.6
Average (−0.6 to +0.6 sd)	7.6–13.3	16.4–22.4	12.7–18.1
Above average (+0.6 to +1.8 sd)	13.4–19.0	22.5–28.4	18.4–23.6
Excellent (+1.8 to +3.0 sd)	>19.0	>28.4	>23.6

*Upper-body strength is expressed in units of newtons per kilogram (N/kg). Values are the mean sum of isometric forces recorded for elbow flexion, elbow extension, and shoulder extension.

Abbreviation: sd = standard deviation.

Adapted from Kofsky PR, Shephard RJ, David GM, et al: Fitness classification tables for lower-limb disabled individuals. *In* Sherrill C (ed): Sport and Disabled Athletes. Champaign, IL, Human Kinetics Publishers, 1986, p 147; with permission.

either to attend a clinic for regular exercise sessions, or to sustain a home exercise program. Thus, there has been great interest in the potential of vigorous sports and recreation as a means of developing strength, coordination, and endurance. Where possible, such conditioning should be pursued on an integrated rather than a segregated basis.[15] Personal training programs may focus upon the cardiovascular or the muscular system.

Each category of disability has its particular program requirements. The cardiorespiratory function of the blind can be developed by adapted running programs using handrails or a sighted guide. Likewise, guide ropes can be fitted to a swimming pool, and visually impaired subjects can also use muscle-building equipment after points of danger have been carefully explained. The difficulty with many sports programs for the blind is that the fitness of the individual shows a rapid regression once the personal guide or the special equipment is no longer available.[37] Programs for the deaf focus particular attention upon activities that are likely to improve balance.[123,124] When training children with cerebral palsy, it is desirable to avoid movements that provoke reflex spasms. If such spasms cannot be avoided, an attempt must be made to build the unwanted movements into the desired sports skill.[1,125] Training in a heated pool may help by encouraging a decrease of muscle tone. A pool is also helpful in providing body support during the training of those individuals with muscular dystrophies.[126] Where aerobic power is limited, it is important to maximize mechanical efficiency and, thus, the use that is made of available physiologic resources. In amputees, much of the emphasis of training is upon improving the mechanical efficiency of movement; Kabsch[127] has argued that the sequence of movements involved in competitive skiing is particularly helpful in this regard.

Cardiovascular Training

For the paraplegic, training in a wheelchair or a wheelchair ergometer (Fig. 35–5) has the merit of specificity relative to both wheelchair sport and everyday ambulation.[128] However, with the exception of a few bursts of anaerobic activity, the heart rate of the wheelchair-confined does not reach the threshold for cardiovascular training during normal ambulation.[76,91,106,109,121] Thus, Kofsky and colleagues[39,40] found no differences in cardiorespiratory condition among mobile, sedentary, and incapacitated wheelchair users. Those who have become accustomed to life in a wheelchair too often tend to avoid strenuous everyday activities,[4,5,129] leading to a vicious circle of decreased cardiorespiratory fitness and further restriction of mobility. The problem is particularly acute in those using motorized wheelchairs. Knutsson and co-workers[130] have commented that many handicapped adults tolerate endurance effort so poorly that it is difficult for them to initiate the prolonged and repeated exercise sessions needed for effective rehabilitation.

Several authors have now made laboratory studies of cardiovascular training responses, particularly in spinally injured subjects. Engel and Hildebrandt[50] noted a decrease of steady-state heart rate for a given submaximal power output when 13 men undertook progressive daily wheelchair ambulation following spinal cord trauma; however, part of the observed response could have been due to routine physiotherapy rather than the prescribed exercise. Ekblöm and Lundberg[131] found significant increases in both mechanical efficiency and physical performance when a group of 24 disabled adolescents with low initial fitness undertook twice-weekly wheelchair training as part of a supplementary physical education program. Glaser and associates[132] recommended interval training as mimicking the normal periodicity of wheelchair propulsion; they were able to increase physical work capacity by almost 30% using such a regimen. Factors modifying the magnitude of the training response include initial fitness,[133–135] age,[41] skill in wheelchair propulsion, obesity, and any "wasted" movements due to spasticity or clonus.[136] Voight and Bahn[51] found that, in individuals with high-level spinal lesions, the limited

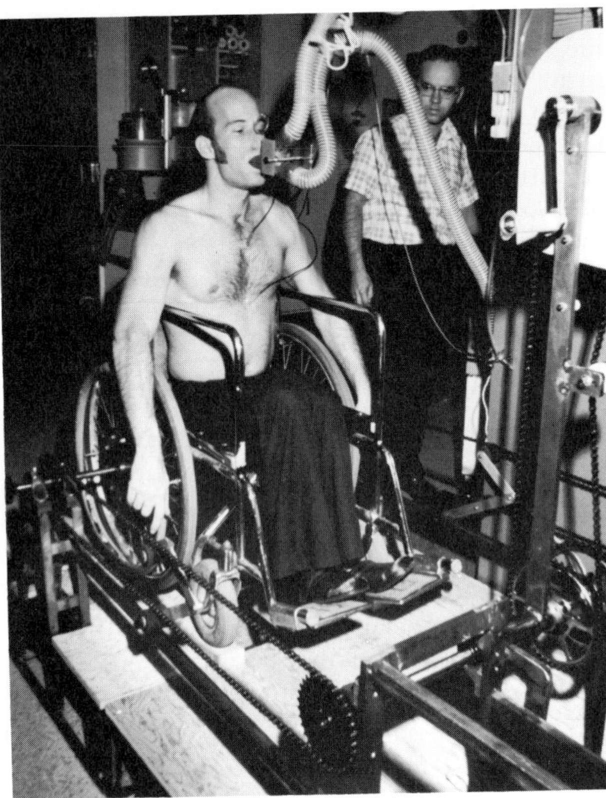

Figure 35–5. One possible design of wheelchair ergometer. (Courtesy of G. R. Ward, PhD, Wollongong, Australia.)

effective muscle mass became fatigued too rapidly to develop a cardiorespiratory training response.

Forearm ergometry (Fig. 35–6) is quite popular in many centers for rehabilitation of the spinally injured because the power output can be monitored precisely, and the device makes an efficient use of space.[49,130,137] Nilsson and colleagues[91] observed a gain in maximum oxygen intake of 12% over 7 weeks of training; Pollock and associates[138] found a 19% response over 20 weeks. The latter authors reported a 37% gain in nondisabled, age-matched controls. They attributed the differential response to (1) a higher intensity of effort in the able-bodied (use of trunk and leg muscles for wheelchair stabilization), (2) a greater habituation of able-bodied subjects who were initially unfamiliar with vigorous arm effort, and (3) a lower peripheral oxygen extraction in the untrained upper-body muscles of the able-bodied.

Davis, Plyley, and Shephard (in press) showed that while training tended to occur faster in those following a regimen with long (40-minute) training bouts at a high intensity of effort (70% of peak oxygen intake), lower-intensity programs (50% of peak oxygen intake) were also able to induce some gains in physical condition over a 24-week period of observation. The response may depend in part upon the usable muscle mass, and some investigators have found only a minimal response to forearm cranking in severely disabled individuals.[138–140]

Muscle Strength Training

The development of arm strength and endurance has considerable practical importance not only for competitions involving speed and power, but also for the daily life of ampu-

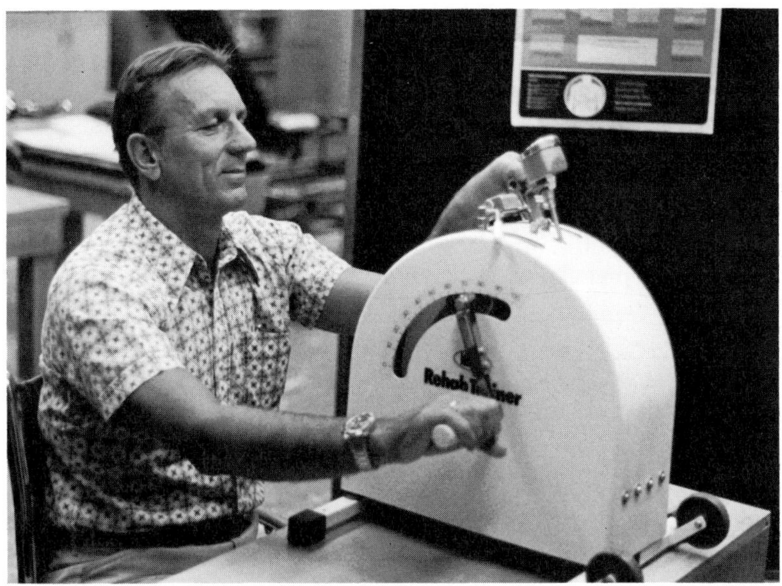

Figure 35–6. A popular type of portable forearm crank ergometer. (Courtesy of M. Durocher, Toronto.)

tees and those confined to wheelchairs. However, there have been relatively few experimental studies of conditioning responses to date.

Cross-sectional comparisons show that relative to their inactive peers, wheelchair athletes have much higher values for both isometric and isokinetic muscle force, this advantage being particularly marked in the muscles used for wheelchair propulsion. However, normal ambulation has little influence upon strength; Gersten and associates[93] could find no difference in triceps function between habitual wheelchair users and recently injured paralytics.

Nilsson and associates[91] noted that upper-arm girth was unchanged following a program of forearm ergometer training, although the dynamic strength and endurance (as assessed by the lifting of free weights) increased by 19% and 80%, respectively. Knutsson and co-workers[130] also observed a 50% increase in forearm physical work capacity when low-level paralyzed patients underwent a 6-week period of weight training and forearm ergometry. Gains were attributed to a strengthening of the active musculature, an increased peripheral oxygen extraction, and an improved cardiorespiratory fitness. Likewise, Davis and Shephard (1990) commented that although their forearm cranking program had been devised primarily to improve cardiorespiratory performance, within 8 weeks there was a 10% to 20% increase of average isokinetic power output at elbow joint velocities of 2.1 to 4.2 radians/sec. Gains of shoulder flexion were also observed, and subjects reported a reduction of fatigue during normal wheelchair ambulation although, as in earlier studies, there was no strong evidence of any increase in muscle dimensions.

In training programs based upon the use of crutches, walking frames, or wheelchairs, there have been less consistent gains of static and isokinetic strength in the arms[141,142]; this probably reflects the specificity of muscular training responses.

Strength training programs have occasionally been applied to those with various forms of muscular dystrophy. Here, the immediate objective is to conserve and maximize function in muscles as yet unaffected by the disorder.[15] As in other types of disability, there is also the more general objective of improving the overall quality of life for the affected individual.

CONCLUSION

The involvement of the disabled in sports is desirable not only for psychosocial reasons, but also because of substantial physiologic dividends which have long-term implications for health and the quality of daily life. A part of the difference between current international competitors and the inactive disabled is admittedly due to competitive selection. Nevertheless, a modest training program can make good as much as a half of the difference of function between the two categories of the disabled. Moreover, with appropriate planning, the medical problems associated with contests for the disabled are no greater than those encountered in competitions for the able-bodied. Physicians should thus actively encourage disabled patients to participate in sports and active recreation.

REFERENCES

1. Sherrill C: Adapted Physical Education and Recreation. Dubuque, Iowa, WC Brown, 1986.
2. Stafford G: Sports for Handicapped. New York, Prentice-Hall, 1939.
3. Dendy E: Recreation for disabled people—what do we mean? Physiotherapy 64:290, 1978.
4. Weiss M, Beck J: Sport as a part of therapy and rehabilitation of paraplegics. Paraplegia 11:166, 1973.
5. Jochheim KA, Strohkendl H: The value of particular sports of the wheelchair disabled in maintaining health of the paraplegic. Paraplegia 11:173, 1973.
6. Jackson RW, Fredrickson A: Sport for the physically disabled—The 1976 Olympiad (Toronto). Am J Sports Med 7:293, 1979.
7. Guttmann L: Reflection on the 1976 Toronto Olympiad for the physically disabled. Paraplegia 14:225, 1976.
8. Hullemann K-O, List M, Matthes D, et al: Spiroergonometric and telemetric investigations during the XXI International Stoke Mandeville Games, 1972, in Heidelberg. Paraplegia 13:109, 1975.
9. Guttmann L: Development of sport for the disabled. *In* Grüpe O (ed): Sport in the Modern World. Berlin, Springer-Verlag, 1973, p 254.
10. Benedick J: Winter sports NHSRA style. Palaestra 1(3):25, 1985.
11. Croucher N: Sport and disability. *In* Williams JGP, Sperryn PN (eds): Sports Medicine, ed 2. London, Arnold, 1976, pp 523–538.
12. Croucher RJ: Outdoor activities. Physiotherapy 64:294, 1978.
13. Birrer RB: The Special Olympics: An injury overview. Physician Sportsmed 12(4):95, 1984.
14. McCormick DP: Injuries in handicapped Alpine ski racers. Physician Sportsmed 13(12):93, 1985.
15. Shephard RJ: Fitness in Special Populations. Champaign, IL, Human Kinetics Publishers, 1989, pp 1–350.
16. Kessler HH: Disability: Determination and Evaluation. Philadelphia, Lea & Febiger, 1970, pp 1–25.
17. Guttmann L: Textbook of Sport for the Disabled. Oxford, HM & M Publishers, 1976, pp 1–731.
18. Simon JI: Emotional aspects of physical disability. Am J Occup Ther 25:408, 1971.
19. Shontz FC: Psychological adjustment to physical disability: Trend in theories. Arch Phys Med Rehabil 59:251, 1978.
20. Vargo JW: Some psychological effects of physical disability. Am J Occup Ther 32:31, 1978.
21. Sherrill C: Social and psychological dimensions. *In* Sherrill C (ed): Sport and Disabled Athletes. Champaign, IL, Human Kinetics Publishers, 1986, p 21.
22. Sherrill C, Rainbolt W, Montelione T, et al: Sport socialization of blind and cerebral palsied elite athletes. *In* Sherrill C (ed): Sport and Disabled Athletes. Champaign, IL, Human Kinetics Publishers, 1986, p 189.
23. Flynn RJ, Solomone PR: Performance of the MMPI in predicting rehabilitation outcome: A discriminant analysis: Double cross-validation assessment. Rehabil Lit 38:12, 1977.
24. Glick SJ: Emotional problems of 200 cerebral palsied adults. Cerebral Palsy Rev 14:3, 1953.
25. Harper DC: Personality characteristics of physically impaired adolescents. J Clin Psychol 34:97, 1978.
26. Harper DC, Richman LC: Personality profiles of physically impaired adolescents. J Clin Psychol 34:636, 1978.
27. Katz S, Shurks E, Florian V: The relationship between physical disability, social perception and psychological stress. Scand J Rehabil Med 10:109, 1978.
28. Lazar AL, Demos GD, Gaines L, et al: Attitudes of handicapped and non-handicapped university students on three attitude scales. Rehabil Lit 38:49, 1978.
29. Davis GM, Kofsky PR, Shephard RJ, et al: Classification of psychophysiological variables in the lower-limb disabled. Can J Appl Sport Sci 6(4):141, 1981.

30. Goldberg G, Shephard RJ: Personality profiles of disabled individuals in relation to physical activity patterns. J Sports Med Phys Fitness 22:477, 1982.
31. Mastro J, French R: Sport anxiety and blind athletes. *In* Sherrill C (ed): Sport and Disabled Athletes. Champaign, IL, Human Kinetics Publishers, 1986, p 203.
32. Nakamura Y: Working ability of the paraplegics. Paraplegia 11:182, 1973.
33. Roberts K: Sports for the disabled. Physiotherapy 60:271, 1974.
34. Ankebrand RJ: An investigation into the relationship between achievement and self-concept of high-risk community college freshmen [PhD thesis]. St. Louis, University of Missouri, Dissertation Abstracts 13(8A):4338, 1972.
35. Dalton RB: Effects of exercise and vitamin B-12 supplementation on the depression scale scores of a wheelchair confined population. University of Missouri, St. Louis, unpublished doctoral dissertation, 1980.
36. American Alliance for Health, Physical Education, and Recreation: Testing for Impaired, Disabled and Handicapped Individuals. Washington, DC, American Alliance for Health, Physical Education, and Recreation, 1975.
37. Lee M, Ward G, Shephard RJ: Physical capacities of sightless adolescents. Dev Med Child Neurol 27:767, 1985.
38. Rhodes EC, MacKenzie DC, Coutts KD, et al: A field test for the prediction of aerobic capacity in male paraplegics and quadriplegics. Can J Appl Sport Sci 6:182, 1981.
39. Kofsky PR, Davis GM, Shephard RJ, et al: Cardio-respiratory fitness in the lower limb disabled. Can J Appl Sport Sci 5(4):1980.
40. Kofsky PR, Shephard RJ, Davis GM, et al: Fitness classification tables for lower-limb disabled individuals. *In* Sherrill C (ed): Sport and Disabled Athletes. Champaign, IL, Human Kinetics Publishers, 1986, p 147.
41. Shephard RJ: Endurance Fitness, ed 2. Toronto, University of Toronto Press, 1977, pp 1–38.
42. Shephard RJ: Human Physiological Work Capacity. London, Cambridge University Press, 1978, pp 1–303.
43. diNatale JM, Lee M, Ward G, et al: Loss of physical condition in sightless adolescents during a summer vacation. Activity Quarterly 2:144, 1985.
44. Hattin H, Fraser M, Ward G, et al: Are deaf children unusually fit? A comparison of fitness between deaf and blind children. Adapt Phys Activ Q 3:268, 1986.
45. Hamill J, Knutzen KM, Bates BT: Ambulatory consistency of the visually impaired. *In* Winter DA, Norman RW, Wells RP, et al (eds): Biomechanics IXA. Champaign, IL, Human Kinetics Publishers, 1985, p 570.
46. Asmussen E, Molbech SV: Methods and standards for evaluation of the physical working capacity of patients. *In* Communication of Testing and Observation Institute, vol 4. Hellerup, Denmark, Danish Infantile Paralysis Association, 1954, pp 1–16.
47. Zwiren L, Bar-Or O: Responses to exercise of paraplegics who differ in conditioning level. Med Sci Sports 7:94, 1975.
48. Wicks J, Lymburner K, Dinsdale S, et al: The use of multistage exercise testing with wheelchair ergometry and arm-cranking in subjects with spinal cord lesions. Paraplegia 15:252, 1977–78.
49. Marincek CRT, Valencic V: Arm cyclo-ergometry and kinetics of oxygen consumption in paraplegics. Paraplegia 15:178, 1977–78.
50. Engel P, Hildebrandt G: Long-term spiro-ergonometric studies of paraplegics during the clinical period of rehabilitation. Paraplegia 11:105, 1973.
51. Voight ED, Bahn D: Metabolism and pulse rate in physically handicapped when propelling a wheelchair up an incline. Scand J Rehabil Med 1:101, 1969.
52. Gass CG, Camp EM: Physiological characteristics of trained paraplegic and tetraplegic subjects. Med Sci Sports 11:256, 1979.
53. Gass GC, Camp EM, Davis HA, et al: The effects of prolonged exercise on spinally injured subjects. Med Sci Sports Exerc 13:277, 1981.
54. Brouha L, Korbath H: Continuous recording of cardiac and respiratory functions in normal and handicapped persons. Hum Factors 9:567, 1967.
55. Gandee R, Winningham M, Deitchman R, et al: The aerobic capacity of an elite wheelchair marathon racer. Med Sci Sports 12:142, 1980.
56. Lundberg A: Wheelchair driving—evaluation of a new training outfit. Scand J Rehabil Med 12:67, 1980.
57. Glaser RM, Bolduc S, Laubach LL, et al: A cardiopulmonary fitness test utilizing the wheelchair ergometer. Fed Proc 37:429, 1978.
58. Glaser RM, Sawka MN, Laubach LL, et al: Metabolic and cardiopulmonary responses to wheelchair and bicycle ergometry. J Appl Physiol 46:1066, 1979.
59. Sawka MN, Glaser RM, Wilde SW, et al: Metabolic and circulatory responses to wheelchair and arm crank exercise. J Appl Physiol 49:784, 1980.
60. Noreau L: Unpublished doctoral dissertation, University of Toronto, 1991.
61. Brattgard S, Grimby G, Hook O: Energy expenditure and heart rate in driving a wheelchair ergometer. Scand J Rehabil Med 2:143, 1970.

62. Glaser RM, Giner JF, Laubach LL: Validity and reliability of wheelchair ergometry. Physiologist 20:34, 1977.
63. Davis GM, Ward GR: Hey coach, what about the disabled? Coaching Sci Update 3:34, 1982.
64. Glaser RM, Sawka MN, Young RE, et al: Applied physiology for wheelchair design. J Appl Physiol 48:41, 1980.
65. Engel P, Hildebrandt G: Wheelchair design—technological and physiological aspects. Proc R Soc Med 67:409, 1974.
66. Kamenetz HL: The Wheelchair Book: Mobility for the Disabled. Springfield, IL, Charles C Thomas, 1969, pp 1–267.
67. Peizer E, Wright D, Freiberger H: Bioengineering methods of wheelchair evaluation. Bull Prosthet Res 1:77, 1964.
68. Gessaroli ME, Robertson DGE: Comparison of two wheelchair sprint starts. Can J Appl Sport Sci 5(4):1980.
69. Higgs C: Analysis of racing wheelchairs used at the 1980 Olympic Games for the Disabled. Res Q 54:229, 1983.
70. Higgs C: Science, research and special populations: The view from biomechanics. *In* Berridge M, Ward G (eds): International Perspectives in Adapted Physical Activity. Champaign, IL, Human Kinetics Publishers, 1987, p 193.
71. Kavanagh T, Pandit V, Shephard RJ: The application of exercise testing to the elderly amputee. Can Med Assoc J 108:314, 1976.
72. Schwade J, Blomqvist CG, Shapiro W: A comparison of the response to arm and leg work in patients with ischemic heart disease. Am Heart J 94:203, 1977.
73. Strauss RH, Haynes RL, Ingram RH, et al: Comparison of arm versus leg work in induction of acute episodes of asthma. J Appl Physiol 42:565, 1977.
74. Bergh U, Kanstrup IL, Ekblöm B: Maximal oxygen uptake during exercise with various combinations of arm and leg work. J Appl Physiol 41:191, 1976.
75. Hjeltnes N: Oxygen uptake and cardiac output in graded arm exercise in paraplegics with low level spinal lesions. Scand J Rehabil Med 9:107, 1977.
76. Glaser RM, Laubach LL, Sawka MN, et al: Exercise stress fitness evaluation and training of wheelchair users. *In* Leon AS, Amundson GJ (eds): Proceedings of the 1st International Conference on Lifestyle and Health. Minneapolis, University of Minnesota, 1978.
77. Glaser RM, Young RE, Surprayasad AG: Reducing energy cost and cardiopulmonary stresses during wheelchair activity. Fed Proc 36:580, 1977.
78. Davis GM, Shephard RJ, Jackson RW: Cardiorespiratory fitness and muscular strength in the lower-limb disabled. Can J Appl Sport Sci 6:159, 1981.
79. Bevegard S, Freyschuss U, Strandell T: Circulatory adaptation to arm and leg exercise in supine and sitting position. J Appl Physiol 21:37, 1966.
80. Bobbert AC: Physiological comparison of three types of ergometry. J Appl Physiol 15:1007, 1960.
81. Wicks JR, Oldridge NB, Cameron BJ, et al: Arm cranking and wheelchair ergometry in elite spinal cord injured athletes. Med Sci Sports Exerc 5:224, 1983.
82. Glaser RM, Sawka MN, Brune MF, et al: Physiological responses to maximal effort wheelchair and arm crank ergometry. J Appl Physiol 48:1060, 1980.
83. Hjeltnes N: Control of medical rehabilitation of para- and tetra-plegics. *In* Natvig H (ed): 1st International Medical Congress on Sports for the Disabled. Oslo, Royal Ministry for Church and Education, 1980, pp 162–173.
84. Heigenhauser CF, Ruff CL, Milter B, et al: Cardiovascular responses of paraplegics during graded arm ergometry. Med Sci Sports Exerc 8:68, 1976.
85. Munro AF, Robinson R: The catecholamine content of peripheral plasma in human subjects with complete transverse lesion of the spinal cord. J Physiol (Lond) 154:244, 1960.
86. Mathias CJ, Christensen NJ, Corbett JL, et al: Plasma catecholamines, plasma renin activity and plasma aldosterone in tetraplegic man, horizontal and tilted. Clin Sci Mol Med 49:291, 1975.
87. Mathias CJ, Christensen NJ, Corbett JL, et al: Plasma catecholamines during paroxysmal neurogenic hypertension in quadriplegic man. Circ Res 39:204, 1976.
88. Bar-Or O, Inbar O: Relationships among anaerobic capacity, sprint and middle-distance running of schoolchildren. *In* Shephard RJ, Lavallée H (eds): Physical Fitness Assessment. Springfield, IL, Charles C Thomas, 1978, p 142.
89. Coutts KD, Stogryn JL: Aerobic and anaerobic power of Canadian wheelchair athletes. Med Sci Sports Exerc 19:62, 1987.
90. Lakomy HKA, Campbell I, Williams C: Treadmill performance and selected physiological characteristics of wheelchair athletes. Br J Sports Med 21:130, 1987.
91. Nilsson S, Staff P, Pruett E: Physical work capacity and the effect on training on subjects with long-standing paraplegia. Scand J Rehabil Med 7:51, 1975.

92. Bar-Or O, Zwiren L: Maximal oxygen consumption test during arm exercise—reliability and validity. J Appl Physiol 38:424, 1975.
93. Gersten J, Brown I, Speck L, et al: Comparison of tension development and circulation in biceps and triceps in man. Am J Phys Med 42:156, 1963.
94. Asmussen E: Correlation between various physiological test results in handicapped persons. *In* Communication of Testing and Observation Institute, vol 27. Hellerup, Denmark, Danish Infantile Paralysis Association, 1968, pp 1–16.
95. Asmussen E, Poulsen E: A battery of physiological tests applied to two different groups of handicapped persons. *In* Communication of Testing and Observation Institute, vol 23. Hellerup, Denmark, Danish Infantile Paralysis Association, 1966, pp 1–13.
96. Asmussen E, Poulsen E, Bogh HE: Measurements of muscle strength necessary for driving a motor car. *In* Communication of Testing and Observation Institute vol 19. Hellerup, Denmark, Danish Infantile Paralysis Association, 1964, pp 1–12.
97. Grimby G: Aerobic capacity, muscle strength and fiber composition in young paraplegics. *In* Natvig H (ed): Proceedings of 1st International Medical Congress on Sports for the Disabled. Oslo, Royal Ministry of Church and Education, 1980, pp 13–17.
98. Davis GM, Tupling S, Shephard RJ: Dynamic strength and physical activity in wheelchair users. *In* Sherrill C (ed): Sport and Disabled Athletes. Champaign, IL, Human Kinetics Publishers, 1986, p 139.
99. Baltzopoulos V, Brodie DA: Isokinetic dynamometry: Applications and limitations. Sports Med 8:101, 1989.
100. Shephard RJ: Physical Activity and Growth. Chicago, Year Book Medical Publishers, 1982, pp 1–340.
101. Shephard RJ, Lavallée H, Jéquier J-C, et al: A community approach to exercise tolerance in health and disease. J Sports Med Phys Fitness 19:297, 1979.
102. Cumming GR, Goulding D, Baggley G: Working capacity of deaf, visually and mentally impaired handicapped children. Arch Dis Child 46:490, 1971.
103. Sündberg S: Maximal oxygen uptake in relation to age in blind and normal boys and girls. Acta Paediatr Scand 71:603, 1982.
104. Jankowski L, Evans JK: The exercise capacity of blind children. J Vis Imp Blindness 75:248, 1981.
105. Sawka MN, Glaser RM, Laubach LL, et al: Wheelchair exercise performance in the young, middle-aged and elderly. J Appl Physiol 50:824, 1981.
106. Hjeltnes H, Vokac Z: Circulatory strain in everyday life of paraplegics. Scand J Rehabil Med 11:67, 1979.
107. Davis GM, Shephard RJ, Leenen FHH: Cardiac effects of short-term arm crank training in paraplegics: Echocardiographic evidence. Eur J Appl Physiol 56:90, 1987.
108. Davis GM, Shephard RJ: Cardio-respiratory fitness in highly active versus less active paraplegics. Med Sci Sports Exerc 20:463, 1988.
109. Grimby G: Aerobic capacity, muscle strength and fiber composition in young paraplegics. *In* Natvig H (ed): Proceedings of 1st International Medical Congress on Sports for the Disabled. Oslo, Royal Ministry for Church and Education, 1980, pp 13–17.
110. Davis GM, Kofsky PR, Shephard RJ, et al: Classification of psycho-physiological variables in the lower-limb disabled. Can J Appl Sport Sci 6(4):141, 1981.
111. Cameron BJ, Ward GR, Wicks JR: Relationship of type of training to maximum oxygen uptake and upper limb strength in male paraplegic athletes. (Abstract.) Med Sci Sports Exerc 9:58, 1977.
112. Wicks JR, Head E, Oldridge NB, et al: Maximum oxygen uptake of wheelchair athletes competing at the 1976 Olympiad for the physically disabled. (Abstract.) Med Sci Sports Exerc 9:58, 1977.
113. Berg K, Isaksson B: Maximal oxygen uptake of cerebral palsied children in relation to body cell mass. *In* Macek M (ed): Proceedings of the Second Pediatric Work Physiology Symposium. Prague, Charles University, 1970, p 89.
114. Taylor AW, McDonnell E, Royer D, et al: Skeletal muscle analysis of wheelchair athletes. Paraplegia 17:456, 1979.
115. Taylor AW: Physical activity for the disabled. *In* Richardson JR (ed): Report on the Research Priority Development Conference, March 1981. Ottawa, Fitness & Amateur Sport, 1981, p 15.
116. Pender RH, Patterson PE: A comparison of selected motor fitness items between congenitally deaf and hearing children. J Spec Educ 18(4):71, 1982.
117. Cratty BJ, Cratty IJ, Cornell S: Motor planning abilities in deaf and hearing children. Am Ann Deaf 131:281, 1986.
118. Winnick JP, Short FX: Physical fitness of adolescents with auditory impairments. Adapt Phys Activ Q 3:58, 1986.
119. deLateur B, Giaconi R: Effect on maximal strength of submaximal exercise in Duchenne muscular dystrophy. Am J Phys Med 58:26, 1979.
120. Bar-Or O, Inbar O, Spira R: Physiological effects of a sports rehabilitation program on cerebral palsied and post-poliomyelitic adolescents. Med Sci Sports Exerc 8:157, 1976.

121. Greenway RM, Houser HB, Lindan O, et al: Long-term changes in gross body composition of paraplegic and quadriplegic patients. Paraplegia 7:310, 1970.
122. Pollock ML, Miller H, Linnerud A, et al: Arm pedalling as an endurance training regimen for the disabled. Arch Phys Med Rehabil 55:418, 1974.
123. Effgen SK: Effect of an exercise program on the static balance of deaf children. Phys Ther 61:873, 1981.
124. Lewis S, Higham L, Cherry D: Development of an exercise program to improve static and dynamic balance of profoundly hearing impaired children. Am Ann Deaf 130(4):278, 1985.
125. Robertson BL: A therapeutic program for the spastic child. Am Corr Ther J 34:102, 1980.
126. Gehlsen GM, Grigsby SA, Winant DM: Effects of an aquatic fitness program on the muscular strength and endurance of patients with muscular sclerosis. Phys Ther 64:653, 1984.
127. Kabsch A: The ski camp as a rehabilitative aspect in the training of the gait of above-knee amputees with a prosthesis. *In* Grüpe O (ed): Sport in the Modern World. Berlin, Springer-Verlag, 1973, p 260.
128. Getman L, Greninger L, Molnar S: Efficiency of wheeling after training. Proc Ann Conv Southern District Am Assoc Health Phys Ed Recreation 7:83, 1968.
129. Clinkingbeard JR, Gersten JW, Hoehn D: Energy cost of ambulation in the traumatic paraplegic. Am J Phys Med 43:157, 1964.
130. Knutsson E, Lewenhaupt-Olsson E, Thorsen M: Physical work capacity and physical conditioning in paraplegic patients. Paraplegia 11:205, 1973.
131. Ekblöm B, Lundberg A: Effect of physical training on adolescents with severe motor handicaps. Acta Paediatr Scand 55:17, 1968.
132. Glaser RM, Laubach LL, Foley DM, et al: An interval training program for wheelchair users. Med Sci Sports Exerc 10:54, 1978.
133. Shephard RJ: Intensity, duration and frequency of exercise as determinants of the response to a training regimen. Int Z Angew Physiol 26:272, 1968.
134. Pollock ML: The quantification of endurance training. Exerc Sport Sci Rev 1:155, 1973.
135. Shephard RJ: Future research on the quantifying of endurance training. J Hum Ergol 3:163, 1975.
136. Gordon E, Vanderwalde H: Energy requirements in paraplegic ambulation. Arch Phys Med Rehabil 37:285, 1956.
137. Hook O: Arm ergometer for patients with paraplegia. Scand J Rehabil Med 3:77, 1971.
138. Pollock ML, Miller H, Linnerud A, et al: Arm pedalling as an endurance training regimen for the disabled. Arch Phys Med Rehabil 55:418, 1974.
139. McDonnell E, Brassard L, Taylor AW: Effects of an arm ergometer training program on wheelchair subjects. Can J Appl Sport Sci 5(4), 1980.
140. Stoboy H, Wilson-Rich B: Muscle strength and electrical activity, heart rate and energy cost during isometric contractions in disabled and non-disabled. Paraplegia 8:217, 1971.
141. Caiozzo VJ, Perrine JJ, Edgerton VR: Training induced alterations of the in vivo force-velocity relationship of human muscle. J Appl Physiol 51:750, 1981.
142. Kanehisa H, Miyashita M: Specificity of velocity in strength training. Eur J Appl Physiol 52:104, 1983.

SUGGESTED READINGS

Davis GM, Shephard RJ: Strength training for wheelchair users. Br J Sports Med 24:25–30, 1990.

Davis GM, Ryley M, Shephard RJ: Gains of cardiorespiratory fitness with arm-crank training in spinally disabled men. Can J Sport Sci. In press.

Noreau L, Shephard RJ: Relationships between physical fitness and the productivity of 74 paraplegic persons. Can J Sport Sci 15:175, 1990.

D

E

F

G

H

J

K

L

M

U

Urticaria, 143

V

W

X

Y

Z